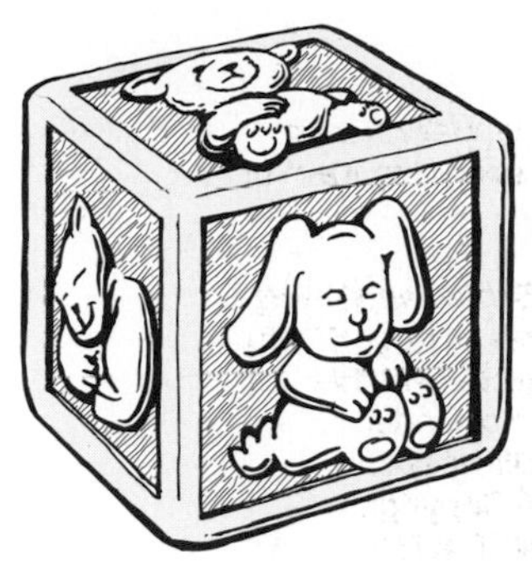

CONTENTS

 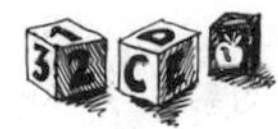

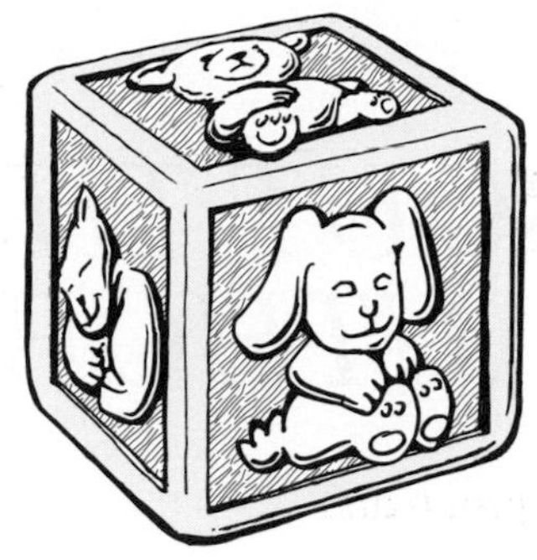

INTRODUCTION

This book has been written for both child-care students and practitioners with the intention of providing a comprehensive guide to all aspects of the development of children from birth to 8 years. The book relates particularly to the syllabus requirements of the CACHE Diploma in Child Care and Education at level 3, as well as the CACHE Certificate in Child Care and Education and the BTEC National Diploma in Early Childhood Studies. The book also covers the requirements for underpinning knowledge for NVQ awards in Child Care and Education. Students on any of the many other courses that require a knowledge and understanding of child development will also find the book useful. Child-care establishments may find the book a valuable addition to their reference shelves and helpful in supporting in-service training.

The book is divided into 11 units, each unit containing one or more chapters covering an area of the DCE. All aspects of child development are presented in a way that is accessible to the reader and the responsibilities of the child-care worker and their role in promoting children's development are emphasised. Case studies help the reader to relate theoretical points to real-life situations and throughout the chapters there are questions to recall knowledge and develop understanding.

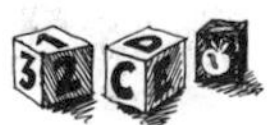

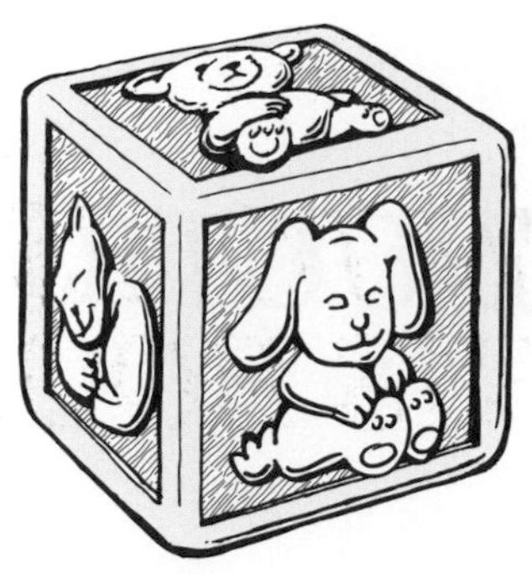

ABOUT THE AUTHORS

Marian Beaver has worked in social work, teaching and early years care and education. She has taught for many years on child-care courses in further education. She continues to work in further education at New College Nottingham, was an external verifier for CACHE, and, as well as writing, she inspects nursery provision for OFSTED.

Jo Brewster has practised as a nurse, midwife and health visitor. She has taught for many years on child-care courses in further education at New College Nottingham, as well as writing, inspecting nursery provision for OFSTED and working as an external verifier for CACHE.

Pauline Jones worked in residential child care and as a social worker before lecturing and managing in further education, including at West Nottinghamshire College, Mansfield. She developed the Diploma in Nursery Nurse Training for profoundly deaf students. She is now a regional manager for SureStart.

Anne Keene comes from a background of nursing, midwifery and health visiting. Until June 1998, she taught and managed child-care programmes at New College Nottingham. She now owns and manages a large private day nursery.

Sally Neaum has taught in nursery classes and across the infant age range. She has taught a range of child-care courses in a college of further education, has been an OFSTED inspector for nursery provision, and now works freelance, writing and teaching.

Jill Tallack has taught in schools across the whole primary age range. She has worked for some years in a college of further education, teaching on child-care programmes. As well as writing, she also inspects nursery provision for OFSTED.

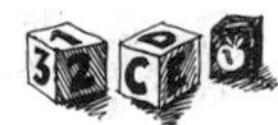

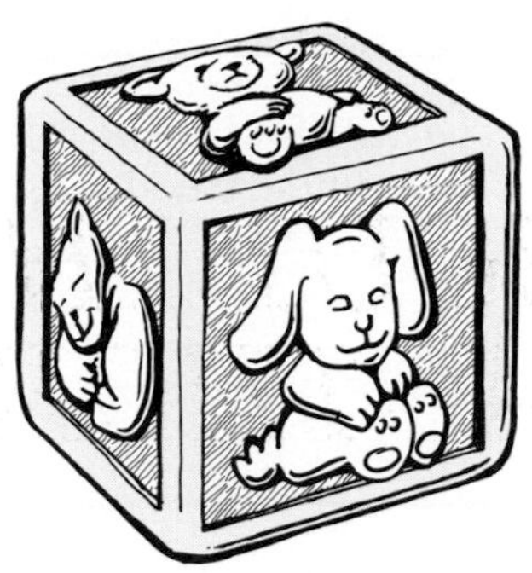

HOW TO USE THIS BOOK

This book has been written and designed to cover the DCE units precisely. It is presented in an attractive, open design for easy reference and all the features are up-to-date and of immediate relevance to the DCE course. The range of features used in the book is described below.

Introduction to each part

The book is divided into units, with each unit title matching one of the units given in the DCE specifications. There is a brief introduction to each unit.

Chapter introduction

Every chapter begins with a summary of its contents, and mentions other chapters that relate closely to those contents.

Definitions

Students can be surprised by some of the technical language included in what they read. Where significant new words are introduced in the text, you will find a clear definition of each word in a box in the margin alongside.

Case studies

New case studies have been developed, showing how an issue can be dealt with in a practical environment. Each is followed by two or three questions to give you practice in problem solving.

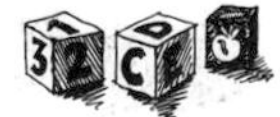

Progress check

At the end of each major section within a chapter you will find a short list of questions. Answering these will confirm that you have understood what you have read.

Key terms

At the end of each chapter, you will find a reminder to go back and read through the information in the key terms boxes to check that you understand each one.

'Now try these questions'

Each chapter finishes with a number of short-answer questions. If you answer these, you will show that you understand the key concepts in the chapter and are able to write about them in your own words.

Glossary

At the end of the book you will find a comprehensive glossary. It explains all the key terms used.

Key skills

Many students studying child care also need to demonstrate their competence in Key Skills. You will find guidelines to five of the level 2 Key Skills on pages ix–xiv. (More detailed coverage will be available from your tutor, assessor or supervisor.)

This book has been written to support the CACHE DCE syllabus, but will also be useful for other level 3 courses. It aims both to provide knowledge and understanding and to enhance practical skills for a range of workers, including NVQ candidates. We are sure that you will like it – and wish you good luck with your studies.

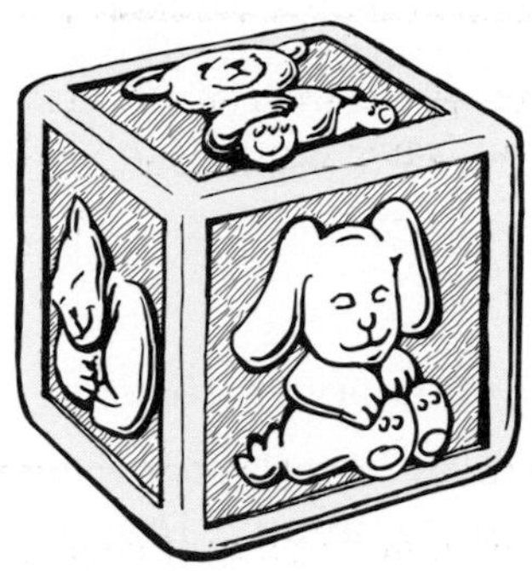

KEY SKILLS GUIDELINES

Communication

Effective communication is at the heart of good working practice. There are many ways in which we communicate at work, through conversations, discussions and presentations. These may be direct, over the telephone, by fax, letter or e-mail. They may involve colleagues, managers, children, their parents and others in the community. When you are caring for children what you say and what you understand can have serious consequences for the children's well-being. Communication includes each of the following areas.

TAKING PART IN DISCUSSIONS

Child-care workers need to be able to speak clearly and listen carefully. In any discussion it is helpful to:

- keep to the subject
- express yourself clearly
- keep the discussion moving forwards.

Discussions take many forms: informal conversations with colleagues, formal meetings such as staff meetings, planned presentations to groups of people or telephone conversations with, for example, a child's parent or carer.

PRODUCING WRITTEN MATERIAL

The benefit of written material is that the opportunity for misunderstanding may be reduced and accurate records kept. Information can also be shared between several people when direct contact is not possible. Once something is written down, however, it is more difficult to amend. Written information needs to be accurate, legible, easy to understand and in a suitable format.

There are many ways in which written material can be produced. You may need to complete a child's record card, send a letter to a parent, produce a report for a nursery manager, apply in writing for a job as a nanny or complete surveys and questionnaires when helping to set up a local playgroup. Spelling, grammar and punctuation should always be checked to ensure accuracy.

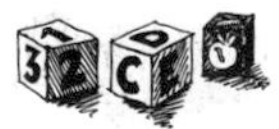

USING IMAGES

You have probably heard the saying that 'a picture is worth a thousand words'. There will be many opportunities in your work in early years care to use pictures and images to communicate.

Choose clear images that are relevant to what you want to say and:

- suited to those who will need to understand them
- recognise and value diversity
- promote equality of opportunity and anti-discriminatory practice.

Images may be nursery floor plans, illustrations for a monthly newsletter for parents, graphs and charts of attendance for use in an annual report, or eye-catching photographs for advertising your facilities. Images can equally well be used to clarify a point in one-to-one or group discussion.

READING AND RESPONDING TO WRITTEN MATERIAL

We are surrounded by written materials: magazines, reports, advertisements, timetables, signs, books and leaflets – the list is endless. It is important to be able to choose the right source of material for your purpose and to be able to get the information you want from it. Once you have chosen your source, you need to be able to extract the relevant information, check that you understand it and that you are able to summarise it.

As a child-care worker you need to understand documents such as the important written policies and procedures of your workplace, the timetable for the children's day, letters from parents or the statutory bodies, and agendas and minutes for meetings. You also need to be able to interpret any pictures and images accompanying written information.

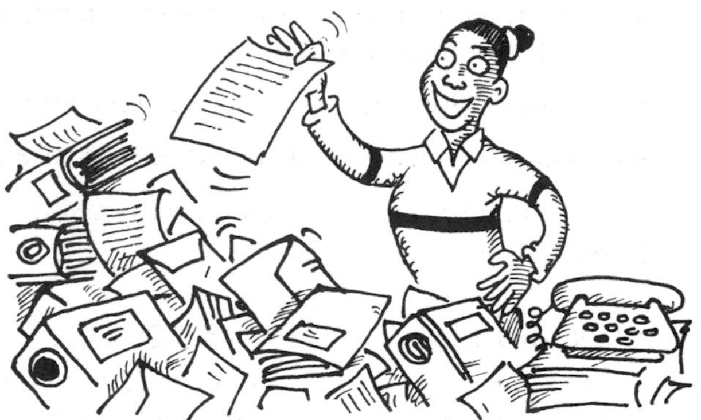

Application of number

It may surprise you how often you will be dealing with numbers, data and mathematical problem solving in your work with children. Dealing with numbers is more straightforward when you understand why you are doing it. Accuracy is important. Application of number includes the following areas.

COLLECTING AND RECORDING DATA

Data is numerical information; you need to be able to collect and record such information. Once you know what kind of information you need, you will have to decide how you are going to collect it, conduct your tasks in the right order and record your results clearly and accurately. You may wish to record information from

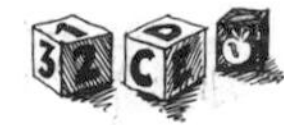

parents at an enrolment interview or record attendance levels at a nursery over a period of weeks. You may need to plan a new home corner, measure up the space available and draw up an accurate plan of your proposals. You may be involved in collecting money from parents and keeping accurate records of how much has been paid to you.

One question you do need to ask yourself when collecting data is how precise you need to be. If you are surveying the arrival times of children at a nursery you may need to be precise only to the nearest five minutes. If you are collecting money from parents, you cannot afford any mistakes at all!

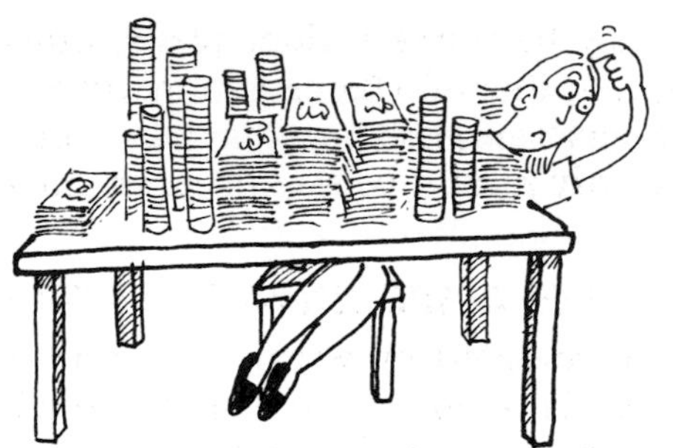

TACKLING PROBLEMS

From time to time you will come across problems at work that will need to be solved using numerical techniques. It is important to choose the correct technique to start with and to make sure that you do everything in the right order. Any calculations need to be accurate and you should check your work to make sure that there are no errors and that your results make sense.

You may need to:

- work out amounts of disposable materials such as paper, paints or clay that will be required for an activity
- account for how money has been spent during a certain period
- help in conducting local surveys for the opening of a new nursery.

All these require their own techniques and the results of each need to be presented appropriately.

INTERPRETING AND PRESENTING DATA

Large amounts of data are impossible to understand unless presented clearly; just as a picture can speak a thousand words, so a graph can present a thousand numbers. It is almost certain that you, or someone else, will be making decisions based on the information you present, so the graphs, charts, tables, pictograms, plans, diagrams or drawings used should be clear and appropriate. You should outline the main features of your data, ensure that appropriate axes or labels are clear and explain how your results are relevant to the problem.

The outcome of a nursery survey may best be presented in graphs, charts and tables, while proposals to change the use of nursery space, for example, will probably use plans and diagrams.

Information technology

Most information is now stored electronically, on an information technology (or IT) system. The strength of such systems is that they can also reorganise, manipulate and provide information and (in theory at least!) reduce the amount of paper used in the workplace. Information technology includes the following areas.

PREPARING INFORMATION

Output information is only as good as the information put in, so all information should be accurate. It is important to plan carefully so that the information you put in is in an appropriate form, and once entered, can easily be edited. You should also save all your information in well-organised files and folders and make back-up copies in case something goes wrong with your centrally stored files.

The names, addresses and postcodes of parents, for example, should be organised so that the information can be easily used for mailings; survey and questionnaire findings should be carefully recorded so that they can be transferred to a spreadsheet and source information for a termly newsletter (text, pictures, tables or graphs) entered so that it can be electronically merged into a single file.

PROCESSING INFORMATION

Entering information onto a system is not, in itself, particularly useful. It is the computer's power to access and select information in different ways, to combine information from different sources and to provide user-friendly output that makes it such a useful tool. Finding, retrieving, editing, combining and reorganising information will help you shape raw data to your needs.

Once properly organised, parental addresses can be used, for example, for mail shots, individual letters, reaching the parents of children within a specific age range or within a particular postal district. The raw data from the survey can be processed into graphs, charts or tables, and the individual parts of the newsletter put into an appropriate format.

PRESENTING INFORMATION

Presenting information clearly and professionally is in your own interests as well as your employer's. Even the best ideas may go unnoticed if poorly presented; people may simply not understand your point. A professional approach is particularly important in working with children, as you may need to win the approval, confidence and support of parents, the local authority and the wider community – as well as your employer.

You should be able to present your processed information in an appropriate way and choose the most effective software to do so. Consistency is important and you should always save your finished work in carefully organised files and make regular back-ups.

You will develop a reputation for thoroughness and professionalism by doing the following:

- consistently and accurately fulfilling and updating your mailings
- producing surveys and other reports in a recognisable form in a common format
- publishing your newsletters to the same high standard every term.

EVALUATING THE USE OF INFORMATION TECHNOLOGY

It is important that you know when information technology can make your life easier – and when it cannot! It is also important to understand the range of software available to you and what its functions and limitations are.

 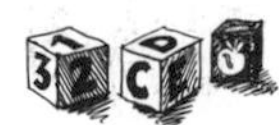

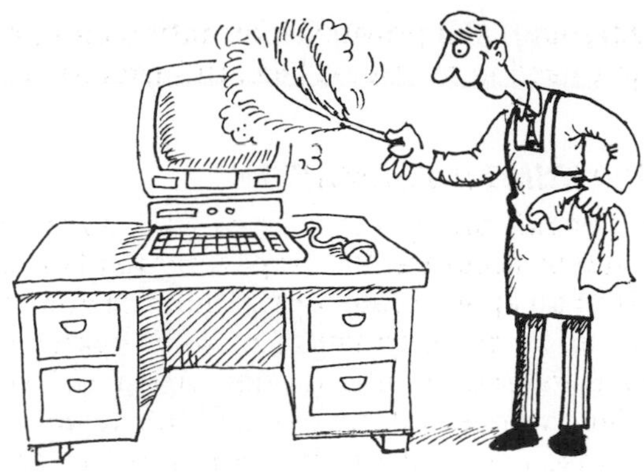

A computer and its software is like any other machine. It needs to be carefully maintained, and faults and problems logged so that they can be dealt with. It is also important that your working practices are healthy and safe, and that you protect yourself and your machine by correctly positioning the keyboard and screen, keeping cables tidy, keeping food and drink away from where you are working, and storing equipment away from sources of heat and other electrical equipment.

Improving own learning and performance

We all have strengths and weaknesses, and to improve our own learning and performance it is important that we can identify them. Setting targets and reviewing progress will help you focus more clearly on what you need to do. Improving own learning and performance includes the following areas.

IDENTIFYING TARGETS

You should be able to identify your strengths and weaknesses and provide evidence to support what you say. You will also need to be able to help in setting short-term targets for your own improvement, in conjunction with your teacher, assessor or workplace supervisor. When targets have been set, make sure that you understand what is required of you!

FOLLOWING SCHEDULES TO MEET YOUR TARGETS

Once your targets for improvement are agreed, you should be able to follow them without close supervision, within the specified timescale. You will, of course, receive support in your work and you should know how to put this to good use in improving your work and meeting your targets.

BEING SMART!

Be	**S**pecific in setting your targets and schedules!
Tackle learning in	**M**anageable chunks!
Make sure your targets are	**A**chievable!
Keep your targets	**R**elevant!
Track progress so you are on	**T**ime in meeting your targets!

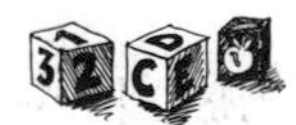

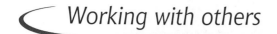

Working with others

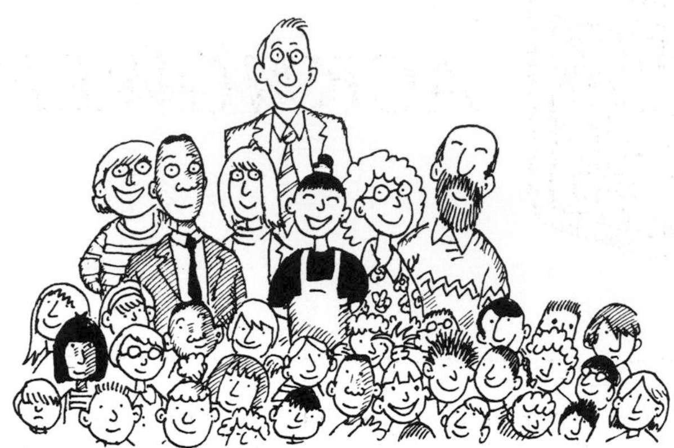

When you work in child care, you are unlikely to work alone. Learning with other people can be a great challenge, but also bring great rewards. Working with others includes the following areas.

IDENTIFYING COLLECTIVE GOALS AND RESPONSIBILITIES

When you work with others you need to be able to identify and agree group goals. You also need to be clear about who is responsible for what and how you are going to organise working together.

WORKING TO COLLECTIVE GOALS

Once you understand your responsibilities you should set about organising your work so that you will be able to achieve your goals on time. You will need to stick to the working methods agreed by the whole group.

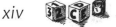

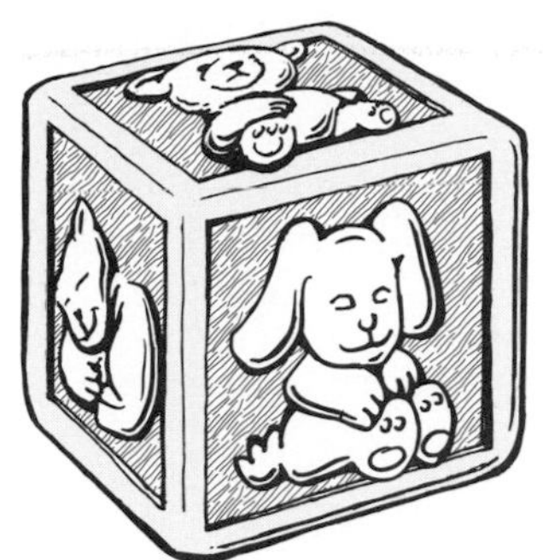

ACKNOWLEDGEMENTS

The authors and publishers would like to thank the following people and organisations for permission to reproduce material in this book:

Photos:
Clockhouse Pre-School Centre, Nottingham, page 495; Sue Didcott, pages 66 and 478; Format Photographers, page 249; Great Ormond Street Hospital for Children, page 303; Sally and Richard Greenhill, pages 57 and 648; The Guardian Newspapers Ltd, page 220; Renate Hallett, pages 114 and 232; Val Jackson, pages 238 and 260; Juliette Khan, pages 230 and 252; Dr S. Lingham, Royston Westgarth/BDA, page 246; The National Eczema Society, page 303; The National Medical Slide Bank, The Wellcome Trust, page 303; Photodisc, pages 416 and 533; Jean Reed, page 631; Jane Rigg, page 210; St John's Institute of Dermatology, page 303; Irene Tipping, pages 362 and 566 and Angela Hampton for the front cover photograph.

Text:
The DfEE for extracts from the *National Literacy Strategy: Framework for Teaching Literacy from Reception to Year 6* (1998) and the *National Numeracy Strategy: Framework for Teaching Mathematics from Reception to Year 6* (1999) on page 384 and the *Qualifications and Curriculum Authority Curriculum Guidance for the Foundation Stage* (2000) on pages 386–88; L. Murray and L. Andrews for an extract from *The Social Baby: Understanding Babies' Communications from Birth* (The Children's Project, London, 2000) on page 499; The National Children's Bureau for an extract from *Young Children in Group Day Care: Guidelines for Good Practice* on page 622 and Ward Lock Educational for an extract from *Listening to Children Talking* by Joan Tough (1976) on page 154.

Every effort has been made to contact copyright holders and we apologise if anyone has been overlooked.

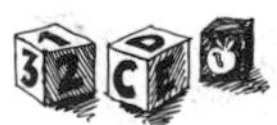

Unit 1: Observation and Assessment

This unit concentrates on developing the important professional skill of observing and assessing children. You will consider what constitutes good practice in observation and how to ensure this in your own work. A range of observation and assessment techniques will be examined and their use will be discussed. As your skills and knowledge develop, you will understand how to analyse and evaluate your observations, and use your findings to enhance your work with children.

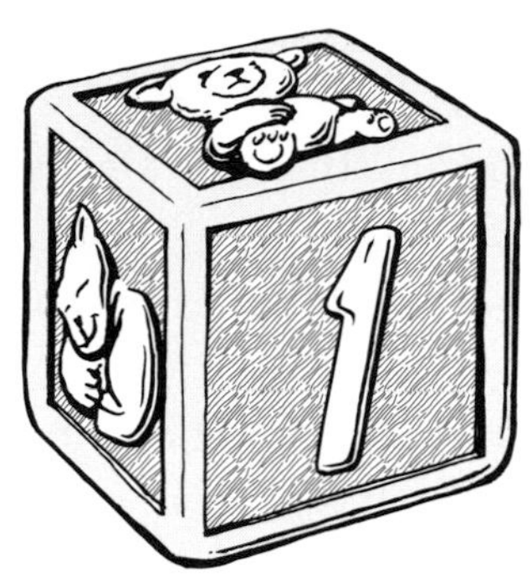

OBSERVATION AND ASSESSMENT

This chapter will cover the following topics:

- *the importance of observation and assessment*
- *good practice in observing and assessing*
- *observation and assessment techniques*
- *evaluating your observations.*

The importance of observation and assessment

During your training, you will spend a significant amount of time learning how to observe children and practising your skills in this area. In order to achieve your qualification, you will need to demonstrate your skill in this important area by submitting a portfolio of observations and assessments of children across the age range from birth to 7 years 11 months, focused on all aspects of development, in different contexts and using a range of appropriate methods of recording. As you work through this chapter you will be able to demonstrate your developing professional knowledge and experience as you draw conclusions from your observations.

key terms

Observation
a record of a child's response to an activity or situation, used by professionals to determine progress and needs

Assessment
matching a child's reponses or performance against a standardised scale, measuring achievements (e.g. SATs) or norms of development

WHY OBSERVE?

Observation is a vital professional tool for child-care workers. We observe children in order to:

- understand the pattern of development
- gather information to make **assessments** about a child's progress in relation to developmental norms
- learn about the interests of a child or group of children
- identify any particular difficulties a child may have
- meet the specific needs of individuals or groups of children
- establish an understanding of children as individuals
- assess what the child has achieved and then plan for the next stage
- record and document any unusual behaviour or any that gives cause for concern
- provide information about the child to parents and to others who have an involvement with the child
- measure the progress and achievements of children against national targets, e.g. SATs (National Curriculum Standard Assessment Tests)
- evaluate the effectiveness of the provision made for children.

Child-care workers make observations and respond to them in intuitive ways all the time – observing that a child has fallen over and offering comfort, observing that the paper tray is empty and refilling it. However, there is a place for observation that is structured, that has a clear aim and purpose and which is recorded appropriately. This will enable conclusions to be drawn about the progress and needs of children and, importantly, recommendations for action to be considered.

Progress check

List some of the reasons why we observe children.

Why is structured, recorded observation helpful to child-care workers?

What is the difference between observation and assessment?

Good practice in observing and assessing

It is important in undertaking observations of children that you comply with the requirements of good professional practice, particularly in recognising and ensuring the rights of children and their families.

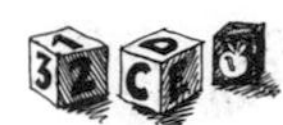

CONFIDENTIALITY

One of the ways in which you show respect for the rights of children is in maintaining confidentiality. In order to provide a full picture of the child or children you are observing, you might record confidential information about a child. When making observations of children for your portfolio, you should conceal the child's identity, usually by using initials or first names only, and you should not identify your placement by name. It is your responsibility to ensure that this information contained in observations is not used in ways that could be harmful or embarrassing to the child or family. In passing on information, your consideration should always be what is in the best interests of the child. If you observe something that causes you concern or that you find upsetting, it will be in the child's best interests that you raise this with your line manager or placement supervisor who will then take appropriate action. In all child-care settings there will be a clear policy about the sharing of confidential information that staff will be required to follow. As a member of staff, it is likely that you will make observations of children that will provide information for other professionals who work with the children, for example social workers, speech therapists or educational psychologists.

During your work placements you will need to obtain permission from your placement supervisor before you make observations of the children you are working with and demonstrate in your portfolio that you have done this. In most settings, staff make it clear to parents that their children will be observed as they play and work in the setting, for the range of purposes described above. In settings where students are trained, staff will explain that students need to make observations as part of their placement and parents will usually agree to their children being observed for this purpose. However, sometimes parents may not agree to this and you should always check that you have permission to observe a particular child. If you use photographs or videotape, where children could be identified, to make a record of your observation, you must make sure you have permission from parents.

SHARING OBSERVATIONS TO INFORM PLANNING AND PROVISION

Observations made of children in the setting will be discussed by staff and used to inform decisions about planning the next steps for individuals or groups of children and to identify any action to be taken. For example, the observation might demonstrate that children found it difficult to have access to some of the play equipment, indicating a need to reorganise the play area. Participating in these discussions as a student, and contributing what you have learned from your own observation, is very worth while, as it will help you to understand the importance of this observation in practice. Often staff share the observations they make of children with parents, providing them with an opportunity to share their own observations of their child at home. This enables staff to gain a more complete picture of the child. It is likely that observations will also be shared with other professionals as part of assessment, monitoring or support procedures.

key term

Objective
free of personal feelings or thoughts

OBJECTIVITY

Observations should be **objective**, that is, free of personal feelings or thoughts. The way that you perceive a child may be governed by:

- previous experience of the child or of others
- your own attitudes and values

- your needs and personality
- comments made by others.

If you approach a child or a situation with a preconceived idea of what you expect to find, this will influence what you see and undermine the validity of your observation. One way of ensuring objectivity in your observations is to record simply what you saw, rather than to make assumptions about the child or his behaviour. For example:

- 'Jamie threw himself on to the floor screaming, kicking his feet and hammering the air with clenched fists' *not* 'Jamie was in a rage'.
- 'Sarah snatched the doll from Nicola, kicked her and then bit her arm' *not* 'Sarah is an aggressive child'.

It will also help you to be objective if you *avoid*:

- jumping to conclusions, e.g. 'he is a naughty boy'
- making generalisations, e.g. 'all children cry when their mothers leave them'
- expressing personal opinions, e.g. 'she is a lovable child'
- labelling children, e.g. 'she is a bully'
- ascribing feelings to children, e.g. 'they were frightened'.

All of the above examples give a subjective view. Describing exactly what you see will ensure objectivity in your observations.

Another aspect of objectivity relates to the possibilities for bias and stereotyping in observations and assessments of children. It may be that you have expectations of children that relate to your own linguistic, cultural or social background, and this may lead you to make assumptions about the development and behaviour of children whose backgrounds are less familiar to you. For example:

- Judging a 4-year-old Pakistani child to have poor self-care and manipulative skills because she finds it difficult to handle a knife and fork at lunchtime. You would need to be aware that using knives and forks at the table is a practice confined mainly to Western societies and that she may be unfamiliar with using these in her home environment.
- Assuming insolence and poor social skills because a child will not make eye contact when you are speaking to him. You would need to know that in some cultures it would be considered very impolite for a child to look directly at an adult.
- Concluding that a child who speaks few words in English has language problems, when in fact he is fluent in his home language. An accurate assessment might be that he needed support in developing his competence in English.

Where children's progress is to be measured using standardised assessments, these tests should be screened for cultural bias. For example, a child with only experience of the Islamic tradition of art, which emphasises pattern and decoration, but not representation of living things, would not demonstrate his abilities accurately against a scale measuring mental age that requires the child to draw a figure and score points for every detail.

LIMITATIONS OF OBSERVATIONS AND ASSESSMENTS

A one-off observation or assessment of a child will not give you a complete and reliable view and you should avoid hasty conclusions on the basis of this. In order to

 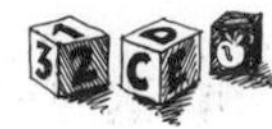

make secure judgements about a child's abilities or progress, or to act on any concerns, you would need to have a fuller picture, perhaps compiled from a number of observations made over a period of time and take into consideration factors that might have an influence on the child's behaviour or responses. For example, a 1-year-old child asked to post some shapes into a sorter by the health visitor during a routine development check might bury her head in her mother's lap. The health visitor would not assume that she was unable to pick up and post the shape, but conclude that she chose not to try, perhaps because of the unfamiliarity of herself and the situation. Assessments of children when they are tired or wary or in unfamiliar surroundings are unlikely to give an accurate picture. (However, there may be situations where you have serious concerns about something you have observed and where the child might be at risk. It is your responsibility to raise this with your placement supervisor who will follow up your concerns and take any necessary action.)

Case study . . .

. . . using observation

Alex had been attending nursery for about 6 months. At this nursery staff make focused observations of individual children on a regular basis and discuss their findings at team meetings. The general feeling was that Alex had settled well and enjoyed most activities. The nursery nurse observed Alex for the whole of a morning session, focusing on his social interactions with other children and on the areas of activity he chose to play in. She found that although he appeared to be part of a group, for much of the time he was watching others play and was not able to take a real part in the activity. He chose a range of activities but during that session avoided painting and craft. This observation was discussed at the team meeting with other staff. They had seen him obviously engrossed in painting and craft on other occasions and did not feel his missing those activities this time was a significant. However, they felt that he did need a chance to break into group play and suggested that a member of staff should play alongside Alex in a group and encourage him to be more assertive. At their next meeting, they would review the situation and decide whether there was still cause for concern.

1. *Why was focused observation useful in this situation?*
2. *What pre-conceived ideas might the staff have had about Alex?*
3. *In your own placement or work setting, what use is made of observation?*

WHAT DO YOU OBSERVE?

- Observe individual children during their play and other activities. You will get the best results from observing children in familiar, naturally occurring, everyday situations rather than those specially set up for the purpose of observation. You may want to focus on an area of development, an aspect of the curriculum or an area of concern. All children will benefit from the attention of observation, not just those about whom you have a concern.
- Observe groups of children and look at interaction and co-operation. Small groups will give you an opportunity to compare skills and responses.
- Look at a piece of equipment or a particular activity and see how children respond to it.

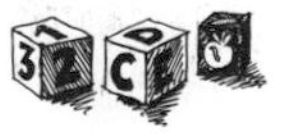

- Observe children over a period of time. Map their pathways around the room. Do they take up all the activities? Are some areas avoided?

WHAT SHOULD YOU LOOK FOR?

Remember to refer to the observation matrix for your course, to ensure that your portfolio covers the required range. You will be expected to complete observations across the age range, on all areas of development, of children with particular needs and in a range of contexts.

WHEN OBSERVING AN AREA OF DEVELOPMENT, LOOK FOR EVIDENCE OF:

PHYSICAL DEVELOPMENT – GROSS MOTOR SKILLS

- Using balancing skill
- Controlling movement in running, skipping, hopping, jumping
- Whole body co-ordination
- Using strength
- Practising a skill

PHYSICAL DEVELOPMENT – FINE MOTOR SKILLS

- Using fine finger movements (manipulative skills)
- Using hand–eye co-ordination
- Placing and positioning skills

COGNITIVE DEVELOPMENT

- Concentration
- Using imagination
- Using memory
- Being creative
- Experimenting and investigating
- Thinking carefully, understanding
- Exploring with senses
- Solving problems
- Using symbols, e.g. a ruler for a sword, a doll for a baby
- Understanding of concepts, e.g. of colour, shape, size, number
- Imitating others, adults or children

LINGUISTIC DEVELOPMENT

- Listening to others
- Thinking out loud
- Discussing ideas
- Following instructions
- Using words thoughtfully, carefully, imaginatively
- Describing an object or event
- Reading or following a plan
- Recording with drawing or writing
- Pronunciation, articulation, intonation
- Non-verbal language
- Grammar, tenses, appropriate use of parts of speech
- Complexity of sentences – one word, simple, complex
- Use of vocabulary
- The purpose of the children's language

SOCIAL DEVELOPMENT

- Relating to friends or relatives
- Relating to unknown adults and children
- Sharing – space, equipment
- Co-operating with others
- Taking turns
- Working in a group, with partners

EMOTIONAL DEVELOPMENT

- Look for demonstration of feelings, e.g. happy, relaxed, confident, amused, pleased, proud, sad, confused, distressed, angry, timid, shy, etc.
- Record how the child deals with those feelings

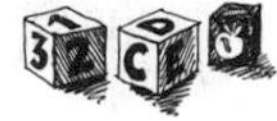

Observing babies under 1 year old

When you observe the development of young babies, you will find it helpful to focus on the following:

- *Gross motor* – large body movements including head control, rolling over, sitting, crawling, pulling to stand and walking.
- *Fine motor* – hand–eye co-ordination including random arm movements, eye contact, focusing, attempts at grasping and manipulating objects.
- *Social and play* – how the baby relates to and interacts with parents, carers, family and others. Look for the beginnings of social behaviour in smiling, laughing, imitation, recognising people and situations.
- *Hearing and language* – how the baby responds to various sounds, cooing, babbling, recognising familiar sounds and voices, understanding language, e.g. responding to 'No' and own name.

Children with particular needs

Children may have a particular need that affects their development. This may be a long-term need – a child with a hearing impairment – or it could be a short-term need, perhaps feeling unsettled following the arrival of a new baby. The focus of your observation will determine whether it is relevant to consider the child's particular need when you analyse your findings. For example, if a child has a particular need concerning her mobility, this would be relevant to an observation on physical development, but probably not if you were looking at language skills.

WHEN CAN YOU OBSERVE?

Observing children is an important part of your training and can only be carried out in your placement. You should discuss what you need to do with your placement supervisor and agree times when you will carry out your observations. Staff will often help you to choose who to observe and in what situation if you explain the focus of your observation.

RECORDING OBSERVATIONS

- Try not to let children know that you are observing a particular child or group of children as this is likely to have an effect on their behaviour.
- If you are not participating in the activity, position yourself unobtrusively so that you can see the child but you are not within the child's personal space.
- Try not to make eye contact with the child as that may encourage the child to come towards you and affect your focus.
- You will need to make notes while you are observing because you may not remember in enough detail. A small notebook is less obtrusive than a heavy ring binder.
- You should write up your notes as soon as you can after the observation or you will forget what any abbreviations and key words mean.
- Sometimes careful preparation will be necessary. For example, if you are observing the spread of children around the classroom, then a sketch of the layout will be required. Checklists can be devised for many purposes. These are straightforward to complete, particularly when you are observing at an activity with a group.

- If you are interested in children's language interaction, you may wish to use a small, unobtrusive tape recorder. (Background noise may be a problem with this method though.)
- Many settings have access to video cameras but filming will raise issues of confidentiality and will probably have an effect on the children's behaviour.

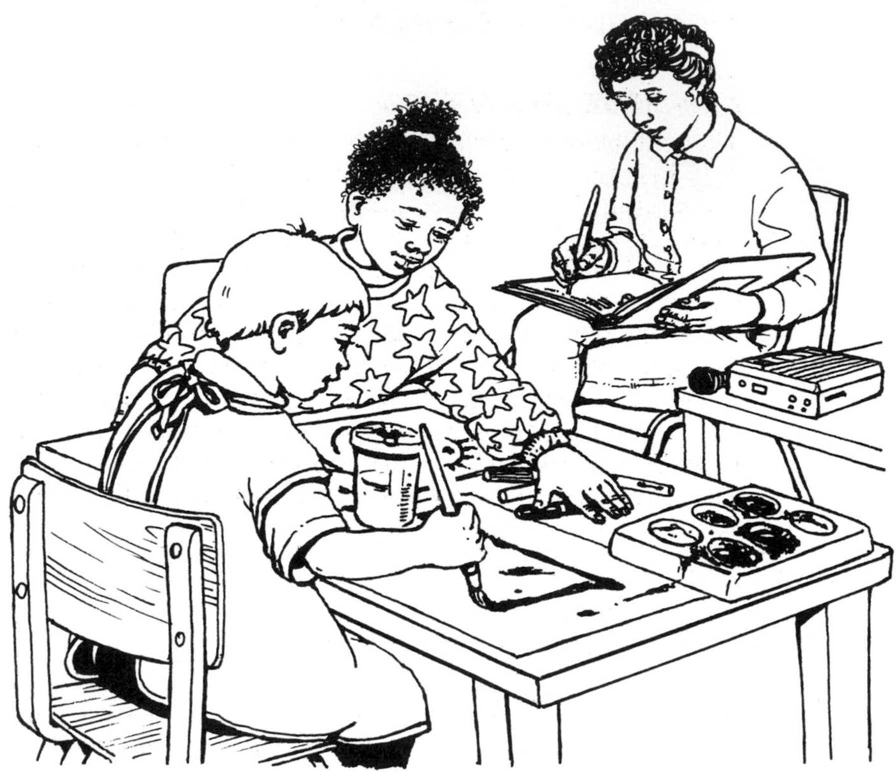

Position yourself unobtrusively, away from the child's personal space

Progress check

1 *How can you ensure confidentiality when you make observations of children?*
2 *Why is it important to be objective in your observations?*
3 *How can observations help with planning for children?*
4 *Describe how you can avoid drawing the wrong conclusions from observations.*
5 *Why should you try to be unobtrusive when making observations of children?*

Observation and assessment techniques

This section will introduce you to a range of different methods to record observations, helping you to choose the technique most appropriate to the focus of any observation. It will also outline the background information that you need to present for every observation you include in your portfolio.

 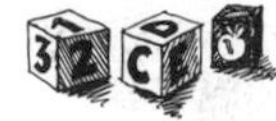

There are a number of techniques that can be used to observe children. During your training you will have the opportunity to practise a range of these. As you become more experienced, you will be able to select or modify a method so that it is appropriate for your intended observation.

Some techniques are listed below and there are many others. Each method will have advantages and disadvantages. Your skill in choosing the best technique for your purpose and identifying its strengths and shortcomings will contribute to the grade you achieve for your portfolio.

NARRATIVE (DESCRIPTION)

This is a prose record of what you observe. It is useful because it can provide a very detailed picture of what is going on. You may find it difficult to write down everything that you see, and using abbreviations and keywords will help here. Another problem might be maintaining your focus. If the purpose of your observation is to find out about a child's gross motor skills, then you must discipline yourself to look primarily for sufficient evidence of these skills and to record this. While you are observing, you should not be sidetracked into recording examples of, say, social behaviour or language, as these are not part of your focus. Choosing the right activity to observe is also crucial to success when using this or any method of observation. If you want to find out about social skills you will need to observe when children have opportunities to engage with one another: observing a silent reading activity would not provide you with much evidence of this.

A narrative observation

AIM – *To observe Ashley during a 'parachute' PE session.*

PURPOSE – *To assess Ashley's gross motor skills.*

The children were standing in a circle, holding hands, around the outside of the parachute, which was spread out on the floor. Ashley was standing up straight holding two of the children's hands either side of him and he was being stretched both ways. Firstly he was pulled to his right and hopped about on his right leg, then he was pulled on to his left leg and shuffled his foot about to keep his balance. The teacher told the children to sit on the floor so Ashley let go of the children's hands and quickly dropped to the floor on his bottom with his right leg already crossed over his left leg. He bent his legs at the knees and crossed them so that the soles of his feet were pointing away from him. He used his large arm muscles to lift them at the shoulders and bend them at the elbows. He crossed his right arm over his left and held on to the tops of each opposite arm.

Next the children were asked to stand up. Ashley unfolded his arms and uncrossed his legs by bringing his right leg over his left. He used his right foot, which was now flat on the floor, to push himself up to a standing position and his left foot quickly did the same. He had used his hands flat on the floor to keep his balance and as he stood up grasped the handle of the parachute and lifted it up with him. The children were asked to gently lift the parachute and lower it again. Ashley lifted his arms up until they were straight and stretched upwards and stood on his tiptoes so that he was at the same height as the two children either side of him. He staggered about a little on his toes trying to keep his balance. After lifting it twice he pulled it up into the air and let go by lifting up his arms and stretching them above his head. He brought his arms down and caught hold of the handle when the parachute came down again.

Ashley's name was called after a few minutes so by lifting his arms quickly and letting go of the parachute he was able to duck under it by bending his head and neck downwards slightly and run to the other side underneath. He ran very fast, on flat feet, bending his knees as he lifted alternate legs. His arms were bent at the elbows and moved back and forth alternately as he ran. Ashley lifted his arms and took hold of a handle again.

Next a ball was put on to the parachute and sent round in a circle as the children lifted and lowered their arms. Ashley was shaking the parachute up and down quickly, by lifting his straight arms at the shoulder and moving them up and down while he was bending and straightening his back and knees. Eventually, he watched the other children who waited until the ball got to them before lifting the parachute, then copied them. They are asked to sit down again and Ashley lifted his right leg bent at the knee and crossed it over his left leg. He quickly dropped to the floor on to his bottom and let his knees relax so that he was sitting cross-legged again. He was still grasping the handle of the parachute with both hands and he sat quite still while children took turns to crawl underneath the parachute to retrieve a beanbag. He was moving his head from side to side as each one went. As Robert ran past him with the beanbag Ashley shouted 'Give me 5' and lifted his arm high in the air with his flat palm facing Robert.

Ashley's name was called and he launched himself under the parachute by lifting both arms high and throwing himself forwards on to his knees in a crawling position. He crawled very fast towards the beanbag by moving one leg after the other at the hip, and moving his arms alternately with his palms flat on the floor for balance. He disappeared under the parachute then came out head first, and still crawling he turned himself over by swinging his left arm backwards over his body and landing on his bottom. His legs were out in front of him, bent at the knees. The class teacher told the children that it was time to go and packed away the parachute.

TARGET CHILD (PRE-CODED)

This method is useful because it enables the observer to record quickly, accurately and unobtrusively, using pre-coded categories. The focus on the target child (TC) is maintained throughout the observation as everything is recorded in relation to that child. To use this method successfully, the observer needs to prepare the recording sheet to fit with the purpose of the observation and be totally familiar with the coding for the categories.

TIME SAMPLING

This method entails observing for a set period at regular intervals, for example for 2 minutes every half-hour during a session. The focus can be a child or a group of children or an activity or piece of equipment. It can be used for a number of purposes. Noting the range of activities chosen by a child would show whether a balanced programme was being taken up. Recording a child's interactions with others might show social skills and friendship patterns. Recording responses to a particular activity would help staff to evaluate the provision. Disadvantages associated with this method are that it requires the observer to be disciplined about recording only that which occurs during the 'watching' slot and it involves watching the clock.

EVENT SAMPLING

This method can be useful for tracking an aspect of behaviour that might be giving cause for concern, over a set period of time, for example, the frequency of a child's temper tantrums over a week. It enables the observer to consider whether there is any recognisable pattern to incidents, to identify possible triggers and to form an overview of the situation. Parents may be asked to record incidents too.

DATE: 16.6.01 METHOD: Target Child pre-coded observation

AIM AND/OR REASON FOR OBSERVATION:

To detect any possible change in behaviour due to birth of new baby

DETAILS OF SETTING:

Nursery class

IMMEDIATE CONTEXT:

N/A

TIME OBSERVATION STARTED: 10.35 am

TIME OBSERVATION FINISHED: 10.44 am

TOTAL NUMBER OF ADULTS IN SETTING: 2

TOTAL NUMBER OF CHILDREN IN SETTING: 20

FIRST NAME(S) OF CHILD(REN) BEING OBSERVED: LUKE

AGE(S): 4:4

GENDER(S): M

MEDIA USED AND JUSTIFICATION (IF NECESSARY):

SUPERVISOR'S SIGNATURE	TUTOR'S SIGNATURE	PERMISSION IF APPLICABLE
C. Clarke	J. Brown	✓

CHILD'S INITIALS: LF SEX: M AGE: 4:4

DATE AND TIME OBSERVED: 16.6.01

ACTIVITY RECORD	LANGUAGE RECORD	TASK	SOCIAL
1 MIN TC at activity table making a model from junk	TC → A 'pass the scissors' A → TC 'when James has finished'	Art	SG
2 MIN TC waiting for scissors	TC humming a song	W	SG
3 MIN TC cutting a large cereal box	TC ↔ C (about the models they are making)	Art	SG
4 MIN TC gluing model	TC → A 'Look at my aeroplane! Can I paint it?'	Art	SG
5 MIN TC goes to paint table to paint his model		Art	SOL
6 MIN TC goes to bathroom to wash hands	TC ↔ C (discussing Neighbours on TV) A watching	D A	PAIR + A
7 MIN TC drying hands	TC ↔ C (continues conversation) A leaves room	D A	PAIR
8 MIN TC & C go outside & chase each other round playground	shouting	I G	PAIR

Codes: TC – Target child, C – Child, A – Adult; W – Waiting, Art – Art activities, D A – Domestic activities; I G – Informal group, S G – Small group, SOL – Solitary

Target child observation

AIM – *to record any occurrence of anti-social behaviour over a period of one week.*

PURPOSE – *to see if there is any pattern to the incidence of this behaviour.*

DATE/TIME	BEHAVIOUR	ANTECEDENT	WHO WAS THERE	CONSEQUENCE
20.6.00 11.05	L had both his hands around A's neck from behind.	The children of class 5 were walking in a singular line into the classroom after playtime.	The other children were following behind L and I was already in the room.	I intervened and comforted A. I subsequently informed the teacher, she immediately confronted L. He admitted saying "it's because she's lying, cause she said I've got sweets and I haven't". L was told to apologise to A and if he has a problem he should talk about it.
21.6.00 10.40	L kicked J on the back of his leg.	Children were tidying the tables before playtime.	J & L were alone at the table. Teacher sat at her desk.	J backed away from L. Teacher called J and L to stay in class as others went out. L was confronted about kicking then said: "he was nicking my pens and rubber". J interrupted saying he was only putting them back into the pencil case. L was told that for whatever reason he should not kick or hurt anyone. He was then kept in at playtime.
21.6.00 10.55	L pushed K from behind and K fell over. L then pointed his finger into K's cheek saying, "You are not in my game".	Playtime and several year I children were playing a game of tiggy scarecrow in the playground and climbing area.	The whole class plus teacher and myself supervising.	Teacher intervened and instructed L to stand with her. K went on to play the game.
26.6.00 1.40	L threw a container of money on to the floor then pushed the table forwards into C's chest.	L and C were playing a shopping game.	They were alone at the table and the teacher was sitting quite close with two other children.	C looked at L's face with his eyes wide and mouth open. Teacher intervened and ordered L to let go of the table then pick up the money. L kicked the table leg then began picking the money up. He then was told to sit next to her while the other children played in pairs.

Event sampling observation

AIM – *to observe E throughout the session, for three minutes every 15 minutes.*

PURPOSE – *to identify any factors affecting his performance and to assess any need for support.*

TIME/SETTING	OTHERS PRESENT	ACTIONS & REACTIONS	LANGUAGE
9.00 Classroom.	Whole class for register and assembly.	Sitting attentively. Hands up to face, starts to look around.	Answers "yes" to name. Body language, leaning across desk.
9.15 Classroom.	Whole class spelling test.	Gets ready with spelling book and pencil.	Waits quietly as teacher reads out spellings group by group.
9.30 Classroom.	Whole class.	E wanders round tables with spelling sheet. Should be in line to take new spellings to cloakroom.	Teacher asks E if he knows what he is supposed to be doing. He smiles at her, and says "yes". Teachers aks E to join the line of children.
9.45 Library, giving me instructions to work Roamer.	E and C.	E very interested, gave me precise instructions of how to use the Roamer.	E said, "To work the Roamer you switch on the button on the side, press CM press one of the arrows, forward press a number and GO."
10.00 Craft table in area between library and classroom.	J and T.	Cutting paper and card for owl nest.	E said, "You give the paper a twist, on the floor of the nest is where the babies play", pointing, "thats their rattle".
10.15 Craft Area	J, P and T.	Standing to table making owls habitat. Stopped working to look at J and P making their nest. E was supposed to be working with T.	Staring at J and P working. Teacher walks through and asks E if he is helping T with their model. E nods his head.
10.30 Classroom milk time	Whole class and a teacher from another class.	Sits drinking juice from flask.	Does not enter any conversation with peers; concentrates on drinking.
10.45 Playtime	In line with whole class, standing between S and T.	Standing between T and C. rocking backwards and forwards, knocking into them.	E smiles, nods head.

Time sampling observation

FLOW CHART

A flow chart enables a child's movements to be tracked and recorded in diagrammatic form. It can be used for a variety of purposes. It will show the choices a child makes in terms of provision, perhaps identifying gaps in what is experienced. It can also indicate social interactions and friendship groups and, if times are recorded, can give an indication of a child's ability to sustain interest in an activity. It is helpful to prepare a plan of the room, indicating what is available during the particular session. As this method records movement and choices, it is not a useful method if children are expected to stay in one place for the period. (Children's movements can be tracked using different diagrammatic forms. The following is an example of one type of chart.)

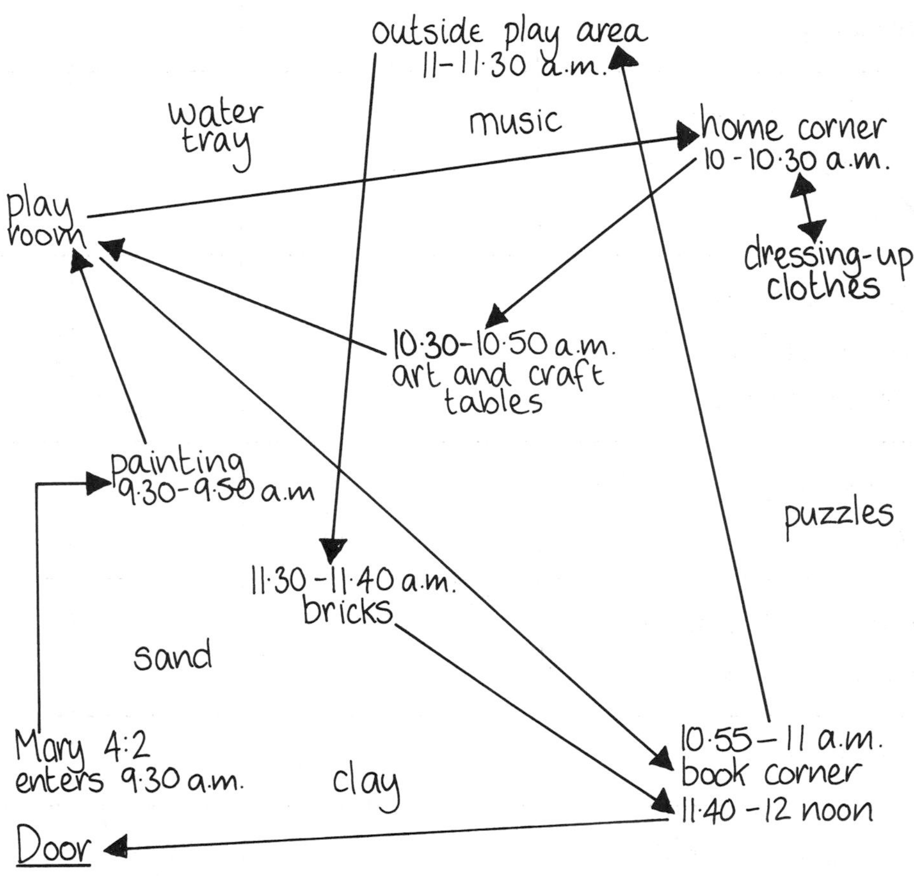

Flow chart observation **Aim** – to record a child's movements during the nursery session.
Purpose – to comment on her choices and preferences in play.

key term

Baseline assessment required assessment of children's skills currently (January 2001) undertaken on entry to school. In future, likely to be applied at the beginning of Year 1

CHECKLIST

This is a useful way of gaining a lot of information in and recording it in a straightforward way, usually by ticking against a chart. Checklists can be used to compare performance across a group of children. You can devise your own checklists perhaps to assess a particular skill or aspect of development, or you can refer to the many published developmental scales and checklists. **Baseline assessment** relies on the use of checklist assessment.

The following example of a checklist provides an opportunity to observe several babies of the same age to compare their developmental progress.

AIM – *to observe a series of babies at 3 months.*

PURPOSE – *to note the similarities and/or differences in their physical developmental achievements.*

PHYSICAL ACHIEVEMENT	BABY A AGE:	BABY B AGE:	BABY C AGE:	COMMENTS
In prone, lifts head and chest supported on forearms				
Sags at knees when held standing				
Smooth, continuous movements of legs and arms				
In ventral suspension, head is held above the plane of the back				
No head lag when pulled to sit				
Holds rattle briefly when placed in the hand				
Finger-play				
Turns head to follow adult movements				

Checklist observation

SNAPSHOT

This is a useful technique for evaluating the provision that you make available to children. It can show which activities are taken up by children, where staff are located and demonstrate how space is used. The following example was compiled to identify the range of opportunities for mathematical learning available during the session. The second sheet shows the student's analysis of the activities and of the areas of mathematics offered. As she also recorded the presence of adults at activities, she could then link this to their role in promoting mathematical understanding.

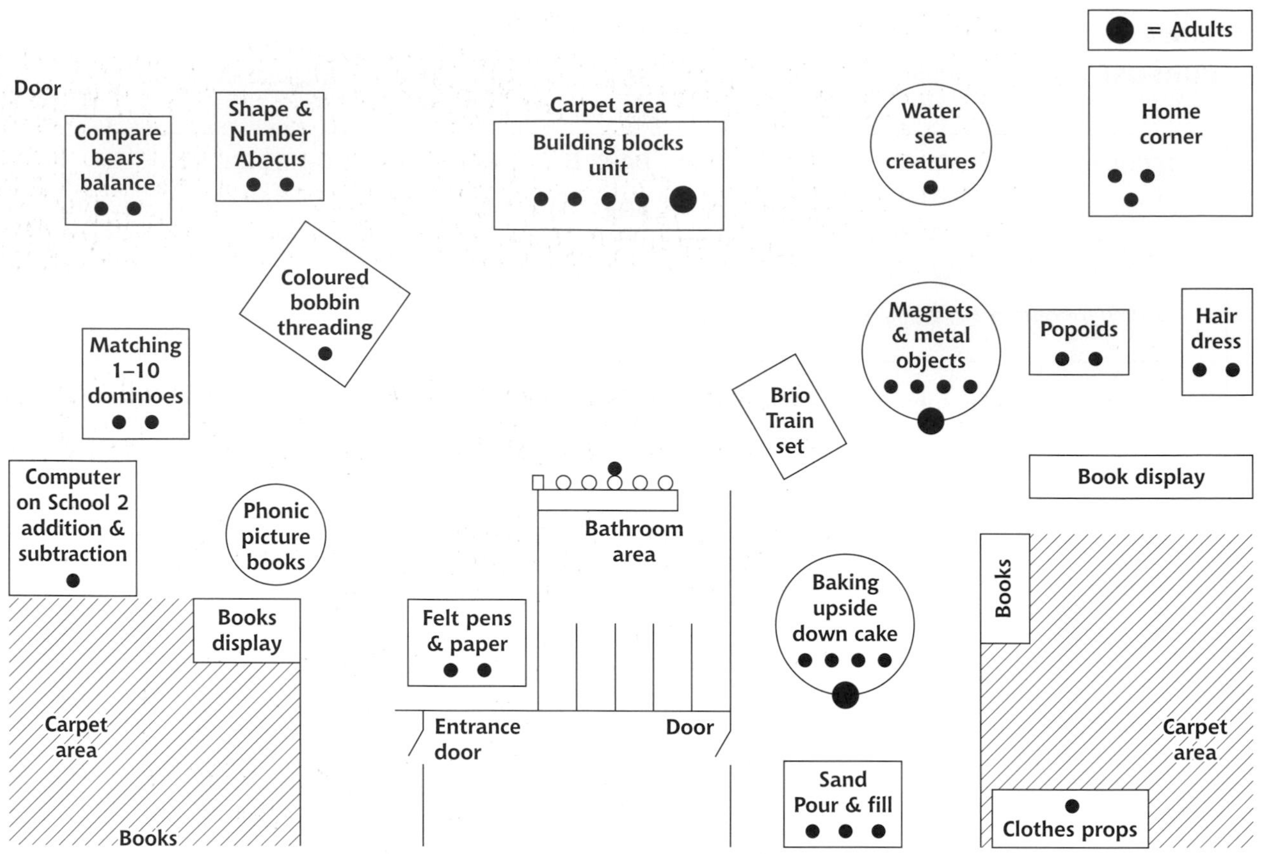

Snapshot observation – (sheet 1) **Aim** – to record the activities available during a session.
Purpose – to identify the range of mathematical opportunities available.

	Blocks	Baking	Computer	Sand	Water	Dominoes	Balance	Abacus	Threading	Home corner
Number										
matching	✓		✓			✓	✓	✓	✓	✓
sorting	✓	✓	✓			✓	✓	✓	✓	✓
one-to-one correspondence		✓	✓				✓	✓		✓
cardinal number	✓		✓				✓	✓	✓	✓
ordinal number	✓	✓		✓		✓		✓	✓	✓
Space										
topological	✓	✓		✓	✓	✓	✓	✓	✓	✓
euclideon	✓			✓		✓		✓	✓	
Time										
personal		✓		✓						
universal		✓		✓						
volume & capacity		✓		✓						
shape	✓			✓		✓		✓	✓	✓
size	✓			✓				✓	✓	✓
area	✓	✓		✓	✓	✓			✓	✓
pattern	✓			✓	✓	✓		✓	✓	
weight	✓	✓		✓	✓		✓		✓	
length	✓					✓			✓	

(sheet 2) Analysis of mathematical opportunities available.

SOCIOGRAM

A sociogram demonstrates friendship patterns within a group in diagrammatic form. You can observe children's friendship choices and plot them on a diagram or you can ask children about their friends. You need to bear in mind that young children may find it difficult to say who their friend is and that friendships in this age group are likely to be fluid. (There are many different formats that can be used to present sociogram observations.)

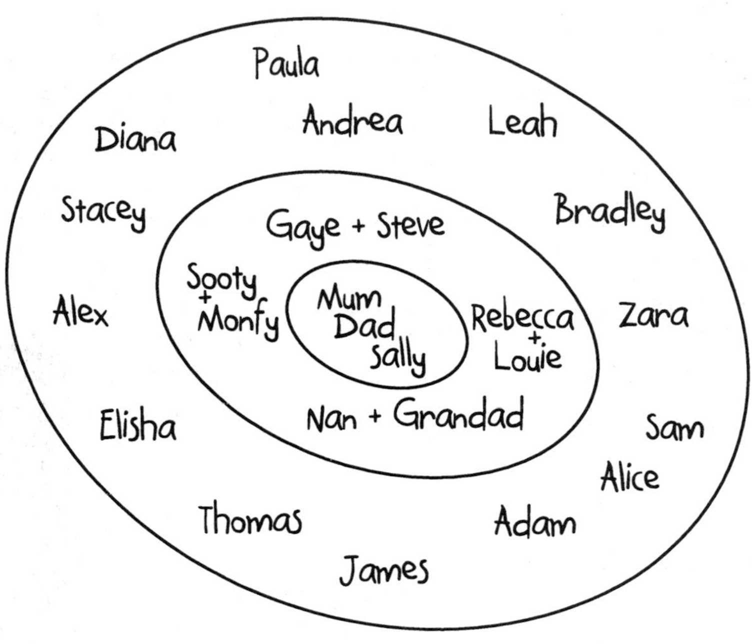

A sociogram observation

In the above example, a group of 7-year-old children were asked to think about the people they were closest to. This child put her closest relatives (Mum, Dad and sister Sally) in the centre. In the next ring she included other relatives, close family friends and family pets. The outer ring showed her classroom friends. All of the children filled in similar diagrams and the child-care worker was able to compare them looking at friendship patterns within the group and seeing whether friendship choices were reciprocated.

BACKGROUND INFORMATION

As a student, for all observations, whatever technique you use, you should record details about the child/children observed, the setting and the context and focus of your observation so that your tutor can make a judgement about what you have observed to assess your progress and grade your work. Some tutors ask for a completed proforma to accompany each observation as a check that everything is included. An example is given here.

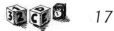

NAME: Jeannie Smith	TUTOR: Mary Brown
OBSERVATION NUMBER: 7	DATE OBSERVED: 15 Jan 2001
TIME STARTED: 9.55am	TIME FINISHED: 10.05am

TITLE: Early Years Curriculum

INDIVIDUAL / GROUP Individual

'I certify that this observation was undertaken as stated and with my permission':
Placement supervisor's signature :

AIM:
To observe Rahila in the role play area (café)

PURPOSE: To comment on Rahila's play in this area, focusing on her language and social skills

TECHNIQUE: Narrative. I chose this method because it enabled me to focus on the child for a short but concentrated period and record her language and interactions with other children in detail.

TYPE OF SETTING: Nursery class (30 place) in a county primary school

PARTICIPATING CHILDREN :

First name	Age (Yrs & months)	Other relevant factors
Rahila	4years 1 month	Rahila's home language is Punjabi. She speaks English at nursery.

ADULTS PRESENT DURING THE OBSERVATION AND THEIR ROLES:
Nursery teacher, 2 nursery nurses and myself (student)

IMMEDIATE CONTEXT / ENVIRONMENT:
The nursery was set up with a range of activities for the children to choose from. The children had been in their groups for circle time and had been asked what they were going to do next. Rahila said that she wanted to play in the café and so did her friend Amy. As circle time finished, she walked over to the café where there were already two children. She picked up a waiter's apron and fastened it.

A proforma to accompany a student's observation

Some of the information included here relates to the assessment requirements of the course you are following, but some background details will be required for any observation of a child carried out in a professional capacity, as follows:

- Time and date establish the currency and validity of an observation. This could be extremely important for any observation used in child protection or other legal proceedings.
- An aim and purpose identifies the focus of your observation. As you record information you should refer to it – it reminds you what you want to investigate. Your aim says what you are going to do – observe James on the climbing frame – and your purpose establishes why you are observing – to find out about his climbing and balancing skills.
- Indicating the child's age is important too. If you are making assessments of a child's developmental progress you will need to know his chronological age so that you can compare it with the developmental norm for that age. With very young babies, you should record the age in weeks.
- You will need to consider what 'other relevant information' to include and this will relate to your focus. In the example above, which is examining the child's language development, it is obviously relevant to record that she is bilingual. There may be other relevant factors to note, depending on what and why you are observing. In some observations, factors such as being new to the setting or some change in home circumstances may have a bearing. Noting these factors will enable you to analyse your observation more accurately.
- Noting the immediate context helps to set the scene for your observation and may include factors that have a bearing on what is to be observed. This could be particularly important when the observation is discussed or referred to away from the setting.

Progress check

1 *Why is a checklist a useful observation technique?*

2 *If you were concerned about an aspect of a child's behaviour, which observation technique might be useful?*

3 *Which technique might be helpful for finding out about children's friendship groups?*

4 *Why should observations have a focus?*

5 *Why is it important to include background information alongside your observations?*

Evaluating your observations

On an individual basis, evaluation of observations will reveal the child's learning potential and can help to assess the progress achieved. More widely, evaluating provision through observation will demonstrate how effectively plans are being implemented and the intended learning objectives being achieved. Staff can then plan for subsequent sessions, making any necessary adjustments in organisation, resources, interaction and expectations on the basis of this.

The evaluation section of your observation is where you can analyse what you have learned about the child/children or the provision on the basis of what you have recorded. Most evaluations will include the following elements:

- interpretation
- assessment
- recommendations
- conclusion/personal learning.

It is not necessary to present your work using the above headings but your evaluation should include all the elements.

At the end of each of the following sections is an example of part of the evaluation from a student's observation. The observation's focus was on the fine motor skills of two children, a 5 year old and a 6 year old.

INTERPRETATION

You will find it helpful to go through the observation and interpret it in the light of your focus. This means looking back and finding how what you have recorded links to your focus. For example, if you wanted to find out about a child's ability to get on with her peers and work as part of a group you would look at the observation and note any examples of sharing, taking turns, discussing, joining in etc. (You might find a highlighter pen helpful to indicate this as you go through your observation.) You can then relate what you have observed to the aspects of social development you were focusing on, for example:

- she played the game and was able to wait for her turn
- she asked her friend to come and play the game with them
- when they came to the end of the game, she organised the clearing away

and so on until you have referred to everything you think is relevant.

If you have used a standardised assessment test or task with the child, your interpretation will involve looking back at the responses and scoring.

'I was looking for T and E's fine motor skills. Both of them demonstrated them well throughout. Both of them listened to the teacher's instructions, showing me that they were alert because they were keen to get on with the task. Both of the children controlled their fine movements well, because they knew how to hold the pencil in their own way, in order to write. E balanced the letters well on the lines provided. T sometimes missed balancing letters on the line, but when he concentrated, his writing skills were good. Some of his letters were slightly crooked. He tended to find writing the letter "p" difficult (he repeated the stem part of the letter, meaning he doesn't lift his pencil to write the rounded part).

Both the children's hand–eye co-ordination was good, because they knew what writing tools to choose and they coloured inside the lines very neatly. After writing for a longer period, I noticed both children tended to press hard. They knew how to tidy up, putting all the stationery in the right boxes, and placing the paper into the middle, the correct way up. This shows good positioning control.'

ASSESSMENT

Now you should be in a position to assess what you have observed, that is to compare your findings to what you might expect for a child of this age. With standardised tests or assessment tasks, you will be able to match the scores you have recorded against tables to give a result. For other observations, you will need to refer to published norms of development and also to compare the child with her immediate peers. You should be wary of jumping to conclusions and making sweeping statements on the basis of one observation and also you should consider any special circumstances that might have a bearing on your assessment. For example, you might expect most 5 year olds to be sociable and able to join in with a group. However, a 5 year old during his first week in a new group might be more reticent. There could be other factors too that might have had an impact on what you have observed; the routine might have changed, the staffing might be different. You should refer to this, too, if you think it might be significant. In this section you will be able to consider theories of child development and the findings from research and studies and compare these with your own findings. (When you make references to published material you should acknowledge these in your writing and provide a bibliography.) A thoughtful and perceptive assessment should provide you with a basis from which you can make recommendations regarding the child or the provision.

> *'I will compare E and T to the rest of the class. All the children knew what tasks they had been asked to do and what writing equipment they needed. T and E knew what they needed as well. I noticed most children are right-handed and so is E. T is left-handed, meaning his left side is more acute. He tends to pick up items with his left hand only. T suffers from hemiplegia (his right side is weakest), and he doesn't tend to put it to use.*
>
> *Most children including E have their hand positioned near the pencil's nib and have their wrists resting on the paper, during writing, making them write more quickly. T's hand was well above the nib and his wrist never rested on the paper, perhaps making it harder to write quickly and making his writing look wobblier than other children's. This could be due to the hand itself not being stable.*
>
> *T can sometimes lose concentration and you have to push him to carry on working. This might be due to his hemiplegia, which causes him to become tired faster than E and other children because one side of his body is weaker. T does put in more effort than some others, even though his writing rate is slower than the average child.*
>
> *Children all develop differently and in various ways. The development scales can only suggest what stage a child should be at according to average development. But because children are all individuals there is no set age for developmental milestones. Children who are slower at developing may need more time. They will reach the scale when ready, and it is down to the education worker and primary carer to notice this and try to support and encourage the child. E and T matched Frankel and Hobart's (1994) scale for 5 years in that they can control the pencil and crayon, copy adult writing and colour pictures in neatly. T had neat colouring due to slow hand movement and correct crayon positioning. E coloured in faster. (But she hasn't got a condition that affects her manipulative skills.) I think that the scale hasn't taken physical disabilities into account, because T, who is 6, can't tie his laces, because he has one strong arm. You need two arms to do this. At 6, children should be able to tie laces, according to Frankel and Hobart (1999). T is a bright child, but his disability will affect his acquiring this skill. Other development scales are different. Another development scale, Sharman, Cross and Vennis (1995), states that children should be able to tie their laces at 5 years. This proves that these scales provide only guidance about children's development.'*

RECOMMENDATIONS

Here you can make suggestions concerning what the next steps should be. This might be in terms of providing particular experiences or activities for a child or a group of children, supporting a particular aspect of development or consolidating a skill or concept. It might be that you have indicated the need for some extra support for a child or that you have a concern that needs to be discussed with the team and perhaps followed through with further observations. In recording your recommendations, you should try to be realistic and sensitive to the feelings of the staff who will be looking at your work. It will not be conducive to a good working relationship if you make remarks such as 'the nursery nurse should pay more attention to T, rather than chat with her colleague' even if you believe this to be so!

'It is clear that both E and T enjoy the written work, because they both started it as soon as the teacher finished discussing it, meaning they are keen. To maintain a good standard of written work, they need to practise writing and holding the tool, to find a comfortable position that will make them feel less tired when writing. Also this regular practice will enable them to become neater. I noticed that when E and T work, they tend to keep their heads down, close to the paper. They should try and keep their back straight and head more upwards, to prevent future neck and back strains.

When E and T knew their spellings, their writing was faster. When they were not sure how to spell a word, they tended to write slower and press much harder on to the paper. Thorough learning of spelling will speed up the rate of writing and therefore they don't tend to press so hard. I think because of T's condition, he should exercise his weaker side, to strengthen his body muscles. Arm rotation and picking up objects with this arm is good to get the muscles working, to prevent his arm drooping with weakness, as it does presently. T can get more tired than other children. He should get plenty of sleep, so he can concentrate and be alert in more intensive tasks but this could also apply to any child of this age.'

CONCLUSION

In this section you can reflect on your own learning from the observation. It might be that you now have a clearer understanding of a particular aspect of child development or it might be specific to the group you have observed, perhaps becoming aware of the range of abilities within a class of 5 year olds. You should also use this section to consider the observation technique that you used in relation to your focus. What were its strengths? What were its limitations? Would another technique have been more revealing? You might also think about whether you should observe the same child or group of children again, perhaps at a different activity or in another situation in order to gain a fuller picture of your focus.

'My observation is narrative. This is a good method because you have to write down all the movements of the children you see. It's like telling a story to a person who didn't see the moves. You are giving them an idea of how far these children are in the development scale of the fine motor skills. However, this method has disadvantages, because in describing all the details you saw in the situation, it is sometimes difficult to put into words that make it clear to the reader. Also it is hard to look and write simultaneously. It is easy to miss a lot of small movements. There are other alternative methods of observation. Two people can observe one child each, then swap papers, to make it easier on the brain and speed up on time. Two people watching one child together is effective, because one person may see different movements to the other. Then you can share notes. (Comparative observation.)

Filming a child enables you to repeat sections over and over, so you can write things you missed. But this requires permission from the parent and placement supervisor. Parents may not be keen on exposing their child's identity. This method doesn't respect confidentiality. I think if I could do another observation based on fine motor skills, I would look at other aspects of the skill. Although watching E and T at these activities met my stated aims, it didn't cover all the aspects of fine motor skills. Seeing their cutting skills and puzzle arrangements as well, would give me a better idea of their overall development in this area as one aspect will not give me a full picture. This would require more time to observe. I would possibly have to ask the teacher to change her plans to include opportunities for the children to demonstrate these skills. I could take the children out of the class to do the activities required, but then they could miss out on the lesson and may fall behind the rest of the class. Also, other children may question why certain children get to try other activities and not others, making the situation more awkward. T and E could feel singled out and this would not be good for them.'

Progress check

What is the purpose of evaluating observations?

How can you go about interpreting your observation?

What should you include in your assessment section?

Why is it helpful to make recommendations based on your observation?

Now try these questions

Why is observation such an important professional skill?

Identify some ways in which you can record observations.

Why is it important to match your choice of technique to the focus of your observation?

How can doing observations contribute to your own knowledge and understanding of child development?

key terms

You need to know what the key terms and phrases in this chapter mean. Go back through the chapter and find out.

Unit 2: Work with Young Children

In this unit you will learn about planning activities, experiences and routines for babies and children. You will learn about the planning cycle: how to plan, prepare and evaluate activities, and ways to interact with the children during the activity.

This unit helps you understand why planning is important and what must be included in your plans. It outlines the role and responsibilities of adults to plan appropriate learning experiences that promote equality of opportunity.

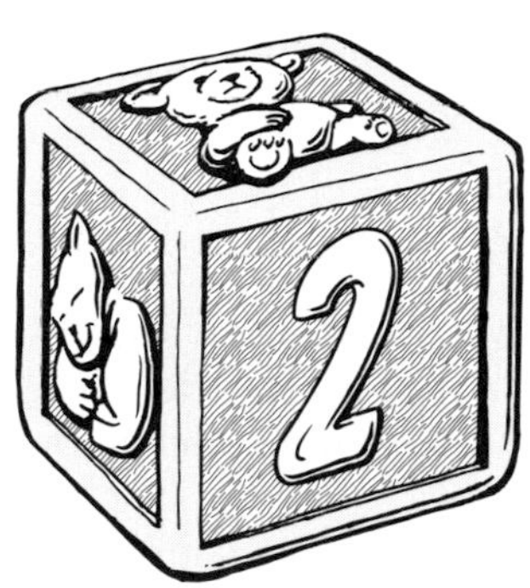

PLANNING AND EVALUATING ACTIVITIES AND ROUTINES

This chapter will cover the following topics:

- *why plan*
- *the planning cycle.*

Why plan

Conclusions from research and an examination of the **nature–nurture debate** indicate that children's learning is significantly influenced by the quality of their environment. Included in any consideration of the environment are the adults who care for children. It is important, therefore, when providing a learning environment for children, that we are aware of how to plan, prepare and monitor children's activities and also how to interact with children during the activities so

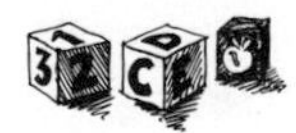

key term

Nature–nurture debate
discussion as to whether genetic factors (nature) or environmental factors (nurture) are more important in influencing behaviour and achievement

that their learning is optimised. Careful consideration of the learning environment provided can contribute to children achieving their potential.

Effective planning also ensures **continuity** and **consistency** in provision and interaction. Planning should always be related to the children's needs. These needs will be constantly changing. This fluidity has to be taken account of when planning. In the planning cycle continuity is evident when the activities planned refer to these needs and either repeat work that requires repetition or move forward to develop further skills and concepts.

Consistency is evident when all the staff are working towards the same goals. Therefore the activity and its focus must be clear in the plans. This is especially important when staff are absent and others have to implement the activity.

The planning cycle

key terms

Continuity
provision of activities and experiences in a logical sequence

Consistency
provision and quality of interaction that is constant (remains the same) regardless of which adults the child is in contact with

Successful planning and interaction with children should start with the children. It begins with an understanding of their needs and interests, then is developed through activities and experiences and, where appropriate, linked to aspects of the curriculum. Monitoring and evaluation of the implementation process will provide a basis for the next stage of planning.

PLANNING

When planning an activity or experience many things need to be carefully considered and in many instances recorded.

The starting point is the children's needs and developmental levels. This information is gathered through evaluation of previous activities and experiences and/or through formal assessment procedures, e.g. baseline assessment, developmental charts, individual education plans (IEPs).

key terms

Rationale
the reason for providing an activity or experience

Learning outcome
a statement of what the children/child will learn from the activity or experience

There must be a **rationale**, or reason, for doing the activity. This is sometimes written as a **learning outcome**, that is, what the children will learn by doing this activity. In nursery settings and schools, what children need to learn is outlined in the National Curriculum both at the Foundation Stage (Early Learning Goals) and at Key Stage One. These curricula should be referred to when planning activities and experiences.

Where these curricula are not relevant, children's developmental needs should be referred to, for example, a baby of 8 months will need stimulation through play and talk (see pages 33 and 34).

Proper resourcing of an activity is central to its success. It is important that all resources are available to enable the children to explore and learn during the activity. When unusual resources are needed these need to be included in the planning documentation so that the staff preparing the activity are clear about what is needed.

Consideration of staffing is essential when planning. The level of interaction needed for the children to achieve the learning outcome identified for the activity must be considered. At times a high level of adult–child interaction will be necessary, while at other times children can explore activities freely.

Preparation

Preparation is based on careful planning so that the environment provided meets the needs of the children across the developmental range. Practical considerations are important when preparing an area. Activities should be presented attractively to encourage the children to participate, for example:

- similar items collected together so that they can be found easily
- plenty of working space around the resources

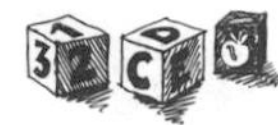

AREA	MONDAY	TUESDAY	WEDNESDAY
Writing table	**ACTIVITY:** Threading beads	**ACTIVITY:** Tracing patterns in sand and on paper	**ACTIVITY:** Writing captions for Autumn display **Red group** observe adult writing **Green group** over highlighter **Blue group** copy printing
	LEARNING OUTCOME: ● hand-eye coordination ● development of fine motor control	**LEARNING OUTCOME:** As Monday and ● left to right orientation **Red group** focus on pencil grip **Blue group** focus on letter formation	**LEARNING OUTCOME:** As for Tuesday and ● awareness of the purposes of writing ● letter formation
	STAFF Sam **RESOURCES** Beads of various sizes	**STAFF** Sam **RESOURCES** Trays and dry sand Paper, pencils, etc.	**STAFF** Betty **RESOURCES** Card for table top display, highlighter pens

This section shows what the children will be doing. Activities are differentiated for children at different stages of development.

This section identifies what the children will learn from doing this activity. Monday's skills are developed in activities throughout the week. A different focus for the activity is identified for children at different stages of development.

An example of a planning document

- all the necessary resources easily accessible
- beginning an activity to demonstrate how resources can be used.

Some activities will need to be introduced formally to ensure that learning is optimised. For example:

- children will benefit from looking at the equipment provided for role play as doctors and nurses and perhaps practising putting bandages on each other
- children will be more successful at weaving and threading if it is demonstrated before they have a go
- children will benefit from knowing how tools on a workbench can be used to assemble and join materials.

Case study . . .

. . . planning and interacting in play

For some time the nursery staff had been concerned about the way that the home corner was being used by the children. Staff observed that children moved rapidly in and out of the area, and rarely became involved in any play that lasted for more than a couple of minutes. They also noticed that a significant number of the children never went into the home corner, ignoring the activity completely. Adults only went into the home corner to find some equipment or to sort out a disagreement.

At the planning meeting, the staff decided that they needed to take positive action to improve the quality of the play in this area. The term's topic was planned around the story of 'The Three Bears' and the home corner was quickly transformed into the bears' cottage in the woods. For some of every session, a member of staff was to be based in the cottage and a number of different, focused activities were planned, all of which linked to the Three Bears theme.

After a week the staff reflected on the changes. All children had visited the bears' cottage and most had participated in a range of planned activities, successfully matching bears to the right-sized bed, laying the table for breakfast, making porridge and so on. They devised their own play too and seemed to be approaching this with more concentration and involvement. Staff agreed that the children were initially attracted by the new focus of the cottage, but felt that as they became used to this it was the presence of an adult in the area that enabled children to develop their play and become immersed in what was happening.

1. *Why do you think the home corner was neglected by the children?*
2. *Why were the staff concerned?*
3. *What was the role of the adult here?*
4. *How might the nursery develop this kind of play in future?*

Interaction

Interaction with the children must take account of their individual developmental needs and of the learning outcome identified for the activity or experience. Some of this information is gathered through observation and must be incorporated into the planning. Practical considerations of adult time are an important issue here.

Interaction can involve:

- talking with children
- asking questions
- offering encouragement
- playing alongside children
- offering suggestions and guidance to extend the children's learning.

Interaction can be within a structured and unstructured framework. Opportunities to interact and develop children's skills will present themselves throughout the day. The adult–child interaction then flows from the child's interests and questions.

Case study . . .

. . . making a grand prix car

Four-year-old Amelia had seen the grand prix on television at the weekend. On Monday she got the car track out and set it up. Unfortunately she could only find motor cars to use on the track and not Formula 1 cars. The childminder suggested that they should make one as they did not have any.

Firstly, they looked in detail at a car and discussed the similarities and differences between that and a Formula 1 car. They considered the design of the car and what they would need to make it. Together they built the car.

Amelia took the car to play with it on the car track. Some time later the childminder joined in the play. While they were playing Amelia commented that the wheels on her car didn't go round like the ones on a real car, and it would be more fun if they did. Amelia and the childminder experimented with a number of different ways of fixing the wheels to the car until they went round successfully.

In this activity the ideas flow from the child's interests and ideas. The childminder picks up on Amelia's interest and provides the time, resources and adult interaction necessary to develop her ideas.

1. *How did Amelia communicate her interest and ideas to the childminder?*
2. *How did the childminder develop these ideas?*
3. *Which skills and concepts could be developed through the activities that the childminder provided?*

At other times interaction will be more formal. This will usually flow from planning. The plans will outline a skill or concept that needs to be developed and the adult–child interaction will be directed towards the child acquiring the necessary skill/concept.

Case study . . .

. . . developing a concept of time

At group time, an adult showed the children four photographs of a baby, a child, a teenager and an adult. They discussed the photographs in terms of which was the baby etc. and how they knew this. The children commented on the size of the people and tried to guess how old they were.

Eventually the adult told the children that all the pictures were of the same person and asked them how that could be possible because they were all different. They discussed their own families and the idea of growing up.

The adult asked the children if they could bring in a photograph of themselves as babies. As children brought in their photographs they were put up on a pinboard titled 'Guess who I am'. The children enjoyed looking at the photographs and guessing.

Some time later the adult went through the pictures with all the children and identified who they were. They discussed how they had guessed who was whom. The children were able to recognise that there were similarities between the babies' and the children's features and that the babies had grown up.

1. *How does the adult interaction during this activity help the children develop a concept of time?*
2. *Why did this concept have to be introduced and taught in a structured way?*
3. *Think of other concepts and/or skills that need to be introduced in this way.*

Observation, monitoring and evaluating

Evaluation of activities and experiences provides valuable information on the success of the activity and what the childen have learned or the skills they have practised and developed. This forms the basis of planning and preparing the area, and also for interaction with the children.

Observation and monitoring can be both formal and informal. Its focus can be the child, the adult and/or the activity.

Formal assessment includes:

- baseline assessment
- written observations
- checklists
- developmental charts.

Informal assessment consists of the things that you notice as you play and interact with the children. It may be facts about the children, the adult and/or the activity. These things may eventually form part of a formal assessment but to begin with they arise naturally and flow from the child's play and talk.

Planning children's experiences and activities is an ongoing process; the areas are interdependent. People who work with young children need to be constantly reassessing what they provide as the children in their care grow and develop. This diagram of the planning cycle shows the ongoing pattern of planning, preparing, interacting and monitoring.

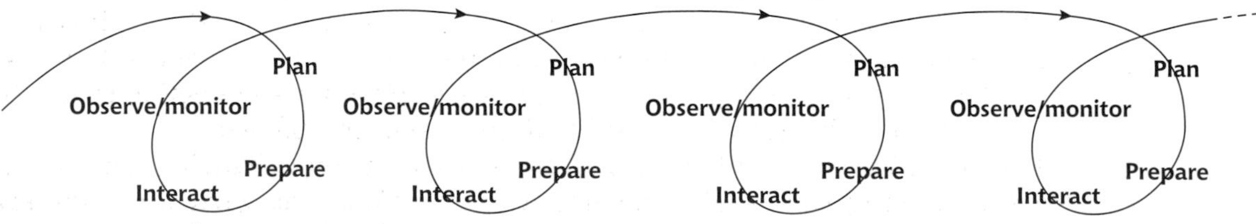

The planning cycle

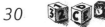

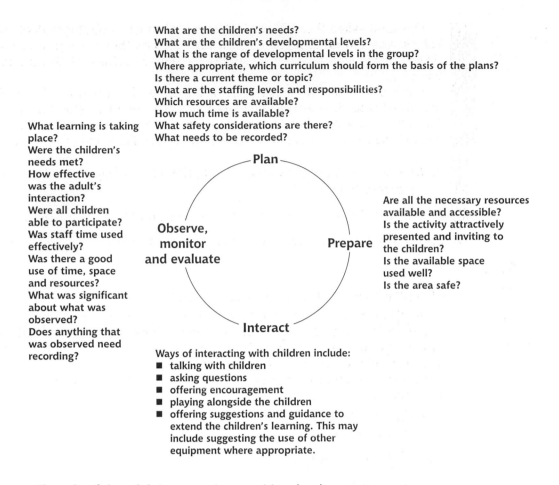

What are the children's needs?
What are the children's developmental levels?
What is the range of developmental levels in the group?
Where appropriate, which curriculum should form the basis of the plans?
Is there a current theme or topic?
What are the staffing levels and responsibilities?
Which resources are available?
How much time is available?
What safety considerations are there?
What needs to be recorded?

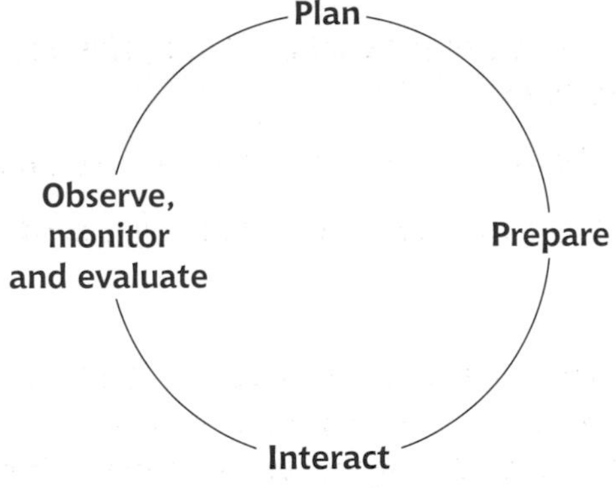

What learning is taking place?
Were the children's needs met?
How effective was the adult's interaction?
Were all children able to participate?
Was staff time used effectively?
Was there a good use of time, space and resources?
What was significant about what was observed?
Does anything that was observed need recording?

Are all the necessary resources available and accessible?
Is the activity attractively presented and inviting to the children?
Is the available space used well?
Is the area safe?

Ways of interacting with children include:

- talking with children
- asking questions
- offering encouragement
- playing alongside the children
- offering suggestions and guidance to extend the children's learning. This may include suggesting the use of other equipment where appropriate.

The role of the adult in promoting cognitive development

PLANNING ROUTINES, ACTIVITIES AND EXPERIENCES FOR BABIES AND VERY YOUNG CHILDREN

Planning

Planning to meet children's needs is the same for babies and very young children as it is for older children. You need to be clear about what you are doing and the reason for doing it. You must prepare carefully, interact effectively and then evaluate how successful it was.

For children aged 0 to 1 plans need to be made for their physical care, for establishing routines and providing experiences to stimulate their senses. Children aged 0 to 1 have many physical needs that must be met by the adults who care for them, for example a balanced diet, cleanliness, rest and sleep and safety. These needs form part of everyday life. However, when planning you need to think about and record how, why and where the children's needs will be met.

It is a similar case with routines, for example nappy changing, bedtime and dressing, where plans need to include why it is important, what the child learns through this experience and how it will be organised. The chart below gives some examples of learning opportunities in routines.

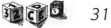

Learning opportunities in routines

- An excellent opportunity to bond with a child, through interaction creating a feeling of being loved, wanted, enjoyed and enjoyable.
- Satisfies a need for physical contact and adult attention.
- Satisfies the need for physical comfort, i.e. warmth, cleanliness, security.
- Provides opportunities for social interaction, for example eye contact and smiling.
- Provides opportunities to hear and respond to language.
- Provides opportunities for the development of gross motor skills, e.g. leg kicking, arm waving, rolling.

key term

Developmental level
the stage of development that a child has reached. This may or may not be consistent with the child's chronological age (age in years)

key term

Key worker
a system of staff organisation where a named member of staff takes responsibility for a group of children

Plans for activities and experiences to stimulate and interest the children need to be linked to the child's **developmental level**. Ask why this activity or experience is being provided for a child at this stage of development. It may be useful to employ the areas of development, such as physical, intellectual, linguistic, emotional and social, to identify needs and to plan appropriate activities. The chart on pages 33–4 provides some suggestions for activities for very young children.

THE ROLE OF THE ADULT

Many centres organise staff in a **key worker** system for babies and young children. This is where one, named person takes responsibility for a group of children. The member of staff and each child are then able to form a close relationship. The adult is responsible for getting to know each child's abilities and their needs and then for planning appropriate activities. Also, the key worker will liaise with parents/carers and, where appropriate, other agencies involved with the child. This system ensures that parents/carers and others have a named person to whom they can talk who knows the child very well.

When planning activities or routines the adult's role is vital and needs careful consideration. Clearly, with routines and the physical care of children hygiene and safety are the adult's responsibility. Why this is important and what the adult needs to do to ensure a clean and safe environment should be included in the plans.

Adults must also interact with children to stimulate their senses. Babies and young children need an environment in which they hear and begin to respond to language and opportunities to interact socially with others.

Effective interaction includes:

- pointing things out and naming them
- providing a commentary on what is being done
- introducing vocabulary
- mirroring (copying) the child's noises and facial expressions
- mirroring (copying) the child's actions
- playing alongside the child to model actions and skills.

Interaction with the child should be included in the rationale of all plans for children aged 0–1, including any particular need identified by the staff and/or the key worker.

STIMULATING ACTIVITIES AT 1 MONTH

All the caring routines should enable the baby to progress physically, to explore their movement and to improve their co-ordination. For example, at changing times and bath times, give the baby space and opportunity to kick safely without nappies or clothing.

- Sensory experiences, such as gentle massage and stroking, help the baby to feel secure and to develop sensitivity to touch.
- Bouncing cradles to transport the baby from room to room with their carer encourage visual skills as they view the world around them. Small toys strung across the chair also increase visual focusing and hand–eye co-ordination.

STIMULATING ACTIVITIES AT 3 MONTHS

- Offer toys that a baby can hold as well as look at, for example brightly coloured rattles made of light, safe materials that produce interesting sounds, or a chiming ball.
- Blowing bubbles fascinates babies at this age as they watch them float and pop.
- Sing songs with actions with the baby sitting on your knee, giving the baby the opportunity to bounce and find their feet.
- Toys attached to a baby gym or strung over the cot will stimulate the baby to reach out with their arms and provide the stimulus for grasping interesting objects.
- Provide the opportunity for exercise – let the baby lie safely on a floor mat without a nappy or clothing so that they can explore their movements and develop further their co-ordination skills. Place the baby in prone position to help them to develop the strength to support their upper body on their forearms and to prepare for rolling their body over.

ACTIVITIES AT 6 MONTHS

- Offer toys that nest and stack, for example round beakers.
- Provide bricks to hold and bang together – adults building with the bricks will encourage the baby to copy the actions and experience delight as the tower falls.
- Offer objects to grasp, for the baby to transfer from hand to hand and which are safe to put in the mouth.
- Offer finger-feeding foods – always with supervision.
- Allow the baby to experience the texture of their food with the fingers.
- Provide sensory experience with the use of bean bags filled with different materials, such as rice or cornflakes.
- Give the baby a plastic mirror to hold and recognise their reflection!
- Encourage the baby to wave goodbye.
- Play clapping games and peek-a-boo.
- Repeat finger rhymes, such as 'This little piggy'.
- Look at picture books and point out familiar objects.
- Encourage the baby to practise drumming, using upturned saucepans and wooden spoons, and to put them in the mouth to explore them.
- If a toy is dropped, the baby will watch where it falls, if it is within sight.
- If a toy falls out of sight, the baby does not look for it. At this age the world ends where the baby can see it!

ACTIVITIES AT 9 MONTHS

- Roll balls for the baby to catch as they sit.
- Strings attached to small, wheeled toys will encourage a pincer grasp as the baby tries to pull the toy towards them.
- Provide bath toys that can be used to pour and squeeze.
- Offer toys and objects that have specific results so that babies begin to learn cause and effect; for example, balls and wheels roll when pushed, bricks stack, some toys squeak when squeezed.

ACTIVITIES AT 12 MONTHS

The following equipment will provide suitable opportunities for developing fine motor skills:

- boxes and containers with small objects to put in and take out
- containers to post round shapes into
- stacking and nesting cups and boxes
- balls for throwing and rolling
- thick, non-toxic wax crayons to make marks on paper
- board books to point at pictures and turn pages
- bricks to practise building.

Remember: at 12 months, babies are still at the oral phase and tend to put objects in their mouths. This is a choking hazard and babies should be supervised at all times.

ACTIVITIES AT 15 MONTHS

Provide:

- large round and cuboid beads to thread with thick laces
- small bricks for building
- crayons and paintbrushes
- books with familiar characters and pictures to point at
- plastic bottles and jars with screw caps to remove and replace
- small-world toys, such as Duplo
- spoon and fork at mealtimes to practise feeding skills.

ACTIVITIES AT 18 MONTHS

Provide opportunities for:

- sand and water play – jugs for pouring, plastic pots to fill
- finger painting and hand and foot printing
- water painting with large brushes and buckets of water
- practising drawing skills with chalk and large crayons
- helping with domestic routines – dusting, vacuuming, etc.
- large-piece jigsaws
- large-piece construction toys with pieces to twist, turn, hammer and push into place
- threading beads
- pushing and pulling toys.

EVALUATING PLANS

All plans need to be evaluated to gather information about the sucess of the activity or experience and to provide a basis for further planning. Questions that need to be asked include the following:

- Did the activity or routine meet the children's needs?
- If not, why didn't it meet their needs and how should it be altered?
- Was it flexible enough to be adapted if necessary?
- Was all the necessary equipment available?
- Was the interaction appropriate?
- If not, how was it changed and/or what needs to be different next time?

THE PLANNING PROCESS

Planning should be meaningful, manageable and useful. Consideration of the following areas will help to achieve this aim.

Planning as a team

All those who work with the children should participate in the planning process. This will help develop a sense of ownership as everyone will have something to contribute and will ensure a consistent approach. It will also mean that preparation tasks and the gathering of resources can be shared. Students should also be encouraged to contribute to planning as an integral part of their training and they may well bring a different perspective to the procedure. To this end, planning meetings should be scheduled at times when everyone involved is able to attend. Someone needs to take responsibility for organising these meetings and ensuring participation. In some centres this will be the role of a senior member of staff; in others this responsibility may rotate.

Case study . . .

. . . planning as a team

The nursery team always got together to plan for their next topic about 2 months before they intended to introduce it. As the nursery had two job-share nursery nurses, planning and team meetings were arranged for their changeover day, which also happened to be a day when a nursery nurse student was there on placement. At a previous team meeting there had been discussion of a number of possible themes and they had settled on using transport as the focus for the half-term's work.

The meeting started with the staff brainstorming ideas and recording these on a flip chart. These suggestions were then mapped to the curriculum areas and looked at carefully. Gaps were identified in some areas and suggestions were made as well as to how the usual activity areas could be used to develop the theme. The group then considered what resources they needed to support the topic. Members of staff volunteered to seek these out, with contacting the library service to order a project collection as a priority. Some trips were suggested and another member of staff said that she would investigate and report back. The nursery nurse student suggested some equipment that she had used at college and said that she would arrange to borrow it and perhaps plan to use it with the children herself. Someone proposed that they reorganise some of the furniture to provide room for another dramatic play area and that was agreed.

New children would be joining the nursery at the beginning of the next half-term and planning for their settling-in period alongside the introduction was also considered. As the meeting drew to a close, the nursery teacher recapped on what had been decided and said that she would provide a copy of the plan for each of the participants and that she would display a version on the nursery notice board for parents to see.

The development of the topic was looked at during subsequent team meetings and weekly breakdowns containing more detailed planning were agreed. As the topic got under way some of the original ideas were modified and others included in response to the children's reactions. Parents became involved through lending resources and generally making suggestions. Several offers of help were received, including one parent arranging to come and talk about his job as a train driver.

1. *Outline the components of planning demonstrated in this case study.*
2. *Why was this planning so successful?*
3. *Examine the planning process in your workplace. Could you suggest ways of making it more effective?*

Planning and flexibility

Planning should not operate as a strait-jacket but should allow for flexibility in responding to children's interests. Sometimes children will respond in a way that you had not anticipated but which is equally valuable. Allow for some spontaneity – the caterpillar truck that comes to dig up the playground provides a stimulus to learning that is too good to miss but you may not have planned for it. Similarly, it would be unwise to deny children the opportunity of playing in the first snow that they have ever seen simply because you had planned something else for that day.

Involving parents

Share your planning with parents. This is particularly important for parents who work alongside you with the children. However, all parents will benefit from knowing what you are working on and may be able to contribute to the learning either with time or resources or by following things through with their children at home. Plans can be displayed in the centre or included in regular newsletters.

Recording planning

Planning needs to be recorded for reference and for accountability. There is no one way of doing this and individual centres will develop ways of recording their planning that meet their own needs.

Long-term planning will be linked to curriculum policy documents, both centre-devised and statutory, and to statements that provide an operational framework for the centre.

Many centres record their medium-term planning on topic webs or on grids. Here the planning will be organised around developmental and/or curriculum areas and linked to specific activities or experiences. This provides a fairly detailed framework of intentions that might be added to or amended as the topic develops.

Weekly or daily planning can be recorded in a variety of ways using grids, webs, charts or notebooks. In these, specific activities will be indicated alongside resources needed, sometimes with the focus of the activity highlighted.

Members of staff will also plan for work with particular children or groups of children on a week-to-week or day-to-day basis. This short-term planning is easily updated if, say, a member of staff is absent or there is an unplanned-for visitor or event. The availability of this planning provides for continuity when regular members of staff are away and someone else takes over the programme.

Evaluation

Evaluation is an essential feature of the planning process. It is through continuous observation of children's responses and progress that staff can assess whether their planning and delivery is meeting the needs of the children. This information will enable staff to plan most effectively to meet these changing needs.

key terms

Equal opportunities all people participating in society to the best of their abilities, regardless of race, religion, disability, gender or social background

Positive action taking action to ensure that a particular individual or group has an equal chance to succeed

Stereotyping when people think that all the members of a group have the same characteristics as each other; often applied on the basis of race, gender or disability

ANTI-DISCRIMINATORY/ANTI-BIAS PRACTICE IN PROVIDING ACTIVITIES FOR CHILDREN

Activities and experiences provided for children can be a powerful tool in promoting **equal opportunities**. Child-care workers have a responsibility to present activities and experiences in a way that includes and enables all children and that reflects the experiences of all sections of society. The planning and delivery of the activities and experiences must provide for equality of opportunity, irrespective of race and culture, gender, socio-economic background or disability. It must also consider how best to develop the potential of children who are more timid or aggressive or more confident than might be expected of the group. Treating all children the same will not provide for equality of opportunity. We need to recognise that some children in our society are more likely to experience disadvantage than others and that some **positive action** might be necessary to enable them to succeed. This is an important consideration when planning the curriculum.

Activities and experiences transmit not just skills and knowledge, but attitudes and values too. The early years are crucial in the formation of children's attitudes about themselves and about the world that they live in. Activities that promote equality of opportunity will enable children to feel positively about themselves and their achievements, to avoid the limitations of **stereotyping** and to value diversity.

Case study . . .

. . . valuing diversity

Karen felt the children in the small, all-white, rural playgroup she ran had a very limited experience of cultures other than their own. As part of their regular listening to music sessions, she played some Indian music to the children. Karen had planned the session carefully and had borrowed a box of Indian instruments from a nearby resource centre. After playing the tape a couple of times, she showed the children the instruments and demonstrated the sounds that they made, passing them round so that the children could try them out for themselves. As she played the tape through again, the children were able to recognise some of the instruments as they appeared in the piece. Once the children had become familiar with the instruments and had been shown how to use them, they were placed alongside the other equipment in the music corner so that they could use them in their own play. Indian music was introduced as part of the playgroup's regular dance sessions and, later on that term, Karen was able to organise a visit to the playgroup by a group of Indian dancers, based at a nearby Community Arts Group.

1. *Why was this a valuable experience for the children?*
2. *How did Karen ensure that this activity would be successful?*
3. *Think of other, meaningful ways in which this group's experience of cultural diversity could be extended.*

Promoting equal opportunities through activities and experiences

This section suggests some practical pointers to promoting equal opportunities through the activities and experiences provided for children. It is important to understand that resources in themselves do not promote equal opportunities. It is up to staff to make an equal opportunities perspective integral to planning and to present activities and resources in a way that develops children's awareness of the issues.

key term

Positive images
the representation of a cross-section of a whole variety of roles and everyday situations, to challenge stereotypes and to extend and increase expectations

For example, in the visual environment:

- Display **positive images** in the setting. Black people, women and people with disabilities are under-represented in the wider visual environment. Choose images that challenge stereotypes, for example a black barrister, a disabled doctor, a woman police officer.
- Give children the opportunity to represent themselves accurately. Provide mirrors and paints and crayons that enable children to match their own skin tones.
- Look at the illustrations in books and posters that you provide. Do they convey a positive image or do you see line drawings of white children shaded to represent black races, girls always in the background taking a supporting role or disabled people portrayed as helpless and reliant on others?
- Visitors in the setting can challenge stereotypes – a father with his new baby, a black dentist, a female electrician.

Choosing toys and planning activities

- Look at jigsaws, games, play figures, musical instruments and their packaging too. Do they reflect cultural diversity? Do they encourage both boys and girls to play? Are children with disabilities represented?
- Provide dolls that represent different racial groups. Do not buy black dolls that have white facial features or hair. Monitor the way that the dolls are played with. Think of the message conveyed when the white dolls are tucked up in prams and the black dolls thrown into a box. Encourage boys to show that they can cuddle and care for 'babies'.
- Home corner play can be a secure and comforting play space. Make sure that your provision of cooking equipment and play food reflects a variety of cultural styles and traditions. If you introduce some new or unfamiliar equipment, such as chopsticks, make sure that the children know how to use it properly.
- Dressing-up clothes give children an opportunity to elaborate their role play. Avoid identifying items as 'for boys' or 'for girls' and encourage children to try out everything. Provide everyday clothes from a range of cultures but do not over-generalise – Pakistani children are as likely to wear tracksuits or jeans as they are shalwar-kameez!
- Mark a range of festivals. Children who celebrate these festivals at home will feel valued: others can gain an insight and understanding of unfamiliar traditions. Care needs to be taken in this area to avoid a **tokenistic** approach which emphasises the 'exotic' aspects of cultural difference. Festival celebrations need to be researched carefully if they are to have any real educational significance. Enlist help from community groups or parents. (Think about the message that you are sending about the relative worth of festivals if you spend 6 weeks building up to Christmas and an afternoon on Diwali.)

key term

Tokenistic
a superficial representation of minority or disadvantaged groups, for example including a single black child in a school brochure, a single woman on the board of directors

- Cooking sessions can present an opportunity to try different recipes and taste a range of foods. They can also provide children with a chance to confront any stereotypical ideas about whose job it is to cook. Again, when talking about cultural preferences in diet avoid over-generalisations. Children from Caribbean families may like to eat rice and peas, but they will also eat pizza and visit McDonald's.
- Make sure that activities are not dominated by one group of children to the exclusion of others. It may be necessary to exclude one group for a while so that others can have a chance to gain confidence and skills.
- Provision for creative activities should reflect cultural diversity. Introduce children to a range of artistic traditions and styles and provide a range of materials for them to work with. Play all kinds of music, provide instruments and this will influence the children's own music-making.
- Make sure that all children can participate in the range of activities, including those with disabilities. This may involve an adjustment to the physical environment, such as moving a construction activity to a table-top so that a child in a wheelchair can reach it or it may mean providing appropriate equipment, such as tactile dominoes so that a child with a visual impairment can be included in the game.

Recognising the power of language

- Value language diversity. Encourage children to listen to languages other than their own. Teach greetings and rhymes and share dual-language books with children.
- Choose books and tell stories that challenge stereotypes and provide positive role models.
- Introduce stories and rhymes from many literary traditions.

Case study . . .

. . . providing for special needs

Rahila had been blind since birth. Her parents were offered a playgroup place for her at a school for visually impaired children when she was 3, but they chose to send her to the nursery class of the local school that both her sisters had attended. At first the staff were apprehensive and concerned that the nursery might not be able to provide a suitable environment for a blind child, but after discussing these concerns with the parents, they agreed that she should attend. The staff spent some time looking at the physical environment and identifying pathways round the nursery that could be indicated with tactile markers for Rahila to follow. They planned activities, ensuring that no child would be excluded from participating.

Rahila made visits to the nursery with her parents prior to starting. The other children were initially curious and asked questions about blindness that were answered in a straightforward way. She settled quickly and confidently into the nursery, participating fully in the activities, sometimes with adult assistance, more often independently.

Equipment and advice were available to the nursery from the local visually impaired unit and from the Royal National Institute for the Blind. Rahila transferred to school at 5, confident and competent, and having benefited greatly from her pre-school experience.

1. *What made Rahila's experience so successful?*
2. *What is the adult's role here?*

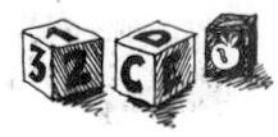

The hidden curriculum; what else do children learn from the activities and experiences provided for them?

key term

Hidden curriculum
messages, often unintended, that are communicated to children as a consequence of the attitudes and values of the adults who deliver the curriculum

Perhaps even more important than the 'official' curriculum in promoting equal opportunities are the attitudes and values of those who work with children and deliver the curriculum. This is sometimes known as the **hidden curriculum** and is communicated to children in the way that we talk to them and in the expectations that we have of them.

Here are some examples of ways in which the hidden curriculum can operate against equal opportunities:

- an expectation and acceptance that boys' play is rougher than girls'
- adults giving more time to boys (many studies show this to be the case)
- having low expectations of the behaviour and achievement of children from minority groups
- regarding particular games and activities as sex-appropriate
- overprotecting children with disabilities
- comments such as: 'Boys don't cry'; 'Here's a picture of a wedding. The girls will like this'; 'Find me two strong boys to move this table'; 'The girls can wash the cups'; 'It's not ladylike to fight'.

Children absorb these messages and they can affect their view of themselves. The attitudes and values of the staff as well as the content of the curriculum need to address the issues of equal opportunities.

Child-care workers are very influential in the formation of children's attitudes and values – children will take their cue from adult responses and reactions. Because of their powerful role, it is important that staff take issues of equality seriously and do not skate over them.

Progress check

Why is equal opportunities an important aspect of what we provide for young children?

How can equal opportunities be promoted through what is provided?

What is stereotyping and why should we challenge stereotypes?

Why is the promotion of equal opportunities an issue for all settings?

How can staff show that they are committed to promoting equal opportunities?

key terms

You need to know what the key terms and phrases in this chapter mean. Go back through the chapter and find out.

Unit 3: Foundations to Caring

This unit will enable you to work safely with children and to provide care and appropriate stimulation in a variety of settings. You will understand your role and that of other professional workers in providing a positive environment, both in indoor and outdoor settings, that will meet the needs, including the nutritional needs, of all the children. You will learn how to identify and understand best practice in the provision of physical care, and to understand the legislation, regulations, policies and professional practice that support this.

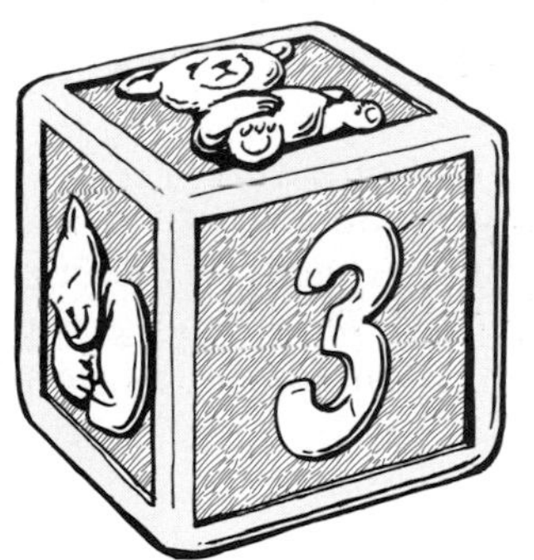

THE CHARACTERISTICS OF A POSITIVE CHILD-CARE AND EDUCATION ENVIRONMENT

Child-care workers should plan and create an environment that is caring, stimulating and attractive to children and one that best meets their needs at different ages. There are many factors involved in creating a stimulating and caring environment for children. It can be achieved by providing a range of age-appropriate equipment and resources, giving careful consideration to the layout and decoration of a room, including safety, through good teaching skills and a caring approach. Displays and interest tables are also an effective way of creating a stimulating and attractive environment for children and enhancing their self-esteem.

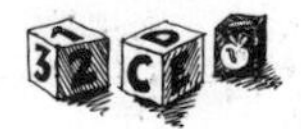

The child-care and education environment may be the only place outside the child's home where a child is left without their main carer. Child-care workers need to provide a reassuring setting for the children in their care. If their needs are met in a friendly and nurturing environment, it will increase their feelings of security and well-being.

This chapter will cover the following topics:

- *the physical environment*
- *creating a stimulating environment for children*
- *a reassuring environment.*

The physical environment

ARRANGING THE AREA

Child-care settings are located in a variety of types of accommodation. Some will be modern and purpose-built, but others will be sited in buildings that were not designed with the needs of children in mind. In a large area, such as a village hall, several activities can be in progress at the same time. In a home environment, the activities may be restricted to one or two at a time, but with changes of scene and other everyday activities, like shopping, planned throughout the day.

Choosing furniture and equipment and planning the layout is important to make the setting welcoming, safe, reassuring and stimulating for the children.

When deciding how to arrange the area, the following factors are important.

Local authority regulations

In order to comply with the Children Act 1989, all social services departments issue guidelines for providers of day care, including childminders. These guidelines cover aspects of child care such as safety, heating, ventilation, hygiene and outside play spaces. **Regulations** also cover the amount of space required for each child and the number of adults required to care for the children. (For more on this, see Chapter 4.)

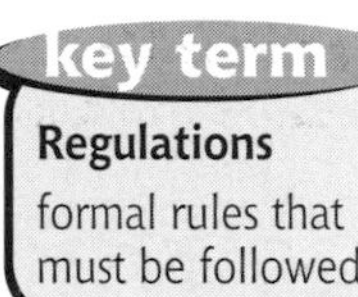

Regulations
formal rules that must be followed

Safety requirements

There should be adequate space, heating, ventilation and lighting. Heating appliances should be properly guarded. Exit doors should be securely fastened and not be capable of being opened by any of the children. Doorways, emergency exits and fire escapes should be kept clear at all times. Staff should be aware of the procedure for emergencies, such as fire, and there should be regular drills and practices.

Feeling secure

Welcoming children into an attractive and thoughtfully arranged environment will help to reassure an insecure child. Child-care settings should be geared to the needs of the children with child-sized equipment, attractive displays and a quiet, calm atmosphere.

Attractiveness

Furniture, carpets and curtains will all help to make the environment a pleasant place for the children to work in. In a child-centred environment, these items should be chosen with children in mind, particularly with regard to size and durability.

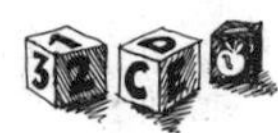

Space

Children need plenty of space to play, but often a large open space is not conducive to the most purposeful types of play. Large spaces should be broken up by moving furniture into smaller areas that offer different types of activities, for example, sand/water/painting/imaginative play/book area. This will enable the children to concentrate more readily and allows for flexibility in the overall makeup of the space.

Outdoors

The outdoor area provides for an important aspect of children's learning and should be planned with care. Eliminate obvious hazards with regard to large equipment, like slides and climbing frames, by paying particular attention to where they are placed and providing adequate supervision. A tarmac or paved space should be available and, where possible, a grassy area and space for growing things.

Comfort

Ensure that the temperature of the setting is kept between 16 and 24°C (60–75°F) and that there is adequate fresh air circulating. Lighting in each part of the setting should be adequate for the activities provided. A quiet area with carpet and/or cushions to settle and look at books or to do a puzzle will encourage children to pick up and look at books and engage in quieter activities.

Working as individuals, in pairs or groups

The environment can be modified to encourage children to work alone, with partners or in groups. A carpeted area is a good idea for bringing the children together for registration, sharing news and at story time. Children may also be encouraged to work in groups by setting small tables with chairs. Individual work, such as reading to the carer and using the computer, can also be managed in this way.

Movement between activities

Adults and children need to be able to access all parts of the setting. Planning the layout of the environment should allow for sufficient space between activities and free access to the cloakroom, toilets and outdoor areas.

Access to equipment

Children thrive on responsibility and being allowed to make their own decisions within a safe framework. Resources should be as accessible as possible to the children so that they can choose which materials they are going to use.

Providing a variety of activities

Child-care workers will need to change the activities on offer, perhaps with the help of the children. Children can be encouraged to be responsible for parts of the setting, putting equipment away, tidying areas of the setting and clearing litter from the outdoor area. Children can also be involved in helping to prepare and give out snacks.

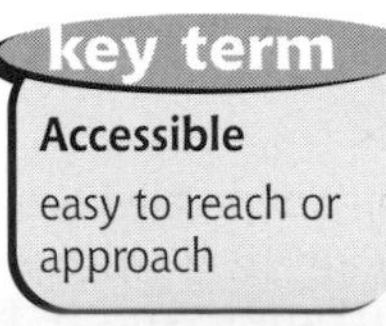

key term
Accessible
easy to reach or approach

ENSURING ACCESSIBILITY

All activities and areas of the setting must be **accessible** to all children. Children with special needs can be welcomed into any setting where thought and consideration is given to their needs. Children with a physical disability may need wider doorways, ramps, larger toilet area and space to manoeuvre around classroom furniture.

Children with a sensory impairment may need equipment to help to increase their sensory awareness. For example, a deaf child may need a hearing aid, good lighting, use of British Sign Language. A visually impaired child will need the floor to be kept clear, and the furniture and activity areas to be arranged in the same way. Any changes to the physical environment should be planned and explained to the child in advance. Large-print books may be helpful and it is important to provide rich and varied tactile experiences.

A CHILD-ORIENTATED ENVIRONMENT

There are several ways of making a child-care environment that is not purpose-built, such as a family home, safer and more child-friendly. Provide:

- small tables and chairs
- small toilets or toilet seats
- steps to make sinks accessible and to enable children to reach things
- stair-gates and fireguards
- high handles on doors where you need to prevent children gaining access to other areas
- locks on cupboards not to be used by the children, and on fridges and upstairs windows
- low cupboards for storing creative equipment/books/activities for the children to select themselves.

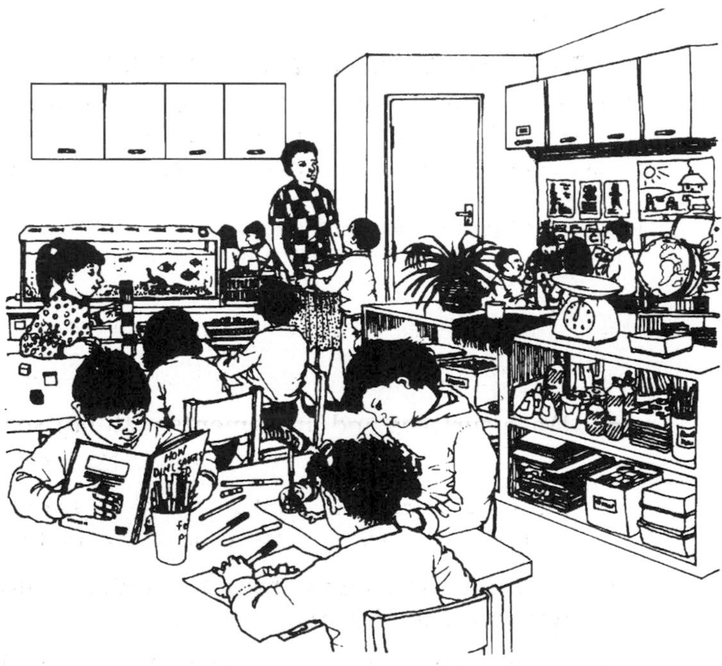

Group activities can be encouraged in a child-centred environment

OUTDOOR PLAY AREA

Children need to be able to be out in the fresh air as much as possible and to be involved in vigorous play activities. The external environment may need to be adapted to allow this, or there may be no garden or outside play space, so the children will need to go out on walks or to local parks or playgrounds. The outdoor play space should be safe and secure. It should provide a variety of surfaces, areas that are covered for use when the weather is wet and shady areas to provide cover on hot days. If possible, there should be trees and plants within the outdoor area. The activities should be planned within the outdoor area to allow for space to run around and use the wheeled toys safely, while still allowing an area to be used for more restful activities.

Case study . . .

. . . playing outside in hot weather

Maria is a childminder and cares for three children each day – Tom and Venus, both aged 3, and Damon who is 4. It is a very hot and sunny day, too hot to be indoors. Maria's house has a garden that the children like to play in; there is some shade in one part of the garden under the tree. Maria is very careful to put high-factor sun cream on the children's skin and she reapplies this regularly. She also makes sure that the children have plenty to drink.

1. *How can the outdoor play be arranged to make it suitable for the children on days like this?*
2. *List three activities that would be suitable for the garden of a family home on a hot day?*
3. *How could you, quickly, create more shade in the garden?*

KEEPING THE ENVIRONMENT HYGIENIC

It is very important that strict hygiene procedures are followed in child-care settings so that cross-contamination and cross-infection can be avoided. (For more on avoiding the spread of infection, see Chapter 16.)

Checklist for a hygienic environment

The environment

- Keep kitchen work surfaces and implements clean.
- Use disinfectant to clean work surfaces regularly.
- Wash surfaces and implements with hot soapy water after they have come into contact with raw food, particularly meat, fish and poultry.
- Wash tea towels, dish cloths and other cleaning cloths regularly on the hottest cycle of the washing machine, or use very hot water if washing by hand.
- Clean children's toys at least each day or after each session with hot, soapy water or disinfectant.
- Keep toilet areas clean. Disinfect the seats, handles, door handles and sink taps at least after each session. Keep rubbish bins securely closed and out of the reach of the children. Nappies and other waste involving bodily fluids must be securely wrapped and disposed of in the designated bins following the policy of the setting. Child-care workers must ensure that they wear latex gloves when handling any waste contaminated with bodily fluids.
- Any spills should be mopped up immediately; separate mops should be assigned to the different areas of the setting.

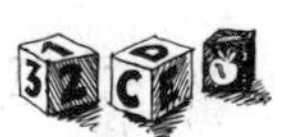

- Any spills or accidents involving bodily waste must be mopped up using a bleach solution, and gloves and aprons must be worn.

Personal hygiene (includes both workers and children)
Hands must be washed before:

- preparing food
- preparing babies' bottles or weaning food
- eating or drinking
- attending to minor cuts or grazes (gloves should also be worn)
- giving children's medicine.

Hands must be washed after:

- going to the toilet
- handling raw food
- changing nappies
- wiping noses
- coughing or sneezing
- touching pets or their equipment.

Animals

- Keep pets free from infection.
- Keep pets out of food preparation areas.
- Wash and store pets' equipment separately.
- Keep pet food and litter trays out of children's reach.

Food preparation

- Ensure that food is handled and stored correctly.
- Prepare food following the instructions on packaging and in recipes.

(For more information on food preparation and handling, see Chapter 7.)

THE NATURAL WORLD

Children learn from and enjoy activities involving growing plants and investigating the living world. Participating in gardening activities has many benefits for children if there is an awareness of their level of development and if expectations are adjusted accordingly. Safety will be an important consideration, and fences and gates must be secure.

The benefits of these activities include:

- an increased knowledge of biological processes and cycles as seeds develop into plants
- a sense of achievement as the children see the plants grow
- an increased awareness of the care of plants, for example the need for regular watering and feeding

- developing language as new words are used to describe the plants, stages of their development and gardening activities
- learning new skills, such as planting, digging, watering, pruning
- an awareness of time during the growth cycle
- learning about safety issues, for example not eating berries or flowers, taking care with gardening tools, hygiene after gardening.

PETS

There may also be an opportunity to keep pets in the child-care setting. This can be an enjoyable way for children to learn about animals and to take responsibility for their care. However, it is important to find out whether any child or member of staff is allergic to any type of pet. Pets must be kept well away from any food preparation areas and children should be taught to wash their hands after touching any pets.

Progress check

What factors are important when deciding the layout of a child-care setting?

What type of equipment would make the environment more child-centred?

How can a child with a physical disability be made to feel welcome and secure in the child-care setting?

How can the environment be adapted to enable a visually-impaired child to make full use of all facilities?

What are the benefits for children of exploring the natural world?

Creating a stimulating environment for children

Displays and interest tables are an effective way of creating a stimulating and attractive environment for children and of enhancing their self-esteem.

THE VALUES OF DISPLAY

Display has many values. It can:

- be used as a stimulus for learning across all areas of the curriculum
- encourage children to look, think, reflect, explore, investigate and talk and respond to their interests
- act as a sensory and imaginative stimulus
- give children ideas, and promote further investigation and research
- encourage parental involvement in their children's learning, and reinforce links with home
- encourage self-esteem by showing appreciation of children's work
- encourage communication with children

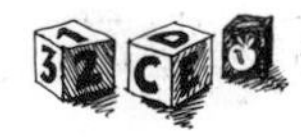

- make the environment attractive, and attract children's attention
- encourage awareness of the wider community, reflect the rich cultural diversity of society and reinforce acceptance of difference.

The length of time a display remains should be considered and planned. Any display that has become old or faded should be replaced. A display should remain only while it bears relevance to the curriculum and is still being referred to. Displays can be used as an integral part of the curriculum, especially to reflect aspects of topic work. Once a new topic is begun, it is important to plan and make new displays.

WHERE TO DISPLAY

Displays should be placed wherever they can be seen easily, or touched if appropriate. It is worth an adult getting down to the child's eye level and viewing the surroundings from that position. The position of the display will affect the size and type of display. A flat wall can be made into a three-dimensional display if there is enough space in front of it. A corner can be made into an imaginative play area with appropriate decoration; the display may be on a table, cupboard or screen.

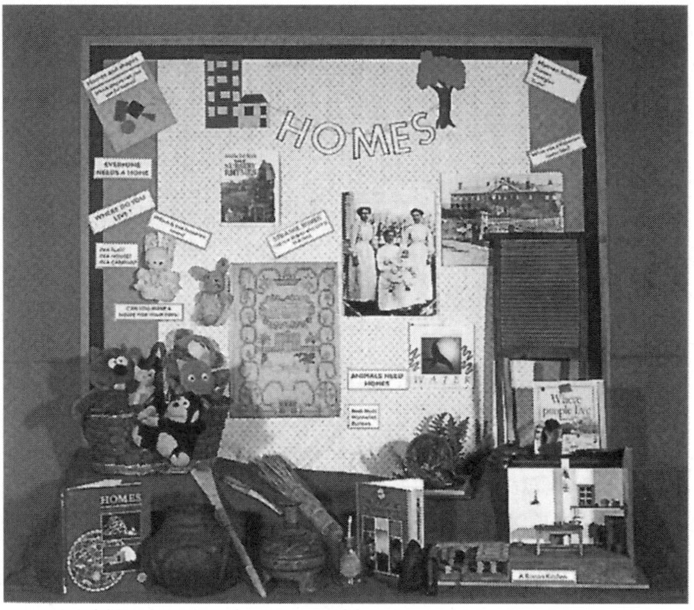

Displaying work encourages children's interest

WHAT TO INCLUDE IN A DISPLAY

Variety makes displays interesting, so it is important to change styles, techniques and content. Displays can include paintings, items of children's individual work, co-operative efforts, natural materials and plants, objects of interest, photographs, pictures, collage, real objects, use of different colours, textures and labelling.

All children should be able to contribute to the displays in their environment. When looking around their room, it is preferable for every child to have at least one piece of their work displayed, or have taken part in a group display.

Children should be involved in the choice of work that will be displayed and, where possible, in the mounting of work and the creation of the display.

 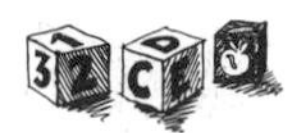

Any labels and captions must be clear, of an appropriate size, in lower-case letters except at the beginning of sentences and proper nouns, and include the home languages of the children in the setting. If labels and captions are hand-written they should be carefully printed, and it is important to practise printing using guidelines to help you until you are confident enough to print free-hand.

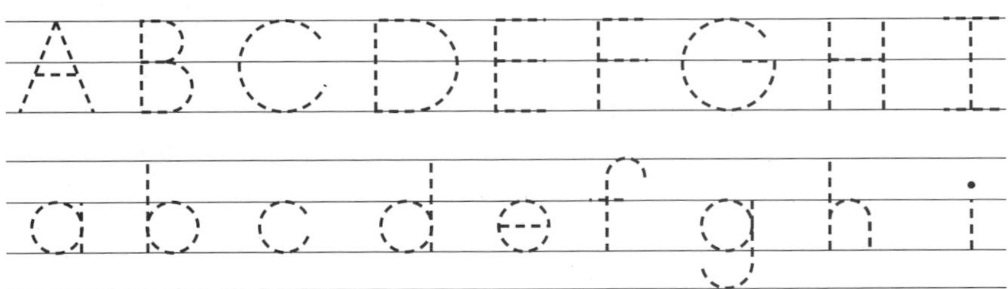

Practise printing using guidelines to help

key terms

Multi-cultural society
a society whose members have a variety of cultural and ethnic backgrounds

Multi-ability society
a society where people have a variety of differing abilities and disabilities

Displays that include people should, wherever possible and appropriate, reflect a **multi-cultural**, **multi-ability society** and be without gender bias. Displays should project positive images in any setting. Black people, women and people with disabilities are usually under-represented in the wider visual environment. When planning displays, workers should choose images that challenge stereotypes. Children should be given the opportunity to represent themselves accurately. Workers should provide mirrors, and paints and crayons that enable children to match their own skin tones. (For more about supporting anti-discriminatory practice and promoting equal opportunities, see Unit Ten.)

The entrance to a centre gives the first impression that parents, children and visitors gain of your work. A welcoming entrance with displays of children's work will contribute to giving a positive impression and demonstrate your professional standards.

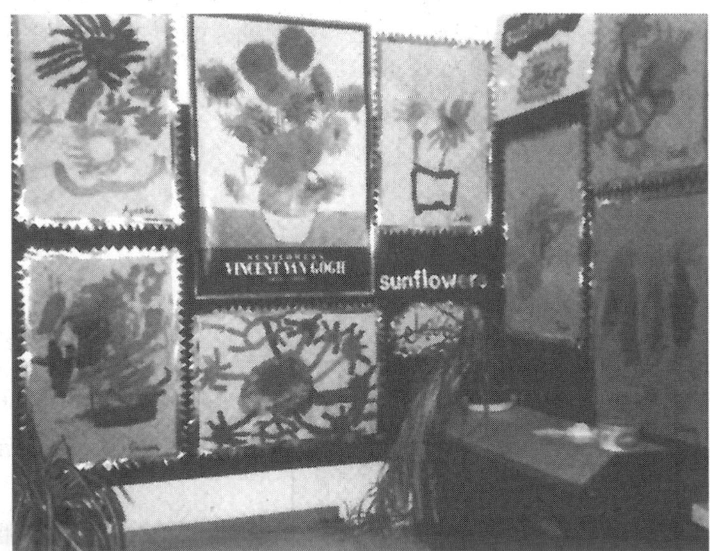

Good planning and presentation are essential for successful displays

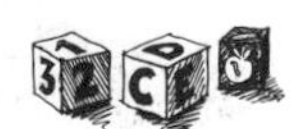

DISPLAY TECHNIQUES

It is important to plan displays, thinking everything through first. Having decided the position, consideration should be given to appropriate colours, backing, drapes and borders.

Good presentation is essential, including good mounting and well-produced lettering. Staples and adhesive materials should be used discreetly.

The use of colour should be carefully considered. There are no rules – bright colours can be effective, but black and white may also be appropriate.

Case study . . .

. . . an outing to the theatre

It is December and the staff of a rural infant school plan to take the children to see a performance for schools of a pantomime at a theatre in a nearby town. On their return a variety of cross-curricula work is planned, including a display showing both the stage and the audience at the theatre.

The outing is very successful for the children. On their return the teacher first discusses what and who they have observed, and establishes they have understood the story of the pantomime. She also finds that they have noticed there were children from different ethnic backgrounds in the audience, and also some children with special needs. As part of the display, in order to make a collage, the children are encouraged to paint a small figure of themselves and also a few paintings of other children in the audience. The children enjoy painting themselves and others, and then cutting around them and helping to stick them on to the display. The result is a colourful, multi-ethnic, multi-ability picture that is a source of much discussion both between the children, and with their parents and other visitors to the classroom.

1. *Why might it be particularly relevant to take children from a rural environment to the theatre in a town?*
2. *Why is it valuable for children to paint pictures of themselves for the display?*
3. *What is the value of the discussion about the people the children had observed in the audience?*
4. *What do you think the children gained from painting other children in the audience?*
5. *Why do you think this display was such a valuable resource for discussion?*

INTEREST TABLES

Interest tables can be used to follow a theme or the class topic, or display work/collections from a recent outing. They should be at the child's height, used to display three-dimensional objects and sited in a quieter area of the setting. The table should be covered and any objects that are not intended to be touched should be placed in a protective container, such as a plastic tank.

Helping children to learn about the natural world is vital – seeing how things grow and develop is part of learning about the world. Children can collect and display their findings – from autumn leaves to sea-life. Health and safety is important when displaying such objects – be aware of the dangers of displaying poisonous berries and plants, or sharp objects. Food on display should be fresh and changed regularly. Reference books should be available on the table for children to look up their areas of interest.

Adding interest to displays

Interest can be added by good use of:

- *colour* – a co-ordinated backing and border can be used to display the children's work to its best advantage; drapes may add interest
- *texture* – include things that are interesting to touch and contrast with each other, for example smooth, shiny pebbles and rough sandpaper
- *movement* – consider hanging displays
- *sound* – crackly paper, shakers and musical instruments made by the children all make appealing displays
- characters with whom the children are familiar from books read at story time; people they have met on a trip or who have visited the establishment.

Benefits to child development of display work

- *Fine motor skills* – placing, cutting, sticking, drawing, painting.
- *Gross motor skills* – co-ordination, reaching, stretching, bending, balancing.
- *Cognitive (intellectual) development* – encourages problem-solving, decision-making and thinking skills, stimulates memory.
- *Mathematical skills* – using and creating patterns, shapes, angles. Measuring, estimating.
- *Language development* – new words and vocabulary, use of reference books, discussion and listening skills, asking questions.
- *Emotional development* – sense of achievement and increased self-esteem, children feel proud of their work displayed for parents to see. Displays that are pleasant and stimulating to look at help children to feel comfortable with their environment.
- *Personal and social development* – encourages teamwork and co-operation between adults and children, sharing of resources and ideas. Provides opportunities to experience new materials and textures, sensory stimulation. Increases awareness and knowledge of cultural diversity.

Progress check

What are the values of good displays?

Why is it important to display children's work?

What do you need to think about before planning a display?

How can interest tables be used?

What are the benefits of display to development?

A reassuring environment

The child-care and education environment may be the only place outside the child's home where a child is left without their main carer. Child-care workers

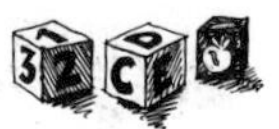

therefore need to provide a reassuring setting for the children in their care. If children's needs are met in a friendly and nurturing environment, it will increase their feelings of security and well-being.

PROVIDING A SECURE ENVIRONMENT

In order to provide adequate and appropriate reassurance for children, child-care workers need to know about typical social and emotional development. Looking at the world from the child's point of view will help to identify their fears. Most babies up to the age of 6 months are usually afraid of loud noises and sudden movements. Fears commonly experienced by toddlers and older children are of separation, loud noises, the dark, spiders, strangers, animals, blood and other anxieties.

All children should be kept physically safe from harm, but they also need to feel safe and secure emotionally. You can avoid physical harm by making adaptations to the physical environment; large areas can be divided into smaller spaces for quieter activities. Pre-school children who are in day care should be offered experiences that are similar to those they would have at home, such as visiting the shops, the park and posting letters. Adopting similar sleep times and daily routines and offering familiar foods will also help a child to feel more secure.

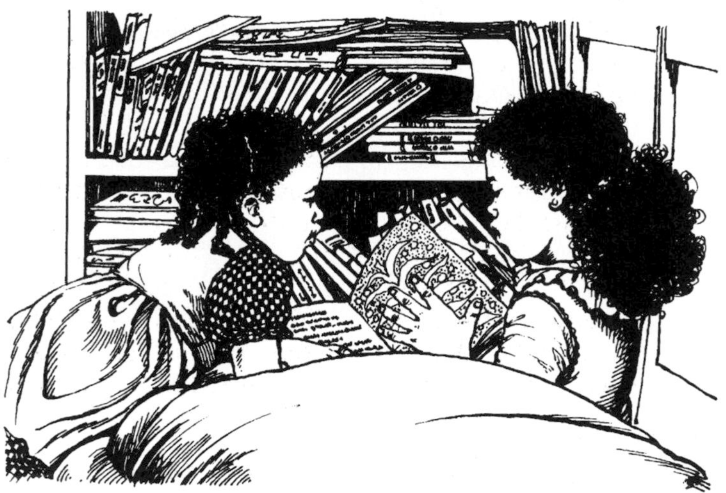

Children feel secure with familiar objects

COMFORTING CHILDREN

Most children who are afraid will cry and seek comfort from a caring adult. Some fears are shown in more subtle ways and a child may show signs of being generally anxious. Children in an unfamiliar environment may react in a variety of ways. They may show their fears by crying, clinging to their parent/carer, being unwilling to try new experiences, losing appetite, having sleeping problems. As children cannot always tell the adult what the source of their anxiety is, the child-care worker must try to identify the cause.

Dealing with the problem depends on the cause of the anxiety. Some children may need more reassurance than anticipated in certain situations, so it is important to know about any special methods for helping individual children. Listening to what parents and carers tell you about this will help. Generally, children will respond positively to the following actions:

- clear and honest explanations about what is going to happen. You may need to repeat these explanations, as young children may not remember or understand what you have said.

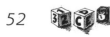

- in the case of an unexpected incident, a clear explanation of what has just happened
- a reassuring cuddle – although some children may not appreciate physical comfort
- encouraging stress-reducing activities like playdough, looking at books, painting
- having their preferred comfort objects, such as a special blanket or soft toy, to hand. This is especially important for the under 2s. Young children should not be discouraged from having their preferred comfort objects as they help to bridge the gap between the home setting and the care environment. They also play an important part in helping children to become more confident and independent in new situations. Comfort objects should be readily available to children. It may be advisable to keep all comforters, labelled with the children's names, in a central location until they are needed. A list of comforters and particular remedies will be useful if this can be displayed where staff can see and readily refer to it.

CHANGES AND UNEXPECTED EVENTS

Children can easily become unsettled and upset if there are changes to their routine or environment. This can be more upsetting if the changes are unexpected or not explained, so it is important that, wherever possible, children have advance warning of any changes that you know about. Telling the children what is going to happen in simple and understandable terms will help to prevent anxiety. It is important for child-care workers to be positive and cheerful about any changes, as this will be reassuring for the children. It will also be necessary to repeat and remind the children about what is going to happen. One of the most upsetting changes for children can be when their child-care worker leaves or is absent because of sickness or holiday. Whenever possible, children should be prepared for changes, but it is not possible to plan for unexpected events so the children will need to be reassured and comforted if they become distressed.

Case study . . .

. . . an unexpected visitor

The children at Fir Tree Pre-school were happily enjoying their mid-morning snack of fruit and milk. Helen, the leader, had opened the outside door as it was a warm day. The children were gathered on the carpet happily discussing the morning's events and sharing news from home. Helen was talking with the children when she noticed that Tom and Tanya were laughing and pointing at the doorway. Helen stood up and at that moment a large dog appeared, barking loudly. Some of the smaller children began to cry and the older ones looked anxious. Leanne, one of the other helpers, rushed to the door and managed to close it, leaving the dog outside. However, the dog continued to bark very loudly and more of the children got upset. Helen and Leanne comforted the children, but they were very relieved when the dog's owner arrived. He apologised, saying that the dog had run off and explained that it was noisy but friendly. He put the dog on a lead and made it stop barking.

1. *What would you do to help the children after the dog had gone?*
2. *What activities might help the children retell the event?*
3. *How would you help the children learn more about dogs and when it is safe to touch them and be friendly?*

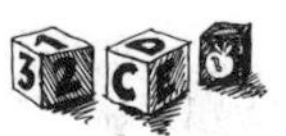

BELONGING

Children need to develop a sense of belonging and will feel more at home in a setting containing objects that are familiar to them from their homes and reflect their culture. Here are some examples:

- The home play area should contain a range of types of cooking equipment – woks, griddles, chopsticks, as well as saucepans, kettles, knives and forks.
- Dressing-up clothes should reflect a diversity of cultures and include saris, head-dresses, veils.
- A wide selection of books should be available showing positive images of different races, cultures and sexes and reflecting equality of opportunity (for more on Anti-discriminatory/anti-bias practice, see Unit Ten).
- Displays should reflect all cultures in society. Children can be encouraged to produce art and/or written work about their homes and families for display.
- Visitors should be invited to come and talk to the children and help them to experience and appreciate social and cultural diversity.
- Coat hooks should be labelled with names and/or pictures.
- Equipment should be personalised – names on cups, flannels, work trays, etc.

OFFERING REASSURANCE

Child-care workers should be warm, caring and responsive. Children easily recognise those who value and appreciate their company and those who have no real interest in them. The following points can help if you are not confident and will give positive messages to the children in your care.

- Be calm and try to speak softly.
- Maintain eye contact when speaking to children and try to get down to their eye level, sit with them or squat down to them if they are playing on the floor.
- Meet their needs quickly. Pick up the non-verbal clues and anticipate their needs; for example the child hopping from one foot to another may need the toilet.
- Be ready to cuddle a young child who is unhappy or upset. On the other hand, never force physical comfort on a child who does not welcome it.
- Encourage conversation and give children time to speak. Ask open questions that will encourage a child to answer with more than a yes or no.
- Always be cheerful, positive and polite. Enjoy your contact with the children in your care.

Progress check

How can child-care workers help children to feel secure?

What are some common fears in young children?

How can adults comfort children who are distressed?

How can a sense of belonging be encouraged in a child-care setting?

Describe how you would explain to a group of children that the fire service will be coming to test the fire hydrants that morning.

Now try these questions

When planning the indoor and outdoor play areas and putting out the equipment, what are the main factors you will need to take into account?

Describe some tasks that would be suitable for children, aged 2–5 years, to encourage a sense of responsibility towards the environment.

How can display work promote children's all-round development?

In what ways can displays be used to promote positive images of society?

Describe the behaviour of a child who is new to your child-care setting and who is anxious about the unfamiliar surroundings. How would you be able to help this child and allay their anxieties?

key terms

You need to know what the key terms and phrases in this chapter mean. Go back through the chapter and find out.

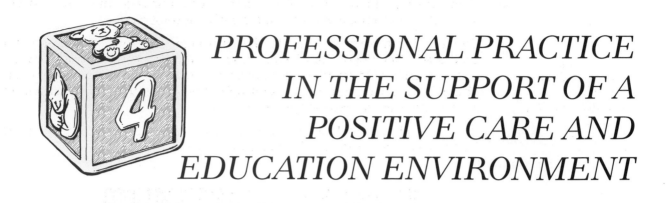

PROFESSIONAL PRACTICE IN THE SUPPORT OF A POSITIVE CARE AND EDUCATION ENVIRONMENT

Providing a positive care and education environment for children will depend on staff commitment to the needs and rights of children, and to their ability and willingness to carry out their duties in a professional way.

This chapter will cover the following topics:

- *the rights and needs of children*
- *professional child-care workers*
- *lines of management and reporting*
- *ways to promote relationships between the care and education setting and the home and family*
- *working as part of a team.*

The rights and needs of children

The following statements, taken from *Young Children in Group Day Care: Guidelines for Good Practice* by the Early Childhood Unit of the National Children's Bureau, outline a challenging set of beliefs about the needs and rights of young children. These statements apply equally well to any care or educational setting.

> **key term**
> **Paramount**
> of first importance

- Children's well-being is **paramount**.
- Children are individuals in their own right, and they have differing needs, abilities and potential. Thus any day-care facility should be flexible and sensitive in responding to these needs.
- Since discrimination of all kinds is an everyday reality in the lives of many children, every effort must be made to ensure that services and practices do not reflect or reinforce it, but actively combat it. Therefore equality of opportunity for children, parents and staff should be explicit in the policies and practice of a day-care facility.
- Working in partnership with parents is recognised as being of major value and importance.

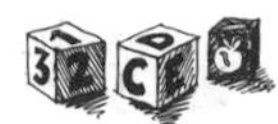

- Good practice in day care for children can enhance their full social, intellectual, emotional, physical and creative development.
- Young children learn and develop best through their own exploration and experience. Such opportunities for learning and development are based on stable, caring relationships, regular observation and ongoing assessment. This will result in **reflective practitioners** who use their observations to inform the learning experiences they offer.
- Regular and thorough evaluation of policies, procedures and practices facilitates the provision of high quality day care.

key term

Reflective practitioners workers who think about what they have done/said, with a view to improving practice

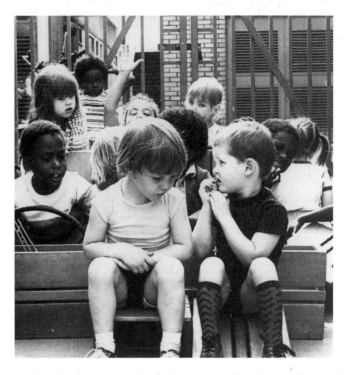

Children learn and develop best through their own exploration and experience

Professional child-care workers

The role of a professional child-care worker involves the following commitments:

- putting the needs and rights of children and their families before your own needs
- respect for the choices and freedoms of others
- respecting the principles of confidentiality
- demonstrating responsibility, reliability and accountability
- being willing to plan, do, record and review
- working in partnership with parents or carers
- being committed to personal development and further training.

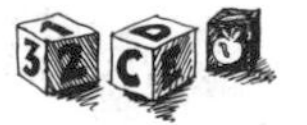

PUT THE NEEDS AND RIGHTS OF CHILDREN AND THEIR FAMILIES FIRST

You will need to meet the needs of children, according to the limits of your work role, irrespective of your personal preferences or prejudices. This will involve recognising the value and dignity of every human being, irrespective of their socio-economic group, ethnic origin, gender, marital status, religion or disability. This is particularly important with young children who may be unable to understand or express their rights and needs fully.

Working with young children may give you a deep sense of satisfaction, but children are not there to provide this for you; you are there to provide for their needs.

Lines of management and reporting

In order to function effectively within an organisation you need to be aware of the people who work there, their role, responsibilities and accountability including their line management. You need to be clear about your own role, responsibilities and accountability.

RESPONSIBILITY, RELIABILITY AND ACCOUNTABILITY

Showing responsibility and accountability involves doing willingly what you are asked to do, if this is in your area of responsibility. You may need to jot down instructions to make sure that you are able to follow them accurately. You then carry out the tasks to the standard required, and in the time allocated, making sure that you are aware of the policies and procedures of your workplace.

You may need to ask your line manager or someone in a supervisory role if you do not understand what to do, or if you think the task is not your responsibility. You may need to refuse to do some tasks until you have been shown how to do them by someone in a supervisory role, or until you have received appropriate training.

If you have any suggestions for changing things, make them to the appropriate person, rather than grumbling or gossiping behind their back. Open communication of positive and negative issues helps staff to develop positive relationships with each other. Assert a point of view, but also be open to the views of other people.

THE PRINCIPLES OF CONFIDENTIALITY

Sensitive information concerning children and their families should be given to you only if you need it in order effectively to meet the needs of the child and family concerned. It should not be given, or received, to satisfy your curiosity or to make you feel superior or in control.

Although the principles of confidentiality may be easy to understand, the practice can be complex and will require self-control and commitment to the welfare of the child and their family.

PLAN, DO, RECORD AND REVIEW

You will need to spend time thinking and planning in advance for your work with young children. A useful way of doing this is to plan, do, record and review. Encourage your colleagues to make comments on your work, as this will give valuable feedback and help you to improve your working practice.

Your aim when planning will be to include all children and make sure that they have full access to the curriculum or activity, irrespective of their **cultural background**, socio-economic group, religion or disability. A further aim will be to avoid repetitive, adult-centred tasks, but rather to help children to develop their creativity and achieve their full learning potential.

> **key term**
> **Cultural background**
> the way of life of the family in which a person is brought up

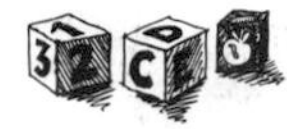

Ways to promote relationships between the care and education setting and the home and family

WORKING IN PARTNERSHIP WITH PARENTS OR CARERS

Professionals recognise the importance of partnership with parents or carers. To carry out your duties in a professional way, you will need to show that you understand the importance of working with parents or carers, respecting their views and wishes, and recognising that, in many instances, they are the ones who know their own children best. In order to do this it is essential to understand and value individual children's cultural background, and take account of their **customs**, **values** and **spiritual beliefs**.

If you have any religious or cultural issues, which may affect your work, you will need to discuss them with your line manager. An example might be if you are unwilling to work on particular days because of your religious practices.

key terms

Customs
special guidelines for behaviour, which are followed by particular groups of people

Values
beliefs that certain things are important and to be valued, for example, a person's right to their own belongings

Spiritual beliefs
what a person believes about the non-material world

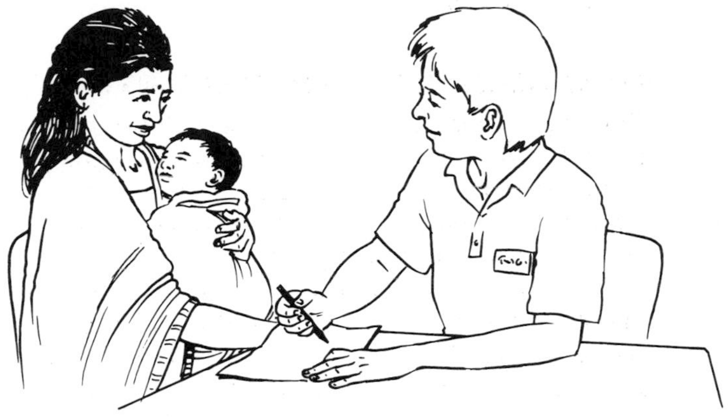

Professionals recognise the importance of partnership with parents or carers

Working as part of a team

In the work setting, child-care workers usually work with colleagues as part of a team. This may be a **multi-disciplinary** team, with representatives from a number of other professional groups, for example teachers and social workers. Those who work as nannies or childminders may find it helpful to see themselves as part of a team with the child's family.

key term

Multi-disciplinary
made up of different professionals

THE ADVANTAGES OF TEAMWORK

The potential advantages of working in a team include the following:

- individual staff weaknesses are balanced by other people's strengths
- members stimulate, motivate, encourage and support one another
- the skills of all members are used to arrive at the best solutions
- a more consistent approach to the task of caring for children and their families is possible
- individual staff feel a sense of belonging and can share problems, difficulties and successes

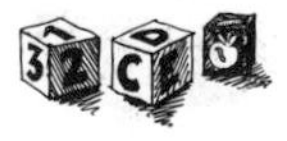

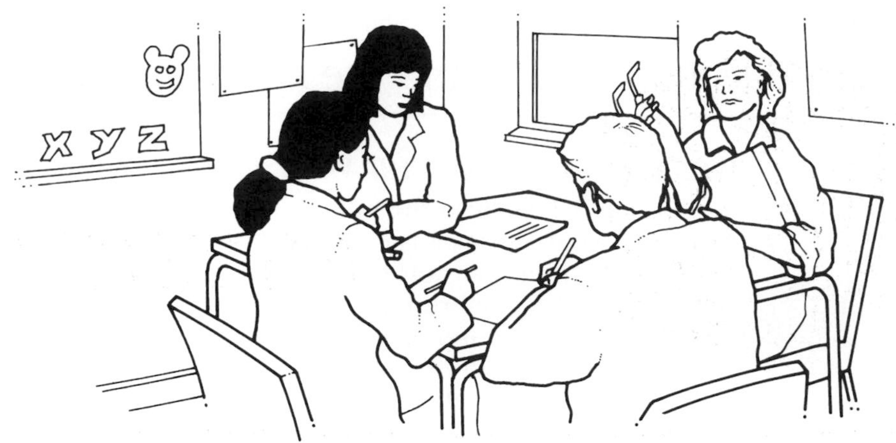

In the workplace, child-care workers usually work with colleagues as part of a team

- responsibility, as well as insight, is shared
- individuals often become more willing to adopt new ways of thinking or working
- team membership satisfies a need to belong and be respected, and have ideals and aims that are confirmed and shared by others
- the children see the benefits of people working together and co-operating with each other.

Progress check

According to the statements of the needs and rights of children, what must always be the most important consideration in the care or education of young children?

When should a child-care worker be given sensitive information about children and their families?

Why may it be necessary to jot down the instructions you are given?

Why may child-care workers need to refuse to do some tasks?

Now try these questions

What are the needs and rights of young children?

Explain the advantages of working with colleagues in a team.

key terms

You need to know what the key terms and phrases in this chapter mean.
Go back through the chapter and find out.

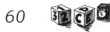

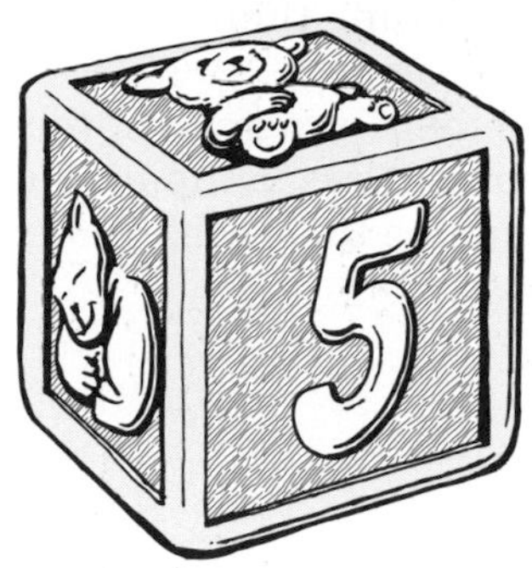

PHYSICAL CARE

All child-care workers recognise that each child is different and that meeting individual needs is the basis of providing for equality of opportunity. This chapter concentrates on some important aspects of the physical care of young children and highlights the particular care they require to promote good health and development.

This chapter will cover the following topics:

- *promoting physical development*
- *exercise*
- *rest and sleep*
- *toilet training*
- *hygiene – care of the hair, skin and teeth*
- *clothing and footwear.*

Promoting physical development

Babies and young children need a safe yet stimulating environment if they are to grow and develop to their full potential. They need space and encouragement to develop new skills, and the opportunity to practise and perfect their technique. A positive atmosphere in which adults praise children's efforts and recognise their achievements will encourage trust and progress.

AGE 1–4

Many babies are mobile by the time they reach their first birthday. This new-found freedom of movement is exciting and should be encouraged, but there is always an element of risk. Babies have no concept of danger and need a watchful adult to ensure their safety. They will fall often, until they can anticipate dangers and avoid obstacles in their path. Their great need to explore and investigate the world should not be prevented, but encouraged in an environment that is safe. They have a desire to find out about everything around them, and an adult who can see the world from the child's point of view will facilitate this discovery. A safe environment to investigate could include containers with safe, but interesting, contents and not random emptying of drawers. A 'safe' cupboard full of exciting things that may be changed frequently will add to the thrill of discovery and learning.

As children get older and their gross motor development progresses, they can run easily, sometimes falling, but less often now. Climbing stairs, jumping, riding a tricycle and gradually beginning to use the pedals are among their achievements.

To stimulate development, carers need to provide:

- space
- opportunity
- freedom to learn from experience
- reassurance
- praise
- access to some equipment.

AGE 4–7

The skills learned in the first 2 years will be perfected as childhood progresses. The hesitant and wobbly runner at 18 months will become a sprinter from 4 to 7 years. The toddler climbing forwards into a chair will eventually perform increasingly hair-raising stunts on climbing apparatus. Skills are being advanced daily and the need to be given the opportunity to practise continues, for example from riding a tricycle, propelling it with the feet, to riding a bicycle without stabilisers, manoeuvring it around obstacles and using the brakes effectively and safely.

When the child has perfected the basic skills of walking, running, climbing, future physical development will depend on the opportunities that are made available to them. Ice-skating, gymnastics, judo, horse-riding and ballet dancing are some of the activities children may enjoy.

Some physical activities may have an element of cost and it may be expensive to provide lessons, but an increasing number of children do participate in them. Some charitable organisations provide funding for children who are skilled in sport, but whose families cannot afford the cost involved in training.

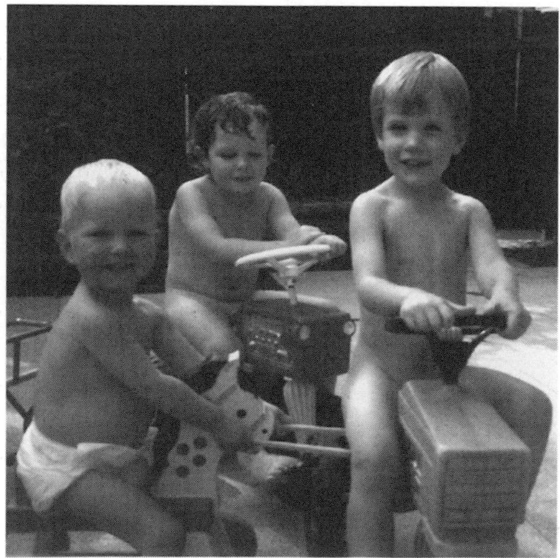

. . . from propelling 3-wheelers with the feet . . .

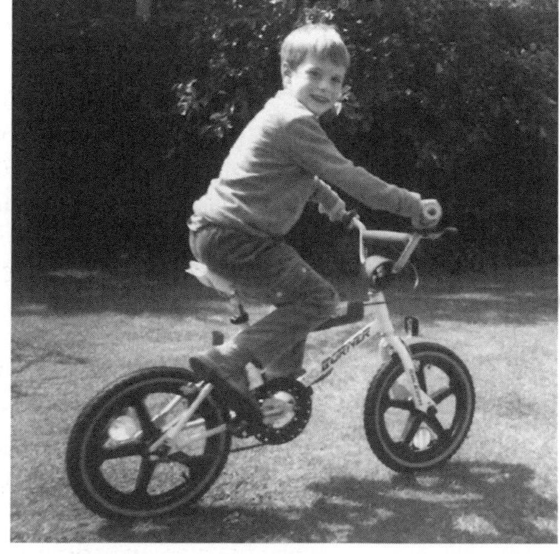

. . . to controlling a bicycle without stabilisers

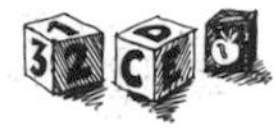

These activities are not a necessary factor in healthy physical development and available opportunities will depend partly on where the child lives and partly on the financial circumstances of the family. For example, a child living in a snowy country may ski, or a child brought up on a farm may ride a horse. The present interests and hobbies of parents or carers may also have an influence on the type of activity offered to a child.

More common activities are swimming, riding a bicycle and football, but they all require practice. This will increase confidence, which in turn will encourage progression. As children get better at a particular skill, their self-esteem will increase. An interested adult who encourages them to repeat a skill, without forcefulness or disappointment if they do not succeed immediately, will help this process.

Not all children enjoy physical activity or exertion. As they get older and develop other interests, like reading, they may prefer not to take part in outdoor pursuits. Gentle encouragement should be used, but without putting undue pressure on the child to participate. Seeing other children's fun and enjoyment will be more of an incentive than a nagging adult.

PHYSICAL DEVELOPMENT AT NURSERY AND INFANT SCHOOL

At nursery and infant school, the curriculum includes the opportunity for physical pursuits of a wide variety. At nursery, outdoor play with tricycles, prams, trolleys, large building blocks, dens, tyres and climbing frames may create an environment for imaginative physical activity. Using music to encourage movement by using the body to interpret the sounds may motivate activity. Group activities may encourage children who lack confidence in themselves.

At infant school, opportunities for exercise should include the following:

- PE, apparatus, dance, music and movement
- football, rounders and other team games, throwing and catching activities, swimming
- Rainbows, Beavers and other clubs for children that provide the opportunity for physical pursuits
- non-stereotypical activities, such as girls playing football and boys using skipping ropes, should be encouraged.

Children with disabilities

When caring for children with disabilities, it is vital to remember that every child is a unique individual with specific needs, which will depend on their own abilities and capacity for independence.

Children with disabilities may not achieve the level of physical competence expected for their age group, so emphasis must be on an individual programme of stimulation which will enable the child to progress at their own pace within the usual sequence of development. They may spend longer at each stage before progressing to the next. Their present developmental achievements must be compared with their past achievements, so that progress can be assessed and improvement recognised.

Remember that children with disabilities are children first. Their special/individual needs must be viewed positively as additional needs to those shared with 'average' children. Each achievement should be encouraged and praised so that they develop a high self-esteem. *They* are important and are not being compared with other children, peers or siblings. Children with disabilities may become frustrated if they cannot achieve a skill quickly, and will require additional, sometimes specialist, help. Adapting the environment to suit their individual needs will help their progress.

Providing a safe environment

Children are the responsibility of the adults who are caring for them. This is often the parents but it may be a nanny, a childminder or playgroup or nursery staff. In the absence of the primary carer, the child is their responsibility. It is of prime importance to keep the child safe and, in doing so, prevent accidents.

An accident is something that happens that is not anticipated or foreseen. This definition is certainly misleading, as it gives the impression that accidents are not preventable, but most accidents that occur to children could be prevented with care and thought. (More about providing a positive environment can be found in Chapter 3 and more about safety can be found in Chapter 6.)

Fresh air

All children need regular exposure to fresh air and preferably an opportunity to play outside. If conditions are not suitable for outdoor play – if it is foggy or raining heavily – the indoor play area should be well ventilated to provide fresh air and to prevent a build-up of carbon dioxide.

The benefits of fresh air are that:

- it contains oxygen; breathing in oxygen gives energy and stimulates exercise
- it contains fewer germs than air indoors; germs are killed by the ultra-violet rays in sunshine
- exposure to sunlight causes the skin to produce vitamin D, which is important for healthy bones and teeth.

Progress check

How can children be encouraged to progress in physical skills?

Which safety factors should be considered when providing the opportunities for physical development for a toddler?

What type of environment must carers provide to stimulate physical development?

What facilities for physical play should be available in a nursery?

How can physical skills affect self-esteem?

How can children with disabilities be encouraged in physical development?

What are the benefits of fresh air?

Exercise

Exercise is a necessary and natural part of life for everyone. It is especially important for young children who need to develop and perfect physical skills.

All physical exercise strengthens muscles, from a young baby kicking on the floor to a 7-year-old child playing football. Encouraging exercise from an early age will lay the foundations for a life-long healthy exercise habit.

It is generally believed that many children do not get enough exercise and will be at increased risk of heart disease and/or other health problems later in life.

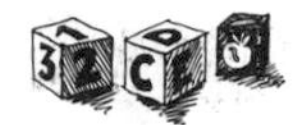

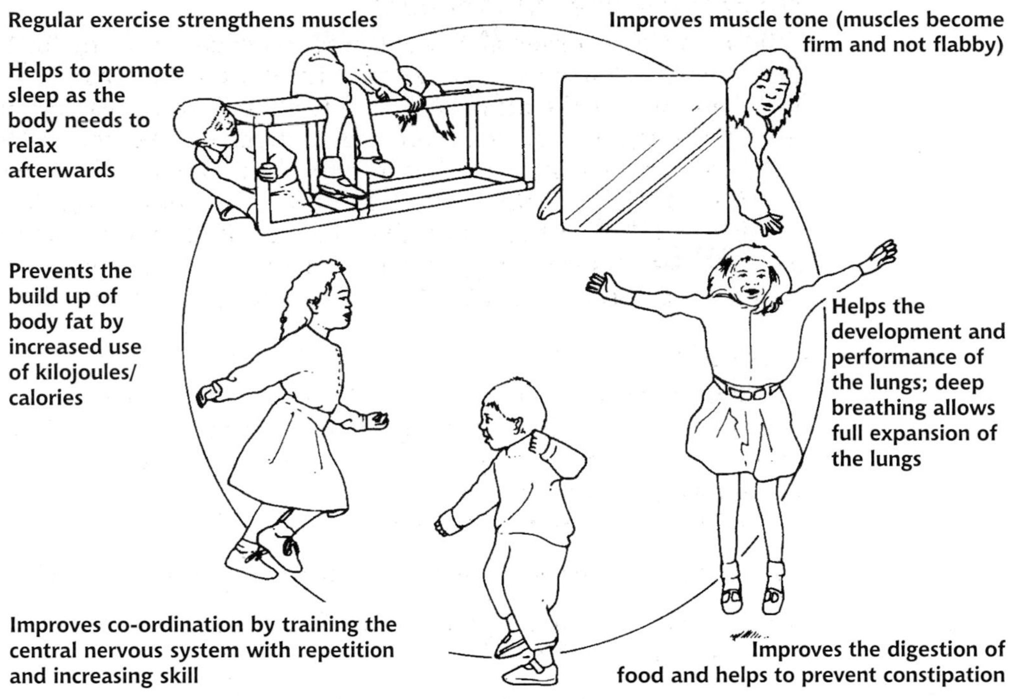

Regular exercise strengthens muscles
Improves muscle tone (muscles become firm and not flabby)
Helps to promote sleep as the body needs to relax afterwards
Prevents the build up of body fat by increased use of kilojoules/ calories
Helps the development and performance of the lungs; deep breathing allows full expansion of the lungs
Improves co-ordination by training the central nervous system with repetition and increasing skill
Improves the digestion of food and helps to prevent constipation

The benefits of exercise

Progress check

Why is exercise important?

What are the benefits of regular exercise?

What illnesses are children at increased risk of developing if they do not get enough exercise?

Rest and sleep

Rest is necessary after physical exercise, and children will know when to stop their vigorous activity as they begin to feel tired.

The benefits of rest are to:

- allow tissues to recover
- eanable the heart rate to fall to its normal level
- allow oxygen to be replaced
- allow the body temperature to drop to its normal level
- allow the central nervous system (CNS) to relax
- enable the body to take in food if required
- prevent muscles from aching and becoming stiff after heavy exercise.

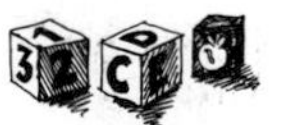

Children should exercise regularly to promote their strength, suppleness and stamina, but they must be allowed to rest – this may be relaxation, sleep or just a change of occupation. One of the values of relaxing or of quiet areas in nursery and school is in providing children with the opportunity to rest and recharge their batteries. A book corner, story time, a home corner, soft cushions and relaxing activities can be provided at nursery and at home. Children need not be challenged all the time; it is sometimes useful for them to be given toys or activities that are relatively easy and do not require deep concentration to complete.

SLEEP

Everyone needs sleep but everyone has different requirements. The sleep needs of children will depend on their age and stage of development, the amount of exercise taken and also their own personal needs.

Sleep is a special kind of rest, which allows the body to recuperate physically and mentally. There are two kinds of sleep:

key terms

Deep relaxing sleep (DRS)
periods of unconsciousness during the sleep cycle

Rapid eye movement (REM)
periods of dream sleep

- **deep relaxing sleep (DRS)**
- **rapid eye movement sleep (REM)**, or dream sleep.

It is generally believed that babies do not dream, but they do have periods of REM, probably when their brains are making sense of all the external stimuli received during the day. Periods of DRS and REM alternate during the sleep period. It is important that periods of REM are completed to awake refreshed. Children who are woken during this period of sleep may be drowsy, disorientated or confused.

Sleep routines

Babies and children need varying amounts of sleep. Some babies may seem to sleep and feed for the first few months, while others sleep very little. Toddlers vary too. Some need a nap morning and afternoon, others need one of these or neither.

Some children wake often at night even after settling late. There is little that can be done apart from following a sensible routine. This will involve:

- patience
- not stimulating the child, remaining quiet, calm, not encouraging interaction

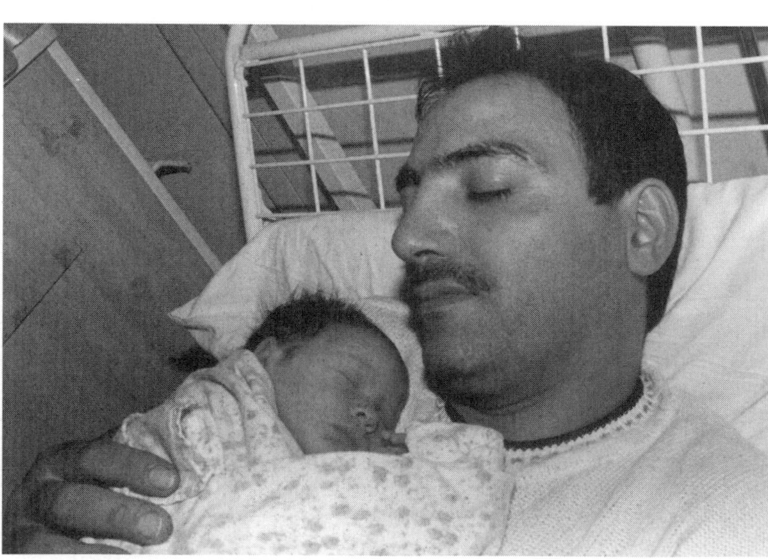

Everyone needs sleep

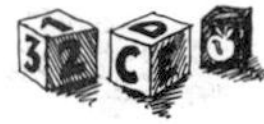

- the child remaining upstairs (do not take the child to where there is any activity)
- encouraging daily exercise
- trying to reduce stress or worries
- being prepared to use the carer's bed – this may resolve waking in the night.

Bedtime routine

Social and cultural expectations of children may include letting them stay up later at night. As long as the child is given the opportunity for an adequate amount of sleep, it should not create a difficulty.

When children need to be at nursery or infant school by 8.45 to 9a.m., their bedtime must be early enough to allow for sufficient sleep. Children who share bedrooms or who live in bed and breakfast accommodation may have more distractions and difficulties sleeping, and these may be difficult to overcome.

> **key term**
>
> **Bedtime routine**
> a consistent approach to putting children to bed, which encourages sleep by increasing security

For successful settling to bed at night, it is important to have a regular **bedtime routine**. The same process each night helps the child to feel secure and comfortable, and so aids sleep. Children need a period of relaxation before going to sleep, and should never be threatened with bed as a form of punishment. This can result in difficulties at bedtime. A suggested routine is as follows:

- A family meal, about 2 hours before bedtime – this is a chance to talk about the day's events. Babies and toddlers enjoy this social occasion too.
- Playtime – with siblings and carers; this is time for individual attention.
- Bath-time – fun, play, relaxation, learning hygiene routines; talking about worries, experiences; this should be one-to-one if possible.
- Offer a drink if required.
- Story time – preferably in bed, after saying goodnight to other family members and cleaning the teeth; story time should be an opportunity for a cuddle, and to snuggle up in bed preparing to sleep.
- Sleep, in a comfortable, warm bed with the light out or night light on if the child requests it.

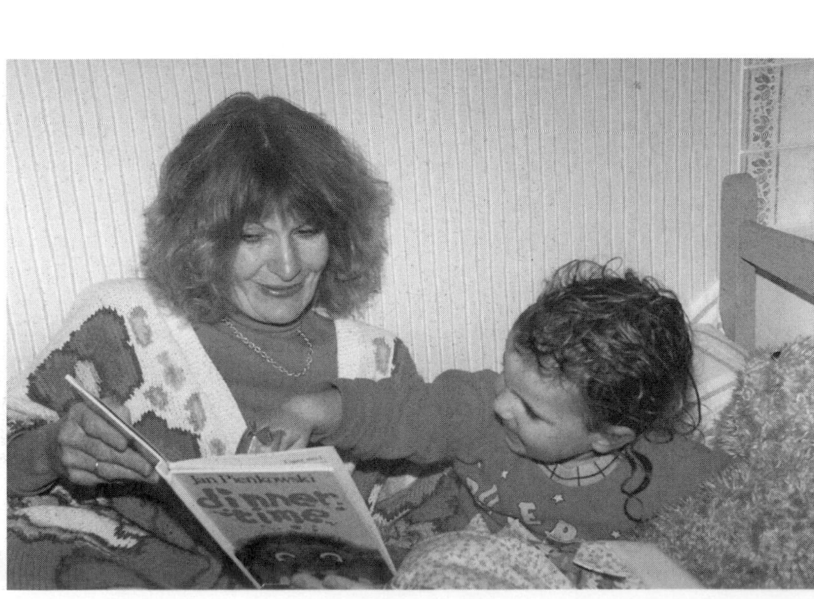

Story time should be an opportunity for a cuddle, and to snuggle up in bed preparing to sleep

Avoid loud noises coming from conversations or the TV which might distract from sleep. This is not always possible and will depend on the housing situation.

Using a familiar routine and reassurance that carers are nearby may encourage children who are unwilling to go to bed to settle more willingly.

Progress check

What are the benefits of rest?

What sort of activities should be available for children to enable them to rest during a busy day?

What factors influence the sleep needs of children?

What are the two types of sleep called?

How can children be encouraged to have a sensible sleep routine?

Toilet training

key term

Toilet training
teaching young children the socially acceptable means of emptying the bladder and bowels into a potty and/or toilet

There are many different theories about **toilet training** – when and how to train babies and children in the use of the potty and the toilet. Some people report that their children were 'trained' before their first birthdays. These are the exception and not the rule! There are wide variations in this area of development, as in all others.

A child will only become reliably clean and dry by the age of 2 to 3 years, at whatever age the potty is introduced. There does not seem to be any point in rushing this skill. It is much more easily achieved if it is left until the child is 2 years at least, unless they show an interest earlier.

GENERAL TOILET-TRAINING GUIDELINES

- The child must be aware of the need to use the toilet or potty. The central nervous system (CNS) must be sufficiently developed for the message that the bowel or bladder is full to be understood by the brain. A baby of 12 to 18 months may know when they are soiled or wet, but are not yet able to anticipate it.
- They must have sufficient language to tell their carer, verbally or with actions, that they need to go.
- Too much pressure at an early age can put the child off the idea completely and create a 'battleground'.
- Wait until the child is ready.
- Make training fun! Carers should be relaxed and not show displeasure or disapproval about accidents, which will certainly happen. The child may be more upset than the adult and deserves understanding.
- Provide good role models. Seeing other children or adults use the toilet will help the child to understand the process.

- In theory, bowel control comes first: the child may recognise the sensation of a full bowel before that of a full bladder. However, most carers report that children are dry earlier than they are clean. This may be because children urinate more often than they have their bowels open, so encourage more practice.
- Have a potty lying around for a long time before it is used. Then it will become familiar and children can sit on it as part of their play.
- Watch for signs of a bowel movement and offer the potty, but do not force it on them. If it is successful then congratulate the child and show them how pleased you are.
- Training is easier in warm weather when children can run around without nappies or pants. They can become aware of what is happening when they urinate or have their bowels open.

key term

Enuresis
involuntary bed wetting during sleep

BEDWETTING

Bedwetting (**enuresis**) is often a hereditary tendency and is particularly common in boys. If it begins after the child has been dry for a long period, it may be due to an infection of the urinary tract or to a stressful event, for example a new baby, moving house or school or the death of a relative or friend. Regression in this area may also be caused by illness.

Children usually become dry at night of their own accord. Accidents are common and should be treated with understanding and not displeasure. There is no need for concern about occasional accidents unless the child is upset. Seeing a sympathetic doctor or health visitor should help.

key term

Encopresis
deliberate soiling into the pants, on to the floor or other area after bowel control has been established

SOILING

Soiling (**encopresis**) may be caused by an objection to using the potty or toilet that grows to an aversion, and the child withholds the motion until they can relieve themselves elsewhere. Soiling may be due to an emotional disturbance, or it may cause one. Children with this difficulty need very sensitive treatment. It can be resolved, often with the help of the health visitor and/or GP.

Progress check

What signs may indicate that a child is ready to be toilet trained?

At approximately what age are children reliably clean and dry during the day?

What is enuresis?

What factors may contribute to enuresis?

What is encopresis?

My best friend's baby is only 9 months old and she is dry now!

She sits there for ages and nothing happens!

Should I tell her off when she has accidents on the floor?

My 2 year old was dry but now that I'm home with the new baby, he is wetting himself again! Why?

At what age should I start training my child to use the potty?

He fidgets all the time and wants to get off!

Watching my big brother might help me understand.

Look for the signs that I'll make when I'm ready: clutching my nappy or looking at you red in the face!

Don't moan if I have an accident. I'm not being naughty!

I mean it, I'll rebel when I'm older if you force me now! Wait until I understand what I have to do!

I'm only 12 months old: you expect too much of me! I can't do it and I'm not just being difficult.

I like training pants. They are easy to move in and get off in a hurry.

Don't nag me and sit me there for hours on end! I don't want to go!

Don't compare me to Jimmy down the road. We are all different!

It's no use putting tights or dungarees on me; you won't have time to get them off!

This potty is too hard. It's a bad shape and it hurts me. No wonder I'm always fidgeting!

I don't mind sitting on the pot for a few minutes after lunch, but give me a toy to play with so that I can relax. . . and if I don't want to go don't leave me there!

I like you giving me sweets for going in the pot, but I've been for 26 little ones today! I've got you on a string!

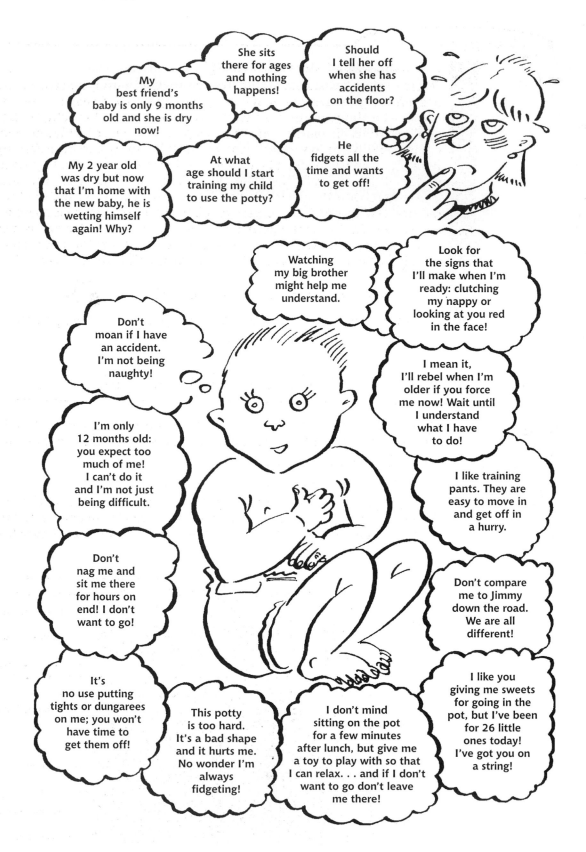

Toilet training: two points of view

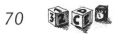

Case study . . .

. . . successful toilet training

Jeremy is just 2 years old and shows no interest in using a potty. His mother, Jane, has left the potty lying around during Jeremy's second year and he is very familiar with it – he always wants to sit on it before he gets into the bath, but has not used it at all! He tells his mother when he has passed urine or had his bowels open in his nappy. Jane is not concerned – she has decided to try and train Jeremy during the family's camping holiday. She explains to Jeremy that he can stop wearing nappies in the daytime while they are on holiday and that she will take the potty everywhere with them. On the beach, Jeremy urinates in the sand frequently for the first few days and then begins to tell his parents when he is about to do so! They encourage him to use the potty and when he does they clap and congratulate him on his clever achievement. Jeremy begins to ask for the potty and despite the occasional 'accident' he is out of nappies by the time the holiday ends.

1. *Why was a holiday 'training' such a success?*
2. *How do you think his parents' attitude helped Jeremy in this process?*

Hygiene: care of the hair, skin and teeth

key term

Hygiene
the study of the principles of health

All children need adult help and supervision in their personal **hygiene** requirements. Good standards of hygiene in childhood are important because they:

- help to prevent disease
- increase self-esteem and social acceptance
- prepare children for life by teaching them how to care for themselves.

To appreciate the importance of hygiene, it is valuable to understand the functions of the skin and hair. The structure of the skin is shown in the figure below.

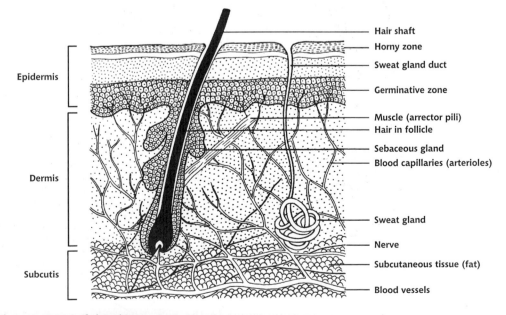

Epidermis
Dermis
Subcutis
Hair shaft
Horny zone
Sweat gland duct
Germinative zone
Muscle (arrector pili)
Hair in follicle
Sebaceous gland
Blood capillaries (arterioles)
Sweat gland
Nerve
Subcutaneous tissue (fat)
Blood vessels

The structure of the skin

FUNCTIONS OF THE SKIN

The skin performs the following functions:

- *protection* – of underlying organs and against germs entering the body
- *sensation* – the skin is the organ of touch, and conveys sensations of hot, cold, soft, hard
- *secretion of **sebum*** – an oily substance, which lubricates the hair, keeps the skin supple and waterproof, and protects the skin from moisture and heat
- *the manufacture of vitamin D* – exposure to ultra-violet rays from the sun synthesises vitamin D, which is necessary for healthy bone growth. (Black children may need a vitamin D supplement in the winter as their skin does not easily make vitamin D.)
- ***sweat*** – the skin excretes sweat and this gets rid of some waste products. Sweating helps to regulate the temperature when the body is hot.

key terms

Sebum
an oily substance that lubricates the skin, it is produced by the sebaceous glands and secreted through the hair shaft

Sweat
liquid produced in the sweat glands and secreted through the pores on to the surface of the skin

GUIDELINES FOR GOOD HYGIENE

Because the skin has so many important functions and because it is the first part of the body to come into contact with the environment, it must be cared for adequately. This does not mean obsessive cleaning of the skin – too much cleaning can be as harmful as too little because it may make the skin dry and sore, and also washes away sebum, which protects it.

- Wash the face and hands in the morning and before meals.
- Wash hands after going to the toilet and after messy play.
- Keep the nails short by cutting them regularly. This will prevent dirt collecting under them.
- A daily bath or shower is necessary with young children who play outside and become dirty, hot and sweaty. Dry them thoroughly, especially between the toes and in the skin creases to prevent soreness and cracking.
- Observe the skin for rashes and soreness. If treatment is prescribed it must be followed.
- Black skin needs moisturising. Putting oil in the bath water and massaging almond oil or coconut butter into the skin afterwards helps to prevent dryness.
- If a child does not require a daily bath, a thorough wash is good enough. Remember to encourage children to wash their bottoms *after* the face, neck, hands and feet.
- Hair only needs to be washed once or twice a week, unless it is full of food or the residue of messy play! Avoid using a hairdryer every time the hair is washed as this can damage the hair.
- Rinse shampoo out thoroughly in clean water. Conditioners may be useful for hair that is difficult to comb.
- Black, curly hair needs hair oil applying daily to prevent dryness and hair breakage. Use a wide-toothed comb.
- Skin needs protecting from the sun to prevent burning and the associated risks of cancer. Use a sunblock or high-factor sun cream and monitor the length of time spent in the sun. Black skin needs the same protection as pale skin.

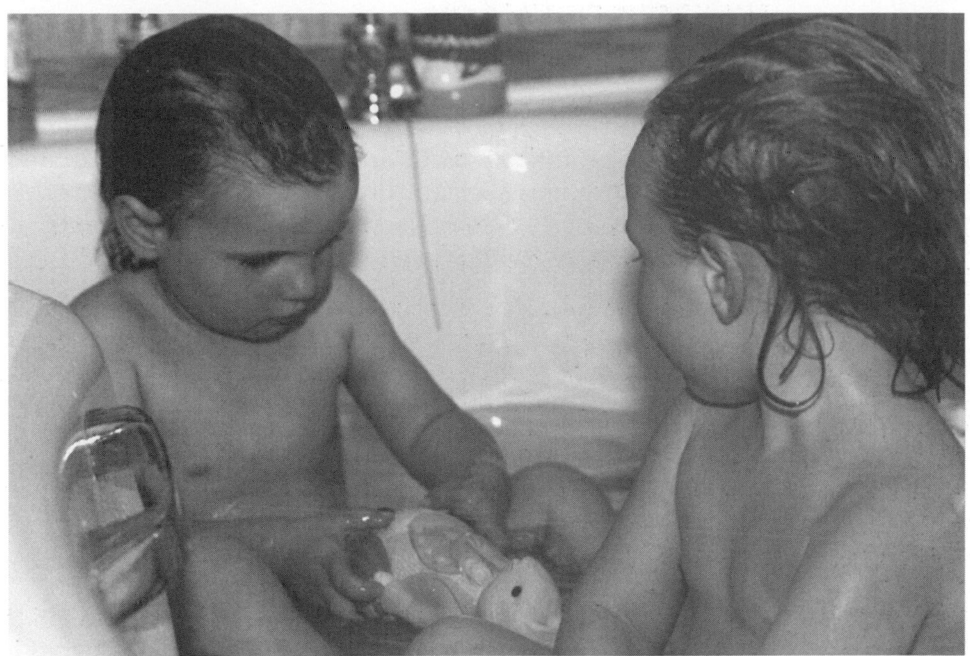

A daily bath is necessary for active toddlers playing outside

Case study . . .

. . . unexpected sunburn

Ashley, aged 4 years, is an energetic child who loves to play outside in all weathers. In the summer his childminder often takes the children to a local outdoor paddling pool where they have a picnic on the grass next to the water – there is a playground nearby where the children also play. She always makes sure that the children are protected by using creams, hats and t-shirts when the sun is shining. One warm but overcast day in May she takes them to the park for a picnic, not expecting them to use the pool. Ashley insists on stripping down to his underpants for a paddle and proceeds to spend 2 hours playing in the water. On arriving home he complains that his shoulders and back hurt. When she looks at them the childminder sees that Ashley's black skin is dark and swollen.

1. *What is the cause of Ashley's discomfort?*
2. *How could this have been prevented?*

The benefits of good hygiene

- Clear, glowing skin and shiny hair are signs of good health.
- The child looks attractive and feels well, and develops a positive self-image.
- Washing is a tonic; children feel healthy as a result.
- Infection is prevented (it can spread from child to child from dirty hands and nails).
- Health is maintained.
- Good habits give a pattern for life.
- It allows the skin to perform its functions.
- It treats skin problems, for example eczema, sweat rash; itchy, sore skin can prevent sleep and make the child irritable and restless. This may affect all-round development.

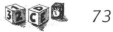

TEETH

key term

Milk teeth
the first 20 (deciduous) teeth

Teeth may appear at any time during the first 2 years of life. It is usually expected that they will begin to erupt during the first year but this is not necessarily so. They usually come through in the same order as shown in the figure below, but variations may occur. The first 20 teeth are called the **milk teeth**, and they will usually be complete by the age of 3 years. From 5 to 6 years, these teeth begin to fall out as the adult teeth come through. There are 32 permanent teeth, and the care they are given in childhood will help them to last a lifetime.

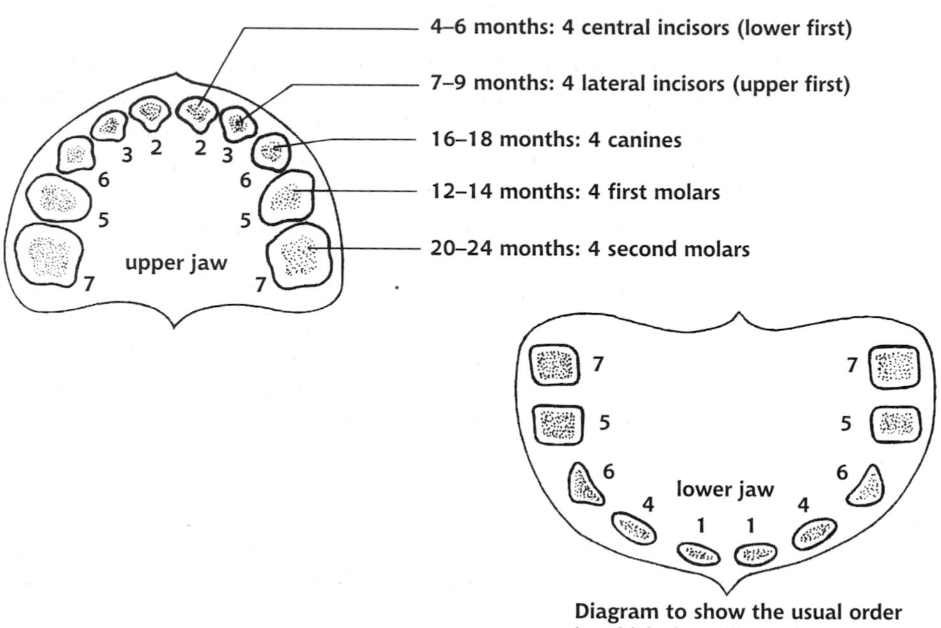

4–6 months: 4 central incisors (lower first)
7–9 months: 4 lateral incisors (upper first)
16–18 months: 4 canines
12–14 months: 4 first molars
20–24 months: 4 second molars
upper jaw
lower jaw
Diagram to show the usual order in which the milk teeth appear

The eruption of the teeth

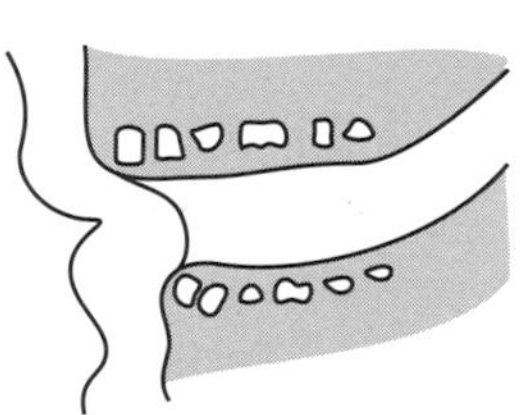

The milk teeth can be seen developing inside the jaw

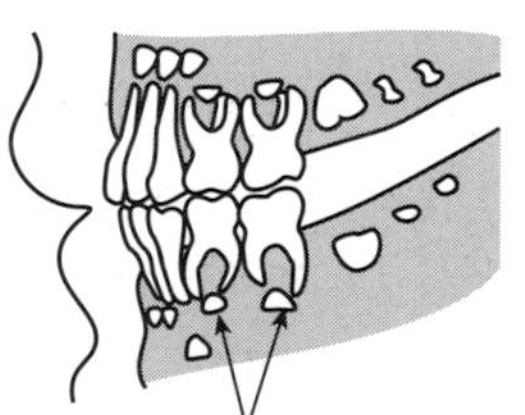

The milk teeth are all through. The permanent teeth are developing underneath

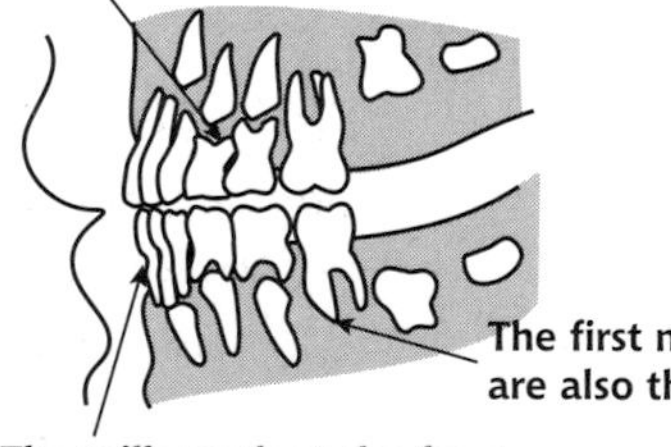

The roots of the remaining milk teeth are beginning to disappear
The first molars are also through
The milk teeth at the front of both jaws (the incisors) have been replaced by permanent teeth

Development of the teeth

Care of the teeth

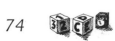

Provide a soft toothbrush for a baby to use and become familiar with. It is not necessary for babies to have teeth to begin oral (mouth) hygiene. They will enjoy playing with the brush, and as they get older, will put it in their mouths to suck it

and to rub their gums. Give them the opportunity to watch adults and siblings clean their teeth. When the first tooth does appear, try to clean it gently with a small, soft brush. If the baby objects, do not force them to have the tooth or teeth cleaned – make it a game and increase their confidence. Teach older children how to clean their teeth. A dental hygienist will be able to offer professional assistance – the dentist will arrange this. Ensure that cleaning the teeth becomes a habit: in the morning after breakfast and after the last drink or snack before bed. Cleaning the teeth after meals should be encouraged, but this may not always be possible.

Diet

Encourage healthy teeth and prevent decay by providing a healthy diet that is high in calcium and vitamins and low in sugar. Avoid giving sweet drinks to babies and children, especially in a bottle or soother; this coats the gums and teeth in sugar and encourages the formation of acid, which dissolves the enamel on the teeth. Sugar can penetrate the gum and cause decay before the teeth come through. This is common in babies and children who are frequently offered sweet drinks.

Children will probably demand sweets. Give them after a meal and then encourage them to clean their teeth. Do not offer sweets and sugary snacks between meals, as this will encourage decay. If you do need to feed a child between meals, provide food that needs to be chewed and improves the health of the gums and teeth, like apples, carrots and bread.

> **key term**
>
> **Fluoride**
> a mineral that helps to prevent dental decay

Fluoride

Fluoride in the water supply has been proven to strengthen the enamel on the teeth, and so prevent decay. In areas where the fluoride content is low, drops can be given daily in drinks. Fluoride toothpaste also helps to prevent decay.

The dentist

Visit the dentist regularly. A baby who attends with an adult, and then has their own appointments, will feel more confident about the procedure. Prepare children for their dental appointments by explaining what will happen and participating in role play. Never pass on any adult feelings of terror, fear or anxiety about the dentist.

ENCOURAGING INDEPENDENCE IN HYGIENE

There are several ways in which carers can encourage a child to develop independence in personal hygiene.

- Provide positive role models.
- Establish caring routines that encourage cleanliness from early babyhood.
- Make hygiene fun: use toys in the bath, cups and containers, sinkers and floaters.
- Provide the child with their own flannel, toothbrush, hairbrush, etc. that they have chosen themselves.
- Allow the child to wash themselves and participate at bath-time. Let them brush their hair with a soft brush and comb with rounded teeth.
- Provide a step so that they can reach the basin to wash and clean teeth.
- Make haircuts fun too: some barbers and hairdressers specialise in children's hair.

Progress check

What are the functions of the skin?

What particular care should be given to black skin?

What are the benefits of good hygiene?

How can independence be encouraged in hygiene routines?

How many milk teeth are there?

How can healthy teeth be encouraged?

Clothing and footwear

Toddlers and children work hard at their play, and this will mean that they get dirty. Although they are often washed for their health and comfort they will soon be dirty again. The attraction of a muddy puddle, digging soil and exploring the sand-pit will see to that! This is all normal behaviour and should be encouraged. Children should not be pressurised into keeping clean or the spontaneity and excitement of play will be lost.

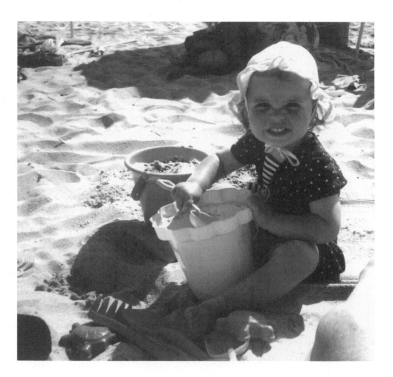

Toddlers will inevitably get dirty when they play

CLOTHING

Clothing must be comfortable and loose enough for easy movement but fitted well enough to prevent loose material from catching and hindering movements.

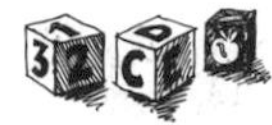

It should be easily washable; children do get dirty. This should be expected and not disapproved of.

Clothes should have fasteners that a child can reasonably manage, for example large buttons, toggles, velcro and zips.

Underwear

- Cotton is preferable, to absorb sweat and increase comfort.
- When babies are in nappies, all-in-one vests prevent cold spots.

General clothing

- Trousers or shorts are best for both sexes when a child is crawling and falling. Dresses often get in the way of active play.
- Stretch tracksuits are ideal.
- Dungarees, except when the child is learning to use the toilet, as they are difficult to remove quickly and replace.
- T-shirts, cotton jumpers.
- Add extra, light layers when it is cold.

Coats

- A showerproof, colourful anorak with a hood is warm and easily washed. Extra underlayers can be added when the weather is very cold.
- Waterproof trousers and wellingtons enable happy puddle splashing.

Pyjamas

- Use all-in-one suits without feet, with correctly sized socks.

FOOTWEAR

The bones of the feet develop from cartilage, and are very soft and vulnerable to deformity if they are pushed into badly fitting shoes or socks. A child may not complain of pain because the cartilage will mould into the shape of the shoe.

Shoes should not be worn unless it is absolutely necessary, and not indoors. Walking barefoot in the house is preferable, partly because babies and children use the toes to balance, and floors can be like skating rinks for a baby or child wearing socks alone. If floors are cold or damp, socks with non-slip soles can be worn. Shoes are not necessary until a child will be walking outside, when they protect the feet and preserve warmth.

Feet grow two or three sizes each year until the age of 4. The primary carer is responsible for making sure that footwear fits correctly. This should be done by regularly checking the growth of the feet. They must be checked every 3 months by an expert trained in children's shoe fitting. Both the length and width are important.

Shoes should:

- protect the feet
- have no rough areas to rub or chafe the feet
- have room for growth
- have an adjustable fastener, for example a buckle or velcro

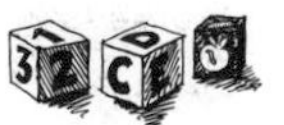

- be flexible and allow free movement
- fit around the heel
- support the foot and prevent it from sliding forwards.

Socks must be of a size to correspond to the size of the shoe. Stretch socks should be avoided.

Progress check

What type of clothing is most suitable for a toddler?

When are shoes necessary?

On average, how many sizes do feet grow in a year until the age of 4 years?

How often should children's feet be measured by an expert?

What are the qualities of a good pair of shoes?

Now try these questions

How can a child-care worker actively promote physical development?

Explain why equal opportunities is important when providing physical care for children.

Why is it important for child-care establishments to provide a variety of activities that offer the children opportunities for exercise and rest?

What positive steps can parents and carers take to ensure a happy transition from nappies to toilet?

How can children be encouraged to develop independence in hygiene routines?

key terms

You need to know what the key terms and phrases in this chapter mean.
Go back through the chapter and find out.

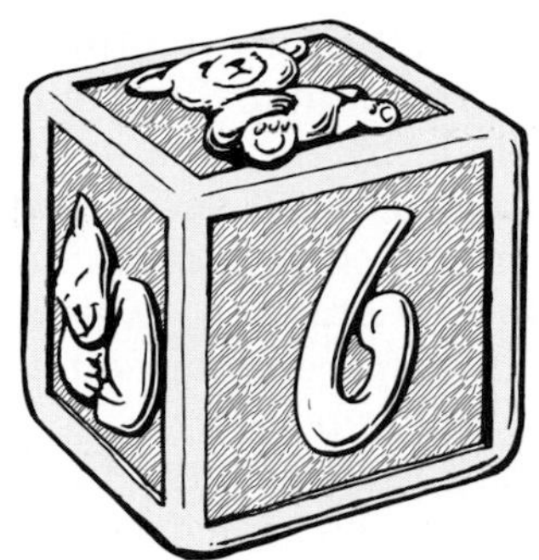

GOOD PRACTICE TO SUPPORT PHYSICAL CARE AND A POSITIVE ENVIRONMENT

Child-care workers have a responsibility to keep the children in their care safe. A stimulating and exciting environment must also incorporate vital safety elements to protect children. Hazardous and dangerous experiences should be anticipated and avoided. The presence of a watchful and vigilant carer at home, in the child-care establishment, on outings and when travelling from place to place is essential if accidents and unintentional injuries to children are to be prevented.

This chapter will cover the following topics:

- *workplace safety policies and procedures*
- *accidents*
- *safety at home*
- *outdoor safety*
- *outings with children.*

Workplace safety policies and procedures

THE HEALTH AND SAFETY AT WORK ACT 1974

The Health and Safety at Work Act 1974 is the principal piece of legislation in this area, and gives general guidance about health and safety. Since the 1974 Act, several regulations (e.g. Control of Substances Hazardous to Health Regulations (COSHH) 1999) have been passed that give more detail about particular situations. Some of these regulations have been introduced to bring UK health and safety law into line with European laws.

Under the 1974 Act both employers and employees have duties:

- Employers must produce a written policy explaining how they will ensure the health, safety and welfare of all people who use their premises.
- Employees must co-operate with these arrangements and take reasonable care of themselves and others.

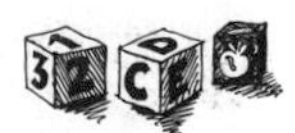

LOCAL AUTHORITY REGULATIONS (CHILDREN ACT 1989)

All child-care settings that care for children for more than 2 hours at a time must register with the local authority and are required by law to maintain certain health and safety standards. All child-care settings must abide by the local authority regulations in order to comply with the Children Act 1989. All social services departments issue regulations for providers of day care, including childminders. These cover aspects of child care such as safety, heating, ventilation, hygiene and outside play spaces. Regulations also cover the amount of space required for each child and the number of adults required to care for the children.

Under the Children Act 1989 local authorities have a responsibility to ensure minimum standards of day care for children under 8 by means of registration and inspection of the care provided. Inspection must be carried out at least once a year. From September 2001 this responsibility will be transferred to the Office for Standards in Education (OFSTED).

> **key term**
>
> **Ratio**
> the numerical relationship or proportion of one quantity to another

The prescribed **ratios** of adults to children for these age groups are:

0–1 years	1 adult to 3 children
1–3 years	1 adult to 4 children
3–5 years	1 adult to 8 children.

These numbers are the minimum requirements. You would expect to have fewer children per adult if some of the children had special needs. Children also need to get out and about to enjoy local outings to the shops or park and you would need more adults in these circumstances.

The required amount of space for each child in these age groups is:

0–2 years	40ft^2 (3.72 m^2)
2–3 years	30ft^2 (2.79 m^2)
3–5 years	25ft^2 (2.32 m^2)

GENERAL CONDUCT

In addition to complying with any local authority regulations all child-care settings will have a health and safety policy that will include:

- clear safety rules for children's conduct, which make it clear what is expected of them and encourage children to behave in a sensible and responsible manner, for example walking and not running along corridors, keeping to the left on corridors and stairs, not shouting, fighting or bullying
- stringent safety precautions, for example space to move around the building and classrooms safely, doors with safety catches, non-slip surfaces, safety glass, safe gym equipment
- procedures for using equipment
- policies for dealing with spills of bodily fluids
- procedures for staff to report potential hazards
- clear rules to ensure that staff practise safety, for example closing and fastening safety gates, reporting any damaged or defective equipment and keeping hot drinks away from children
- policies for collecting children.

SECURITY IN ESTABLISHMENTS

Many child-care establishments have introduced stringent security measures in recent years. These may include locked doors when the children are inside the

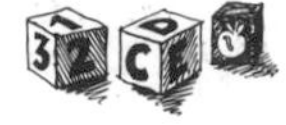

building and name badges for all staff and students. Door entryphones and bells give the staff the opportunity to enquire about the nature of the business of any visitors before allowing them to enter the building. It is always advisable to make an appointment before visiting a child-care establishment to show respect for the establishment's security policies. Staff supervise the children during outdoor play times to ensure their individual and group safety.

Home times

Child-care workers must be vigilant to ensure that children are collected by adults who are known to the staff. Many settings will have a policy that only allows children to be collected by a named adult. Parents should inform staff about who will be collecting the child if they cannot do so themselves. It is preferable for children to remain inside the building to await collection at home time. Every establishment should have a procedure for collecting children.

EMERGENCY PROCEDURES

All establishments should have:

- written emergency procedures
- staff who have been trained in first aid
- first aid equipment
- an accident book for accurate recording of all incidents requiring first aid
- regular review of incidents of accidents to highlight areas of concern
- planned programme of accident prevention.

EVACUATION AND FIRE PROCEDURES

Evacuation and fire procedures must be clearly displayed and communicated to anyone who comes into the building. Regular practices are required by law and all staff must be familiar with evacuation procedures. A fire officer will make regular checks.

Progress check

How can children's safety be ensured at home times?

Which emergency procedures should be in place in all child-care establishments?

How can accidents be prevented in child-care establishments?

Case study . . .

. . . safety on the roads

Josie is a childminder who looks after two children under the age of 5 years during the day. She always pays great attention to safety and her home is regularly inspected by an officer from the Under Eights Unit at the local social services department. The officer notes the safety equipment and its use, for example a fireguard and a stairgate.

Josie also collects two children from infant school and takes them home with her until their parents finish work and are able to collect them. Walking with four children is an enormous responsibility and, although Josie does not have to cross any busy roads, she is very aware of the children's safety on the pavement and when crossing minor road junctions. The two youngest are strapped into the double buggy. Naomi and Kylie, both aged 7, walk together in front of Josie and the other children. They are not allowed to rush off alone, but walk at a steady pace and stop at kerbs so that the whole goup can cross the road together.

1. *Josie uses a stairgate and fireguard. What other safety measures should she take to protect the children in her home?*
2. *How does she ensure the children's safety on the journey to and from school?*
3. *Can you think of any other safety measures that Josie could take to protect the children on the pavement and road?*

Accidents

ANTICIPATING ACCIDENTS

Children are born with no awareness of danger. They are totally dependent on their carers for protection and survival. Carers need a sound knowledge of child development to be able to anticipate when an accident may occur due to a child's increasing physical skills or curiosity. For example, a baby of 4–5 months may seem quite safe lying on the sofa, until the day they roll over and off on to the floor. Or the young baby sitting on a carer's knee as they drink a cup of tea may seem to have no interest or curiosity about the cup or its contents until the day their co-ordination allows them to grab the cup and scald themselves. Babies and children are constantly changing. It may be surprising when they do things for the first time, but their increasing abilities should be expected. Carers should anticipate and avoid dangerous situations.

PROTECTING CHILDREN FROM ACCIDENTS

Babies and toddlers cannot remember what they have been told from one moment to the next. Saying 'No!' as they crawl towards the open fire may stop their progress for a moment, but they will soon be off again. They are not being naughty or disobedient; they are naturally curious and need to investigate. They have lots of energy and will keep trying until they succeed. This is usually encouraged by adults, so babies will be confused and upset when they are discouraged from an unsafe situation, for example trying to pull at that tempting wire hanging from the kitchen work-top, emptying kitchen cupboards, or grabbing a pan handle when it is on the hob. The carer must try to make all situations safe, while leaving children space to explore.

As children get older and their memory develops, their awareness of what is dangerous increases. They will begin to remember what *hot* feels like, that it hurts, and they will avoid touching the oven door or radiator. They are beginning to protect themselves. As they mature they may begin to protect other, younger toddlers, giving them some of the benefit of their own experience.

It is still necessary to provide a balance between protecting the child from danger, yet allowing them the space and opportunity to explore and develop at their own pace to their full potential. Achieving this balance will require an adult to provide a safe environment for exploration. The home, the nursery, the car, the school, the playground must be as child-safe as possible. A watchful adult presence is always necessary.

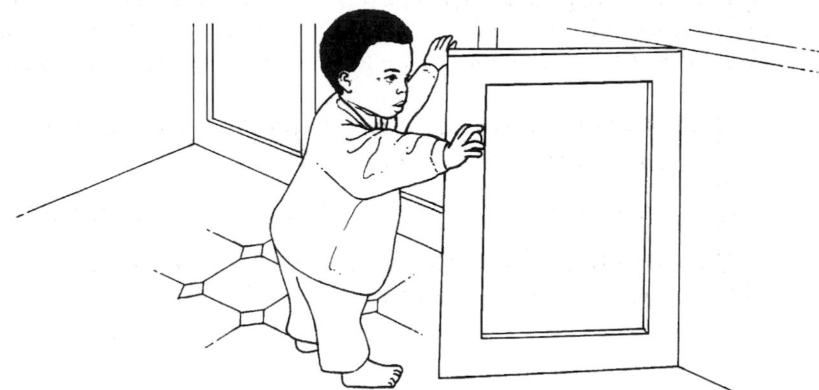

Children love to explore

ACCIDENT STATISTICS

Unintentional injuries (accidents) are the greatest cause of death in children over 1 year old. Most accidents happen at home, and 1 to 4 year olds are most at risk.

The causes of unintentional injuries are directly related to:

- the developmental age/stage of the child
- the child's changing perception of danger
- the degree of exposure to different hazards at various ages.

Social class can affect the chances of an accident occurring – some injuries are up to six times more common in the poorest areas of the UK compared to the most affluent.

Attitudes to child care can also affect this, for example:

- how much independence children are allowed
- supervision travelling to and from school
- opportunities to play safely outdoors – children may be allowed to play on the street and to cross the road before they are old enough to judge traffic safely.

COMMON FACTORS IN ACCIDENTS

All carers are human, and there may be times when they are less vigilant than others, but when caring for children constant awareness is essential. Children may take more risks when adults are distracted, or when they have seen other children do dangerous things. Accidents may occur in the following situations.

Stress

When adults or children are worried or anxious, they may be less alert or cautious. Carelessness creates dangerous situations.

Haste

When late for school or an appointment, anyone may take less care in keeping safe; someone may, for example, rush across the road.

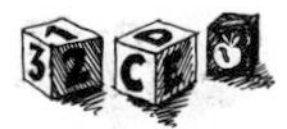

Tiredness

Tiredness makes everyone less alert. Adults may be pleased that children are quietly playing, which allows them to rest. They may be unaware that the garden gate is open, or that the children have wandered on to the balcony of the flat.

Remember that when children are unusually quiet in their play, they have probably found something that fascinates them. Check that they are not playing with a dangerous object or in a potentially dangerous situation.

Under-protection

Children who are not supervised by caring adults are more likely to have accidents. They have not been made aware of dangers and are allowed to play in hazardous situations.

Over-protection

Children who are so protected that they are not allowed to explore are less likely to be aware of danger when they are left alone. They may be determined to do something usually disallowed.

Progress check

Why is it important for adults to be aware of safety when working with young children?

How can attitudes to child care influence the accident statistics?

When are accidents most likely to happen?

How can adult tiredness increase the risk of accidents to children in their care?

Where do most accidents take place?

PREVENTING ACCIDENTS

The successful prevention of accidents depends largely upon the following.

Role models

The most important way of reducing risk is by setting a good example to children. Children copy adult actions so adults have a responsibility to teach them how to be safe in, for example, crossing the road, wearing a seat belt, closing the door.

Modifying the environment

Make sure that the home, and other areas used by children, are as safe as possible, while still allowing them to become independent and learn for themselves.

Education

Children need to be educated about safety. Many national campaigns, for example Play it Safe, Green Cross Code, Stranger Danger, have aimed at increasing awareness of safety issues. Children can be taught how to avoid dangers and how to cope if a hazardous situation occurs. Adults also need educating in these areas: this means child-care workers, teachers, parents, health professionals and those who design environment areas such as shopping centres, parks or roads.

Product safety

All equipment should be safe for use with children and preferably approved for safety and display, for example, the BSI kite-mark, European standards markings, the BEAB Mark of Safety (see page 472).

> **key term**
> **Safety legislation** laws that are created to prevent accidents and promote safety

Legislation

Pressure on local and national government may encourage them to make and enforce **safety legislation,** which supports the prevention of accidents and the promotion of safety.

Progress check

How can the child-care environment be modified to make it as safe as possible for a child?

Which national campaigns have helped to increase awareness about safety issues?

How can adults ensure the safety of products that they buy for children?

Safety at home

Everyone is relaxed at home, and may feel safe because they are at home. This is clearly not true. It is interesting to note that most home accidents occur during the summer months, especially in July. Children most at risk are those between 1 and 4 years old, because they are mobile and want to explore, but they cannot yet anticipate danger. Accident figures indicate that boys are more at risk than girls. Causes and ways of preventing home accidents are given below.

FIRE

House fire is the commonest cause of death by fire. Death usually results from inhaling poisonous fumes given off from furniture.

Prevention

> **key term**
> **Flammable** material that burns easily

- Reduce the source of fire, for example do not leave matches in children's reach, restrict smoking, use a fireguard (it is illegal to leave a child under 12 in a room with an open fire), avoid using chip pans, store petrol and other **flammable** (burnable) materials correctly.
- Reduce the risk of materials such as night-wear and soft furnishings catching fire by ensuring that children wear night-clothes made from low-flammable material and by ensuring that any soft furnishings are made with fire-retardant fabric and foam – modern furnishings should have labels stating this (old furnishings are a particular fire risk).
- Restrict the possible spread of fire by the use of fire doors (which should always be kept closed), fire extinguishers and fire blankets.

- The use of an early warning system such as a smoke alarm will give the extra minutes needed to escape from a fire. All houses should have at least one, especially if children live there.

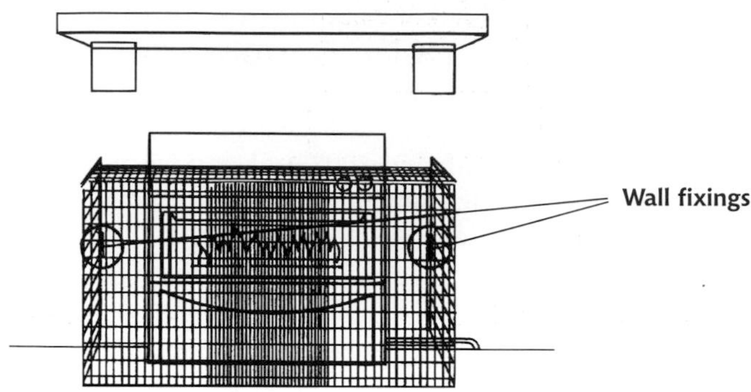

A fireguard correctly fitted

FALLS

Half of all domestic accidents involving children are due to falls, and toddlers are most in danger. Some dangerous situations are:

- a baby in a baby bouncer or carrycot placed on a high surface such as a table or bed
- the baby placed on a high surface
- toddlers in a house with unguarded stairs, open unprotected windows, balconies or bunk beds.

Prevention

- Never leave babies unattended on a high surface; lie them on the floor instead.
- Use stairgates at the top and bottom of stairs, to prevent babies and toddlers from entering the kitchen unattended, or getting out of the back or front door.
- Teach children to use the stairs safely, how to crawl up and down with supervision. This will increase their confidence and reduce fear. It should help to prevent a fall if the stairs are accidentally left unguarded. Ensure that banister rails are close enough to prevent a young child climbing through.
- Use childproof window locks or latches.
- Move furniture away from windows so that children will not be so tempted to climb up.
- Avoid baby walkers. These are very dangerous and cause many accidents. Babies do not need them; they will learn to walk when they are ready.
- Use reins in the pram, pushchair and supermarket trolley.
- Place garden climbing equipment on safe surfaces such as grass or wood chippings.

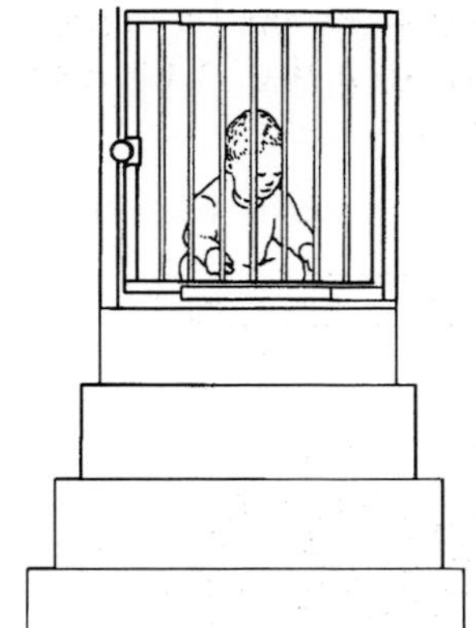

Always use a stairgate

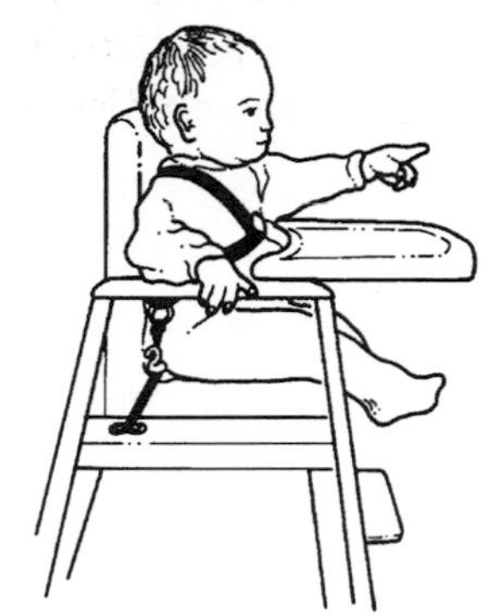

Children must be safely strapped into highchairs

BURNS AND SCALDS

Burns and scalds occur most commonly to babies and toddlers. The causes may be:

- the bath-water too hot
- hot drink spilling on to the child
- pulling the kettle flex
- hot fat from cooking or chip pan
- contact burns from fires, radiators, irons, etc.
- playing with matches.

Prevention

- Use a playpen if you are cooking and prevent toddlers entering the kitchen with a safety gate.
- Use a coiled kettle flex.
- Use a cooker-guard and turn pan handles inwards.
- Do not keep matches where a child can find them. They should be safely locked away.
- Use non-flammable clothing.
- Teach children the dangers of fire.
- Keep children away from bonfires and fireworks, except at safe, public displays.
- Put cold water in the bath first.

CHOKING

Each year children die as the result of a choking accident. It is the largest cause of accidental death in children under 1 year. At 6 months, babies can grasp objects and put them in their mouths to explore them. Small objects such as marbles, Lego, peanuts, sweets, buttons, bottle and pen tops must be kept out of their reach.

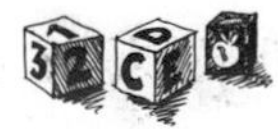

Prevention

It is the responsibility of the carer to remove all potentially dangerous items from the child's reach.

- Dummies must meet safety standards with holes in the flange, in case it is drawn to the back of the throat.
- Never leave small items lying around at home.
- Do not use toys with small parts that are unsuitable for young children.
- Do not give the child peanuts, nor have them available.
- Do not allow the child to play when they are eating.

> **key term**
> **Suffocation** stopping respiration

SUFFOCATION

Suffocation occurs when the airways are covered and the passage of air to the lungs is obstructed. Hanging and strangulation will also cut off the air supply.

Prevention

- Some household items are dangerous for babies and young children, for example, plastic bags, cords around the necks of clothing and pillows.
- Never prop-feed a baby (i.e. do not prop the bottle so that the baby sucks without being held).
- Make sure that there are no jagged edges on the cot or pram that could trap the clothing and strangle the baby as he moves.
- Do not use baby-nests, unless the baby is actually being carried in one.
- Avoid using quilts with young babies under 1 year.
- Warn older children of the dangers of ropes, strings, and dangerous places such as old fridges, freezers and cupboards, where they could get trapped inside.

CUTS

Cuts are usually caused by ordinary items such as glass, sharp knives or tin cans; there are also dangers from items such as gardening equipment, or broken windscreens, windows, etc.

Prevention

- Keep knives out of reach.
- Use plastic drinking cups and bottles.
- Use safety glass in doors or cover glass with safety film.
- Put stickers on large glass areas such as patio doors, so that it is obvious when they are closed; it is much safer to board up low-level glazing such as this.

ELECTRICITY AND ELECTROCUTION

The most likely cause of electrocution in the home is toddlers sticking objects into electrical sockets. Electrical equipment in a bathroom can cause death and it is against the law to have any sockets there, other than those for shavers or electric toothbrushes. Faulty electrical appliances are lethal.

 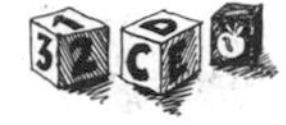

Prevention

- Use safety sockets, to prevent investigation with small fingers or objects.
- Use circuit breakers, which will instantly cut off the electricity supply when there is a short circuit.
- Switch sockets off when not in use.
- Do not use a hair dryer or any other electrical equipment in the bathroom.
- Check all electrical equipment for safety, for example check for worn flexes.

Case study . . .

. . . promoting home safety

'Safety First' is a voluntary organisation created by parents living in a deprived area of a Midlands city, with the aim of reducing the number of accidents involving children in their area. The Children's Accident and Emergency Department at the city's hospital conducted a 'Geography of Accidents' study, which showed that 30 per cent of all accidental injuries presented in casualty involved children who lived within their postcodes. With the co-operation of the local council and the health authority, the group have successfully applied for a grant from the European Social Fund (ESF). They have also been allocated some financing from a manufacturer of home safety equipment. Parent volunteers visit families with children under 5 who live in the area, and offer them the opportunity to purchase safety equipment (stairgates, window locks, cooker-guards, socket covers, smoke alarms and fireguards) at 50 per cent of the retail price. Because the volunteers are local and understand the particular difficulties faced by the families, they are generally well accepted. Families who are dependent upon social security benefits are given the necessary equipment free of charge.

1. *Why are socket covers, smoke alarms and fire guards important safety items?*
2. *What other forms of support (apart from safety equipment) could be offered to families in the interests of child safety?*
3. *Do you think that this type of community action should be encouraged? If so, why do you think it is important?*

POISONING

Many children each year are admitted to hospital after taking a poisonous substance. Those most at risk are between the ages of 2 and 3. They are exploring the environment and will taste anything that appears to be eatable. Many tablets look like sweets and dangerous fluids can resemble soft drinks. There may be easy access to poisons, such as adult medicines, bleach or cleaning fluids that are improperly stored.

Prevention

- Use child-resistant containers.
- Close all containers after use.
- Store medicines in a high, preferably locked cupboard. If there is no lock, use a child-proof latch.

- Put child-resistant locks on all cupboards.
- Do not store dangerous substances in the cupboard under the sink. Find a safer storage area.
- Keep chemicals in their original containers. Do not store them in old drink bottles or jam jars that may look attractive to young children.
- Prevent children eating berries or seeds from the garden or park.

Progress check

How can fires be prevented?

Which children are most at risk of falling?

What may cause burns and scalds?

How can the home be adapted to reduce the risk of burns?

How can choking accidents be prevented?

Outdoor safety

PLAY AREAS

Children should be supervised by a responsible adult during outdoor play. A responsible adult should:

- ensure that all the equipment and the play area has been checked before allowing the children out to play
- encourage co-operative play
- discourage aggression
- ensure climbing equipment is sited on suitable soft landing surfaces with space around it
- lock all external gates and ensure that children cannot leave the play area unsupervised
- remove potential hazards, for example broken equipment, sharp edges, dangerous litter
- ensure that play equipment is appropriate for the age group
- allow children to return to the indoor play area at will, with supervision
- provide areas for alternative play, for example wheeled toys, ball play, obstacle course.

ROAD SAFETY

Children are at risk on the road as pedestrians and as passengers in motor vehicles. Child-care workers can help to ensure their safety as pedestrians by:

- setting a good example when crossing the road

- discouraging parents from allowing children under 8 years to cross roads alone
- only allowing children to leave their establishment with a responsible adult who is known to them
- ensuring the adult–child ratio is within the prescribed limit when going out on trips and visits
- having and using a crossing patrol outside schools
- talking to children about road safety and teaching them the Green Cross Code. The Tufty Club may generate interest in road safety for young children
- discouraging children from using roads and pavements as play areas.

Outings with children

Child-care workers must be able to plan appropriate outings for children and to ensure their safety at all times. Choosing an outing that is consistent with the age/stage of development of the children must include an awareness of the statutory requirements and the safety issues involved.

The following factors are of paramount importance when considering taking children on an outing:

- safety
- appropriate clothing
- food/refreshments
- necessary equipment
- involving parents.

PLANNING AN OUTING

An outing is any trip away from the usual care and education setting. It can range from a visit to the shops to a whole day away. With thorough planning, it will be an enjoyable and educational experience for the children. The benefits of outings are wide-ranging because they give children the opportunity to:

- benefit from new and unfamiliar experiences
- learn about the environment generally or a specific area
- follow up an interest or educational topic
- meet new people.

CHOOSING WHERE TO GO

It may be a straightforward process to decide on where to take the children – there may be a local venue that has been visited successfully by previous groups of children from your setting. However, when planning any trip, remember to consider the following:

The age and stage of development of the children

There are differences in physical capabilities between average children aged from 1 to 7 years, as well as variations in concentration levels and intellectual skills. Choose a destination that meets the needs of all the age groups you are taking. Think about what you want the children to learn (learning outcomes) from the trip, whether it is a trip to the library or a day at a farm.

Adult help

A general guide for ratios on trips away from the setting is:

1 adult to 1 child 0–2 years
1 adult to 2 children 2–5 years
1 adult to 5 children 5–8 years.

It is essential to arrange to have a higher adult–child ratio on any outing away from the establishment because of the increased risks. Risks could include:

- traffic
- a new environment with no physical boundaries
- a different routine for the day and the extra people needed to carry any equipment, for example first aid box, picnic/snacks/educational resources, etc.

Distance of the destination

This can mean the difference between a morning, afternoon or whole day trip. It is vital to make sure that the time spent at the venue will be of value. Children do not like spending a disproportionate amount of time travelling.

Cost

If there is an entry fee or travelling costs, it may not be open to all children in the establishment if some families cannot afford to pay. Check whether there is enough funding to cater for all the children.

Transport

Is the venue within walking distance? If not, can people offer lifts? Do they have child restraints in their cars?

Is there an establishment minibus? Are drivers insured?

If arranging transport with an outside organisation, make sure that:

- they are insured
- the vehicle is large enough to seat everyone – adults and children
- there are sufficient child restraints, booster seats, seat belts, etc.
- the vehicles are safe.

STAGES IN THE PLANNING PROCESS

1 The local authority may have regulations that cover outings and it is important to find out about this so that any arrangements comply with these requirements.

2 Research into the destination, for example opening times and accessibility for children. It may be possible to visit to find out. Are there toilet facilities? Picnic areas? Refreshments? First aid provision?

3. Prepare a timetable for the day. Everyone will need to know times of departure and arrival. Ensure that your programme is practical and that there is enough time to do everything that you have planned for.
4. Plan to take all the necessary equipment with you, for example emergency contact numbers, mobile phone, registers, the first aid kit, camera, money, and audiotapes. Ask children to bring items with them, for example a packed lunch, wet weather wear, pencils/paper, sun hats, suncream.
5. Consult parents. Is it necessary to get written consent from parents to go on any trip away from the establishment? They will need to know about the cost, the day's programme, transport arrangements, special requirements – lunch, clothing, etc. A letter home with a consent slip is the best way to achieve this.
6. For child protection reasons, most settings do not use name labels for the children.
7. Prepare the children for the trip. Discuss the trip and explain what will be happening. Talk about safety issues, such as staying with the adults and not speaking to strangers. Show them pictures or leaflets about the venue. Discuss any activity related to the trip.

Progress check

What are the benefits of taking children on outings?

Why do you need to provide a higher adult/child ratio on outings?

What are the stages in the planning process for an outing?

Which important safety issues are involved in arranging transport for an outing?

Now try these questions

How can adults protect children from unintentional injuries in the home?

What can a child-care worker do in an establishment to keep the children safe?

What is the role of the child-care worker in organising an outing for children?

Explain why children under 1 year of age are most at risk of choking and how this can be prevented.

key terms

You need to know what the key terms and phrases in this chapter mean. Go back through the chapter and find out.

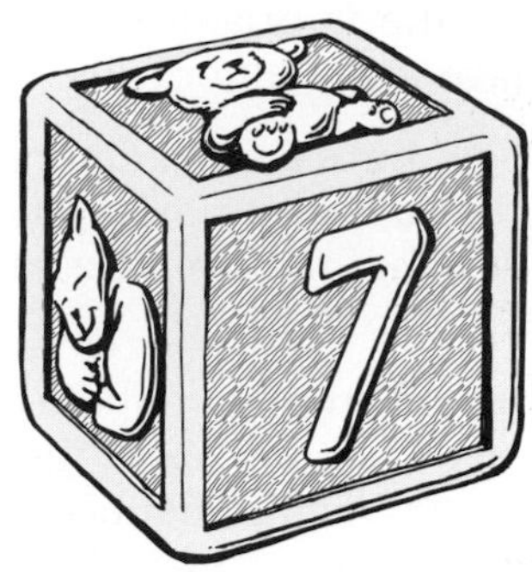

DIET, NUTRITION AND FOOD

Good nutrition is essential for general good health and well-being. We need food for four main reasons:

- *to provide energy and warmth*
- *to enable growth, repair and replacement of tissues*
- *to help fight disease*
- *to maintain the proper functioning of body systems.*

The food we eat each day makes up our diet and contains the nutrients we need. Before these nutrients can be used, food must be digested by the body. Digestion is the process that breaks down food into smaller components that the body can absorb and use.

Inadequate dietary intake is still the most common cause of failure to thrive. Good eating habits begin at an early age and child-care workers need to ensure that children establish healthy eating patterns that will promote normal growth and development.

This chapter will cover the following topics:

- *digestion*
- *the nutrients in food and drink*
- *a balanced diet*
- *diets of different groups*
- *the social and educational role of food*
- *problems with food*
- *food safety.*

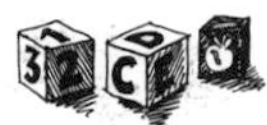

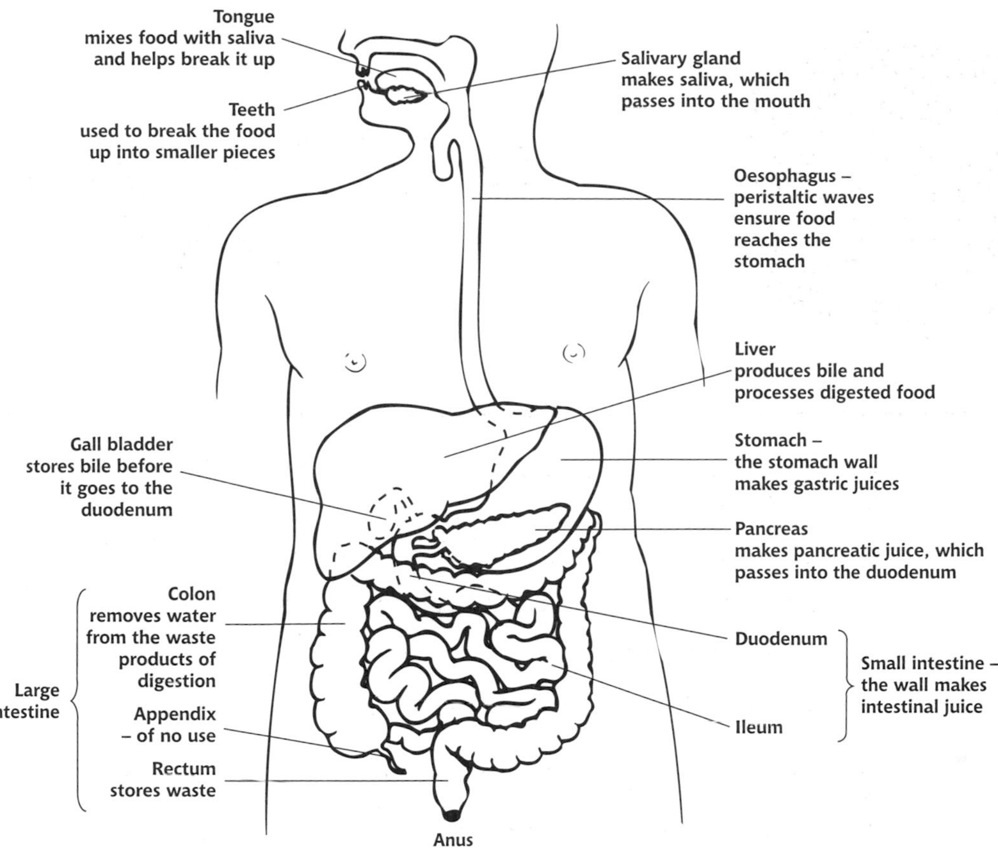

The alimentary canal and the process of digestion

Digestion

key term

Digestion
the process of breaking down food so that it can be absorbed and used by the body

Digestion of food takes place in the alimentary canal. This is a long muscular tube made up of the:

- mouth
- oesophagus (gullet)
- stomach
- small intestine
- large intestine
- rectum
- anus.

key terms

Enzyme
a substance that helps to digest food

Oesophagus
the top of the digestive tract, leading from the mouth to the stomach

THE PROCESS OF DIGESTION

In the mouth

The food is chewed to break it up into small pieces. At the same time it is mixed with saliva. **Enzymes** in the saliva start to work on the food. The food is then swallowed and passes down the **oesophagus** into the stomach.

In the stomach

Food is churned up and mixed with the gastric juices that continue the process of changing and digesting the food.

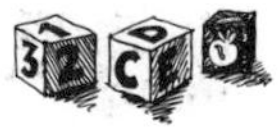

In the small intestine

Digestive juices containing enzymes from the pancreas, gall bladder and intestine are mixed with the food and further digestion takes place. The components of the digested food are absorbed into the body through the walls of the small intestine.

In the large intestine

Materials remaining after absorption in the small intestine are mainly water and fibre. Water is absorbed in the large intestine, and the remaining fibre, bacteria and some water form the waste products that pass into the rectum and out of the body via the anus.

Progress check

Define digestion.

What are the different parts that make up the alimentary canal?

What do the digestive juices contain?

The nutrients in food and drink

key term

Nutrient
a substance that provides essential nourishment

To be healthy, the body needs a combination of different **nutrients**. These nutrients are:

- protein
- carbohydrate
- fats
- vitamins
- minerals
- water
- fibre.

key terms

Complete protein
a protein containing all the essential amino acids; also called first-class proteins

Incomplete protein
a protein containing some essential amino acids; also called second-class proteins

Protein, fat, carbohydrates and water are present in the foods we eat and drink in large quantities. Vitamins and minerals are only present in small quantities, so it is much more common for those to be lacking in a child's diet.

PROTEIN

Protein foods are essential for:

- growth of the body
- repair of the body.

Protein foods are divided into **complete proteins** (first-class proteins) and **incomplete proteins** (second-class proteins). Complete protein comes from animal sources. These include:

- meat
- fish

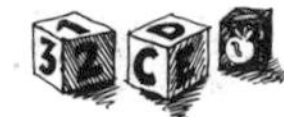

- chicken
- cheese
- milk and milk products.

Incomplete protein comes from vegetable sources. These include:

- nuts and seeds
- pulses (for example, black beans, chick peas, lentils, soya beans, kidney beans)
- cereals (rice, cornmeal, oats) and cereal-based foods (such as bread, pasta, chapattis, noodles).

key term

Amino acid
part of a protein

Protein foods are made up of **amino acids**. There are ten essential amino acids. Complete protein foods contain all of them; incomplete protein foods contain some. If protein in the diet is wholly restricted to vegetable sources, care will need to be taken that a variety of vegetable proteins are used. This will ensure that all ten essential amino acids are included in the diet.

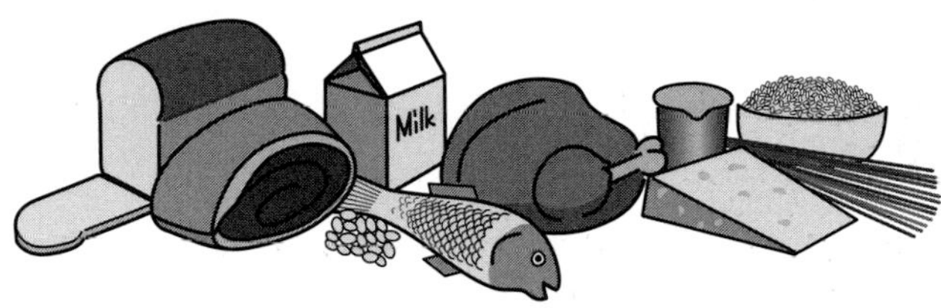

Some sources of protein

CARBOHYDRATES

Carbohydrate foods are divided into starches and sugars, which provide energy for the body. Sources of starch include:

- cereals
- beans
- lentils
- potatoes
- plantain
- pasta
- yams.

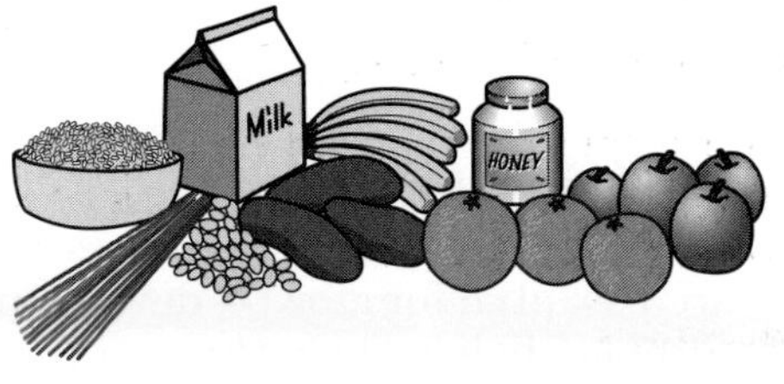

Some sources of carbohydrate

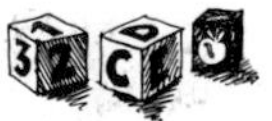

Sources of sugar include:

- sugar from cane or beet
- fruit and vegetables
- honey
- milk.

Carbohydrates are broken down into glucose before the body can use them. Sugars are easily converted and give a quick source of energy; starches take longer to convert to glucose so they provide a steadier, longer-lasting supply of energy. That is why marathon runners often eat large quantities of pasta the night before they race.

FATS

Fats provide energy for the body and contain essential vitamins. They also make food more pleasant to eat and aid its passage through the digestive tract. Fats are divided into **saturated fats** and **unsaturated fats**. Sources of saturated fat include:

- butter
- cheese
- milk
- lard
- meat
- palm oil.

Sources of unsaturated fat include:

- fish oil
- olive oil
- sunflower oil
- corn oil
- peanut oil.

key terms

Saturated fats
solid at room temperature and come mainly from animal fats

Unsaturated fats
liquid at room temperature and come mainly from vegetable and fish oils

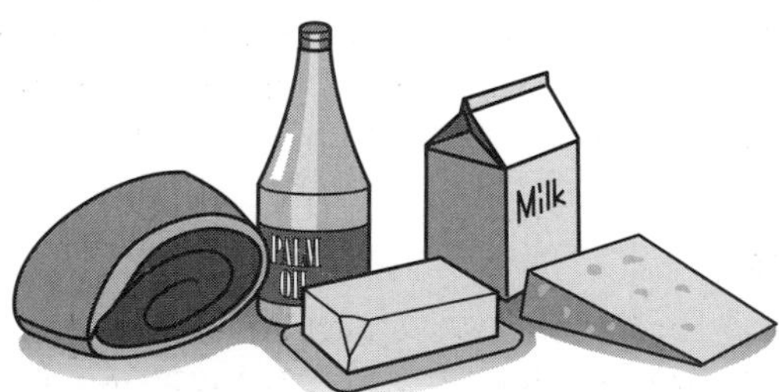

Some sources of fat

VITAMINS AND MINERALS

Vitamins and minerals are only present in small quantities in the foods we eat, but they are essential for growth, development and normal functioning of the body.

The tables below show the main vitamins and minerals, which foods contain them and their main functions in the body.

 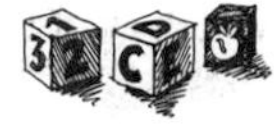

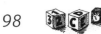

The main vitamins

Vitamin	Food source	Function	Notes
A	Butter, cheese, eggs, carrots, tomatoes	Promotes healthy skin, good vision	Fat-soluble, can be stored in the liver; deficiency causes skin infections, problems with vision
B group	Liver, meat, fish, green vegetables, beans, eggs	Healthy working of muscles and nerves; forming haemoglobin	Water-soluble, not stored in the body so regular supply needed; deficiency results in muscles wasting, anaemia
C	Fruits and fruit juices, especially orange, blackcurrant, pineapple; green vegetables	For healthy tissue, promotes healing	Water-soluble, daily supply needed; deficiency means less resistance to infection; extreme deficiency results in scurvy
D	Oily fish, cod liver oil, egg yolk; added to margarine, milk	Growth and maintenance of bones and teeth	Fat-soluble, can be stored by the body; can be produced by the body as a result of sunlight on the skin; deficiency results in bones failing to harden and dental decay
E	Vegetable oils, cereals, egg yolk	Protects cells from damage	Fat-soluble, can be stored by the body
K	Green vegetables, liver	Needed for normal blood clotting	Fat-soluble, can be stored in the body

A well-balanced diet, which includes a variety of foods, will provide all the vitamins and minerals required for the efficient functioning of the body. It is only when diet becomes restricted in illness or because of food shortages or poor choice of foods that shortages of essential vitamins and minerals will occur.

FIBRE

Fibre in the form of cellulose is found in the fibrous part of plants. It provides the body with bulk or roughage. Fibre has no nutritional value, as it cannot be broken down and used by the body. It is, however, an important part of a healthy diet. Fibre adds bulk to food and stimulates the muscles of the intestine, encouraging the body to eliminate the waste products left after digestion of food.

WATER

Water is a vital component of the diet. It contains some minerals, but its role in maintaining a healthy fluid balance in the cells and blood stream is crucial to survival.

The main minerals

Mineral	Food source	Function	Notes
Calcium	Cheese, eggs, fish, milk, yoghurt	Essential for growth of bones and teeth	Works with vitamin D and phosphorus; deficiency means risk of bones failing to harden (rickets) and dental caries
Fluoride	Occurs naturally in water, or may be added artificially to water supply	Combines with calcium to make tooth enamel more resistant to decay	There are different points of view about adding fluoride to the water supply
Iodine	Water, sea foods, added to salt, vegetables	Needed for proper working of the thyroid gland	Deficiency results in enlarged thyroid gland in adults, cretinism in babies
Iron	Meat, green vegetables, eggs, liver, red meat	Needed for formation of haemoglobin in red blood cells	Deficiency means there is anaemia causing lack of energy, breathlessness; vitamin C helps the absorption of iron
Sodium chloride	Table salt, bread, meat, fish	Needed for formation of cell fluids, blood plasma, sweat, tears	Salt should not be added to any food prepared for babies: their kidneys cannot eliminate excess salt as adult kidneys do; excess salt is harmful in an infant diet

Other essential trace minerals include:
potassium, phosphorus, magnesium, sulphur, manganese, zinc.

Progress check

Name two sources of complete protein.

Name two sources of incomplete protein.

Why are starches a more valuable source of carbohydrate than sugars?

What are the essential differences between saturated and unsaturated fat?

What is the advantage of a vitamin being fat-soluble?

What is the function of:
(a) vitamin C? (b) vitamin D? (c) vitamin K? (d) iron? (e) calcium?

Which vitamin helps the absorption of iron?

Why is excess salt harmful in an infant diet?

What is the essential function of water in the diet?

What is the essential function of fibre in the diet?

A balanced diet

key term

Fat-soluble vitamin
a vitamin that can be stored by the body, so it need not be included in the diet every day

A balanced diet means an intake of food that provides the nutrients the body needs in the right quantities. There are many nutrients that the body is able to store (**fat-soluble vitamins** are an example of this), so nutrients can be taken over several days to form the right balance.

A diet that includes a selection of foods is likely to be nutritious. Different combinations of vitamins are found in different foods, so a varied selection of foods will ensure an adequate supply of all the vitamins needed. Offering a variety of foods gives children an opportunity to choose foods they like. It also encourages them to explore other tastes and to try new foods and recipes.

PROPORTIONS OF NUTRIENTS

Children are growing all the time, so they need large amounts of protein to help the formation of bone and muscle. They are also using a lot of energy, so they need carbohydrate in the form of starches that they can use during the day to sustain their activities. In addition, they will need adequate supplies of vitamins and minerals.

Suggested daily intakes are as follows:

- two portions of meat or other protein foods, such as nuts and pulses
- two portions of protein from dairy products (for vegans substitute two other protein foods from plant sources)
- four portions of cereal foods
- five portions of fruit and vegetables
- six glasses of fluid, especially water.

key term

Calorie
a unit of energy

Although children are small in size they need a considerable amount of food. The table below shows the number of **calories** recommended for children and adults. The energy value of food is measured in calories: a medium egg, for example, is about 75 calories. Comparing the requirements of children and adults gives some idea of portion size. A child of 2 or 3 needs roughly half the amount of food, in terms of calories, of an adult.

The required number of calories for children and adults:

Age range	Energy requirements in calories
0–1 year	800
1–2 years	1,200
2–3 years	1,400
3–5 years	1,600
5–7 years	1,800
7–9 years	2,100
Women	2,200–2,500
Men	2,600–3,600.

Once children are weaned, they can eat the same food as adults. More information about early infant feeding and weaning can be found in Unit Seven.

Progress check

What is the best way to provide a balanced diet?

How many portions of protein should be included in a child's daily intake?

What is the advantage of a fat-soluble vitamin?

What is the calorie requirement of a 2-year-old child?

How many portions of fruit and vegetables should a child have each day?

Diets of different groups

Each region or country has developed its own local diet over many years. Diets have evolved based on available foods, which in turn depends on climate, geography and agricultural patterns, as well as social factors such as religion, culture, class and lifestyle. Each diet contains a balance of essential nutrients.

When people migrate, they take their diet with them and generally wish to recreate it as a familiar feature of their way of life. The psychological importance of familiar food should never be overlooked.

RELIGIOUS ASPECTS OF FOOD

For some people, food has a spiritual significance. Certain foods may be prohibited and these prohibitions form a part of people's daily lives. Adhering to religious food restrictions should not be taken as being difficult about food. Respecting an individual's culture and religious choices is part of respecting that individual as a whole. Talking to parents and carers about food requirements is important for child-care workers, especially when caring for a child from a cultural or religious background different from your own.

Religious restrictions may affect the diets of Hindus, Sikhs, Muslims, Jews, Rastafarians and Seventh Day Adventists. Members of other groups may also have dietary restrictions.

People are individuals and will vary in what they eat and what restrictions they observe; you should be aware of this when discussing diet with parents or carers. It is not possible to make blanket statements about the diets of different groups, only to suggest possibilities and factors that may be important and that child-care workers may find it useful to know about.

- Many devout Hindus are vegetarian. The cow is sacred to Hindus and eating beef is strictly forbidden. Alcohol is also forbidden.
- Sikhism began as an offshoot of Hinduism. Some Sikhs have similar dietary restrictions to Hindus. Few Sikhs eat beef and drinking alcohol is not approved.
- Muslim dietary restrictions are laid down by the Holy Qur'an and are regarded as the direct command of God. Muslims may not eat pork or pork products and alcohol is strictly prohibited. Other meat may be eaten provided it is *halal* (permitted). Healthy adult Muslims fast during the month of Ramadan.

- Jews may not eat pork or pork products, shellfish, and any fish without fins or scales. All meat eaten must have been killed in a special way so as to be *kosher* (fit). Milk and meat may not be used together in cooking.
- Most Rastafarians are vegetarian, but some may eat meat, except pork. No products of the vine, such as wine, grapes, currants or raisins are eaten. Some Rastafarians will only eat food cooked in vegetable oil. Whole foods are preferred.
- Seventh Day Adventists do not eat any pork or pork products.

OTHER DIETARY RESTRICTIONS

- Vegetarians do not eat meat and restrict their intake of other animal products in different ways.
- Vegans do not eat any animal products at all. A vegan diet needs careful balancing if it is to be followed by children, to ensure that they get the right nutrients to sustain normal growth.

It is very important to take account of these points when preparing activities involving food. If you are setting up a baking activity, for example, it would be best to make sure that you use vegetable fats, as these are generally more acceptable. Many more people today are moving towards a vegetarian diet or a diet that restricts the intake of animal products.

Progress check

What dietary restrictions may be followed by:

(a) vegans? (b) Muslims? (c) Rastafarians?

(d) Jews? (e) vegetarians? (f) Sikhs?

The social and educational role of food

Children like to take part in cooking and food preparation at home and in nurseries. These activities can create learning opportunities and enhance developmental skills.

PHYSICAL DEVELOPMENT

Gross motor skills are developed through mixing and beating. Manipulative skills are improved by cutting and stirring. Hand–eye co-ordination is improved by pouring, spooning out and weighing ingredients.

COGNITIVE DEVELOPMENT

Scientific concepts are learnt by seeing the effects of heat and cold on food. Mathematical skills are developed by counting, sorting and grading utensils, laying the table for the correct number of people and weighing and measuring the ingredients. Children can be encouraged to plan and make decisions about what they will eat.

LANGUAGE DEVELOPMENT

Conversation and discussion can be encouraged at mealtimes. Adult interaction will promote and extend vocabulary. Children and adults can share their ideas and experiences of the day.

EMOTIONAL DEVELOPMENT

Eating food is often a comfort, and sharing and preparing food for others provides pleasure. Helping to prepare a meal for themselves and others will give children a sense of achievement.

SOCIAL DEVELOPMENT

Children can learn the skills of feeding independently. They can share with others and learn about appropriate behaviour at mealtimes. Mealtimes are a good opportunity for families and other groups to exchange their news and ideas.

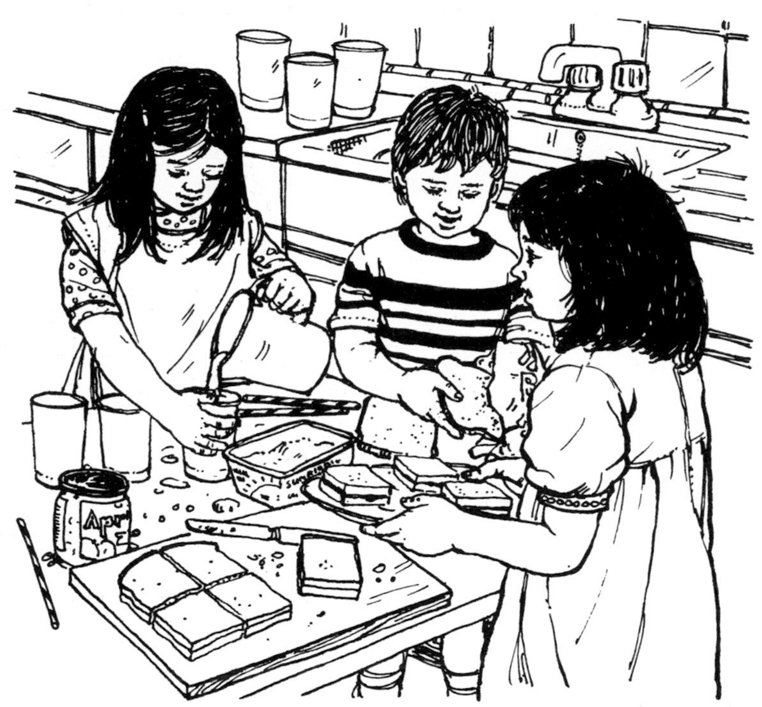

Activities can create learning opportunities

Problems with food

Food allergy and food intolerance have received a lot of publicity. Only a small number of reactions to food are true allergic responses, involving the immune responses of the body.

FOOD INTOLERANCE

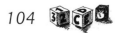

Food intolerance is a condition in which there are specific adverse effects after eating a specific food; this may be caused by an allergic response or an enzyme deficiency. The removal of foods from a child's diet must be carried out with medical supervision. If the suspected food source is a major source of nutrients, for example milk, then alternatives must be included to make good any deficiency. Conditions such as phenylketonuria (PKU) and coeliac disease require very specialised diets. There is more information about these conditions in Chapter 21.

FOOD REFUSAL

Toddler food refusal is common. If the child is of normal body weight and height, is thriving and no medical condition is identified by the doctor, then carers should be reassured. It is important that mealtimes should not become a battleground. The child should be offered food at mealtimes and allowed to eat according to appetite. Any remaining food should be removed without fuss. The next meal is offered at the usual time and no snacks or 'junk food' given between meals. It is important that the child participates in family meals rather than eating in isolation. Allow the child to feed himself and don't fuss about any mess if he is just learning to do this. The child should see eating as a pleasurable and sociable experience and be encouraged to enjoy mealtimes with the family or in other groups.

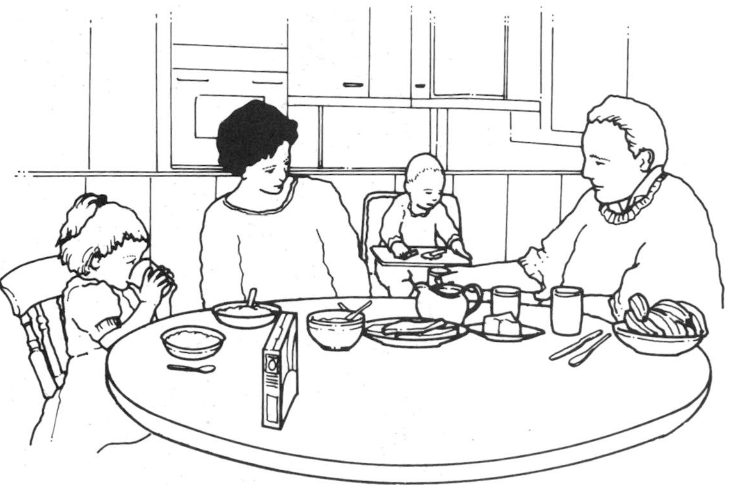

Eating should be a sociable experience, with the family or other groups

Case study . . .

. . . *food refusal*

Joanna is a nanny who looks after Joshua, who is 2 years 6 months old and Anna who is 6 months old, while their parents are at work. Joshua is a lively, happy little boy who knows Joanna well, as she was his nanny before Anna was born.

Joanna has continued to care for him and also his sister when their mother returned to work 4 weeks ago. Joshua seems well and healthy, but for the last week or two he has been refusing to eat his meals. He has become very upset and on one occasion threw his plate on to the floor when Joanna insisted that he eat his dinner. As his nanny, Joanna has decided that she must take some action.

1. *What should Joanna do first?*
2. *What steps should Joanna then take to try to re-establish Joshua's previous good eating patterns?*

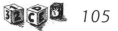

FOOD ADDITIVES

Additives are added to food to:

- preserve it for longer
- prevent contamination
- aid processing
- enhance colour and flavour
- replace nutrients lost in processing.

Care should be taken with additives in children's diets because:

- they often eat more foods with additives, for example drinks and sweets
- they are smaller and the amount they take is, therefore, greater in proportion to their size.

To reduce additives in the diet:

- use fresh foods as often as you can
- make your own pies, cakes, soups, etc.
- avoid highly processed foods
- look at the labels; the ingredients are listed.

Case study . . .

. . . labels on food

Anne is a childminder who looks after Holly, who is 4, and Emma, who is 2, every day. Anne is out shopping at the supermarket, as she needs to give lunch to Holly and Emma today. Holly's family are vegetarian and Emma is allergic to food colourings. Anne has brought home a tin of baked beans from the supermarket that will be part of the girls' lunch. This is a copy of the nutritional information on the label.

Baked beans
Nutritional information

Typical values	**Amount per 100 g**	**Amount per serving 150 g**
Energy	*75 cal.*	*113 cal.*
Protein	*4.7g*	*7.1g*
Carbohydrate	*13.6g*	*20.4g*
Fat	*0.2g*	*0.3g*
Fibre	*3.7g*	*5.6g*
Sodium	*0.5g*	*0.7g*

No artificial colourings

1. *What does the label tell you about the content of the food?*
2. *Will Anne be able to give the food to Holly?*
3. *Will Anne be able to give the food to Emma?*

E numbers

Permitted food additives are given a number. If the number has been approved by the European Union (EU), as well as the UK, there is an E in front of the

key term

E number
a number given to an additive approved by the EU

number – an **E number**. A category name such as 'preservative' must come before the additive number to tell you why it has been included, for example preservative E200.

Food additives and behaviour

Some children may have erratic behaviour after taking, for example, orange squash or coloured sweets, and behaviour improves when these colourings are avoided. Avoiding additives need not affect the nutritional value of the diet, but any regime that leads to a nutritionally inadequate diet should not be followed. Hyperactivity as a medical condition will be diagnosed by a paediatrician, a doctor who specialises in caring for children. Dietary manipulation, for example elimination diets, must be prescribed by a paediatrician and supervised by a dietician. Behaviour and hyperactivity problems are, however, rarely caused solely by food additives and, there are, usually, other contributing factors.

FOOD AND POVERTY

Research has shown that food is one of the first things people cut back on when they are short of money. This can have a serious effect on the nutritional quality of the diet of families managing on a low income.

There may be other problems that contribute to this: cooking facilities may be limited, or impossible if, for example, the family live in bed and breakfast accommodation and much of the food eaten has to be brought in ready cooked. Fuel costs for cooking will also be an important consideration if money is tight. Shopping around for food to get the best bargain or selection may not be possible if bus fares are needed or food has to be carried a long way.

In these circumstances, knowing about food and the nutrients that are essential to provide an adequate diet is very important. Help needs to be concentrated on achieving an adequate diet within the budget and ability of the family. Knowing which cheaper foods contain the essential nutrients will enable sensible advice to be offered.

Progress check

How can you know that a food additive has been approved by the European Union?

What are the main reasons for including additives in food?

Describe two examples of food intolerance.

What strategies would you use to deal with food refusal?

Food safety

Food is essential to good health and survival, but it has to be looked after to avoid contamination with harmful bacteria that could cause food poisoning. Since January 1991 there have been stricter laws about storage and handling of food in shops and restaurants. These laws help to keep food safer and cleaner. Once food has been bought, it must be stored safely and prepared hygienically in order to prevent food poisoning.

BUYING FOOD

- Check the 'use by' dates.
- Take chilled and frozen food straight home and use an insulated bag.
- Make sure you buy from a shop where cooked and raw foods are kept and handled separately.

STORAGE AT HOME

- Put chilled and frozen foods into the fridge or freezer as quickly as possible.
- The coldest part of the fridge must be between 0 and 5°C, and the freezer temperature below 18°C: use a fridge thermometer to check the temperature.
- Keep raw meat and fish in separate containers in the fridge and store them carefully on the bottom shelf so that they do not touch or drip on to other food.

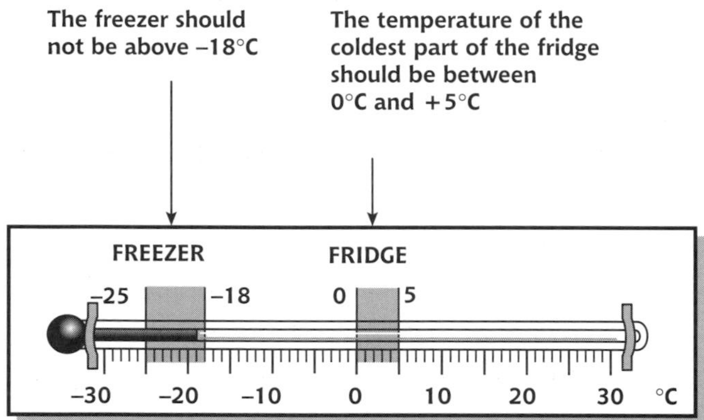

Temperatures for home storage in the fridge or freezer

IN THE KITCHEN

- Always wash your hands well before touching food.
- Cover any cuts with a waterproof dressing.
- Wear an apron and tie hair back when preparing food.
- Avoid touching your nose and mouth, or coughing and sneezing in the food preparation area.
- Kitchen cloths and sponges should be disinfected and renewed frequently.
- Disinfect all work surfaces regularly and especially before preparing food.

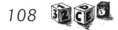

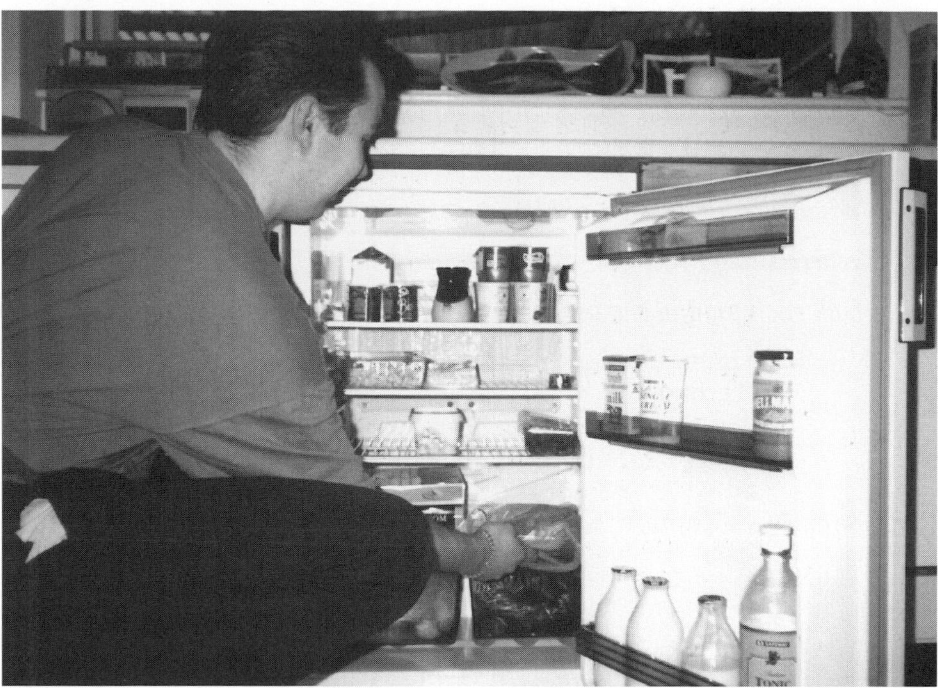

Store raw meat and fish on the bottom shelf of the fridge

COOKING

The following guidelines should always be followed when preparing and cooking food:

- Defrost food thoroughly before cooking.
- Make sure all food is thoroughly cooked – chicken and meat need special care, and must be cooked through to the centre.
- Prepare raw meat separately – use a separate board and knife.
- Cooked food should be cooled quickly and then refrigerated or frozen.
- Cover any food standing in the kitchen.
- Eggs should be thoroughly cooked before eating. For babies and small children, cook the eggs until the white and yolk are solid.
- Cooked food should only be reheated once – reheat until piping hot all the way through.
- Reheat cooked chilled meals properly.
- Pregnant women and anyone with a low resistance to infection should not eat pâté, nor soft cheeses of the Brie or Camembert type.

Children are particularly vulnerable to infection, so it is important to make sure that food is prepared and handled safely. It is also vital that children learn the basic rules about handling food. Always make sure that they wash their hands before eating. If children prepare food as part of a learning activity, the food safety rules should always be followed. Children need to understand why this is important, so that they develop important life skills.

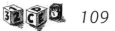

Progress check

What are the basic rules of food handling?

If you buy chilled or frozen food, what is the best way to transport it?

What temperature should the coldest part of the fridge be?

Where should you store raw meat and fish?

Link each food in the table below with the vitamins and minerals it contains.

Vitamin/mineral	*Food*
B group	Egg
A	Vegetable oil
C	Carrot
D	Liver
Calcium	Cabbage
Iron	Cheese
E	Pineapple
K	Green vegetables
Fluoride	Milk
Sodium chloride	Water

Now try these questions

What are the essential nutrients in a balanced diet? Give examples of foods containing these nutrients.

What would you include in a day's menu for a 3-year-old child? Show how you have ensured a balanced diet.

How would you make mealtimes a pleasurable experience for a 4-year-old child?

What are the important points to bear in mind to ensure that food is safe to eat?

What influences might poverty have on a child's diet?

key terms

You need to know what the key terms and phrases in this chapter mean. Go back through the chapter and find out.

Unit 4: The Developing Child

Understanding how children develop is a key requirement for all those working in early years. Your learning in this unit will underpin much of the work you carry out and a great deal of the content of other units.

This unit covers the development of children from 0 to 7 years 11 months. It will assist you with the requirements for many of the units within the National Occupational Standards.

On completion of this unit you will be able to show a basic and broad understanding of the stages of children's physical, intellectual, emotional and social development, and of their cognitive and language development. You should be able to understand the role of adults in the development of the child and understand the uses and limitations of methods of measuring development. You should be able to identify the consequences of development outside the accepted norm and be able to implement basic techniques for managing behaviour.

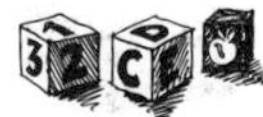

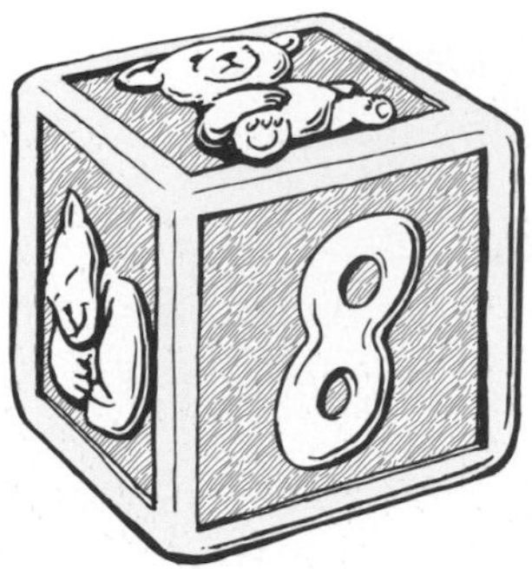

THE GENERAL PRINCIPLES OF CHILD DEVELOPMENT

Adults have a crucial role to play in promoting children's development. Without contact with others, children fail to develop. Children have the need for positive, caring relationships to ensure their healthy development.

Although the family is usually the primary provider of care, all young children eventually spend time with substitute carers, whether at school, in nurseries, or with nannies or childminders. The role of child-care workers in providing substitute care means that it is essential that they have a knowledge and understanding of the different stages of children's development. Child-care workers have an important role in promoting healthy development. It is important that workers support and nurture the children for whom they care.

This chapter will cover the following topics:

- *theoretical perspectives of development*
- *measurements and milestones.*

Theoretical perspectives of development

key terms

Theories of development
ideas about how and why development occurs

Learning theories
children develop as they do because they have contact with other people and learn from them

It is very useful for anyone involved in the care of children to consider why development occurs. There are two basic **theories of development**. A theory is an idea about why something happens.

The two basic theories of development are as follows.

- Development happens because human beings are genetically programmed to develop in a certain way. These are called **biological theories** (the nature or heredity idea).
- People learn their responses and skills. These are called **learning theories** (the nurture or environment idea).

People tend to use a combination of these ideas, or theories, to guide their understanding and practice with children. An awareness of these theories can help carers to find the most appropriate way to respond to and care for children.

Physical development is influenced relatively more by biology and maturation than emotional and social development at the other end of the scale. However, in all areas of development stimulation and learning are essential.

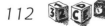

key term

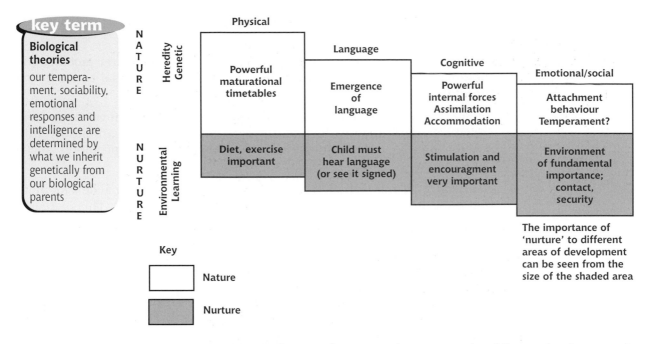

Biological theories
our temperament, sociability, emotional responses and intelligence are determined by what we inherit genetically from our biological parents

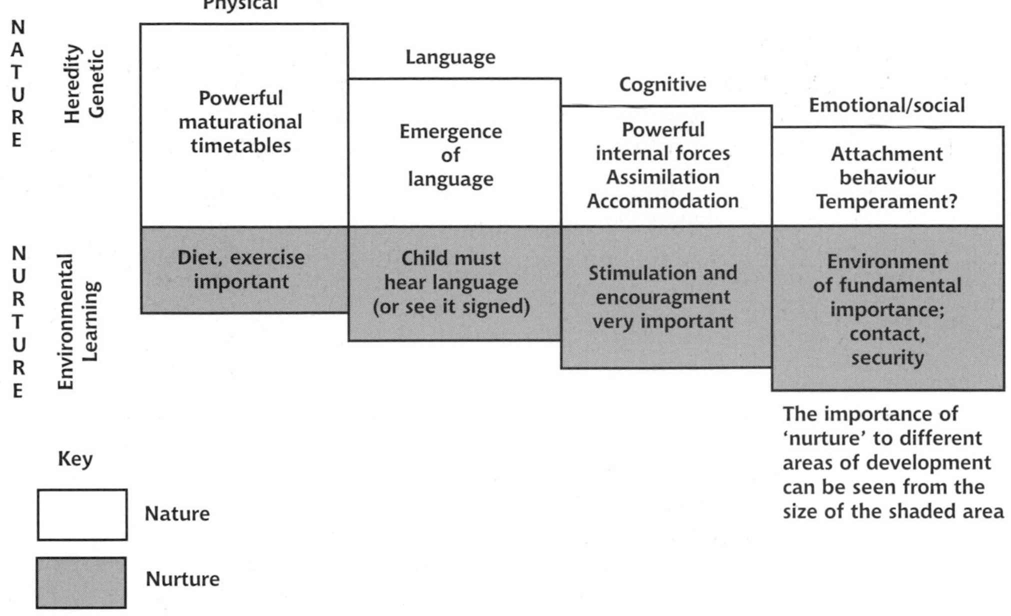

This shows the relative influence of nature and nurture on the different developmental areas

THE INFLUENCE OF OTHER FACTORS ON DEVELOPMENT

The role of social, cultural, religious, economic and environmental factors in the promotion of development, and the provision for children whose development falls outside the accepted norms is covered as appropriate in Chapters 9 to 12 of this unit.

Progress check

What is a theory?

What are the two contrasting ideas about why development occurs in the way that it does?

What are the relative influences of nature and nurture in the different areas of development?

Measurements and milestones

key terms

Maturity
being fully developed and capable of self-control

Independence
the development of skills that lead to less reliance on other people for help or support

THE PATH OF DEVELOPMENT

Children's development in all areas follows a path towards **maturity** and **independence**. Maturity means being fully developed and capable of control. Achieving independence involves the development of skills that gradually lead to less reliance on other people for help or support.

THE LINKS BETWEEN DIFFERENT AREAS OF DEVELOPMENT

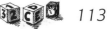

For the purposes of this unit the different areas of development are separated, but in fact all areas of development are linked. They affect and are affected by each other. Some examples of the close links that exist between different areas of development are:

- *walking* – this milestone of physical development gives greater mobility and therefore independence, which then increases possible social contacts and therefore promotes social development
- *talking* – language development enables children to move from non-verbal communication with close carers to being able to communicate with other people in more complex ways and therefore also promotes social development
- *adjusting to separation from main carer(s)* – a stage of emotional development that presents a wider range of experiences and relationships. This increases children's opportunities for play and learning and therefore their intellectual development.

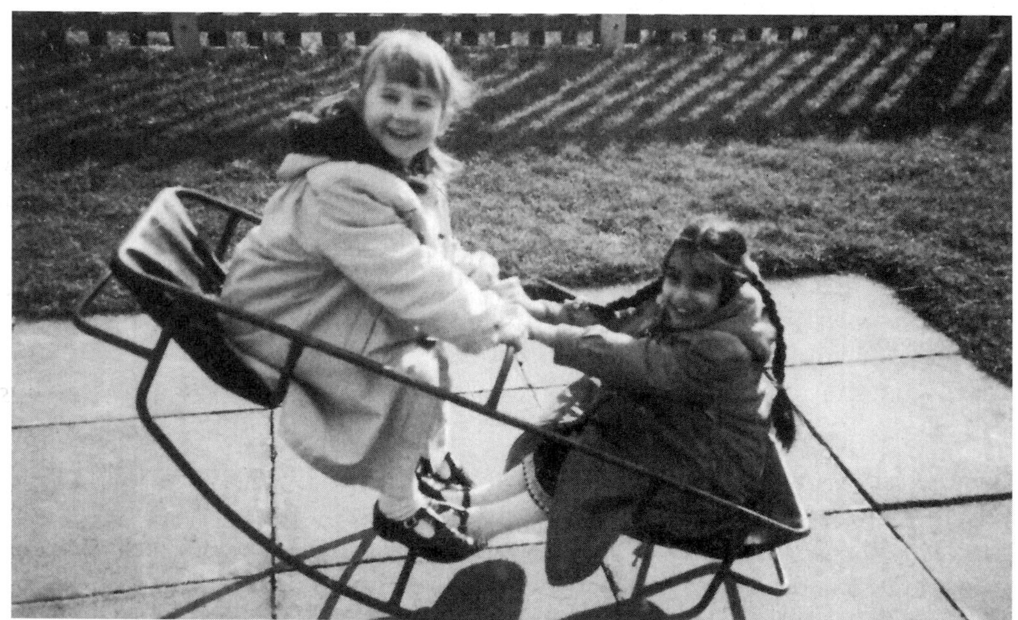

There are close links between the different areas of development

key term

Chronological age
the age of a child in years and months

USE OF MEASUREMENTS AND MILESTONES

There is wide variation in the **chronological age** at which children reach different developmental milestones. Some of the most important things to remember when considering ages and stages of development are as follows:

- There are recognisable stages of development that children reach.
- Children pass through them at different ages – one child will be able to do things at an earlier age than another. The fact that one child is younger than another when they reach an observable stage need be of no significance at all; it does not necessarily mean that there are any developmental problems.
- The development of any skill depends both on the maturation of the nervous system and the opportunity to practise that skill.

Variations in ages of achievement

key term

Average
a medium, a standard or a 'norm'

From observations of children, it is clear that they vary in their rates of development and the age at which they reach different stages of development. It is nevertheless useful to describe an **average** age at which children might be expected to reach a specific developmental stage.

When children's development is what we would expect at their age it is acceptable to describe it as 'age appropriate', and children whose development is not what we would expect at that age or behind the average as 'not having reached the stage of development expected at their age'. It is *not* helpful to use the word 'normal' to describe development, even though the word 'normal' is linked to that of a norm or average, because anything that does not fit this pattern might then be described as 'abnormal' and this is not an appropriate or acceptable term to use to describe developmental delay.

Case study . . .

. . . playing together

Aisha and Jenny are 4 years old. They live next door to each other and frequently play in each other's houses and gardens. One of their favourite games is making a tent from old covers and having a picnic. Sometimes they argue and a parent intervenes to help them to solve their problems. Recently Aisha's little brother Jamil, who is 2 years old, has joined them in their play. Jamil keeps taking their picnic things and filling them with sand; he screams if they try to stop him and throws himself on the ground when his mother comes to see what the noise is. Aisha says he can play with them but only if he does as they say.

1. *List all the examples in this story of children's behaviour that is age appropriate.*
2. *Are there any examples of developmental delay?*

NORMATIVE MEASUREMENTS

key term

Normative measurements
an average or norm against which any individual child's development can be measured

In order to establish average ages for development, the observations of many people in different professional fields have been put together. These have been used to describe an average or norm against which any individual child's development can be measured. These measurements are called **normative measurements**. For example, the many observations of children's first social smiles have led to the understanding that the average age for this to happen is around 6 weeks. There are advantages and disadvantages of using normative measurements, as outlined below.

Advantages of using normative measurements

Using averages or norms of development is useful because:

- it satisfies the curiosity of carers about what a child should be doing at a given age, and it helps them to know what to expect
- it gives background information and a framework within which to assess developmental delay
- it helps people to assess a child's progress after an injury or illness, and can be used to decide whether the child needs additional help and stimulation.

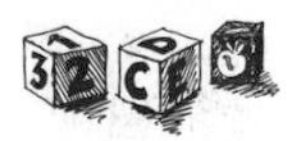

Disadvantages of using normative measurements

The disadvantages of using norms of development are:

- carers may be tempted to think that children are 'good' when they are level with the norm and 'bad' if they fall behind it
- carers and other people may wrongly think a child has an impairment, when in fact they are simply slow to develop in some way.

Progress check

Why is it not helpful to talk about 'normal' development?

What is a normative measure of development?

What are the advantages and disadvantages of using average measurements of development?

Now try these questions

Why does the chronological age at which children reach certain developmental stages often differ?

Describe the relative significance of nature and nurture in the different areas of development.

key terms

You need to know what the key terms and phrases in this chapter mean. Go back through the chapter and find out.

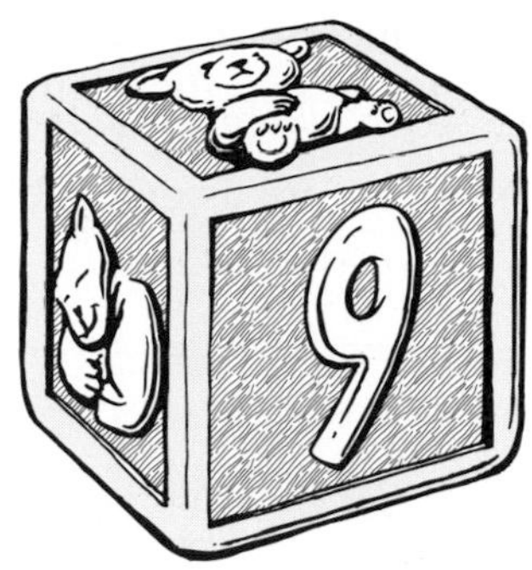

COGNITIVE DEVELOPMENT

In this chapter you will learn about aspects of cognitive development: imagination, creativity, problem-solving, concept formation, reasoning, memory and concentration. The developmental sequence of children's cognition is outlined. The chapter looks at Piaget's theory of cognitive development, assessing its influence alongside criticisms of his findings and conclusions from other studies in this area. It concludes by examining how carers can support and encourage children's cognitive development.

This chapter will cover the following topics:

- *what is cognitive development?*
- *access to learning experiences for all children*
- *Piaget's theory of cognitive development*
- *the role of the adult in promoting cognitive development.*

What is cognitive development?

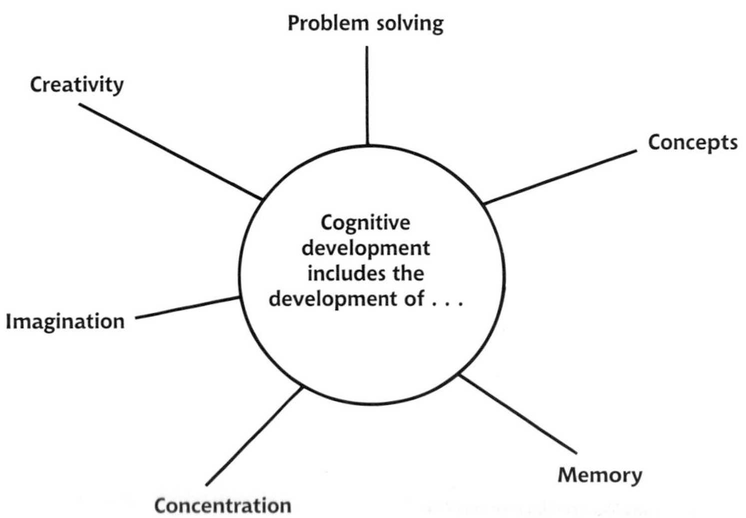

What is cognitive development?

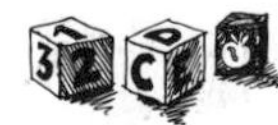

key term

Imagination the ability to form mental images, or concepts of objects not present, or that do not exist

IMAGINATION

Imagination is the ability to form mental images, or concepts of objects not present, or that do not exist. It is fairly easy to conjure up images of, for example, a beach, outer space, grandparents, school or chocolate.

The imagination is the basis for many of the activities we regard as enjoyable:

- books
- films and television
- dance
- art
- music
- design.

These are part of the culture of a society. They are often the basis for activities that people choose to be involved in, in their own time. They provide relaxation and add to the quality of life.

Imagination is also part of the following activities:

key term

Problem-solving the ability to draw together and assess information about a situation in order to find a solution

- **problem-solving**
- innovative and original thought.

Change comes about through new and innovative ideas, and by finding solutions to problems. Imagination is an important aspect of ideas. The idea might be an invention, for example the telephone, television, the car, the aeroplane. All these started as ideas in someone's imagination. The idea might also be a solution to an existing problem, which might be an everyday or individual problem, scientific or medical problem, society or world problem. The process is the same: solving problems in new or unusual ways requires imagination.

Imaginative play in young children also contributes to the development of other important skills. Through using their imagination to play, children develop the ability to use one object to represent another, for example, using a doll to represent a baby, using a pan to represent a hat, using sand and toy cars to represent a race track. This is called symbolic play: one object is being used as a symbol for another.

This skill is transferable. If a child can use symbols in a play situation, they can transfer this skill to learning to read and to write, as reading and writing involve use of the same skill of using symbols, in this case letters and words to represent the spoken word (see Chapter 10, for more on language development).

Children and imagination

Children do not need to be taught to be imaginative. Their play is full of examples where they are using their imagination. Here are some examples; there are many more:

key term

Role play involves acting out being somebody, or something, else

- during creative activities such as painting or collage
- being someone, or something, else in **role play**
- creating an object or design
- thinking up a story or poem
- creating objects from large empty boxes
- moving to music or dancing
- making music
- listening to stories.

 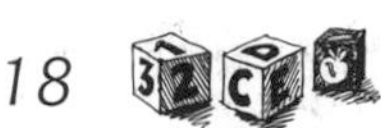

It is important that these imaginative skills are nurtured, which means giving children the opportunity to express and develop their ideas. Your role is to provide the time, space, materials and encouragement to enable the children to do this.

Role play

Role play involves the child becoming somebody or something else. Imagination is an important part of this play. The child may be imitating someone, or something, that they have seen, for example a shop assistant, a doctor, a waiter or a television character. Children also create new, sometimes unique, characters or situations in their play. They create these new characters and situations in their imagination.

Role play of all types is important as it enables the child to try on different roles, for example:

- create imaginary characters and try out new and different roles
- imitate people that they have seen
- act out situations that they have been involved in
- create new characters and situations.

Role play enables children to discover, enquire, organise and make sense of their environment. They can practise and develop their communication skills; feelings can be explored. All this can be done in a safe environment because they can opt out of the play at any time. This is an important part of their all-round development.

Progress check

What is imagination?

Name some things that imagination is needed for.

Explain why imagination is important.

What is symbolic play?

Why is symbolic play important?

How does the ability to symbolise help children to read and write?

What is role play?

Name two ways in which children are involved in role play.

What are the benefits of role play?

key term

Creativity
the expression of ideas in a personal and unique way

CREATIVITY

Creativity is the expression of imaginative ideas in a personal and unique way. When people write books, make films, play or write music, act, dance, paint, create beautiful buildings or gardens or find innovative solutions to problems, we say that they have been creative.

There is a lot of debate about what creativity is and whether it is taught or innate. It is hard, therefore, to say precisely what is and what is not creative, but for something to be described as creative it should have a number of the following features:

- use of the imagination
- begin with an open-ended outcome
- be a personal expression of ideas
- be unique in its process and product
- have the process as equally important as the product.

Children and creativity

Creative activities for children provide the opportunity for them to think beyond what is obvious and to develop their own ideas. This is an important skill for later learning. Children do not need to be taught to be creative. They need the time, space, materials and encouragement to develop their own ideas. This is important: being creative is the expression of personal ideas, not copying or imitating someone else's ideas.

Sometimes it is enough to provide children with the opportunity to be creative and allow them to play without any intervention, for example putting out a range of different sizes and shapes of boxes, and letting the children develop their own play themes and ideas.

At other times, adults may have more influence in the activity by providing a framework for it. It is important that the framework still allows the child the opportunity to develop their own ideas. Frameworks can be provided in many different ways:

- by the type of materials provided
- by the introduction of a theme for the activity
- by suggestion while the child is engaged in an activity
- by the siting of the activity
- through group work – the child works within the framework agreed by the group.

Case study . . .

. . . children and creativity

Catherine, aged 4, was fascinated by woods and forests. She had seen a spectacular bluebell display in a wood while out with her parents. The following day she came into playgroup eager to get to the painting easels. As she painted she provided a running commentary to a member of staff about the trees, squirrels and flowers. She took great care with the details and choice of colour. When she was satisfied that she had everything that she wanted in the scene, she covered the whole of her picture with a thick layer of black paint. She explained that it was so dark in the wood, as the trees were very close together, that the sunshine couldn't get through. Catherine was very pleased with her painting.

1. *Why did the member of staff stand back and watch when Catherine covered her picture with black paint?*
2. *Why do you think that Catherine was pleased with her painting?*
3. *In what ways is this a creative activity?*

Progress check

What is creativity?

List some activities that require a person to be creative.

What features should a creative activity have?

Do children need to be taught to be creative?

How can you provide a framework for a creative activity?

Why is copying not creative?

key term

Concentration the skill of focusing all your attention on one task

CONCENTRATION

Concentration is the skill of focusing all your attention on one task. It is necessary for successful learning to take place. Children need to be encouraged to focus their attention and therefore develop their skills of concentration and perseverance. Children will be encouraged to concentrate at activities when:

- the activities are at an appropriate level
- they are attractively presented
- an adult joins the activity to offer praise and make suggestions.

Young children are likely to have relatively short concentration spans. This needs to be taken into account when planning activities. However, it is also important to be aware that children need to develop their skill of concentration, and to plan and organise activities that stretch their ability. This can be achieved in many ways, such as by:

- encouraging children to listen to a story all the way through without interruption
- encouraging children to complete an activity, for example a jigsaw
- playing board games through to the end
- providing group activities where children co-operate to complete a task, for example, building the train track
- joining in an activity to encourage and develop the play sequence, for example, being a customer in the café
- providing a focus for an activity, for example, asking children to listen carefully to a story so that they can retell it using puppets.

Progress check

What is the ability to concentrate?

Why is it important?

How can an adult help a child to concentrate?

MEMORY

There are three basic stages in learning:

- Taking in information – we do this through our five senses.
- Storing the information – this takes place in our memory.
- Recalling the information – information is retrieved from our memory, we call this remembering.

Learning requires all three stages to be completed. For us to successfully store information in our memory and remember it when appropriate, activities and experiences have to meet certain criteria:

- the concept or skill to be learned should be at an appropriate level for the learner
- the information should be presented in a relevant way for the learner
- the learner should have some previous learning that the information can be linked to
- the information usually needs to be repeated, and/or used in context, for it to be stored and recalled successfully.

The following case study shows this process for a young child.

Case study . . .

. . . learning and memory

Hannah, a nursery nurse, planned a series of activities to enable the children in the nursery to recognise written numbers to 10.

She knew that the children knew many number rhymes and songs, so that they could say numbers to 10. Over a period of weeks activities were introduced to the children to develop their understanding of written numbers:

- As the children sang number rhymes and songs, for example, 'Five little ducks went swimming one day', she held up the relevant number for the children to see.
- As the children began to recognise the numbers they held up the relevant numbers as they sang the song.
- Daily activities using numbers were provided, for example, number jigsaws, lotto, writing numbers in the sand and making them out of dough. Staff drew children's attention to the numbers during the activities.
- Gradually, the activities were extended during group time, for example, the children lined themselves up according to the number card that they held and the other children checked to see if it was correct, the children put the correct number against a collection of items.
- Hannah also created a number table where children sorted items into numbered boxes.
- The children went on a walk in the local environment to see where numbers were written; on their return they painted pictures of what they had seen and made a display.

This series of activities meets the criteria for learning, that is, storing the information in the memory and recalling it when appropriate. They are at an appropriate level for the children and they are presented in a relevant way. The children have previous knowledge of numbers to draw on, and the staff provide opportunities for the children to repeat and use the information in different ways.

1. *Why did Hannah choose these activities?*
2. *What is the role of the child-care worker in supporting children's developing memory skills?*
3. *Suggest some other activities that would reinforce the concept of number recognition.*
4. *List some other concepts that could be learned in a similar way.*

Progress check

What are the three stages in learning?

Why is memory an important part of learning?

What are the criteria for successful learning?

Give an example of this process for young children.

PROBLEM-SOLVING

The ability to solve problems is another aspect of cognitive development. Problem-solving does not just mean complex problems; it also includes everyday problems that all people come across, for example which route to take on a journey or how to put objects into a bag so that they all fit. Experience of the world and of how things work means that most problems are quickly solved.

When older children and adults are faced with a problem, they draw together all that they know about a situation to enable them to solve it. Logic is used to assess possible solutions: for example, to fit things into a bag you need to know about, sizes, shapes, capacity, tessellation (how items fit together) and rotation. You will very quickly be able to assess the problem and come up with a range of ideas to solve it. Children need to develop these skills. Their knowledge and experience of the world is more limited than that of older children and adults, so they have less information to draw on to enable them to solve a problem that they face.

There is a developmental sequence in children's ability to solve problems. **Trial-and-error** learning is the earliest stage in development. The child is trying out solutions to a problem in a random way and will try and fail, try and fail, until they arrive at a solution. This will probably involve returning to the problem many times. At this stage the child is not able to identify clearly the problem that they are attempting to solve. Trial-and-error learning can be very frustrating for a child and in this case careful adult intervention is needed to suggest ways forward for the child.

The next stage in development is a growing ability to identify the problem facing them and work out a possible solution before they try anything out. Children begin to be able to predict what might happen. This **hypothesis** is based on their increasing knowledge and experience of the world. The greater their knowledge and experience the more accurate the hypothesis becomes.

key terms

Trial-and-error learning
the earliest stage in problem-solving. Young children randomly try out solutions to a problem, often making errors, until finding a solution or giving up

Hypothesis
the provisional explanation or solution to a problem reached by assessment of the observed facts

Progress check

What is problem-solving?

What is trial-and-error learning?

What is a hypothesis?

What is the developmental sequence in problem-solving skills?

Suggest reasons for the difference in how young and older children solve problems.

SEQUENCE OF COGNITIVE DEVELOPMENT: BIRTH TO 7 YEARS

Birth

- Are able to explore using the senses.
- Are beginning to develop basic concepts such as hunger, cold, wet.

1 month

- Will begin to recognise main carer and respond with movement, cooing.
- Will repeat pleasurable movements, thumb-sucking, wriggling.

3 months

- Are more interested in their surroundings.
- Begin to show an interest in playthings.
- Begin to understand cause and effect – if you move a rattle, it will make a sound.

6 months

- Expect things to behave in certain ways – the jack-in-the box will pop up but is unlikely to play a tune.

9 months

- Recognise pictures of familiar things.
- Watch a toy being hidden and then look for it (object permanence established).

12–15 months

- Explore objects using trial-and-error methods.
- Begin to point and follow when others point.
- Begin to treat objects in appropriate ways – cuddle a doll, talk into a telephone.
- Seek out hidden objects in the most likely places.

18 months – 2 years

- Refer to themselves by name.
- Begin to understand the consequences of their own actions, for example pouring the juice makes a wet patch.
- Might show the beginnings of empathy (an understanding of how others feel), for example, by comforting a crying baby.

3 years

- Can match primary colours.
- Can sort objects into categories, but usually by only one criterion at a time, for example all the cars from a selection of vehicles, but not the cars that are red.
- Ask lots of 'why' questions.
- Can recite the number words to 10 but are not yet able to count beyond 2 or 3.
- Begin to understand the concept of time – talk about what has happened and look forward to what is going to happen.
- Can concentrate on an activity for a short period of time, leave it and then go back to it.
- Begin to understand the concept of quantity – one, more, lots.

4 years

- Can sort with more categories.
- Can solve simple problems, usually by trial-and-error, but begin to understand 'why'.
- Adding to their knowledge by asking questions continually.
- Memory skills developing, particularly around significant events, for example holidays and birthdays, and familiar songs and stories.
- Includes representative detail in drawings, often based on observation.
- Will confuse fantasy and reality – 'I had a tiger come to tea at my house too'.
- Understands that writing carries meaning and uses writing in play.

5 years

- Have a good sense of past, present, future.
- Are becoming literate – most will recognise own name and write it, respond to books and interested in reading.
- Demonstrate good observational skills in their drawings.
- Understand the one-to-one principle and can count reliably to 10.
- Concentration is developing. At an appropriate task, can concentrate without being distracted for about 10 minutes.

6 years

- Begin to understand the mathematical concept of measuring – time, weight, length, capacity, volume.
- Are interested in why things happen and can formulate and test a simple hypothesis, for example, that seeds need water to grow.
- Begin to use symbols in their drawing and painting – the radial sun and the strip sky appear now.
- Many children will begin to read independently, but there is a wide individual variation in this.
- Can concentrate for longer periods of time.

7 years

- Are able to conserve number reliably and will recognise that a number of objects remains constant, however they are presented. May be able to conserve mass and capacity.
- Begin to deal with number abstractly, can perform calculations involving simple addition and subtraction mentally.
- May be able to tell the time from a watch or clock.
- Are developing an ability to reason and an understanding of cause and effect.

Remember, particularly with the later examples, that children's demonstration of these indicators of cognitive development will be dependent on the expectations a society has of them. For example, all children will develop the cognitive skills required for reading relating to perception and an ability to understand the use of symbols, but they will only learn to read in a society where literacy is valued and the associated skills are taught.

Access to learning experiences for all children

For an establishment to include disabled children, certain aspects need to be considered. Detailed information and training on inclusion of disabled children is available from condition- or impairment-specific voluntary organisations and self-help groups, but outlines of general principles for good practice are listed in Chapter 4. Establishments including disabled children need to provide:

- equipment that all children can use – much equipment produced for disabled people is inclusive: ramps, lifts, adjustable tables, automatic doors, long-handled taps, touch-sensitive controls, large print and grab rails can be used by all children
- a range of options such as tapes, Braille and print versions of documents
- a range of seat and table sizes and shapes
- empty floor space that is kept uncluttered
- flexible, adjustable equipment, for example a sand tray that comes off the stand, high-chairs with removable trays
- sturdy versions of 'ordinary' toys and furniture

- a range of scissors, knives and other implements
- soft play areas for activities such as crawling, jumping, climbing
- extra adult supervision to facilitate integration
- some equipment for individual children to facilitate integration – there should be discussions with the child and full-time carers about what to buy before expensive purchases are made
- spacious toilet facilities designed for wheelchair users that can then be used by all children
- private age-appropriate toilet or changing area
- disability awareness and equality training for all staff.

ACCESS FOR CHILDREN WITH SENSORY IMPAIRMENTS

Children with impaired sight

The following aspects need to be considered in order to include blind and partially sighted children. Establishments will need to provide:

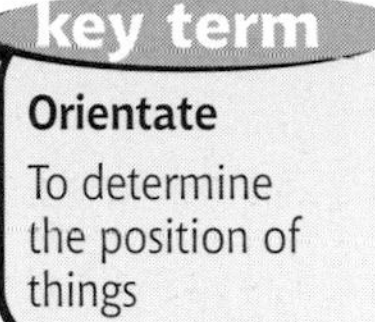

Orientate
To determine the position of things

- opportunities to explore the environment and people using touch, smell, hearing and any residual sight
- the opportunity for children to **orientate** themselves physically (this may involve visiting the setting when few people are present)
- stability and order, a place for everything and everything in its place; the child will need to be informed and shown any changes
- plenty of light
- a hazard-free environment, or an indication of hazardous things such as steps or sharp corners
- information about other children's needs, for example a child with a hearing loss who may not respond to them
- some specific items such as books in Braille, toys or board games that are especially designed to be inclusive.

Children with impaired hearing

The following points need to be considered by an establishment including deaf and hearing-impaired children:

- Hearing impairment is largely invisible; even a mild hearing loss is significant in a noisy, crowded room.
- A child with impaired hearing cannot tell you what they missed!
- Hearing aids are not a replacement for hearing and may be of little use to some children.
- Deaf children's greatest special need is access to language and communication; complete access can only come about through universal use of language and communication accessible to deaf children. This will often mean British Sign Language, which will need to be used by everyone in the setting.
- Deaf children need to communicate with other children as well as adults.
- Deaf children have a range of intellectual ability as all children do; if we deny them access to language we create a learning difficulty for them.

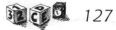

Case study . . .

. . . inclusive education

'Lake View Primary School's brochure states that they provide education for all children in the locality aged 3–7 years. I don't think they realised what a challenge it would be, when they offered my daughter, Emily, a place in the nursery.

Before Emily started, we went to visit for a session. The other children were curious and asked me why Emily had a funny face and couldn't talk properly. After our visit, the staff decided to prepare the children before Emily started properly. They had to search hard for suitable books to read to the children, but finally found Letterbox Library. The staff were willing to learn; they asked me questions about Emily and had a couple of sessions with a disability equality trainer.

Emily was very clingy and demanding at first. Staff couldn't manage her with 35 other children, so the school employed a special needs support assistant for part of the time, to help Emily integrate with the other children. They approached the local college and a student with learning difficulties came to the school on work placement. Emily latched on to him and it seemed to increase his self-confidence, as well as Emily's.

Whenever the children ask what is wrong with Emily, staff explain that she has Down's syndrome. They always answer the children's questions honestly, even when they are funny, like "Is it catching?"

The nursery staff say they have learned so much from having Emily and now do some things differently for all the children.'

1. *Why did Emily's parents want her to go to the local school?*
2. *How did the nursery staff prepare for Emily's admission?*
3. *Why did staff explain Emily's condition using the proper name?*
4. *Why did staff seek out a student with learning difficulties to help in the nursery?*

Progress check

In what formats should written documents/information be produced to ensure their accessibility to parents/carers who may themselves be disabled?

What will be needed to facilitate children's integration in the setting?

How should a setting decide what to purchase to support a disabled child?

What should be provided for all staff?

What creates a learning difficulty for deaf children?

Piaget's theory of cognitive development

Piaget's work on the development of children's thinking is the basis for the way that we provide care and education for young children. His theory looked at the way that children process their everyday experiences and build up an understanding of the world. He demonstrated that the child passes through particular and distinct stages on the way to an ever more complete and complex understanding of their surroundings. Using information gathered from observation of children, he identified the kind of learning that the child is capable of at each of these stages, emphasising that children's thinking is fundamentally different to that of adults.

Some of Piaget's findings have been challenged by more recent psychological studies but, nevertheless, there is still much in his work that enables us to understand the development of children's thinking. It is his work that has been so significant in influencing the child-centred, 'learning by doing' approach that characterises much early years provision.

Case study . . .

. . . understanding right and wrong

The following situation was presented to Laurie, aged 4: 'Mummy asked Peter and Patsy to help by putting some plates away into the cupboard. Patsy said that she was too busy and didn't want to help, but Peter started moving the plates. Mummy went out of the room but Peter carried on. He picked up too many at once and dropped them, smashing all six plates. Patsy liked the noise of the plates breaking and, picking up one for herself, she threw it on to the floor and smashed it.'

Laurie was asked if she thought that either of the children had been naughty. She replied, yes, that Peter had been naughty.

1. *Why do you think Laurie decided that Peter had been naughty?*
2. *What aspects of Piaget's theory does this example illustrate?*
3. *What can this tell about how children of this age understand notions of right and wrong?*

PIAGET'S STAGES

Piaget identified four distinct stages of cognitive development, each with its own characteristics. It is important to remember that the ages given are approximate and are intended only as a guide.

1 Sensory-motor (birth – 2 years)

At the sensory-motor stage the child:

- learns principally through the senses of sight and touch and through movement
- is **egocentric**, that is, can only see the world from their own viewpoint
- processes information visually, as images
- becomes aware that objects continue to exist when not in view **(object permanence) –** this awareness occurs at around 8 to 12 months
- uses abilities intelligently and begins to learn through trial-and-error methods.

key terms

Egocentric
seeing everything only from your own viewpoint

Object permanence
an understanding that objects continue to exist when not in view

2 Pre-operations (2–7 years)

This encompasses the pre-conceptual stage and the intuitive stage. It is during this period that children's language abilities develop rapidly, enabling them to represent and process information and to think in more complex ways.

At the pre-conceptual stage (2–4 years) the child:

- still processes information visually, as images, but as language develops, it makes possible representation of information in other ways
- gathers information through the senses of sight and touch, although hearing becomes increasingly important
- uses symbols in play, for example a doll for a baby, a lump of playdough for a cake
- has a tendency to see everything from their own point of view
- believes that everything that exists has a consciousness, even objects (**animism**). At this stage, the child may blame the table that they have bumped into.

key term

Animism
the belief that everything that exists has a consciousness

By the intuitive stage (4 – 7 years), the child:

- is involved in more complex symbolic play
- is still likely to see things only from their own point of view
- increasingly uses language to process and order information
- uses hearing to gather information
- will find abstract thought difficult and be dependent on immediate perceptions
- understands right and wrong in a simplistic way, often in terms of the most obvious factors. (See the Case study 'Which has more in it?' below.)

3 Concrete operations (7–11 years)

By this stage, the child:

- can see things from another's point of view, that is, can **decentre**
- is capable of more complex reasoning but needs concrete objects to assist this process, for example, uses apparatus to solve mathematical problems
- knows that things are not always as they look, understands **conservation**
- knows the difference between real and pretend
- can understand and participate in play with rules.

key terms

Decentre
being able to see things from another's point of view

Conservation
an understanding that the quantity of a substance remains the same if nothing is added or taken away, even though it may appear different

4 Formal operations (12 years to adult)

Characteristics of this stage include:

- the ability to think logically
- abstract thought with no need for props.

The stage of formal operations represents the most complex level of thinking and understanding that Piaget identified. However, research has shown that progression to this stage is not universal and that many adults function capably in the world without ever reaching this level of thinking.

PIAGET'S STAGES AND PLAY

Recognition of Piaget's stages can help us plan and provide for the kinds of play experiences that are most appropriate for each stage of development.

SENSORY MOTOR STAGE, 0–2 YEARS

Children gather information predominantly through their senses of sight and touch

Children process information imagistically

Sensory motor stage, 0–2 years

Children have a tendency to be egocentric, seeing the world from their own viewpoint

Children use trial and error as their main tool of discovery.

Children in this age range have a limited language ability, therefore senses other than hearing are predominant in gathering and processing information. Sight and touch are vital senses in enabling a child to gather the information in his/her environment. This information is then processed as images, similar to, but more sophisticated than, pictures or photographs. This processing system is inflexible and has limited use. For example, how would you store the concept of justice in this way? Children, therefore, need to acquire language. It thus becomes immediately obvious, even at this early stage, that there is an important link between language and intellectual development. It is an interdependent relationship.

PRE-OPERATIONAL STAGE, 2–7 YEARS

Children continue to gather information, predominantly through the senses of sight and touch but hearing becomes increasingly important

Initially children's information processing is predominantly imagistic. However, it gradually becomes mediated by thought processes as language develops. These are still basic and very dependent upon immediate perceptions of the environment

Children still have a tendency to be egocentric

PRE-CONCEPTUAL STAGE, 2–4 YEARS

Children begin to play symbolically, using one object to represent another, for example a bag as a hat, a doll as a baby

Children believe that everything has a consciousness, for example, teddies have feelings, chairs are naughty

Hearing gradually becomes an important sense for information gathering

Thought processes are increasingly mediated by language as it develops

Children are still dependent upon immediate perceptions of the environment and find abstract thought difficult

INTUITIVE STAGE, 5–7 YEARS

Symbolic play continues

Children still have a tendency to be egocentric

As language develops children increasingly use this to gather and process information. Language is a complex system of representation and therefore enables a child to develop more complex ways of gathering and processing information. Again the link between language and intellectual development is shown to be vital in children's learning.

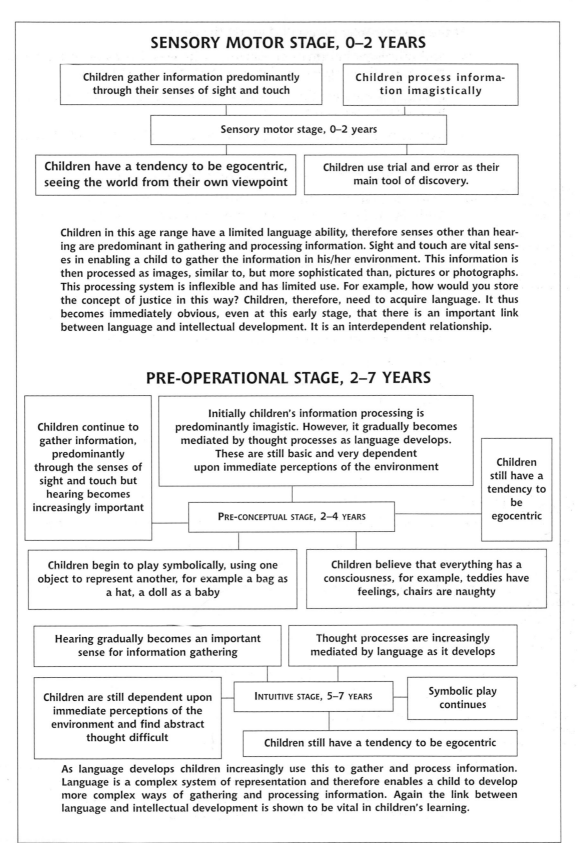

The main features of Piaget's sensory motor and pre-operational stages

At the sensory-motor stage, play involves:

- using the senses
- being self-absorbed
- movement
- lots of practice, often of the same skill. Piaget used the term 'mastery' to describe the child's need to persevere and achieve.

Play for children at the pre-operational stage involves:

- using symbols, for example a cardboard box for a house
- using language to communicate, with oneself, with others, with objects
- make-believe and fantasy
- beginning to play games with simple, straightforward rules
- being alone sometimes, more often with others.

By the concrete operations stage, play involves:

- more complicated rules
- taking responsibility and roles
- an awareness of the difference between fantasy and reality
- an ability to consider the needs and feelings of other people
- working with others, sharing decisions.

key term

Schema
Piaget's term for all the ideas, memories and information that a child might have about a concept or experience

PIAGET AND THE DEVELOPMENT OF CONCEPTS

Piaget uses the term **schema** to describe the skills and concepts that children acquire through the following processes as they interact with their environment:

- *accommodation* – the way in which children take in information from their experiences
- *assimilation* – the process of fitting what the child has learnt from new experiences into their existing concepts or schemas
- *adaptation* – occurs as a result of the interaction between accommodation and assimilation: the child now knows more about certain aspects of the world and can act upon this knowledge.

Piaget used the term equilibrium to describe the stage at which the child has successfully incorporated new understanding into an existing schema. Similarly, disequilibrium occurs when something unfamiliar is presented, requiring the schema to be modified. Piaget considered that the experience of disequilibrium was a crucial motivation to learning, whereby the child needs to make sense of their environment by incorporating new experiences into existing knowledge. These processes are not confined to children's learning. As adults, we are constantly adapting existing concepts as we accommodate and assimilate new information.

A schema for bricks

The following is a simplified example of these terms in context, showing how a child's schema or concept about the physical characteristics of bricks might develop. The same schema is presented in diagrammatic form below.

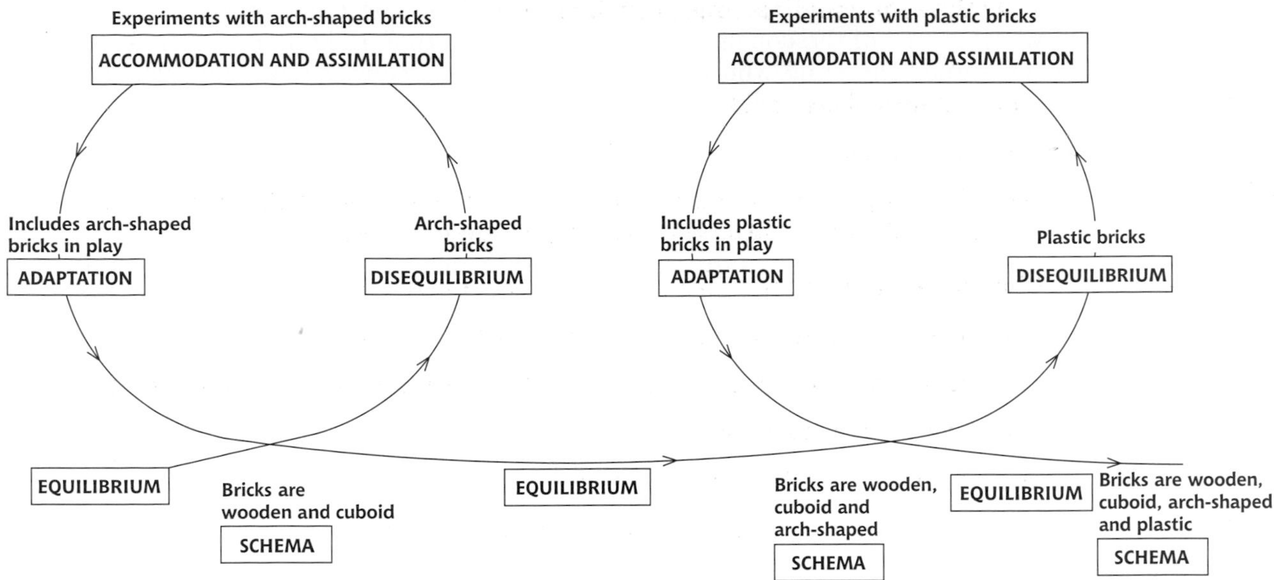

An example of a child developing a schema for bricks

Anna is used to playing with bricks. Her present schema for bricks tells her that they can be different sizes and different colours but that they are all the same shape – cuboid – and that they are wooden (equilibrium). One day some arch-shaped bricks appear in the brick box (disequilibrium). She investigates these new additions, playing with them alongside the more familiar bricks (accommodation). She soon discovers that she can use these new toys in much the same way as the bricks she already has (assimilation), but that the different shapes present her with new possibilities and problems in her building (adaptation). Her schema for bricks is once again in a state of equilibrium. The next time that she gets out the box some plastic bricks have been added (disequilibrium) and as she incorporates these into her play, she moves through the process again. As a result of these additions, the child's original schema for bricks has developed considerably.

EXPERIMENTS IN THINKING

Piaget derived his theory of cognitive development from his observations of children who were asked to solve particular problems. If we pose similar problems to children their responses will identify their stage of cognitive development. The tests most often used are the test for conservation and Piaget's test for decentring, the mountain test.

Conservation

Piaget argued that a child at the pre-operational stage does not understand that a quantity of a substance can be presented in a variety of different ways and, provided that nothing is added or taken away, the amount remains the same. Children at this stage are likely to be tricked by the visual appearance of the substance and say that the amount has changed. They are unable to conserve. There are a number of ways of testing for conservation. Here are some examples.

Conservation of mass

Playdough is used to make two balls of the same size. The child is asked if there is the same amount of playdough in each ball. If the child agrees that the amounts are the same, the adult rolls one of the balls of dough into a sausage shape, making sure that the child can see what is happening. The child is then asked again whether one of the dough shapes has more in it than the other, or if they are both the same. The child who has not yet learned to conserve will be misled by the appearance of the dough and will say that there is more in one than the other.

Conservation of number

Two equal rows of counters (or buttons or sweets) are set out in front of the child. She agrees that each row contains the same number of counters. When the adult, again in full view, moves the counters so that one line is longer than the other, the child who is unable to conserve number is likely to say that the longer line contains more counters.

Conservation of capacity

Conservation of capacity can be demonstrated in a similar way, by using the same amounts of liquid in a tall, thin beaker and a short, squat one.

Case study . . .

. . . which has more in it?

Paul, aged 3, observed his father filling two identical bottles of water. They talked about the bottles and Paul agreed that they were both the same size and had the same amount of water in them. Paul watched while his father emptied each bottle, in turn, into a different container. One container was tall and thin; the other was wide and shallow. Paul agreed that no water had been spilt during pouring. His father then asked whether one container had more in it than the other or if they both contained the same. Paul answered straightaway that the tall, thin container had more in it. When his father asked him why he'd come to that conclusion, he replied that the tall one was bigger.

1. *Why did Paul's father ask questions about the size of the bottles and whether any had been spilt?*
2. *Why do you think Paul chose the tall, thin container?*
3. *Where, in Piaget's stages of cognitive development, would you place Paul?*

Decentring

Piaget's test to show whether a child was able to take another's point of view – the ability to decentre – was his famous mountain experiment. A model comprising three mountains with different features was placed before a 5-year-old child. The child was asked to describe the model from their point of view saying which mountain was furthest away, closest, and so on. A doll was then placed alongside the model, with a different perspective from that of the child. The child was then asked to describe the mountain scene from the point of view of the doll (see the figure below). Piaget believed that the inability of the child to describe the mountain scene from the doll's perspective showed that they could not yet decentre.

More recent research has re-evaluated Piaget's findings from this test and criticised some of his methods.

PIAGET EVALUATED

Piaget's work remains important and his influence on early years provision is significant. However, research by the Edinburgh group in the 1970s, led by Margaret Donaldson, has questioned some of his assumptions. In particular, there

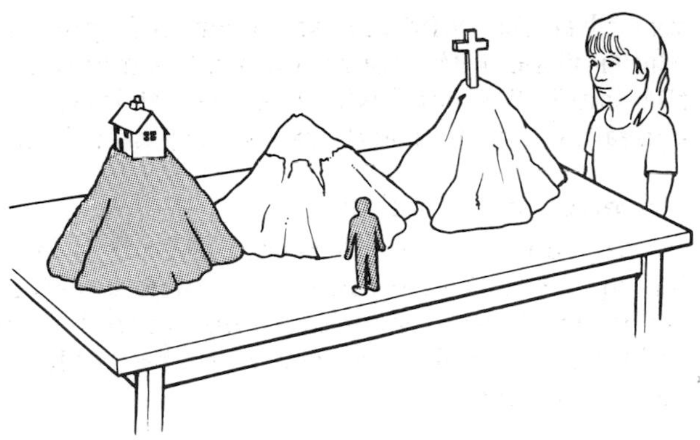

Piaget's mountain test for decentring

has been some criticism of his questioning techniques and of the design of some of his experiments. Donaldson's group held that pre-school aged children respond better to questions that are posed as they arise naturally in a meaningful context, rather than in the artificial environment of the laboratory. They devised a number of tests, used a more child-friendly questioning format and came to different conclusions. The most significant of these was Martin Hughes's reworking of Piaget's mountain test for decentring.

Martin Hughes's model (see the figure below) contained two dolls, a policeman (in a fixed position) and a boy (who could be moved). The child was asked to move the boy doll to a position where the policeman could not see it, thus looking at the model from the policeman's point of view. Children who were unable to see Piaget's mountain from the doll's point of view had much more success in hiding the boy doll from the policeman. It is thought that Piaget's task seemed irrelevant to the children and that they did not understand what they were being asked to do. Hiding the doll from the policeman seemed much more straightforward and showed that, if there was enough reason to do so, children could decentre and see the world from another's perspective.

Piaget's theory of cognitive development has been constantly re-examined and modified. Piaget stressed the importance of the environment in children's learning, seeing children as instinctively and actively curious about their surroundings. His belief that children learn most effectively through first-hand

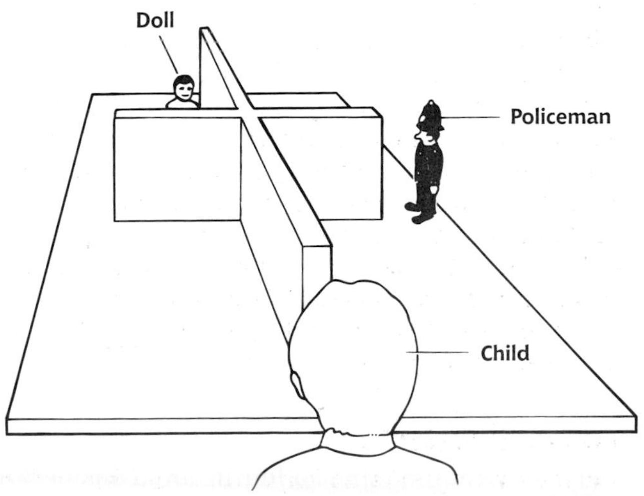

Hughes's policeman doll

experiences has provided the rationale for the discovery learning, or 'learning by doing', child-centred approach to education. The child is seen as an individual who, through interaction with an environment that provides the right kind of learning experiences, progresses according to his stage of development.

Vygotsky's studies on the ways that children learn emphasised not just the individual child but the social context of learning. His findings showed that children had a great deal to learn from each other through interaction and communication. Unlike Piaget, Vygotsky felt that the child's level of ability should not be judged merely on what they could do alone but on what they were capable of with help. He used the term **zone of proximal development** to explain those tasks that might be beyond the child's capability alone, but that were possible with assistance. The child would then be provided with a more challenging and stimulating environment than if left to discover and learn alone.

> **key term**
>
> **Zone of proximal development**
> Vygotsky's term for the range of learning that the child is incapable of achieving alone but that is possible with assistance

The work of Jerome Bruner pays particular attention to the role of the adult in children's learning. He sees the adult's role as not merely to provide a rich environment for children to discover, but to have an active part to play alongside them through scaffolding, that is, providing a structure that supports this learning. There are links here with Vygotsky's work, but the emphasis in Bruner's work is on the skilled adult, tuned in to the child's capabilities, who can offer support that enables the child to break out of a repetitive activity, consolidate what has been learned and move on to the next step.

Recent studies have found that there are aspects of children's learning that Piaget did not give significant consideration to in his initial work on cognitive development. The effects of social interaction with other children and the involvement of skilled and sensitive adults have been shown to have a significant bearing on the way that children learn.

Progress check

Identify the stages in Piaget's theory of cognitive development.

According to Piaget, what kind of play is developmentally appropriate for:
(a) 2 year olds? (b) 5 year olds?

Describe the process through which children develop schema.

Why do young children understand most effectively through a 'learning through experience' approach?

Why have some of Piaget's initial findings been criticised?

What influence does Piaget's work have on the provision of services for young children?

The role of the adult in promoting cognitive development

Conclusions from research and an examination of the nature–nurture debate indicate that children's learning is significantly influenced by the quality of their environment. Included in any consideration of the environment are the adults who care for children. It is important, therefore, when providing for children's cognitive development, that we are aware of how to plan, prepare and monitor children's activities, and also how to interact with children during the activities so that their learning is optimised. Careful consideration of the environment provided for children can contribute to them achieving their potential.

This is an ongoing process; the areas are interdependent, as illustrated by the figure below.

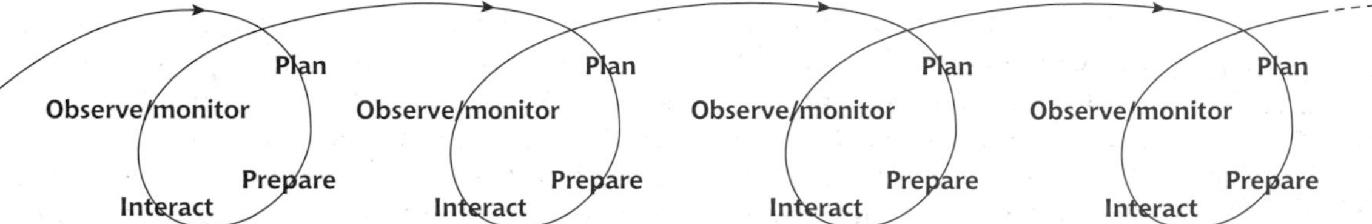

The planning cycle

- Planning is based on observation and monitoring of the children's needs and development. It is also based on observation of practical considerations concerning the use of space, time, equipment and staff.
- Preparation is based on careful planning so that the environment provided meets the needs of the children across the developmental range. Again, practical considerations are important when preparing an area.
- Interaction with the children takes account of their individual developmental needs. Some of this information is gathered through observation and must be incorporated into the planning. Practical considerations of staff time are an important issue here.
- Observation and monitoring provide valuable information on the children. This forms the basis of planning and preparing the area and also for interaction with the children.

Research has shown that the quality of adult–child interaction is a crucial factor in promoting children's cognitive development and that play experiences that are accompanied by a high level of adult-to-child involvement optimise learning. An adult will encourage children to persevere at a task and will extend understanding on an individual basis by presenting a new task or exploring another aspect of the original one. Skilful questioning and the posing of problems by an adult can enable a child to move from one level of understanding to the next. This is not to say that children do not benefit from the opportunity to play alone and uninterrupted, but without the active involvement of sensitive adults who know the children and are aware of their developmental needs, play activities can become circular, repetitive and lack intellectual challenge.

Progress check

Name the four elements of the planning cycle.

Why should we see the planning cycle as a continuous process?

Why is the quality of adult–child interaction important in promoting children's cognitive development?

What do you understand by the term 'circular play'?

Why is it important that adults know the capabilities of the children that they work with?

How can adults present children with intellectual challenge?

Now try these questions

Describe what is meant by the term cognitive development by including reference to all its aspects.

Why is creativity an important aspect of children's cognitive development?

How has Piaget's work influenced our understanding of children's cognitive development?

What are the features of Piaget's stages of cognitive development?

How can the adult make a positive contribution to children's cognitive development?

Give examples of ways in which provision can be differentiated to meet the developmental needs of all children.

key terms

You need to know what the key terms and phrases in this chapter mean. Go back through the chapter and find out.

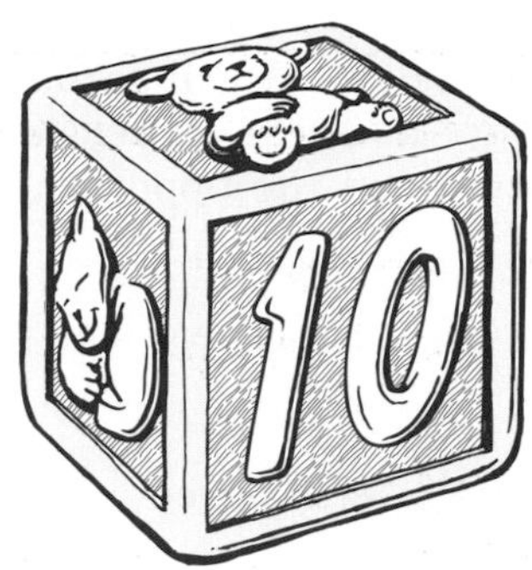

LANGUAGE DEVELOPMENT

In this chapter you will learn about how language develops and how to interact with children to ensure that their potential is realised. You will also learn about the different aspects of language, such as listening, thinking, talking, reading and writing. The chapter outlines the particular needs of children who use more than one language and highlights the effects of language delay.

This chapter will cover the following topics:

- *what is language?*
- *bilingualism*
- *psychology and language development*
- *sequence of language development*
- *talking with children*
- *planning for and monitoring children's language development*
- *factors affecting language development.*

What is language?

Language is the main way in which human beings communicate. We are the only species that has the ability to use language. Other species do communicate, but in ways specific to their needs, for example by making their fur stand on end to communicate danger, by spraying their territory with urine to mark it out or by growling to deter attackers.

Humans live in a very complex world and need a complex system of communication. Language is this complex system. Language is also needed to satisfy the human need to communicate feelings, complex needs, thoughts and ideas.

Spoken language is a structured set of sounds; written language is a structured set of symbols. These symbols are shared and understood by everyone who speaks the same language. For example, consider the word *pain*. In English, this means suffering or distress. In French (and pronounced *pan*), it means bread. Therefore, what the symbols *pain* mean to an individual, and how the word is pronounced, depends upon which language the individual has been brought up to speak.

Language is learned, and the ability to operate well within society is affected by the ability to use language effectively.

There are different forms of language (see the figure below), which are used at different times for different situations. The ability to use all these expressions of language requires a high level of skill. Young children need the opportunity to acquire these skills.

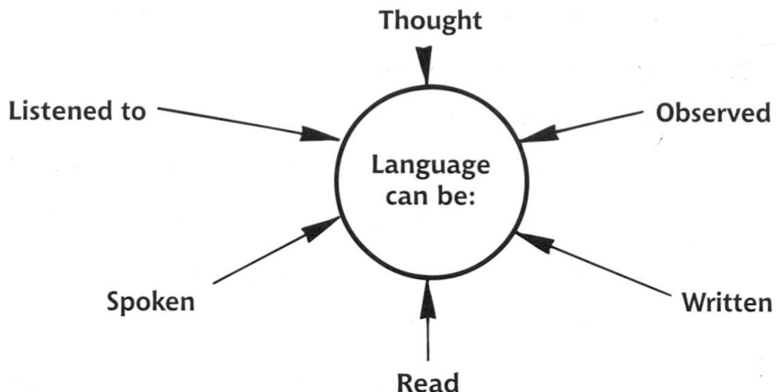

The forms of language

SPOKEN LANGUAGE

The raw materials of spoken language are sounds. These sounds come together to form words. Combinations of words are brought together in special and complex ways to form sentences. The meaning in a sentence is communicated by the way in which words are combined. Look at these sentences:

'The dog bites the man.'

'The man bites the dog.'

The same words are used each time, but because the order of the words is altered in the second sentence, so the meaning is altered.

To ensure that there is a shared understanding of what is being said, there are some rules that everyone needs to learn and use. These include pronunciation and grammar.

Pronunciation and grammar

- *Pronunciation* – this is the way that words are said. It may vary depending on which part of the country a person comes from. These accents add interest and diversity to language, and the variations are not usually so different that people cannot be understood.
- *Grammar* – to be able to communicate exactly what is meant, the speaker must normally use the correct grammar.

For most children, the ability to pronounce words correctly and to use appropriate grammar are acquired in the same way as other language skills. Children need good role models, the opportunity to use their language skills and positive feedback to adjust and refine these skills. Occasionally, however, some children have difficulties with pronunciation which may require help from a speech therapist. It is important to be aware of these children's needs and to seek help for the child.

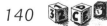

NON-VERBAL COMMUNICATION

When people are speaking and listening, there are many clues besides the actual spoken words that are picked up to help us interpret the interaction:

- tone of voice
- body posture (how and where we stand or sit)
- gesture, body movements (such as a shrug)
- facial expression
- eye contact.

This non-verbal communication may have several functions. It may:

- replace speech, for example a finger on the lips
- signal an attitude, for example yawning when someone is talking to you
- aid verbal communication, for example pointing when saying 'that one'
- express emotion, often evident in facial expression.

As with other aspects of language, there is a general shared understanding of non-verbal signals. However, they are often sent out, received and understood without us being consciously aware of them.

Case study . . .

. . . non-verbal communication

As nursery began, Ruby burst into the room. 'I'm 4,' she shouted. The nursery nurse went over to Ruby and knelt down beside her. He spent a few minutes talking to her about her birthday, her presents and the party she was going to have later that day.

1. *Why was it important that the nursery nurse knelt down to talk to Ruby?*
2. *How else, non-verbally, might he have communicated his interest in what Ruby had to say?*

It is important to realise that there are some cultural differences in non-verbal communication that could result in misunderstanding. In some cultures, for example, children are expected to avoid eye contact when being addressed by an adult, whereas other cultures might interpret such behaviour as insolence on the part of the child.

LISTENING

Although most people are born with the ability to listen and take it for granted, it is in fact quite a complex skill. Listening involves sifting out and selecting relevant information from all the sound around us.

Like all other skills, children need to practise listening carefully. This demands good powers of concentration. This skill is often called active listening.

Case study . . .

. . . developing listening skills

Amarjit planned a story session based on 'Goldilocks and the Three Bears'. She planned to read the story to the children and then retell it using a storyboard.

First, she read the story all the way through. Then, she showed the children the storyboard pictures and characters: Goldilocks, three bears, three bowls, three spoons, three chairs and three beds.

Then she read the story again and asked the children to look out for the bears, bowls, chairs, etc. As the children identified them, Amarjit put them on the storyboard, sequencing the story.

Finally, Amarjit asked the children to tell her the story using the storyboard.

1. *How did Amarjit encourage the children to listen carefully?*
2. *How did she check that the children were listening carefully and selecting the relevant information?*

THINKING

Language is the main tool that human beings use for thinking. Thinking can be done without language, but at a very simple level: we can recall pictures, images and tactile sensations. However, these ways of thinking and recalling information are not complex enough for all that is demanded of human beings. A more flexible and efficient way of using and manipulating information in many different ways is needed: language is this flexible and efficient way of thinking. Language development and cognitive development are therefore very closely linked.

WRITTEN LANGUAGE

Letters, words and sentences are symbols used to represent the spoken word. The understanding of these symbols has to be shared with people who speak and write in the same language. For example, in English this combination of symbols:

APPLE

is used to represent this object:

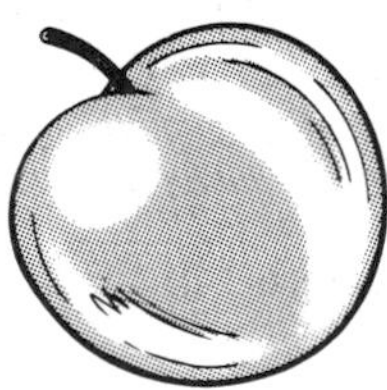

In Punjabi, this combination of symbols: ਆਪਲ is used to represent this object.

So that there is a shared understanding of how to write, there are rules that everyone needs to learn. In English, the following rules apply:

- You write on each line from left to right.
- You start at the top left-hand corner.
- The spacing between the letters in words and between the words in sentences is standardised.
- Words are spelled in the same way each time they are written down.
- Appropriate punctuation and grammar are usually necessary.

Other languages will have different rules.

Before a child can begin to learn to write, they need to develop a wide range of concepts and skills. These include:

- *fine motor control* – good hand–eye co-ordination and manipulative skills
- *visual discrimination* – the ability to see similarities and differences
- *auditory discrimination* – the ability to hear similarities and differences, especially between alphabet sounds
- *sequencing* – sorting, matching, patterning and sequencing items and pictures will eventually enable a child to do the same with letters and words
- an awareness of the need for writing and reading
- *an ability to symbolise* – this is the ability to use one thing to represent another. Children develop this skill in their play – they may use a doll to represent a baby, cuddling and feeding it, or a box to represent a car or a spaceship. Eventually, this skill can be transferred to writing, which is using squiggles (symbols) on a page to represent the spoken word.

Play activities in the nursery enable children to develop these skills and concepts. Children need plenty of opportunities, practice and encouragement to achieve this, before beginning to write.

As children's understanding about writing develops, many will begin to make writing-type marks on a page and will often tell you what it says. This is sometimes called emergent or early writing. This is an important stage of development and provides evidence that children have acquired many of the skills and concepts outlined above.

Case study . . .

. . . developing writing skills

As part of the nursery's topic on 'Our Town', the role-play area was a hairdressers. As well as all the equipment that a hairdresser needs, the staff had provided an appointments book and cards.

Naomi, a trainee in the nursery, became involved in the children's play by going to the hairdressers to book an appointment. She asked for an appointment and encouraged Tim, a child playing in the area, to look in the appointments book, identify a time and write down her name. She then asked for an appointment card so that she did not forget the time that she should come. Again, Naomi encouraged Tim to write this down.

1. *When did Tim use his early reading and writing skills?*
2. *How did Naomi encourage Tim to use these skills?*
3. *What was Tim learning about the needs and uses of reading and writing?*

READING

Once language is written down, it can be read by making sense of the symbols. As with writing, there is a range of skills and concepts that children need to acquire before learning to read. Many early skills and concepts are common to both reading and writing:

- visual discrimination
- auditory discrimination
- an ability to sequence
- an awareness of the needs and uses of reading and writing
- an ability to symbolise.

In addition, a child who is learning to read needs to be able to listen to, share and enjoy stories and to understand how books are organised. For example, young children need to understand that:

- the reader progresses from left to right
- the top left-hand corner is the starting point

and later that:

- there are patterns in words that reflect sound (phonics) and shape (look and say)
- punctuation ensures that the text makes sense.

These rules are learned over a period of time and children need plenty of practice at them.

It is important to note that these rules do not apply to all languages, and that bilingual and multilingual children may be learning to read and write languages with different conventions.

Progress check

Identify the different aspects of language development.

How do children learn appropriate grammar and pronunciation in their spoken language?

What is non-verbal communication and why is it important?

How can children be encouraged to listen carefully?

Why do we need language to think and to store information?

Identify the skills and concepts that children need before they begin to read and to write.

List some play activities that could be provided to develop and refine these skills.

What are the standardised rules in reading and written English?

Why is it important that children learn and understand these rules?

Bilingualism

Many children in the UK today come from families that are **bilingual** or **multilingual,** where English is not the first or the only language used. A child may grow up in an environment where English is never spoken, where English is sometimes spoken or where English is used between some members of the family, while others converse in one or more other languages.

key terms

Bilingual
speaking two languages

Multilingual
speaking many languages

key terms

British Sign Language (BSL)
the visual, gestural language of the British deaf community

Makaton
a system of simple signs used with people who have limited language skills

In order to participate fully in any experiences offered, the child will need to develop confidence and fluency in the language used in the child-care setting. This can only be achieved if child-care workers have an awareness and understanding of the child's linguistic (language) background. With this sensitivity, appropriate provision can be made for the development of language skills in English, while recognising those that the child has already achieved in their first or home language.

Language is an integral part of the cultural heritage of any group. In some situations, a family may use English for all their daily needs and not use the language of their cultural heritage on a regular basis. However, to ensure that the next generations understand and appreciate the breadth and depth of their culture, some minority groups encourage their young people to learn the language.

Children who are deaf, or who have members of their family who are deaf, may have **British Sign Language (BSL)** as their first or preferred language. This is a distinct, visual, gestural language which has a structure and grammar that are quite different from those of spoken English. As BSL does not have a written form – although line drawings of individual signs can be found in some children's books – BSL speakers use English in its literate forms, i.e. for reading and writing. BSL should not be confused with **Makaton**: BSL is a sophisticated language form that allows discussion of complex and abstract issues; Makaton is a system of simple signs used for communication with people with learning disabilities linked to very limited language skills.

Case study . . .

. . . bilingual situations

1. Seven-year-old Shahnaz's grandparents settled in the UK from Pakistan in the 1960s. She has grown up in an extended family where her parents speak to her in English, and where she converses with her grandparents in Punjabi. At school, she talks in English with teachers and sometimes in Punjabi to her classmates. After school, she also learns to read and write in Arabic, the language of the Qur'an.
2. Dieter is the 4-year-old son of a German student on a 2-year study programme. He attends a suburban playgroup where the playgroup workers are encouraging him to use his few words of English. His mother usually speaks to him in German, but is also introducing more English at home.
3. Anna, a 6-year-old girl from Manchester, has moved to rural mid-Wales where her parents have opened a restaurant. All of the children in her class speak Welsh as their first language and, although there are some lessons in English, Welsh is the main language of the school and of the playground.
4. Dinh is 3 years old. His family are refugees from South-East Asia, housed in temporary bed-and-breakfast accommodation. Dinh attends a local authority day nursery and is very withdrawn. His parents communicate with the staff through an interpreter, but this service is not often available.
5. Maria's parents are profoundly deaf. She is hearing, but she uses BSL with her parents at home and with their friends at the Deaf Club. At nursery and with her brother, she communicates in spoken English.
6. Raheel is a 5-year-old boy from a Bangladeshi family. He has recently moved to a small village school from a large city school where many languages were spoken and valued. His last teacher felt that he was progressing well. In his new school, he is the only child for whom English is a second language. There is no ESL (English as a Second Language) support for him and he is slipping behind in his school work.

1. *What similarities are there in the experiences described above?*
2. *What differences are there?*
3. *Consider each individual child. What are the needs of each one?*

IDENTIFYING THE NEEDS OF BILINGUAL CHILDREN

It is neither helpful nor accurate to categorise all bilingual children as having the same needs or experiences. What they do have in common is the experience of using and needing to use more than one language, but there will be other factors that may be quite different.

MEETING THE NEEDS OF BILINGUAL CHILDREN

It is important that the needs of children whose first language is not English are understood and met in the child-care setting. All children will experience some feelings of anxiety on the first days in an unfamiliar setting, such as school or playgroup. These anxieties are bound to be increased if the child is surrounded by an unfamiliar linguistic environment as well. If such children are to benefit from their experiences in nursery, school or day care, staff need to make sure that they understand, build on and value the children's first language (home language or mother tongue) capabilities. In order to help, you need to remember the following points:

- Many children who do not speak English fluently are very capable in their first language.
- Do not label children who speak little or no English as having language problems or language delay. Their lack of competence is in English, not language.
- A child may be able to use language to conceptualise in their first language, but not in their second language.
- The non-verbal language of English (the intonation, rhythm, use of gesture and eye contact) may be quite different from that of the child's first language.
- A bilingual or multilingual child will thrive in an atmosphere where language diversity is valued.
- Speaking more than one language is a positive attribute and should be regarded as such.
- Fluency in a spoken language does not necessarily imply literacy in that language. Many people may not be able to read and write in a language that they can, nevertheless, speak fluently.

Any child unable to communicate in the language of the child-care setting (English, in most of the case studies listed above) will be disadvantaged. Specialist help needs to be available to ensure that the child learns and practises English. Given the right kind of support and an attitude of understanding from the staff, the child will soon acquire the necessary skills in English that are needed to take full advantage of all that is going on.

In our enthusiasm to get children competent in their second language, we should ensure that the development of the first language is fostered too. Studies show that children who are given an opportunity to develop their first language to an advanced level can transfer reading and writing skills to their second language quite readily. However, children who are required to tackle the complex skills of reading and writing in a language that they do not understand will often have difficulty in making similar progress.

SUPPORT FOR BILINGUAL CHILDREN

The kind of support available for bilingual children varies a great deal from one area to another. Here are some examples of the kinds of support that might be available:

- *English as a Second Language (ESL) staff* – these are teachers and classsroom assistants, often nursery nurses, who work alongside members of staff in schools and nurseries where there are children who would benefit from a one-to-one relationship and small group work to develop English skills. Where there are substantial numbers of children whose first language is not English, a member of an ESL team may be assigned to a particular establishment. In other cases, where there are fewer such children, a number of sessions per week might be allocated.
- *Mother tongue (or home language) teachers/assistants/language instructors* – some local authorities employ staff whose job is to support and encourage the acquisition of the child's first (or home) language. This builds on the process that has already begun at home and allows for the growth of confidence and skills in language and in thinking.
- *Bilingual assistant (often a nursery nurse)* – these assistants are usually employed in an establishment where many of the children have a common first language. The assistant works alongside the other staff, translating instructions and information for the children, and also sharing stories, nursery rhymes or games, allowing the child access to the whole curriculum. The bilingual assistant can provide reassurance for the child and can be helpful in supporting a flow of information to and from parents, particularly when settling children into new situations.
- *Saturday or community schools* – these are usually run by members of a local community, including parents, who are anxious that the cultural identity of the community is maintained by keeping the language alive. This is particularly true for children who are the second generation of their family to have been born in the UK. These schools sometimes have a role in religious instruction too.

Case study . . .

. . . valuing language diversity

The playgroup reflected the cultural diversity of the local community in its intake of children, and within the group there was a substantial number of children whose first language was Gujerati, alongside an English-speaking majority. The playgroup made links with a local Asian Women's Project and were offered the services of Nialah, a trained Gujerati-speaking worker, for some weekly sessions.

Initially, Nialah concentrated on those children who spoke Gujerati, presenting activities and sharing stories with them in their own language. As their confidence grew, she worked alongside them in activities that were presented in English, developing and supporting their understanding in their second language. At carpet time, Nialah sometimes told a story or taught a rhyme in Gujerati for all the children to hear. Nialah's presence was very helpful to Gujerati-speaking parents, particularly when their children first started at the group and they wanted to ask questions or pass on information. After only a few weeks, the playgroup staff noted the difference that Nialah's sessions had made both in terms of the children's confidence and learning and in the involvement of the Gujerati-speaking parents with the playgroup.

1. *How did Nialah's involvement help the Gujerati-speaking children in the playgroup?*
2. *What benefits did the children's parents gain from Nialah's work in the playgroup?*
3. *What did all the children gain from being introduced to stories and rhymes in Gujerati?*

LANGUAGE DIVERSITY

We are part of a world where there are many different languages, accents, dialects and other ways of communication, both written and spoken. It would be limiting for children only to be aware of their own language and ignorant of the existence of others. By promoting a positive atmosphere that celebrates language diversity, we can enhance the language experience of all children, while at the same time valuing that of the bilingual child. This is an enriching experience for all children and is of as much benefit to the child in the monolingual environment as it is to the child who is already surrounded by many languages.

The following ideas are suggested for promoting language diversity in a child-care setting. It is important to value language diversity everywhere, not just in establishments where a variety of languages are spoken.

key term

Language Acquisition Device (LAD) the name Chomsky gives to our innate physical and intellectual abilities that enable us to acquire and use language

- Present welcome signs and greetings in a variety of languages.
- Choose dual-language books for your book corner (include sign language too). Draw children's attention to the differences in text and script.
- Teach songs and nursery rhymes in a number of languages. Get help from parents and friends if you need it.
- Make books for children in their own language.
- Listen to tapes of songs and poems and stories in many languages.
- Make a display of printed materials containing as many different languages and scripts as you can find. Get children to help by bringing in things from home.
- Choose stories from all around the world. Find someone who can tell the story in another language; tell the English version alongside this.
- Encourage children to learn simple greetings in languages other than their own.

Try to think of some more ideas to add to this list.

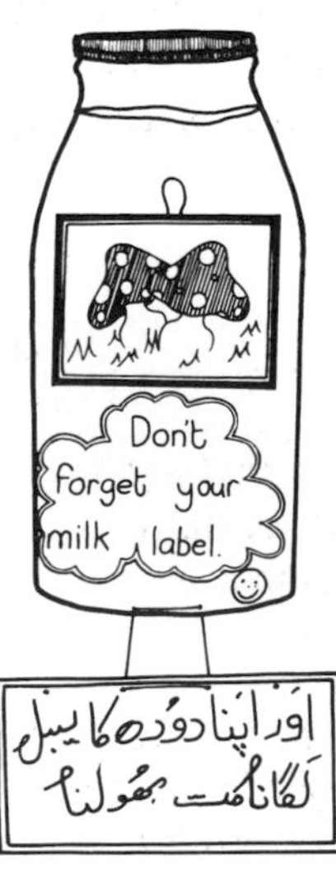

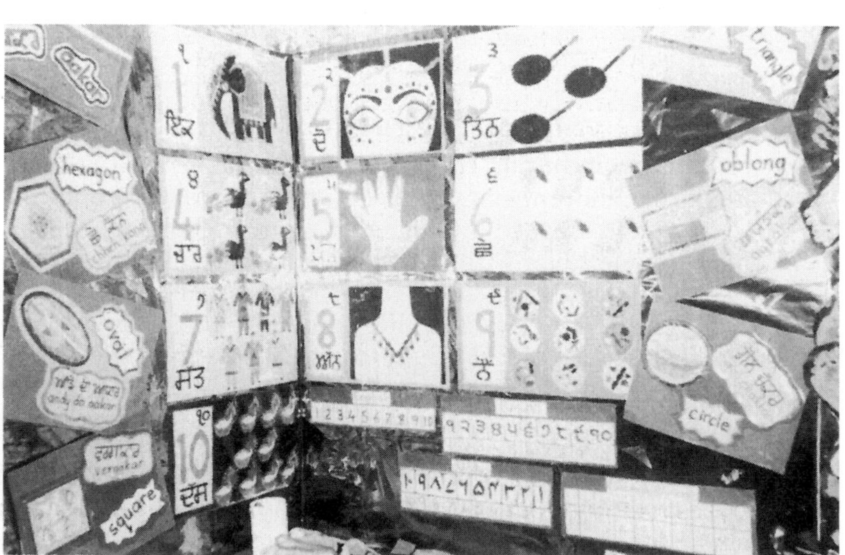

Promoting language diversity in the child-care setting

Progress check

1. *What do you understand by the terms bilingual, multilingual and monolingual?*
2. *What is the role of language in maintaining the cultural identity of a community?*
3. *How can the child-care worker help to meet the needs of children whose first language is not that of the setting?*
4. *What kind of support is available to young children who speak English as a second language?*
5. *Why is it important for child-care workers to value and promote language diversity as part of their work with children?*

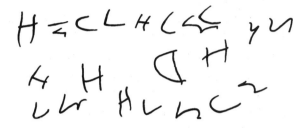

Vygotsky observed that children progress from drawing things to drawing speech

Psychology and language development

Many psychologists have studied and researched how human beings acquire language. Some have concluded that language is predominantly a genetically inherited skill. Others believe that language is learned after a child is born. This is part of the nature–nurture debate.

The nature–nurture debate on language is inconclusive. It seems likely that learning language has elements of both nature and nurture: there is some genetic sensitivity to language, but that children's experiences after birth are very important in their development of language.

NATURE	*NURTURE*
Our ability for language is genetically determined.	Language is learned after we are born through a process of reinforcement.
Noam Chomsky	**B.F. Skinner**
Chomsky believes that we are born with all the appropriate physical and intellectual capabilities for the acquisition of language:	When children utter sounds and words that are part of the language they will eventually speak, they are greeted with a positive

continued

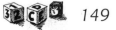

The nature–nurture debate on language continued

NATURE	NURTURE
• speech-producing mechanisms, i.e. tongue, lips, palette, breath control • the intellectual ability to understand complex grammar • parts of the brain that enable understanding of language. He calls this a **Language Acquisition Device (LAD).**	response. This positive response is the reinforcement. It encourages the child to repeat the sound or word. Sounds and words that are not part of the language that the child will eventually speak are not reinforced and are therefore extinguished. This is called operant conditioning. Social interaction is important in the acquisition of language skills. **L.S. Vygotsky** Vygotsky stressed the importance of the relationship between speech and writing. He saw children's early attempts at writing as significant. Children progress from drawing things to drawing speech. This will not initially be recognisable as writing, but conceptually children have understood what writing is: the setting down or drawing of speech. This development occurs through interaction and communication with other people.

Progress check

What is the nature argument for language acquisition?

What is the nurture argument for language acquisition?

How does operant conditioning relate to language acquisition?

Why is children's drawing important in the development of language skills?

Read about the nature–nurture debate on language acquisition again. What are the problems associated with each argument?

Decide for yourself what you think is the combination of nature and nurture in children's language acquisition. Give reasons for your answer.

Sequence of language development

Children's language develops through a series of identifiable stages. These stages are sequential, as outlined in the table below. The level of children's development depends partly on their chronological age, but their experience of language from an early age is, however, just as important a factor. If children are exposed to a rich language environment, this will be reflected in their language development. Children who have not had this opportunity will not have had the same chances for development. It is important to take this into account when assessing a child's stage of language development.

Children who are bilingual may develop their languages at a slightly slower rate than children who are monolingual. This is to be expected as they have much more to learn. Given an environment that promotes language development, bilingual children will become proficient in both languages.

The sequence of language development: birth to 5 years

Approximate age	Developmental level
Birth	Involuntary cry
2–3 weeks	Signs of intentional communication: eye contact
4 weeks onwards	Cries are becoming voluntary, indicating, for example, unhappiness, tiredness, loneliness Children may respond by moving their eyes or head towards the speaker, kicking or stopping crying
6 weeks onwards	Children may smile when spoken to Cooing and gurgling begin in response to parent or carer's presence and voice, also to show contentment
1–2 months	Children may move their eyes or head towards the direction of the sound
3 months	Children will raise their head when sounds attract their attention
4–5 months	Playful sounds appear: cooing, gurgling, laughing, chuckling, squealing; these are in response to the human voice and to show contentment Children respond to familiar sounds by turning their head, kicking or stopping crying Shout to attract attention
6 months	The beginning of babbling: regular, repeated sounds, e.g. gegegegeg, mamamam, dadada; children play around with these sounds. This is important for practising sound-producing mechanisms necessary for later speech Cooing, laughing and gurgling become stronger Children begin to understand emotion in the parent or carer's voice Children begin to enjoy music and rhymes, particularly if accompanied by actions
9 months	Babbling continues and the repertoire increases Children begin to recognise their own name May understand simple, single words, e.g. No, Bye-bye Children continue to enjoy music and rhymes and will now attempt to join in with the actions, e.g. playing pat-a-cake
9–12 months	Babbling begins to reflect the intonation of speech Children may imitate simple words. This is usually an extension of babbling, e.g. dada Pointing begins. This is often accompanied by a sound or the beginnings of a word. This demonstrates an increasing awareness that words are associated with people and objects

continued

The sequence of language development: birth to 5 years continued

Approximate age	Developmental level
12 months	Children's vocabulary starts to develop. First word(s) appear, usually names of people and objects that the child is familiar with. They are built around the child's babbling sound repertoire Children understand far more than they can say. This is called a *passive* vocabulary. Spoken words are referred to as an *active* vocabulary They begin to be able to respond to simple instructions, e.g. 'Give me the ball', 'Come here', 'Clap your hands'
15 months	Active vocabulary development remains quite limited as children concentrate on achieving mobility Passive vocabulary increases rapidly Pointing accompanied by a single word is the basis of communication
18 months	Children's active vocabulary increases; this tends to be names of familiar things and people Children use their language to name belongings and point out named objects Generalisation of words is difficult, e.g. cat can only be their cat, not the one next door One word and intonation is used to indicate meaning, e.g. cup may mean, 'I want a drink', 'I have lost my cup', 'Where is my cup?'. The intonation (and possibly the situation) would indicate the meaning to people who are familiar with the child Children will repeat words and sentences
21 months	Both passive and active vocabularies rapidly increase; the passive vocabulary, however, remains larger than the active Children begin to name objects and people that are not there: this shows an awareness of what language is for Sentences begin. Initially as two-word phrases, e.g. 'Mummy gone', 'Coat on' Gesture is still a fundamental part of communication Children begin asking questions, usually 'What?', 'Who?' and 'Where?'
2 years	Both active and passive vocabularies continue to increase Children can generalise words but this sometimes means that they over-generalise, e.g. all men are daddy, all furry animals with four legs are dog Personal pronouns (words used instead of actual names) are used, e.g. I, she, he, you, they. They are not always used correctly Sentences become longer although they tend to be in telegraphic speech, i.e. only the main sense-conveying words are used, e.g. 'Mummy gone work', 'Me go bike' Questions are asked frequently, 'What?' and 'Why?'
2 years 6 months	Vocabulary increases rapidly; there is less imbalance between passive and active vocabularies Word use is more specific so there are fewer over- and under-generalisations Sentences get longer and more precise, although they are still usually abbreviated versions of adult sentences Word order in sentences is sometimes incorrect *continued*

The sequence of language development: birth to 5 years continued

Approximate age	Developmental level
2 years 6 months continued	Children can use language to protect their own rights and interests and to maintain their own comfort and pleasure, e.g. 'It's mine', 'Get off', 'I'm playing with that' Children can listen to stories and are interested in them
3 years	Vocabulary develops rapidly; new words are picked up quickly Sentences continue to become longer and more like adult speech Children talk to themselves during play: this is to plan and order their play, which is evidence of children using language to think Language can now be used to report on what is happening, to direct their own and others' actions, to express ideas and to initiate and maintain friendships Pronouns are usually used correctly Questions such as 'Why?', 'Who?' and 'What for?' are used frequently Rhymes and melody are attractive
3 years 6 months	Children have a wide vocabulary and word usage is usually correct; this continues to increase They are now able to use complete sentences, although word order is sometimes incorrect Language can now be used to report on past experiences Incorrect word endings are sometimes used, e.g. swimmed, runned, seed
4 years	Children's vocabulary is now extensive; new words are added regularly Longer and more complex sentences are used; sentences may be joined with because, which demonstrates an awareness of causes and relationships Children are able to narrate long stories, including the sequence of events Play involves running commentaries The boundaries between fact and fiction are blurred and this is reflected in children's speech Speech is fully intelligible with few, minor incorrect uses Questioning is at its peak. 'When?' is used alongside other questions By this stage children can usually use language to share, take turns, collaborate, argue, predict what may happen, compare possible alternatives, anticipate, give explanations, justify behaviour, create situations in imaginative play, reflect upon their own feelings and begin to describe how other people feel
5 years	Children have a wide vocabulary and can use it appropriately Vocabulary can include colours, shapes, numbers and common opposites, e.g. big/small, hard/soft Sentences are usually correctly structured, although incorrect grammar may still be used Pronunciation may still be childish Language continues to be used and developed, as described in the section on 4 year olds; this may now include phrases heard on the television and associated with children's toys Questions and discussions are for enquiry and information; questions become more precise as children's cognitive skills develop Children will offer opinions in discussion

LANGUAGE DEVELOPMENT: 5–8 YEARS

Between the ages of 5 and 8 years children use, practise, adapt and refine their language skills. Language is used for a wide range of purposes. Joan Tough in her book, *Listening to Children Talking* (Ward Lock Educational, 1976), identifies seven main uses of language. They provide a useful tool for observation and analysis of children's development. The uses are hierarchical, that is, that children progress through the seven stages in this order. The early stages will be observed in most children before the age of 5.

Joan Tough's seven uses of language

Use	Using language to
1 Self-maintaining	1.1 Protect oneself: *Stop it.* *Go away.* *You're hurting me.* 1.2 Meet physical and psychological needs: *I'm thirsty.* *You're hurting me.*
2 Directing	Direct the actions of self and others: *You push the lorry round the track.* I just need to put this brick here, then I've finished.
3 Reporting	3.1 Label the component parts of a scene: *There is a car, a lorry and a bus.* 3.2 Refer to detail, the colour, shape, size or position of an object 3.3 Talk about an incident: *I fell out of bed last night.* 3.4 Refer to a sequence of events: *We walked to the bus stop and then caught the bus to school.* 3.5 Reflect on the meanings of experiences, including feelings: *I like playing in the shop, especially with Sarah.*
4 Towards logical reasoning	4.1 Explain a process: *I made some tea. First I put the teabag in the pot, then I poured boiling water on to it.* 4.2 Recognise causal and dependent relationships: *You have put sugar in this tea so it doesn't taste very nice.* 4.3 Recognise problems and their causes: *This box isn't big enough to put all these cars in. We need a bigger box.* 4.4 Justify judgements and actions: *I didn't want to go out because I hadn't finished my drawing.*
5 Predicting	5.1 Anticipate or forecast: *We're going to have a hamster and it will have to have a cage with a wheel.* 5.2 Predict the consequences of actions or events: *That propeller will fall off if you don't stick it on properly.*
6 Projecting	6.1 Project into the experiences, feelings and reactions of others: *He was stuck in there and didn't know how to get out and he was frightened.* 6.2 Project into a situation never experienced: *I wouldn't like to be a rabbit and live in a cage, would you?*
7 Imagining	In an imagined context: *Hello, this is Hot Scissors hairdressers. Would you like to make an appointment?*

Progress check

What are the important factors in children's language development?

What is a rich language environment?

Why is it impossible to give an exact age for each stage of development?

Talking with children

The most important factor in children's language development is interaction with other people. It is important that people who work with young children adopt practices that contribute positively to children's language development. There is a recognised link between the quality of adult input and the quality of children's language. Listed below are some important points to remember when talking with children. However, these are only practical points. A sensitivity towards children's needs and knowledge of them as individuals are the basis of positive interaction.

When talking to children, remember . . .	
The tone of your voice	Does it convey warmth and interest in the child?
How quickly you speak	Do you speak at a pace that is appropriate for the child or children you are talking with?
Listening	How do you show the child that you are listening? Eye contact and getting down to the child's level show that you are listening. Becoming involved in the conversation also indicates that you are listening and interested.
Waiting	Do you leave enough time for the child to respond? Young children may need time to formulate their response. It is important to remember that pauses and silences are part of conversation.
Questions	Do you ask too many questions? This may make the conversation feel like a question-and-answer session, especially if your response is 'That's right'. What type of questions do you ask? Closed questions require a one-word answer and do not give the child the opportunity to practise and develop their language skills. Open questions have a range of possible answers and do give the child the opportunity to practise and develop their language skills.
Your personal contribution	Do you contribute your own experience and/or opinions to the conversation? Conversation is a two-way process. It involves both people sharing information. This should be the same with children. It is important that the choice of what to talk about is shared.

continued

When talking to children, remember . . . continued	
What do you talk about?	How much of what you say is management talk? How much is conversation and chatting? How much is explaining? How much is playful talk? Children need to be involved in a wide range of language experiences to enable them to practise and develop their own language.
Developing thought	Do you ask for and give reasons and explanations when talking with children? Do you encourage the child to make predictions in real and imaginary situations? Do you encourage the children to give accounts of what they are doing or have done? Children's language and cognitive skills can be developed in this way.
Who do you talk to?	You must talk to all children within the group. All children need the opportunity to practise their language. There will be a range of developmental levels within every group of children and it is important that each child's needs are met.

Progress check

Why is it important that people who work with young children know how to interact effectively with children?

What is the basis for positive interaction with children?

Identify some of the ways in which adults can interact with children effectively.

Planning for and monitoring children's language development

Children learn and develop their language skills through interaction with other people. Adults therefore have a vital role to play in children's language development through talking and listening to them. Careful consideration also needs to be given to the activities and experiences provided for children. Appropriately planned activities or experiences provide the opportunity for children to use their existing skills and develop others.

Before planning it is necessary to assess each child's level of development. This can be done through careful observation of the child. Once the level is established, relevant experiences and activities can be planned to meet the child's needs. During the experience or activity the adult needs to adopt a variety of strategies to promote each child's language development.

The monitoring, planning, preparation and interaction with children is a continual process. As children develop their language skills the adult needs to respond to their changing needs.

The child/children:

- What language is being used?
- Are the children's needs being met?
- Are all children able to participate in a group situation?
- Was there anything significant about what was observed?
- Does anything need recording?

The activity or experience:

- Are the activities or experiences provided appropriate for child/children?
- Were the adults involved clear about the focus?
- Was the timing appropriate?
- Was there anything significant about what was observed?
- Does any information need recording?

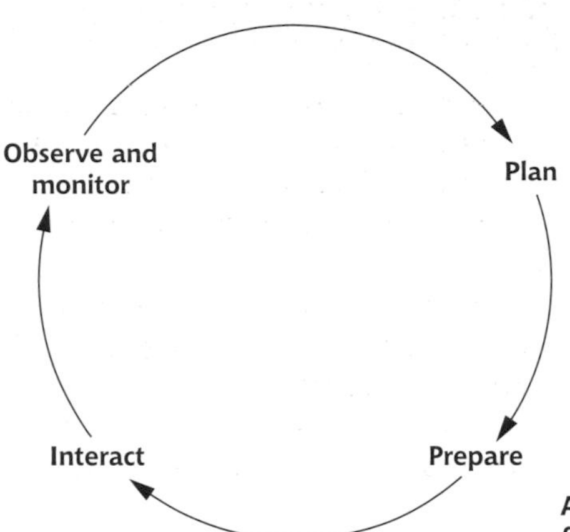

What are the child/children's language needs?
What are the child/children's development levels?
What is the range of development levels?
What time is available?
What are the staffing levels and responsibilities?

Are the staff aware of the focus of the activity or experience?
Are all the necessary equipment and materials available?

Strategies for interaction with the child/children include:

- discussing events with the child/children
- providing a commentary on what is happening
- describing events
- asking open-ended questions
- introducing new vocabulary
- suggesting ideas for extending the experience or activity.

Planning and monitoring children's language development

MONITORING CHILDREN'S LANGUAGE DEVELOPMENT

A key aspect of effective planning and interaction with children is monitoring their developmental level. In this way the activities and experiences can be made relevant to the children's needs. Monitoring development, in all areas, is an ongoing process. It can be done in many ways. However children's development is monitored, ways need to be found to incorporate this information into the planning process, so that provision is relevant to the children in the group.

Effective child-care workers informally monitor children's development through their daily interaction with the children. Their intimate knowledge of individual children enables them to identify when progress has been made, and when a child may need support. This can be particularly effective where there is a key worker system in place. This information should inform the planning process, and interaction should be adjusted accordingly.

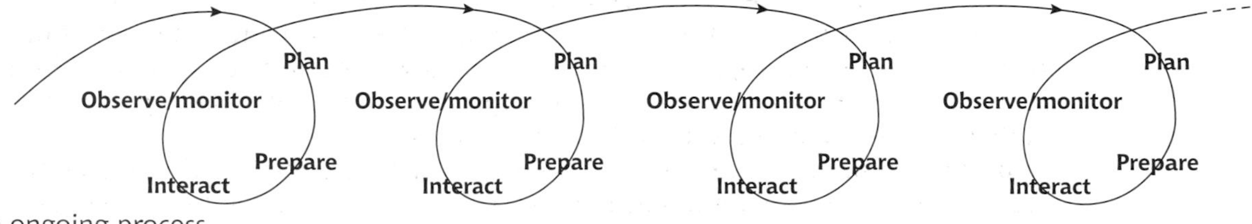

The ongoing process

Some establishments also monitor children's language development formally. They may use a checklist, developmental chart or diary. In this way, a written record of each child's development is available to inform planning and interaction.

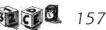

It is important to be aware, when assessing children's language developmental level, that there is sometimes a difference between a child's actual language ability and their ability to use expressive (spoken) language. For example, some children whose grasp of language is excellent may be quiet in a group of children. This is not a reflection of their language ability, but of the way in which they operate socially. Similarly, bilingual children may be very competent in their first language and passively understand most things in their second language. Their apparent lack of expressive skills is not necessarily an indication of their language developmental level.

Progress check

Why is it important for an adult to be aware of each child's level of language development?

What is involved in monitoring children's language use and developmental level?

What is involved in planning experiences or activities to promote language development?

Why is it important that all the adults involved with the child are aware of the focus of the language work?

List the ways in which an adult can interact with a child to promote their language development.

Factors affecting language development

To develop language successfully children need a rich, stimulating environment that provides the opportunity for experiences appropriate to their level of development. There are a number of factors that influence the quality of the language environment:

- the presence of positive role models
- the opportunity for the children to practise their language skills
- positive feedback to enable the children to pick up language and to adjust and refine their language skills.

THE EFFECTS OF TELEVISION

Television, video and computer games are enjoyed by many young children. They have a useful role to play in broadening children's experience, bringing the wider world within their reach, and they provide very good entertainment. However, there are some concerns that long spells in front of the television, video or computer can have a detrimental affect on children's language development. For children's language to develop successfully, they need to practise their skills with someone who knows them and is aware of their capabilities and needs. They rely on feedback that is individual and immediate to encourage them to respond and develop their skills. The point is not that television in itself is harmful to children's language development, but rather that it is no substitute for the carer who is 'tuned in' to the child and can plan for and meet the child's language needs. There are also concerns that too many hours in front of the computer screen can interfere with children's abilities to use language socially in face-to-face situations.

SUPPORTING CHILDREN WITH LANGUAGE DELAY

All children come to a care setting with different experiences. This includes their experience of language. Because the experiences that a child has had are so influential in their development, the pace at which children develop language is not uniform. Within any group of children there will be a wide range of proficiency in language. This could include children who have delayed language development in relation to the expected range of norms; it could also include children who are beyond the expected range of norms. It is important that each child is treated as an individual and that their needs are assessed and met.

When a child's language development is delayed, there are a number of agencies who may be involved in meeting the child's needs. The extent of provision for children with language delay will vary from area to area. Some of the agencies who may be involved are:

- health visitor
- speech therapist
- portage worker
- language unit
- nursery staff
- individual classroom support
- support from charitable organisations, for example Barnardos, NCH Action for Children
- local initiatives, including self-help groups.

Progress check

List the factors that contribute positively to children's language development.

Why might television and videos have a detrimental effect on children's language development?

What do you understand by the term 'language delay'?

Name four agencies that might be involved in supporting children with language delay.

Now try these questions

What is meant by the term language development?

How can the carer support the language development of:
(a) a 1 year old? (b) a 4 year old?

How can the child-care setting meet the needs of bilingual children?

Describe the adult's role in planning and monitoring children's language development.

How can the child-care worker contribute positively to children's language development?

key terms

You need to know what the key terms and phrases in this chapter mean.
Go back through the chapter and find out.

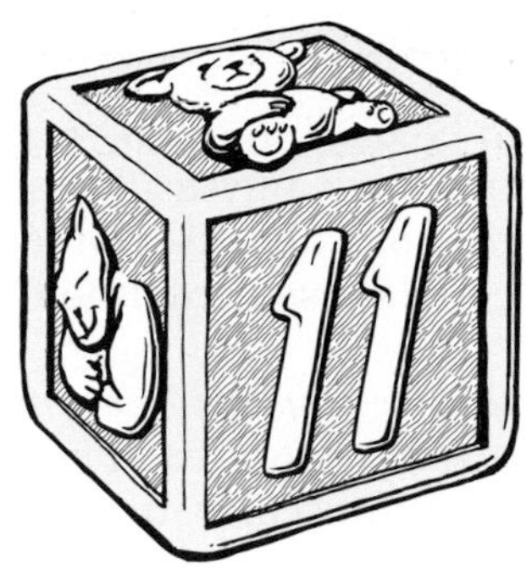

PHYSICAL DEVELOPMENT

In the first year of life physical and cognitive development are closely related, and the achievement of landmark skills are thought to be an indication of the child's intellectual maturity. Delay in the development of physical skills at this age can indicate learning difficulties. As the child gets older, physical development continues at a slower pace, but the achievement of skills is still dependent upon maintaining health and preventing illness. This chapter includes a brief introduction to physical development, followed by detailed descriptions of the average physical achievements to be expected at various ages.

This chapter will cover the following topics:

- an introduction to physical development
- the capabilities of the neonate
- physical development at 1 month
- physical development at 3 months
- physical development at 6 months
- physical development at 9 months
- physical development at 12 months
- physical development at 15 months
- physical development at 18 months
- physical development at 2 years
- physical development at 3 years
- physical development at 4 years
- physical development at 5 years
- physical development at 6 years
- physical development at 7 years
- variations in developmental progress
- the role of the adult.

An introduction to physical development

key terms

Skill
an ability that has been practised

Motor development
the process of muscular movements becoming more complex

Physical means anything to do with the body and can be used in a wide range of contexts, from how people look physically to how they move physically.

Development means a change in performance and is usually associated with progression, becoming more complicated or skilful. It could also be defined as an increase in complexity.

With these two definitions you can see that the phrase *physical development* means the way that the body increases in **skill** and becomes more complex in its performance. This will involve movement. The progress of muscular movement is called **motor development**.

DEVELOPMENTAL NORMS

key terms

Norm
developmental skill achieved within an average time-scale

Fine motor skills
hand–eye co-ordination

Gross motor skills
whole body movements

There is a recognised pattern of physical development that children are expected to follow. These are known as the developmental **norms**. Norm should not be confused with normal, a word that is not encouraged when describing physical development because there is such a wide range of normal (i.e. acceptable or satisfactory) development. It is dangerous to assume that children are abnormal if they do not all progress in exactly the same manner. Variations will always exist, since each child is an individual developing in their own unique way.

A likely expectation is that babies will be mobile (rolling, crawling, creeping, bottom-shuffling or walking) by the time they reach their first birthday. However, a baby may have been concentrating on acquiring **fine motor skills**, social skills or language skills and may have advanced beyond the average in one or more of these developmental areas. In the development of **gross motor skills**, they may not have progressed beyond sitting, but have been absorbing huge amounts of information from the world around them. Examining only their lack of mobility could make the examiner assume that their development was delayed, but the overall picture is of a child who has not yet seen the need for mobility but can do many other things in advance of their age.

Nevertheless, knowledge of these patterns of expected development does help us to look at the child as a whole, and to measure their progress as an individual.

HUMAN ATTRIBUTES

The human animal (we are all animals) has several biological attributes, different from most other animals, which make it easy to separate the different areas of development:

- the ability to stand on two legs and walk, leaving the hands free for more complicated tasks – a gross motor skill
- the use of the hands and flexible fingers in co-ordination with the eyes – fine motor skills
- possession of a spoken language, and the ability to translate non-verbal messages, allowing communication between people
- the evolution of complicated social structures for the benefit and protection of all individuals.

The first two human characteristics are relevant to the study of physical development because they concern movement, so it is necessary to look at them separately and in more detail.

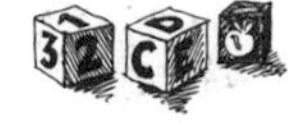

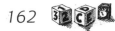

Gross motor skills

key term

Posture
position of parts of the body

The ability of the human animal to use two legs and walk involves the whole body. These whole-body movements are described as gross motor skills. Sometimes they are referred to as **posture** and large movements. These terms have the same meaning and cover the stages a child goes through in developing control of the body:

- learning to support the head
- rolling over
- sitting
- crawling
- pulling to stand
- walking
- running
- climbing the stairs
- hopping
- playing football
- skipping
- riding a tricycle and a bicycle
- standing on one leg
- swimming
- climbing

are examples of gross motor skills. They all require strength, stamina and suppleness to increase co-ordination, balance and judgement.

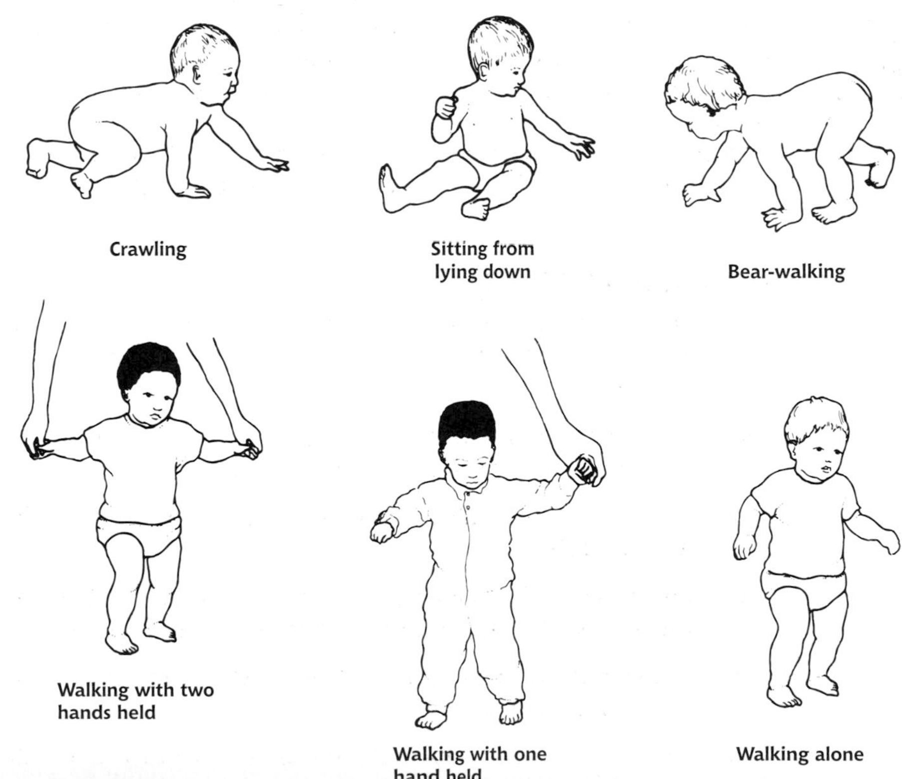
Crawling
Sitting from lying down
Bear-walking
Walking with two hands held
Walking with one hand held
Walking alone

Examples of gross motor skills involved in the development of walking

Fine motor skills

The second human characteristic is the use of the hands in co-ordination with the eyes. This allows human beings to perform very delicate procedures with their fingers, with the eyes influencing the precise movements of the fingers. These manipulative aspects of physical development are called fine motor skills, and include aspects of vision and fine and delicate movements.

The role of those who monitor the physical development of children is to know whether a child can easily perform a certain skill or whether it is a new skill for them and they require further practice.

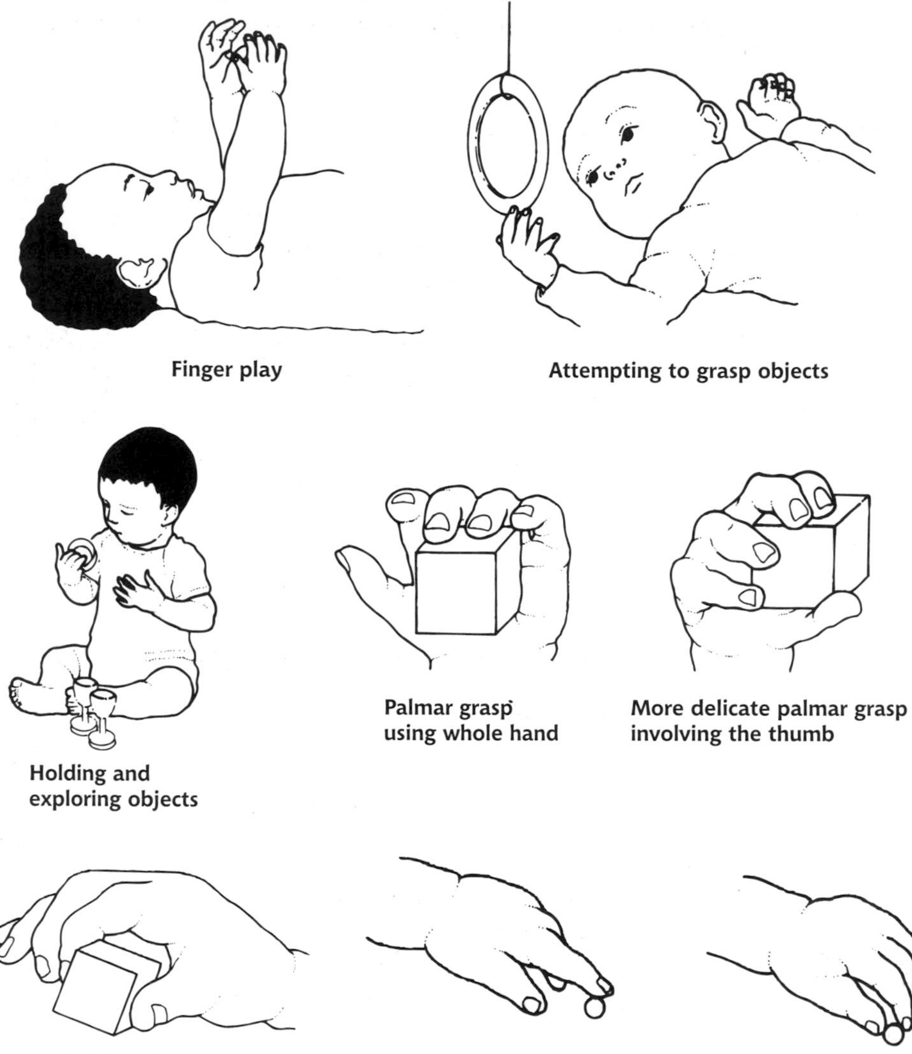

Development of manipulation (fine motor skills)

Progress check

What does motor development mean?

Why should you beware of using the word 'normal' in describing development?

What are the four characteristics that make humans different from most other animals?

The neonate

key term
neonate
a newborn baby

The newborn baby in the first month of life is often called the **neonate**, which means newly born.

New babies have an attitude of flexion, which means that they are curled up, with arms and legs bent inwards towards the body. They maintain this fetal position (the position they were in inside the womb), but gradually extend (straighten) the arms and legs. A baby who was in the breech position may lie with the legs straight up, one each side of the face, if this was the position in the womb.

Descriptions of the typical postures of neonates are shown below.

key term
prone
lying face down

GROSS MOTOR DEVELOPMENT

Prone

- The baby lies with the head turned to one side resting on the cheek.
- The body is in a frog-like posture with the bottom up and the knees curled up under the tummy.
- The arms are bent at the elbows and tucked under the chest with fists clenched.

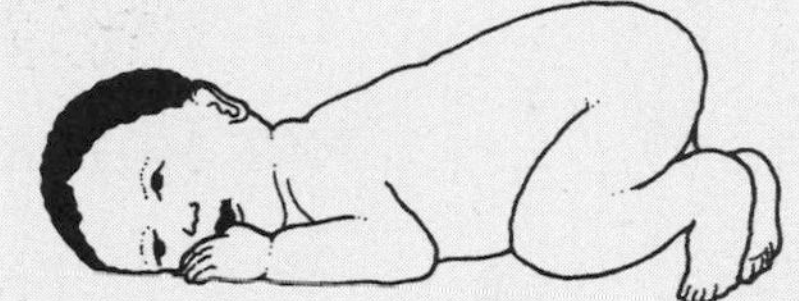

key term
supine
lying on the back

Supine

- The baby lies with the head to one side.
- The knees are bent towards the body, with the soles of the feet touching.
- The arms are bent inwards towards the body.
- Jerky, random, asymmetrical kicking movements can be seen.

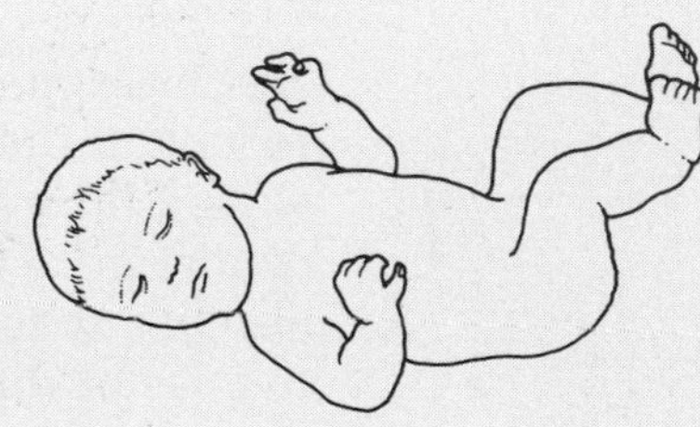

key term
ventral suspension
when the baby is held in the air, face down

Ventral suspension

- The head and the legs fall below the level of the back, so the baby makes a complete downwards curve.

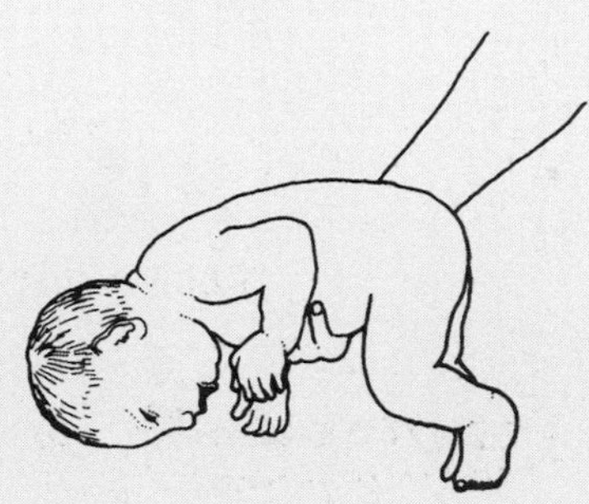

The neonate (continued)

Sitting

key term

head lag
The baby's head falls back when pulled to sit

- When the baby is pulled upwards into a sitting position there is complete **head lag**. The head falls backwards as the body comes up and then flops forwards on to the chest.
- If the baby is held in a sitting position, the back is completely curved and the head is on the chest.

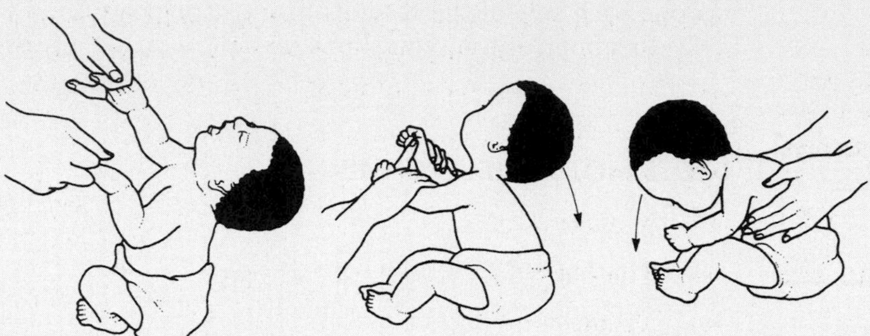

FINE MOTOR DEVELOPMENT

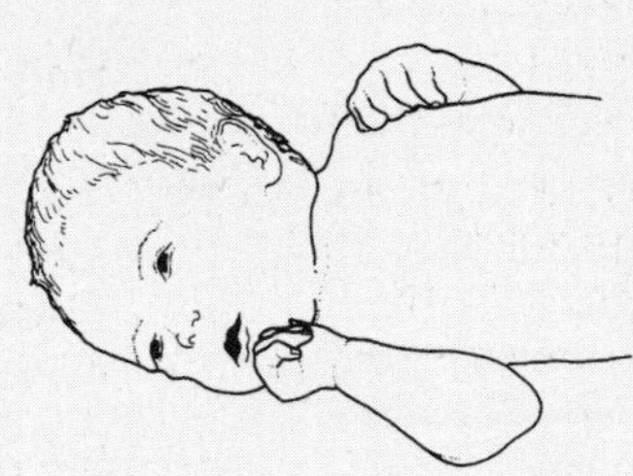

- The fists are clenched.
- The baby can focus 15–25 cm and stares at brightly coloured mobiles within visual range.
- The baby concentrates on the carer's face when feeding.

VISION

Neonates can focus on faces close to their own, and research shows that they prefer to look at the human face. They have skills of imitation and may try to copy facial expressions and movements, for example sticking the tongue out. These are not deliberate actions. Eye contact with parents helps to establish interaction. Babies also like to look at brightly-coloured objects – red, green, blue, yellow – rather than the pastel shades that are often used for nursery equipment. Flat pictures will not generate as much interest as three-dimensional, 'real' objects, such as toys and rattles with faces, mobiles and baby gyms.

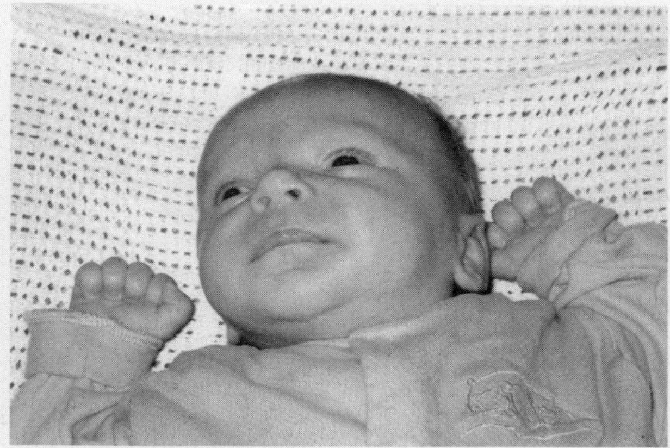

Fine motor development. Fists are clenched

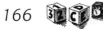

The neonate

PRIMITIVE REFLEXES

A **reflex** action is an automatic, involuntary movement made in response to a specific **stimulus**. Testing the presence of reflexes in babies, children and adults can help doctors to assess the health of the **central nervous system** (CNS). Everyone should have a range of protective reflexes, like blinking, coughing and sneezing. New babies have a range of other survival reflexes, called the **primitive reflexes**, which are only present during the first few months of life. After this they are replaced by actions which the baby chooses to do – **voluntary actions**. The primitive reflexes are a reminder of how the human race has evolved over millions of years. They are:

- rooting reflex
- sucking reflex
- grasping reflex
- placing reflex
- walking reflex
- Moro (startle) reflex.

key terms

reflex
an involuntary response to a stimulus

stimulus
something that arouses a reaction

central nervous system
the brain, spinal cord and nerves

primitive reflex
an automatic response to a particular stimulus in a neonate

voluntary action
an intentional act that a child chooses to do

Rooting reflex

- Stimulus: brushing the cheek with a finger or nipple.
- Response: the baby turns to the side of the stimulus.

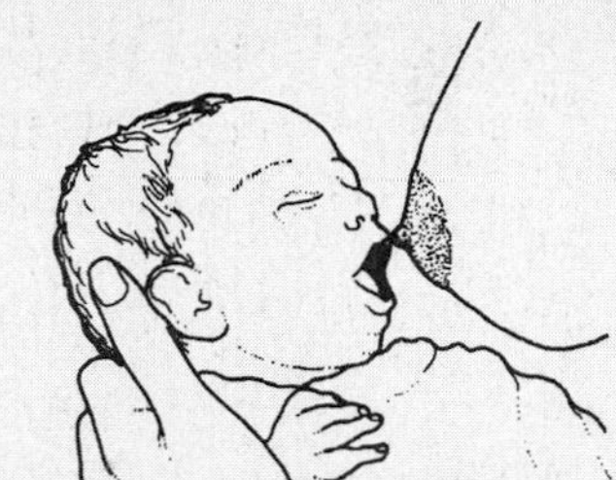

Sucking reflex

- Stimulus: placing nipple or teat into the mouth.
- Response: the baby sucks.

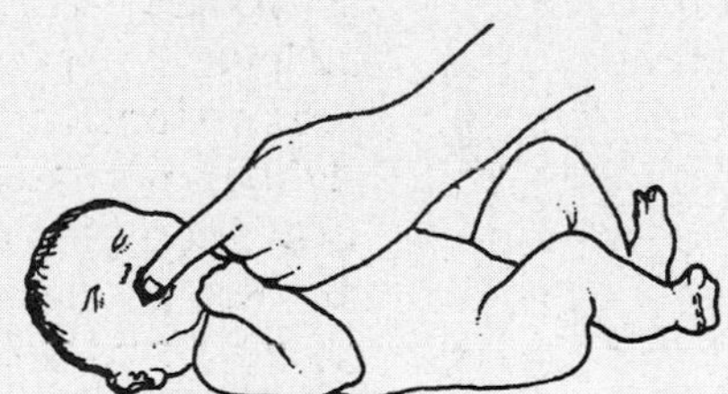

Grasping reflex

- Stimulus: placing object into baby's palm.
- Response: the fingers close tightly around the object.

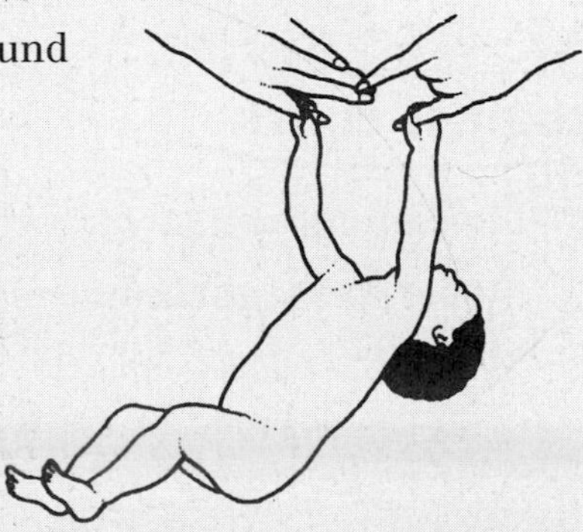

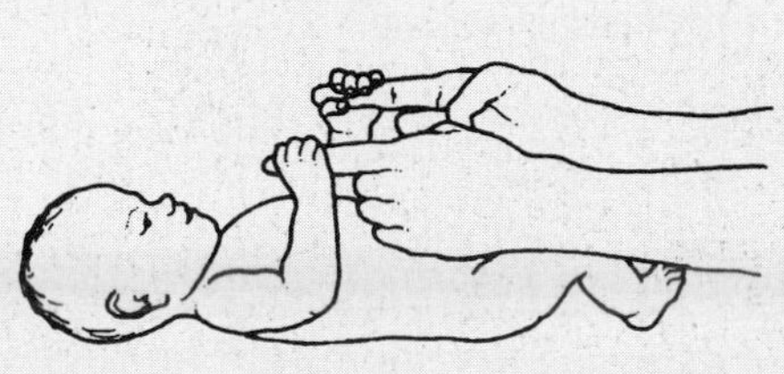

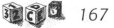

The neonate (continued)

WHY PRIMITIVE REFLEXES ARE IMPORTANT

The presence or absence of these reflexes in a new baby can measure the maturity of the baby and the health of the central nervous system. For instance, a baby born prematurely may not have developed full reflex action. If these reflexes continue for longer than the first few months of life, it can mean that the child has some form of developmental delay and should be examined by a paediatrician.

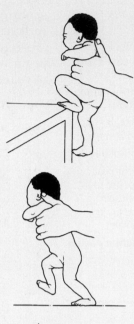

Placing reflex

- Stimulus: brushing top of foot against table top.
- Response: the baby lifts its foot and places it on a hard surface.

Walking reflex

- Stimulus: held standing, feet touching a hard surface.
- Response: the baby moves the legs forward alternately and walks.

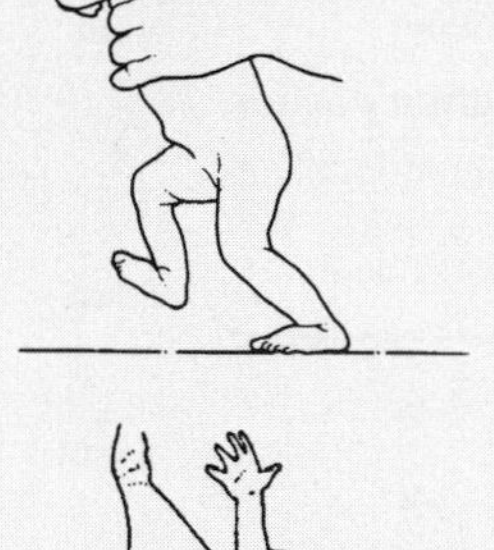

Moro (startle) reflex

- Stimulus: insecure handling or sudden loud noise.
- Response: the baby throws the head and the fingers fan out; the arms then return to the embrace posture and the baby cries.

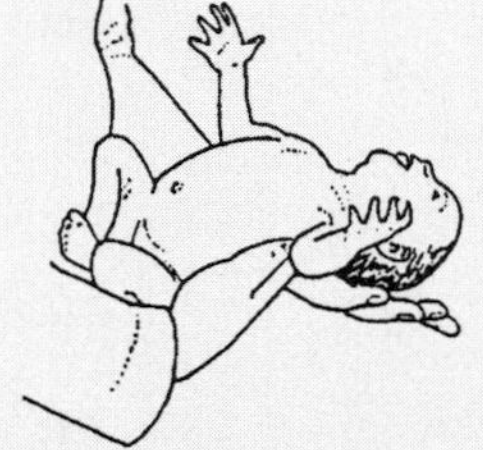

TESTING THE PRIMITIVE REFLEXES

Examination should only be performed by a qualified doctor, midwife or health visitor. The best time to observe and test these reflexes is when the baby is awake but not hungry, quietly lying with the eyes open and with or without arm and leg movements. A crying baby who is hungry, uncomfortable or unhappy, or a baby who is tired or drowsy, will not perform well. It may be possible to accompany a parent for the baby's 6-week check and observe the doctor testing the reflexes.

Progress check

What is the posture of a neonate in prone and supine?

What does ventral suspension mean?

What is a reflex?

Describe the reflex, stimulus and response of six primitive reflexes.

Why are these reflexes important in assessing development?

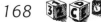

1 month

The infant continues to sleep for long periods between feeds, but is wakeful for varying lengths of time. She enjoys being played with, physical contact and cuddles. Crying is still the main form of communication for letting carers know that the baby's needs must be met, for example hunger, thirst, discomfort due to position, temperature or a desire for physical contact. Making throaty noises of pleasure when being spoken to and enjoying caring routines and attention, the baby will begin to coo at 5 to 6 weeks. The baby maintains an attitude of flexion, but the limbs are beginning to extend, with large jerky movements. Support for the head when being carried, bathed and dressed is very important.

GROSS MOTOR DEVELOPMENT

Prone

- The baby lies with its head to one side but can now lift its head to change position.
- The legs are bent, no longer tucked under the body.
- The arms are bent away from the body, the hands usually closed.

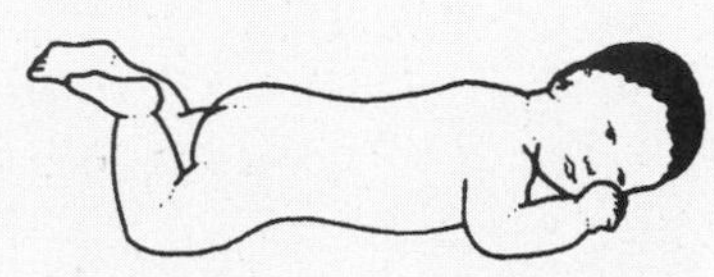

Supine

- The head is on one side.
- The arm and leg on the side the head is facing will stretch out.
- Both arms may be bent, with legs bent at the knees, the soles of the feet facing each other.

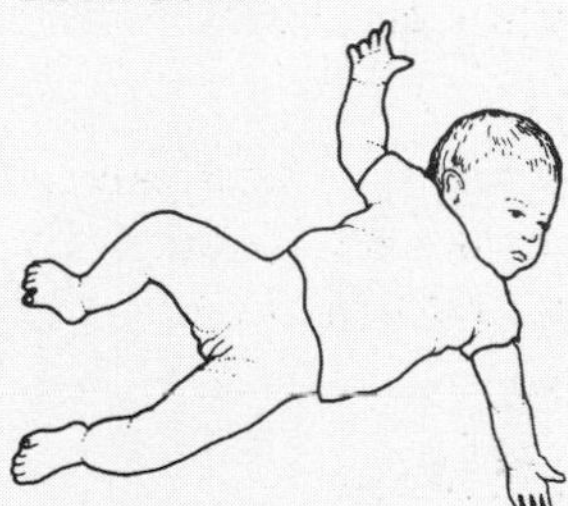

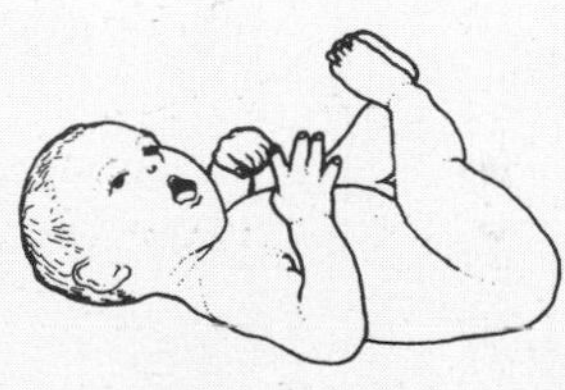

Ventral suspension

- The head is on the same level as the back and the legs are coming up towards the level of the back.

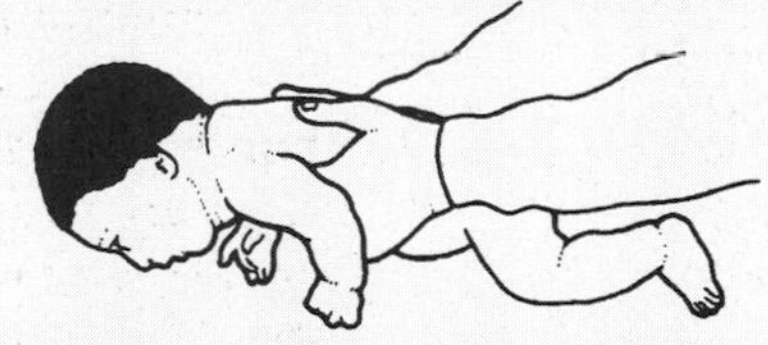

Sitting

- If the baby is pulled to sit the head will lag, falling backwards, but will remain steady for a moment as sitting position is achieved, then it will bob forwards again.
- The back is a complete curve when the baby is held in sitting position.

Note:
The head should be supported at all times.

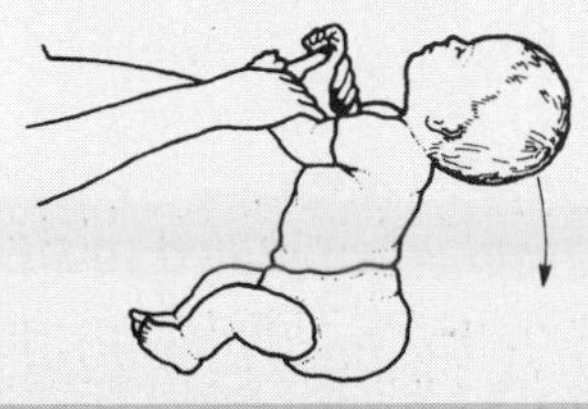

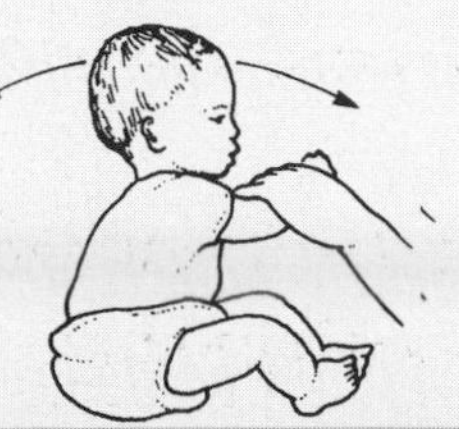

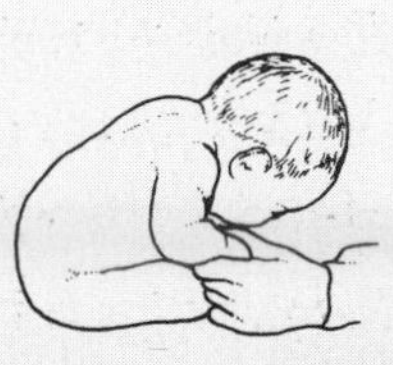

1 month

FINE MOTOR DEVELOPMENT

- The baby turns its head towards the light and stares at bright, shiny objects.

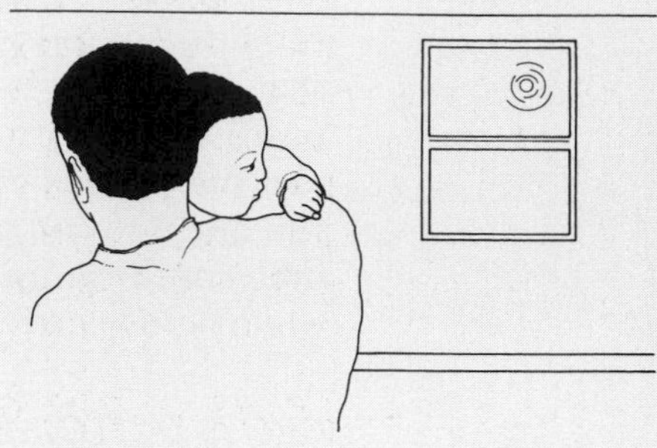

- The baby is fascinated by bright shiny objects and follows moving objects within 5–10 cm from the face.

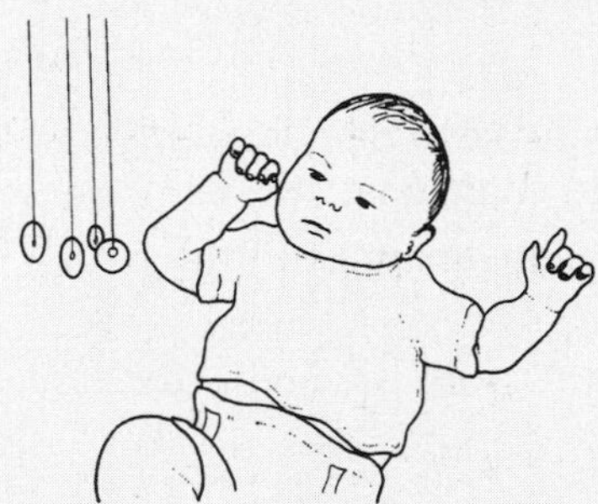

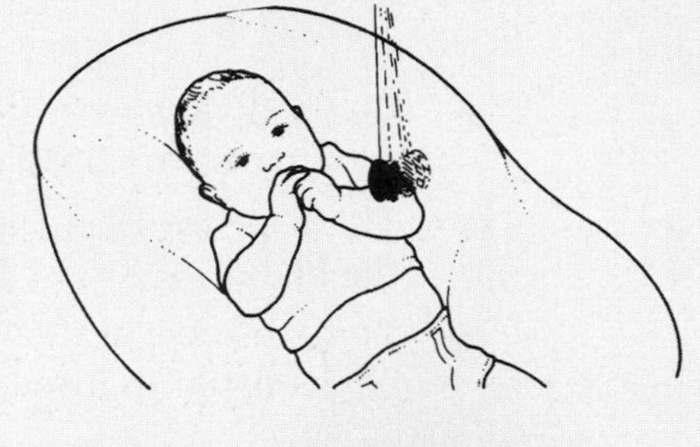

- The baby gazes attentively at carer's face while being fed, spoken to or during any caring routines.
- The baby grasps a finger or other object placed in the hand.

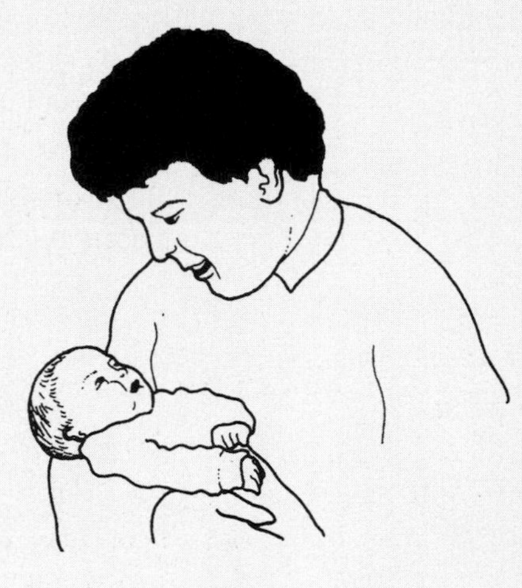

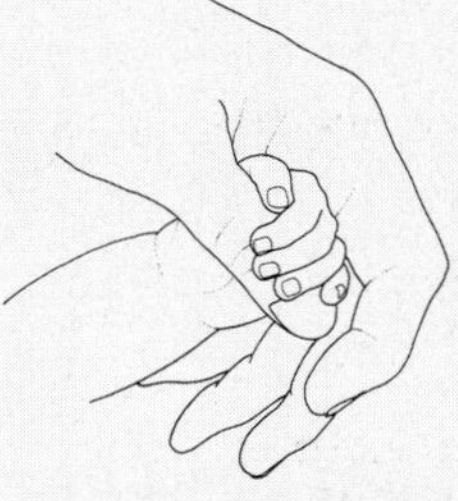

- The hands are usually closed.
- All primitive reflexes are still present.

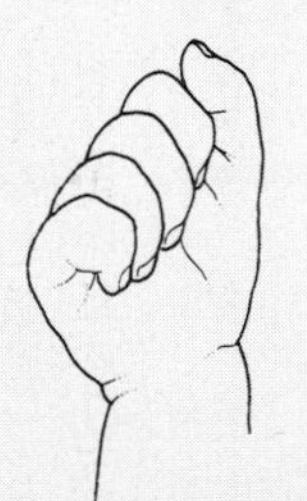

Progress check

Describe the typical position in prone of a baby aged 1 month.

Describe the typical position in supine of a baby aged 1 month.

What is meant by head lag?

At this age, how does the baby control its head when pulled to sit?

What is the position of the head in relation to the back in ventral suspension at 1 month?

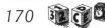

3 months

By now, most babies are developing voluntary movements to replace the primitive reflexes. They are wakeful for longer periods of time and show awareness of familiar situations by smiling, cooing and by excited limb movements when, for example, they hear the bath water running or see the breast or bottle. Babies enjoy all the contact and stimulation of the caring routines of bathing, feeding and changing. They need support at the shoulders during bathing and dressing, even though head control should be fairly well established. They may hold objects briefly, but are unable to co-ordinate hands and eyes yet.

GROSS MOTOR DEVELOPMENT

Prone

- The baby can now lift up the head and chest supported on the elbows, forearms and hands.
- The baby may scratch at the floor and bob the head in a rocking movement.
- The bottom is flat now, with the legs straighter and kicking alternately.

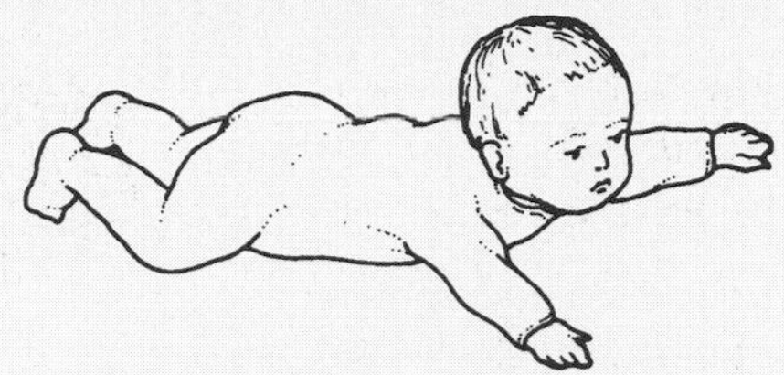

Supine

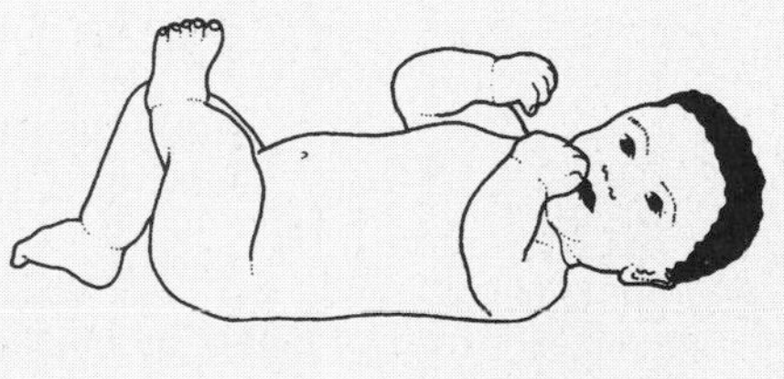

- The baby usually lies with the head in a central position.
- There are smooth, continuous movements of the arms and legs.
- The legs can kick strongly, sometimes alternating and sometimes together.
- The baby waves the arms symmetrically and brings hands together over the body.

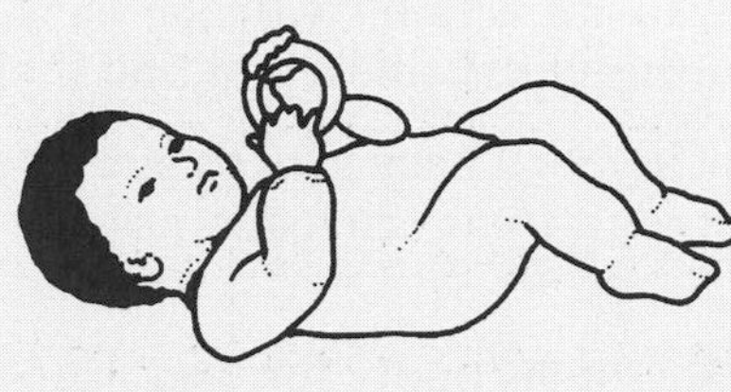

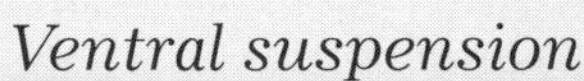

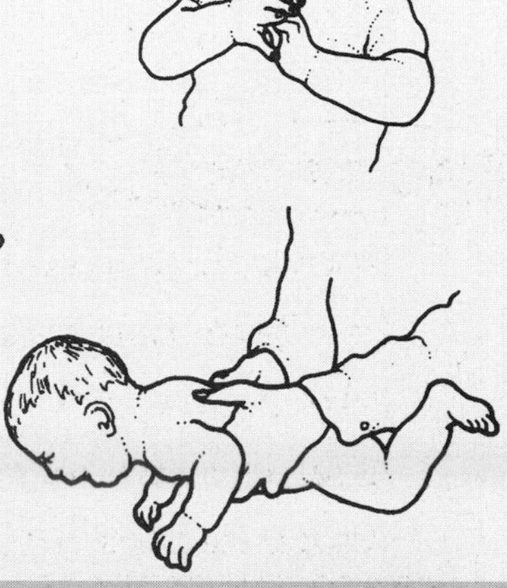

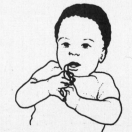

Ventral suspension

The head is now held up above the level of the back, and the legs are also on the same level.

3 months (continued)

Sitting

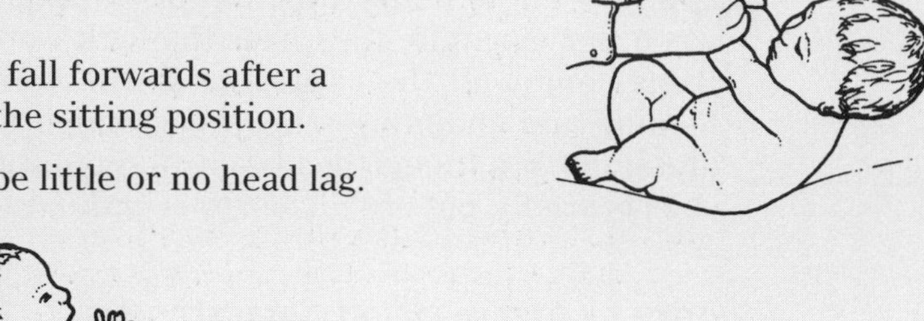

- When the baby is pulled to sit, the head should come forwards steadily with the back.
- The head may fall forwards after a short time in the sitting position.
- There should be little or no head lag.

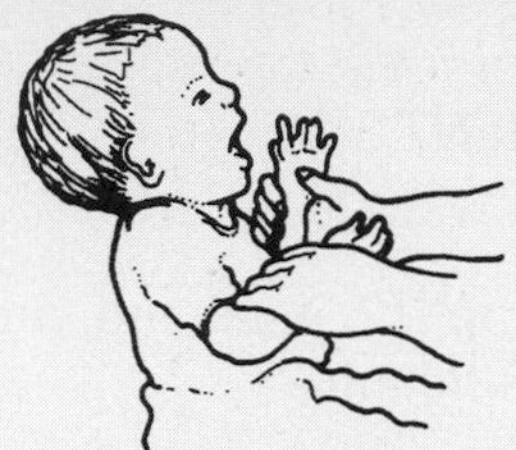

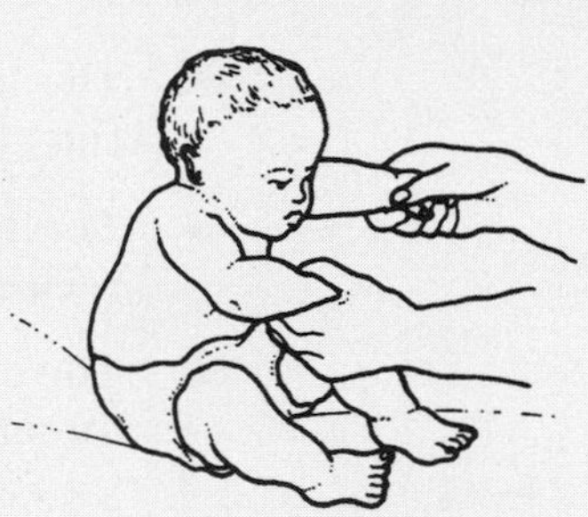

- When held in a sitting position the back should be straight, except for a curve in the base of the spine – the lumbar region.

Standing

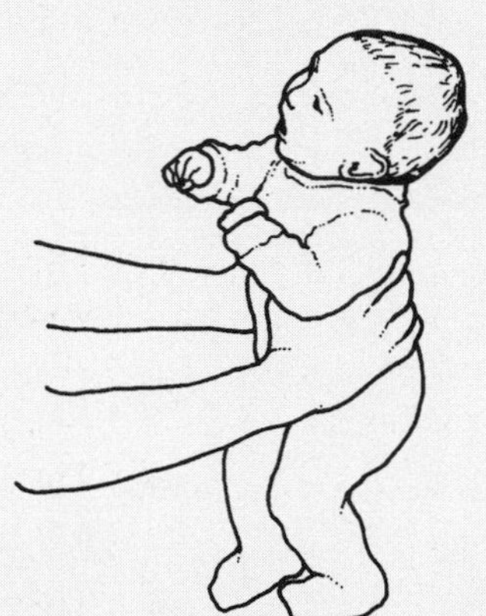

- The baby will sag at the knees when held in a standing position.
- The placing and walking reflexes should have disappeared.

STIMULATING ACTIVITIES AT 3 MONTHS

- Offer toys that a baby can hold as well as look at, for example brightly coloured rattles made of light, safe materials which produce interesting sounds, or a chiming ball.
- Blowing bubbles fascinates babies at this age as they watch them float and pop.
- Sing songs with actions with the baby sitting on your knee, giving the baby the opportunity to bounce and find their feet.
- Toys attached to a baby gym or strung over the cot will stimulate the baby to reach out with their arms and provide the stimulus for grasping interesting objects.
- Provide the opportunity for exercise – let the baby lie safely on a floor mat without a nappy or clothing so that they can explore their movements and develop further their co-ordination skills. Place the baby in prone to help them to develop the strength to support their upper body on their forearms and to prepare for rolling their body over.

3 months

FINE MOTOR DEVELOPMENT

- Finger-play – the baby has discovered its hands and moves them around in front of the face, watching the movements and the patterns they make in the light.

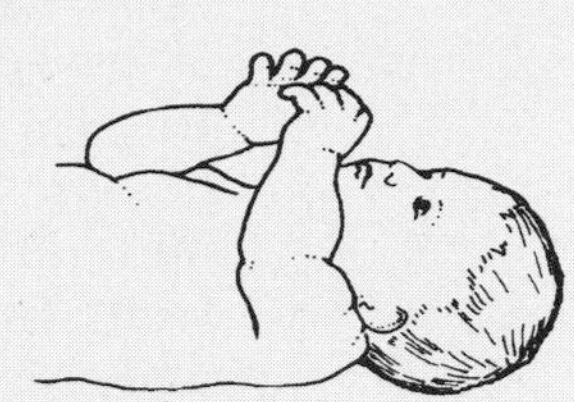

- The baby holds a rattle or similar object for a short time if placed in the hand. Frequently hits itself in the face before dropping it!

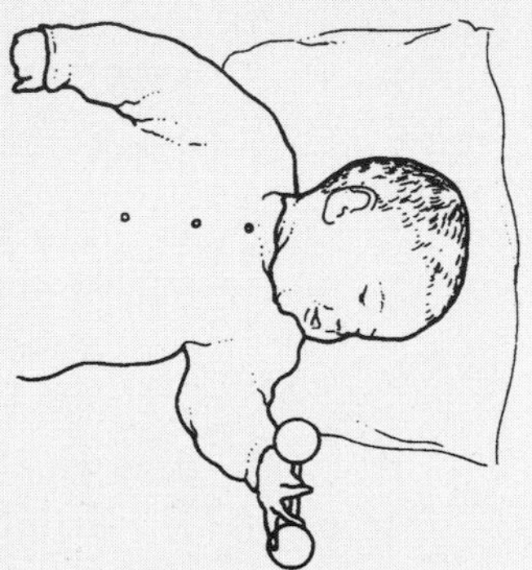

- The baby recognises the bottle or the breast and waves the arms around in excitement.

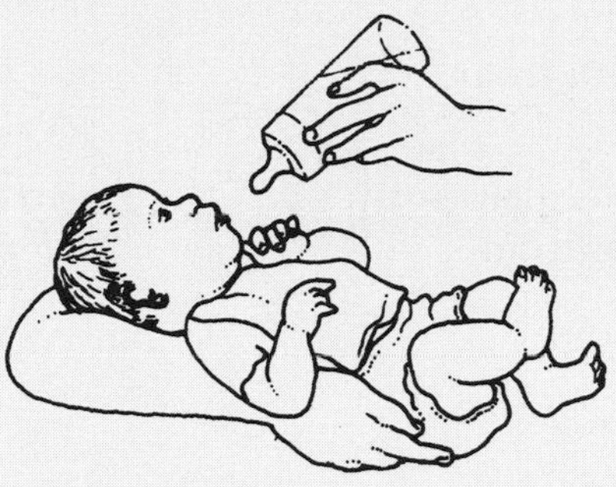

- The baby is now very alert and aware of what is going on around.
- The baby moves its head to look around, and follows adult movements.

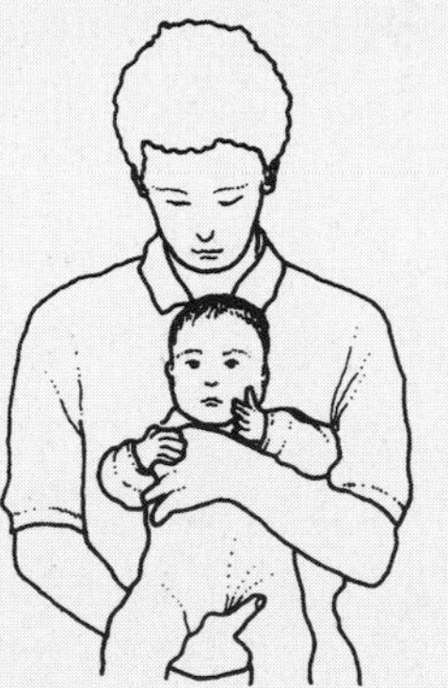

Progress check

What is the position of the baby in ventral suspension at:
(a) birth? (b) 1 month? (c) 3 months?

What are three major elements of gross motor development at 3 months?

Describe three fine motor achievements at about 3 months.

How can physical development be stimulated between birth and 3 months?

Which reflexes should have disappeared by 3 months?

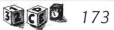

6 months

The baby at 6 months is usually lively and sociable, not yet wary of strangers but welcoming of all friendly interest, usually responding with laughs and loud, tuneful vocalisations. Babbling with double syllables, for example *dada*, *nana*, begins, accompanied by a developing understanding of commonly used words and phrases, for example 'No'. The routine screening hearing test is conducted from 6 months onwards. Physical skills are quite extensive and may include rolling and grasping.

GROSS MOTOR DEVELOPMENT

Prone

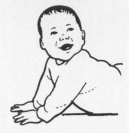

- The baby can now lift the head and chest well clear of the floor by supporting on outstretched arms. The hands are flat on the floor.
- The baby can roll over from front to back.
- She may pull the knees up in an attempt to crawl, but will slide backwards.

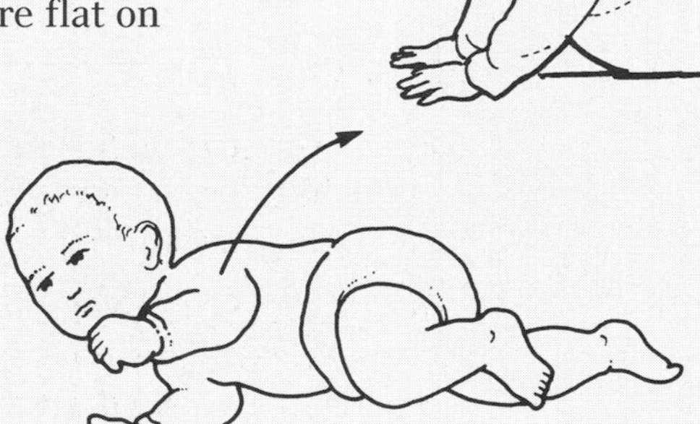

Supine

- The baby will lift her head to look at her feet.
- She may lift her arms, requesting to be lifted.

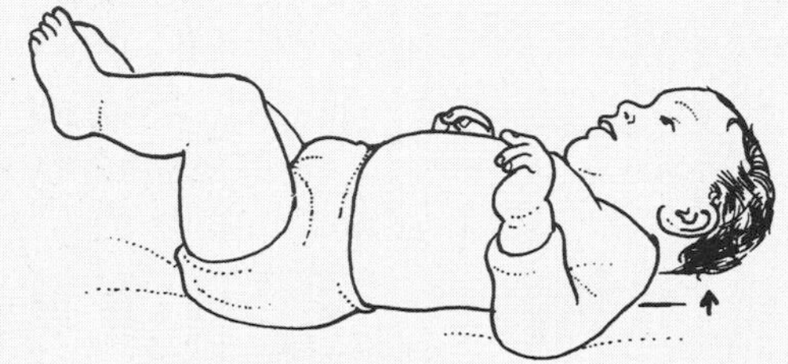

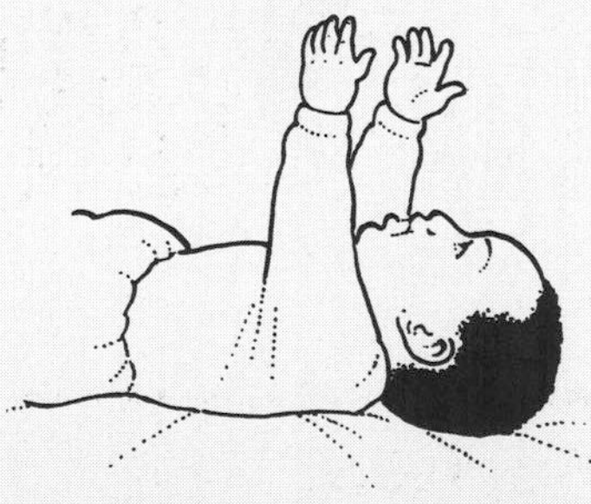

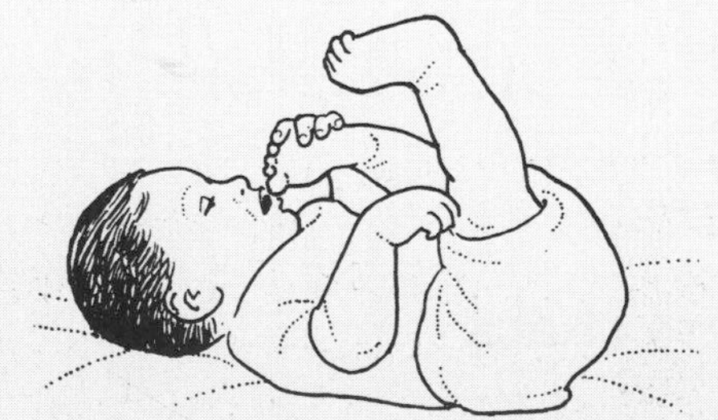

- She may lift up her legs, grasp one or both and attempt to put them in her mouth, often successfully.
- She may roll over from back to front.
- She will kick strongly, enjoying the exercise.

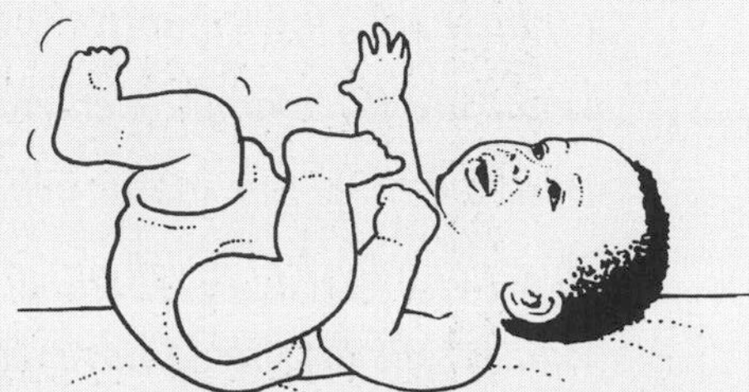

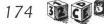

6 months (continued)

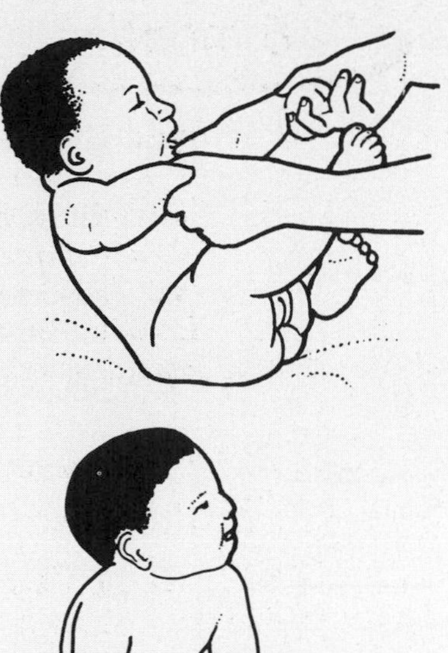

Sitting

- If pulled to sit, the baby can now grab the adult's hands and pull herself into a sitting position; the head is now fully controlled with strong neck muscles.
- She can sit for long periods with support. The back is straight.
- She may sit for short periods without support, but will topple over easily. She cannot yet put an arm out to break the fall.

Standing

- If the baby is held standing she will enjoy weight bearing and bouncing up and down.
- The baby may also demonstrate the downward parachute reflex: when held in the air and whooshed down feet first, the legs will straighten and separate and the toes will fan out.

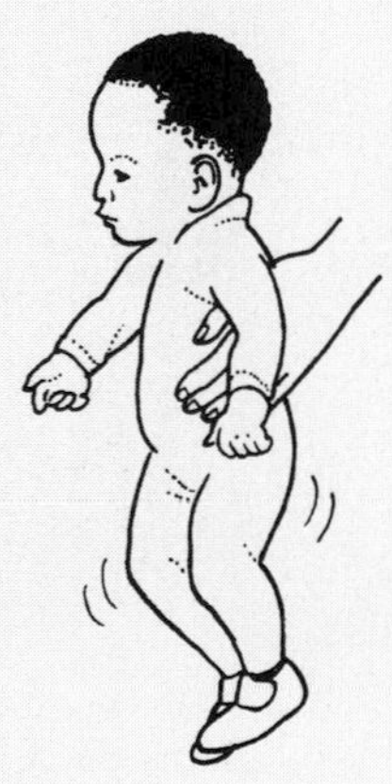

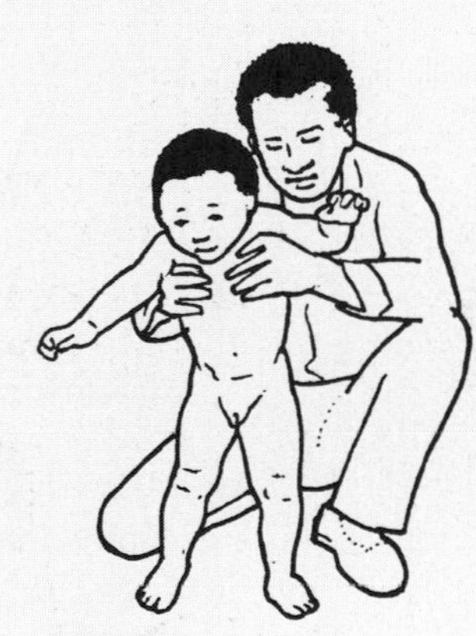

Case study . . .

. . . physical development at 6 months

Jacob was born at term weighing 3.4kg. He is now 6 months old, and the health visitor is very pleased with his progress. He completed his primary course of immunisations at 4 months. Weaning has commenced and, although he is taking an increasing variety of foods from a spoon and has begun to finger-feed, he still enjoys small breast feeds several times a day. At his recent hearing test, the health visitor conducted a routine developmental assessment and confirmed that he is achieving his physical milestones.

1. *Which gross motor and fine motor skills do you think Jacob is displaying?*
2. *What sorts of activity will promote and extend these areas of development?*

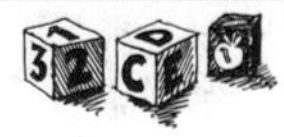

6 months

FINE MOTOR DEVELOPMENT

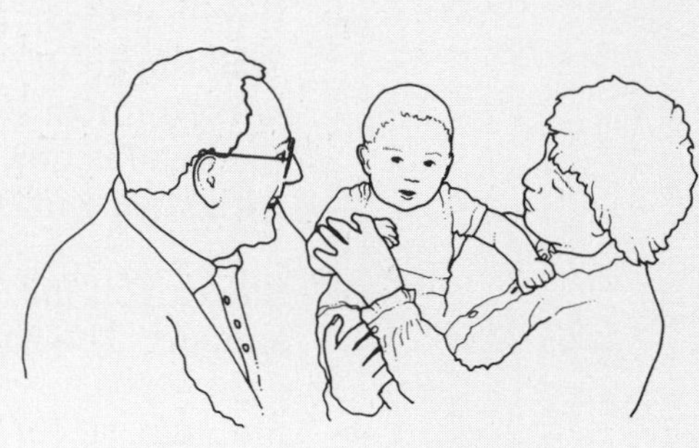

- The baby is bright and alert, looking around constantly to absorb all the visual information on offer.
- She is fascinated by small toys within reaching distance, grabbing them with the whole hand, using a **palmar grasp**.
- She transfers toys from hand to hand.

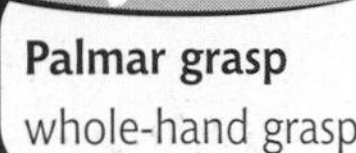

Palmar grasp
whole-hand grasp

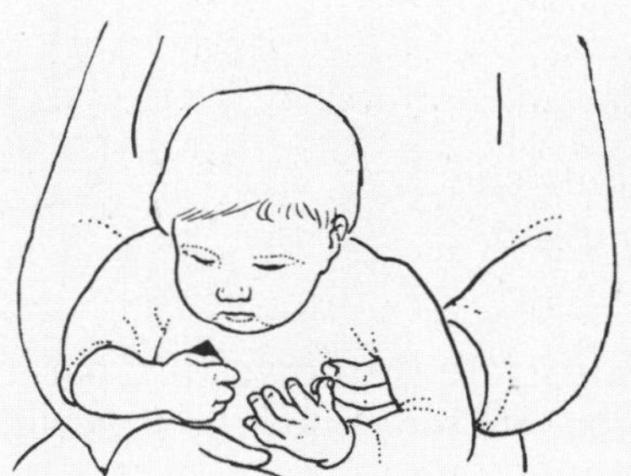

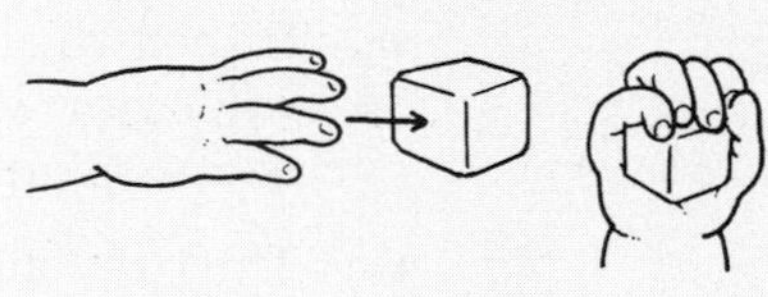

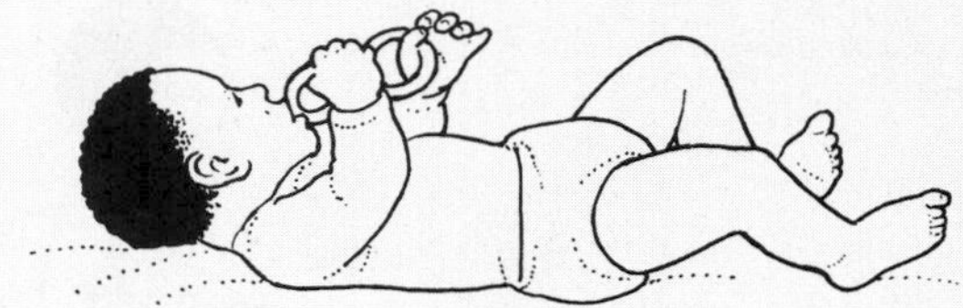

- She puts them in the mouth to explore them.
- If a toy is dropped, the baby will watch where it falls, if it is within sight.
- If a toy drops out of sight, the baby does not look for it. At this age the world ends where the baby can see it!

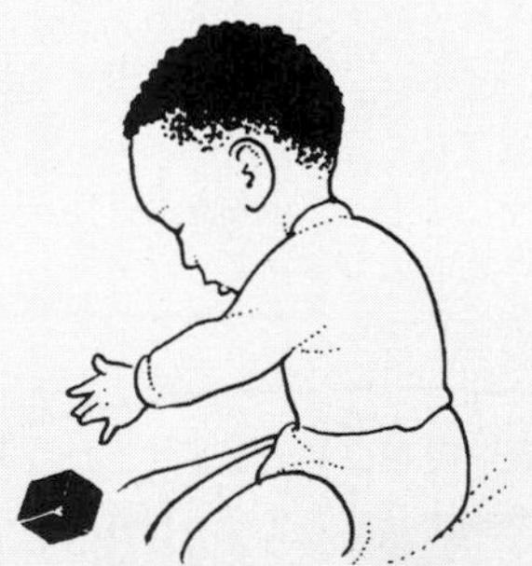

Progress check

Describe the process of head control in the first 6 months of life.

When should the baby have developed a palmar grasp?

Describe the posture of the typical 6-month-old baby in supine and prone.

What is the downward parachute reflex?

9 months

Many babies are mobile by 9 months, with a desire to explore and an increasing curiosity about the world. Mobility does not include common sense, and babies at this age are unlikely to recognise danger. This means that constant vigilance is required to keep them safe. Now stable sitters, they are beginning to balance and develop increasingly complex fine motor skills as they examine objects and investigate their properties. Understanding has increased and the baby is beginning to recognise more words, including their own name.

GROSS MOTOR DEVELOPMENT

Prone

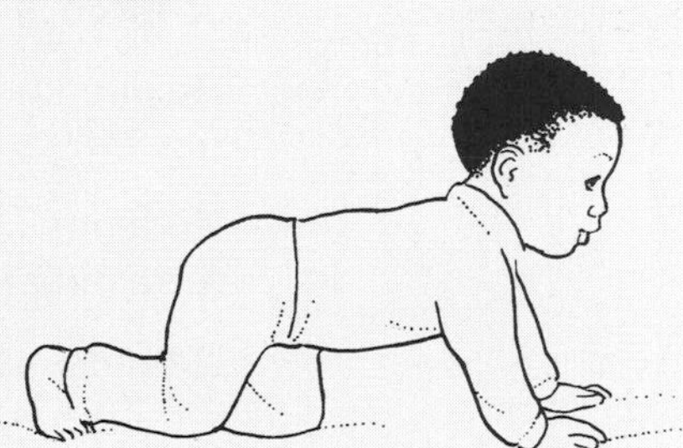

- The baby may be able to support his body on knees and outstretched arms.
- He may rock backwards and forwards and try to crawl.
- Moving backwards in the crawling position precipitates forward movement.

Supine

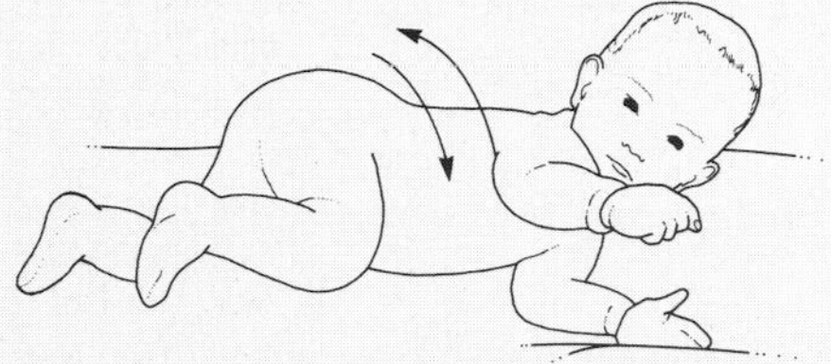

- The baby rolls from back to front and may crawl away, roll around the floor or squirm on his back.

Standing

- The baby can pull himself to a standing position, supporting first on the knees.
- When supported by an adult he will step forward on alternate feet.
- He supports his body in the standing position by holding on to a firm object.
- He may begin to side-step around furniture.

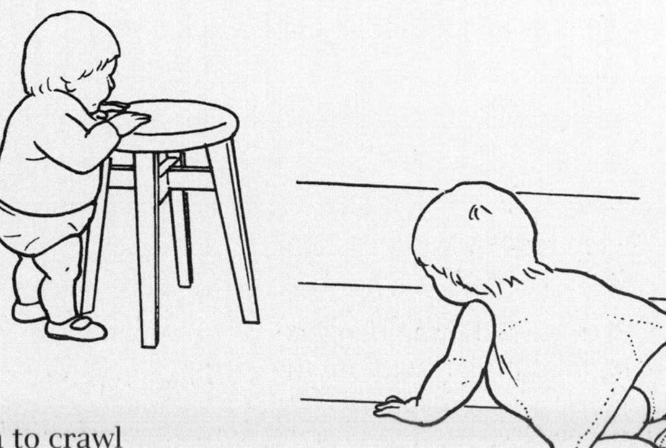

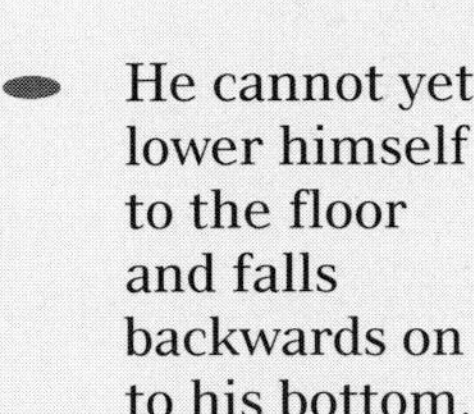

- He cannot yet lower himself to the floor and falls backwards on to his bottom.

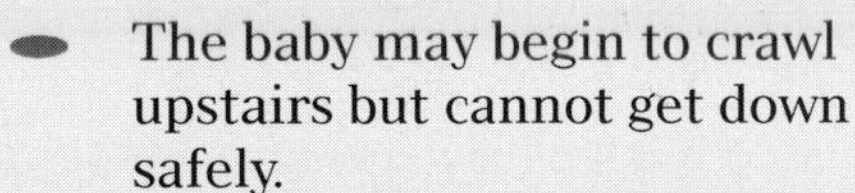

- The baby may begin to crawl upstairs but cannot get down safely.

9 months (continued)

- The forward parachute reflex: when the baby is held firmly during a controlled forwards fall (head first), the arms will shoot out and straighten and the fingers will fan out.

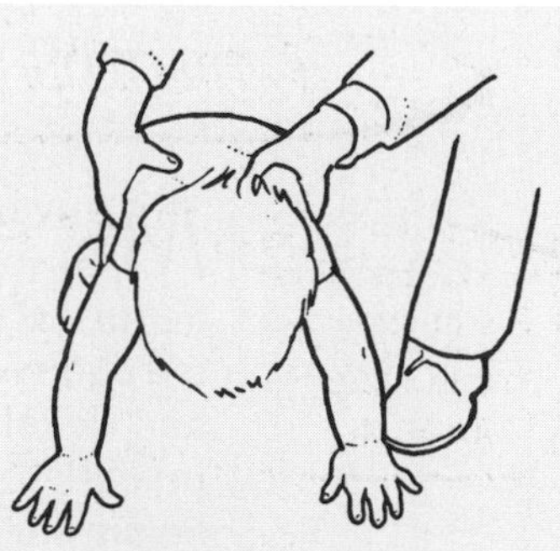

Sitting

- The baby is now a secure and stable sitter – he may sit unsupported for 15 minutes or more.
- He can keep his balance when turning to reach toys from the side.
- He leans forward to retrieve toys, returning to an upright sitting position.
- He puts out his arm(s) to prevent falling.

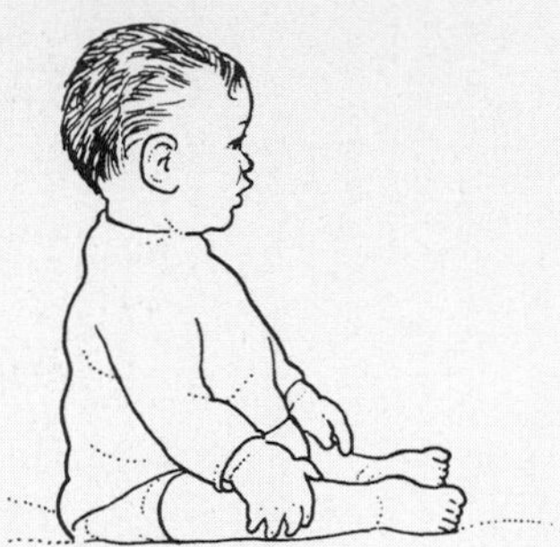

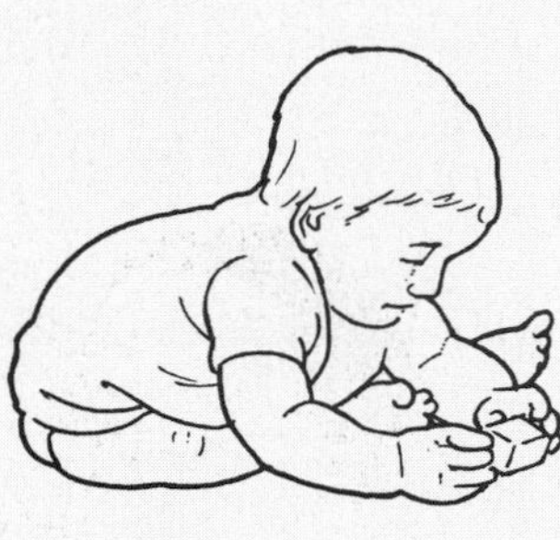

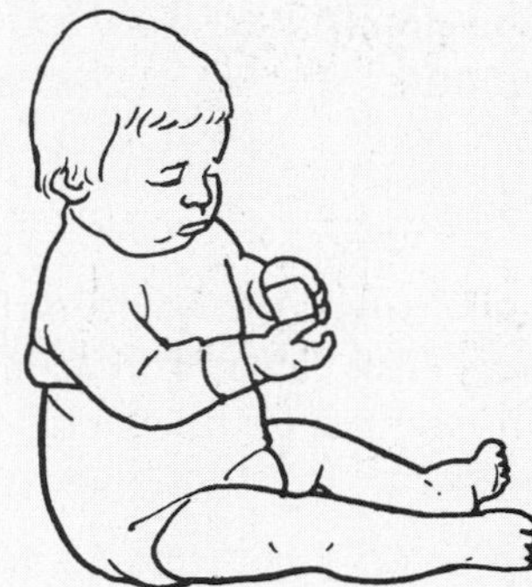

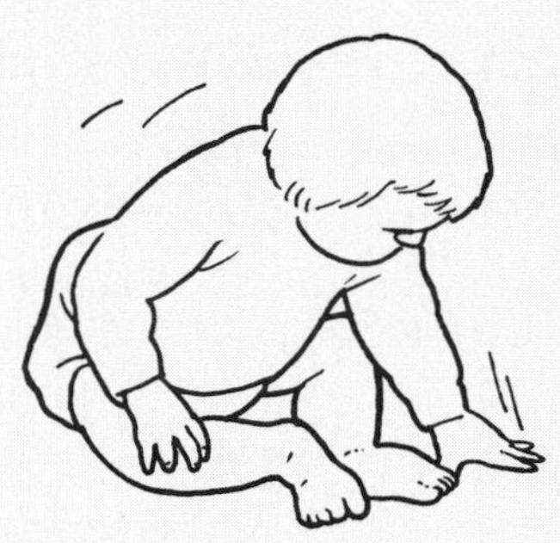

- Some babies may begin to bottom-shuffle, moving around the floor in the upright, sitting position using the legs to propel them.

SAFETY

As babies begin to move, their safety is of paramount importance. They will no longer remain safely in the place they were put. At all times, they require the watchful attention of a responsible adult who is aware of the stages of development.

Remember:

- A baby will put small items in their mouth and this is a potential choking hazard.
- Never leave a baby alone when they are eating finger foods.
- Never use a babywalker. They are dangerous and completely unnecessary – babies will learn to walk without them.
- When babies learn to crawl up the stairs, teach them how to come down safely backwards.
- Remove tempting dangers, for example hanging wires that may be pulled and saucepan handles projecting from the cooker.
- Make sure that fireguards and stairgates are fixed in position.
- When using a high-chair, pram or pushchair, make sure that the baby is safely strapped in.
- A forward-facing baby car seat may be used if it is safely anchored in the car.

9 months

key term

Pincer grasp
thumb and first finger grasp

FINE MOTOR DEVELOPMENT

- He uses the inferior **pincer grasp** with index finger and thumb.
- He drops objects or bangs them on to a hard surface to release them – he cannot let go voluntarily yet.
- He looks for fallen objects out of sight – he is now beginning to realise that they have not disappeared for ever.
- Visually alert and curious, the baby is exploring objects before picking them up.

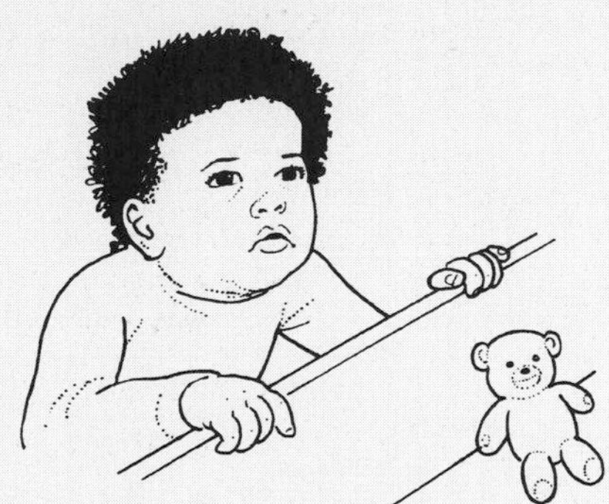

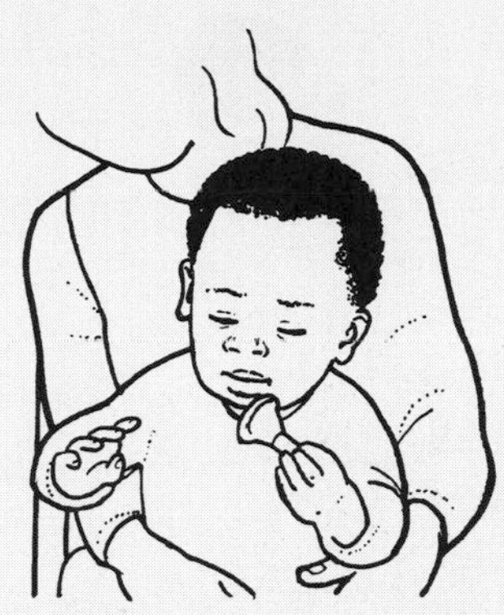

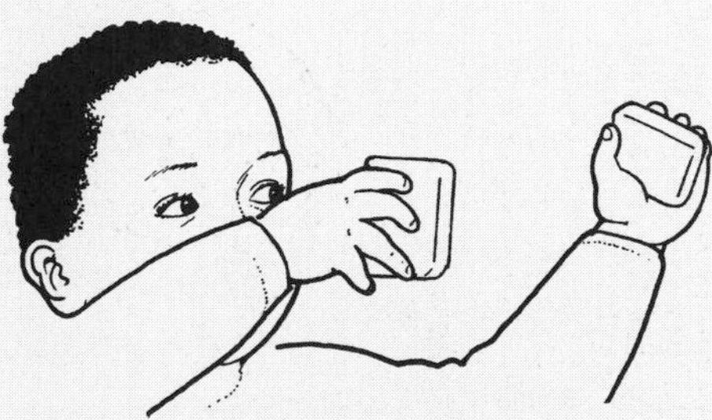

- He grasps objects, usually with one hand, inspects with the eyes and transfers to the other hand.
- He may hold one object in each hand and bang them together.
- He uses the index finger to poke and point; this finger starts to straighten and play a greater role.

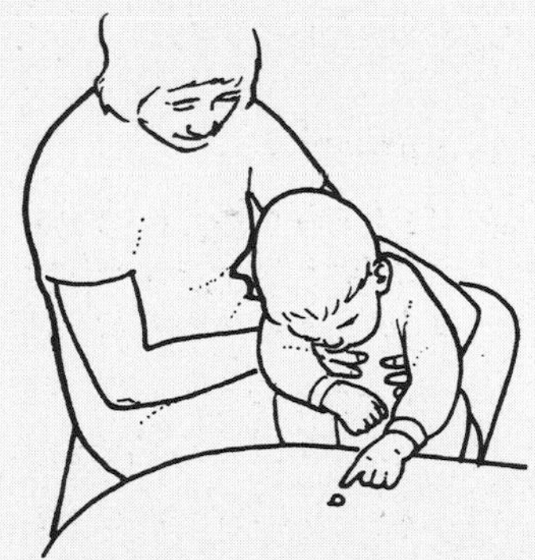

Progress check

How can you stimulate a baby to develop a pincer grasp?

Name three ways in which a baby may be mobile at around 9 months.

What is the forward parachute reflex?

How could you ensure the safety of a baby of this age?

12 months

By 12 months, babies are transformed from the helpless creatures they were just a year before. They are usually mobile and use a delicate pincer grasp to pick up tiny objects from the floor as they travel. A preference for one hand may now be clear, and the baby can use both hands co-operatively, beginning to place objects down with increasing control. With a developing understanding of language, they are often able to say two or three recognisable words and make their needs known by sound and gestures.

GROSS MOTOR DEVELOPMENT

Sitting

- The baby can sit alone indefinitely.
- She can get into sitting position from lying down.

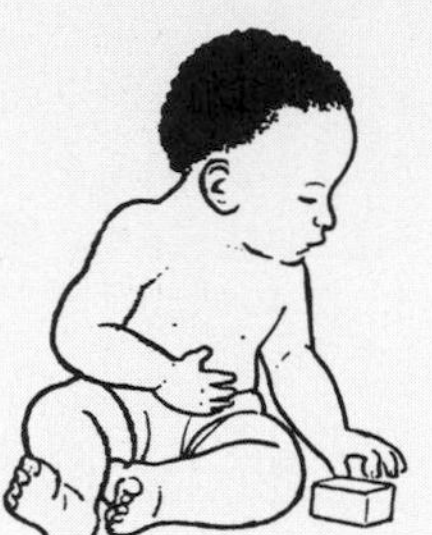

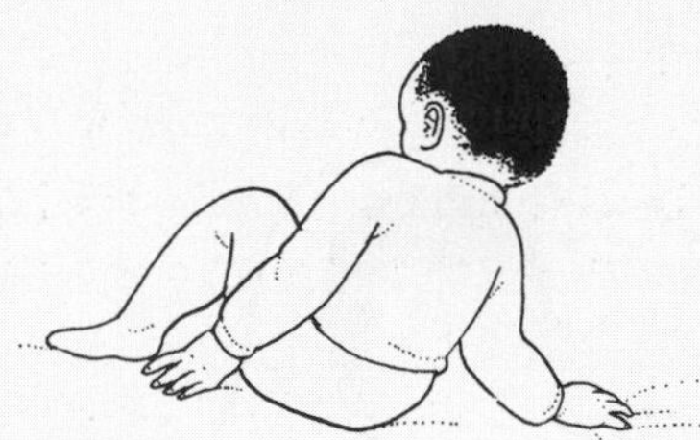

Standing

- The baby pulls herself to stand and walks around the furniture.
- She can return to sitting without falling.
- She may stand alone for a short period.

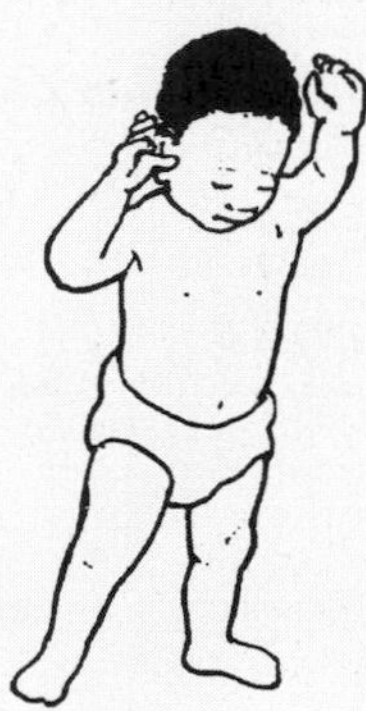

Mobility

- The baby is now mobile by crawling, bottom-shuffling, bear walking, walking alone or with one or both hands held.
- She may crawl upstairs forwards and downstairs backwards.

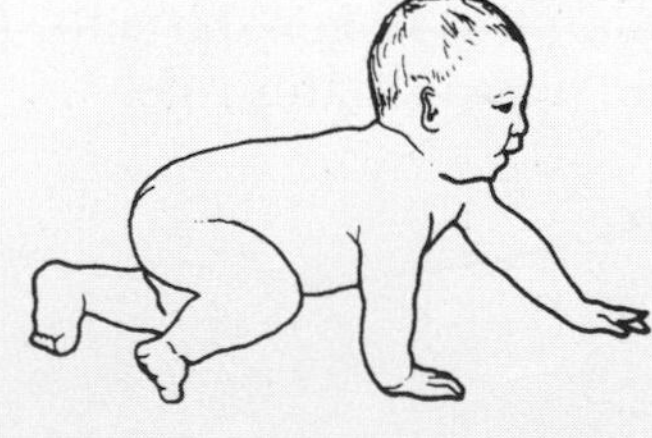

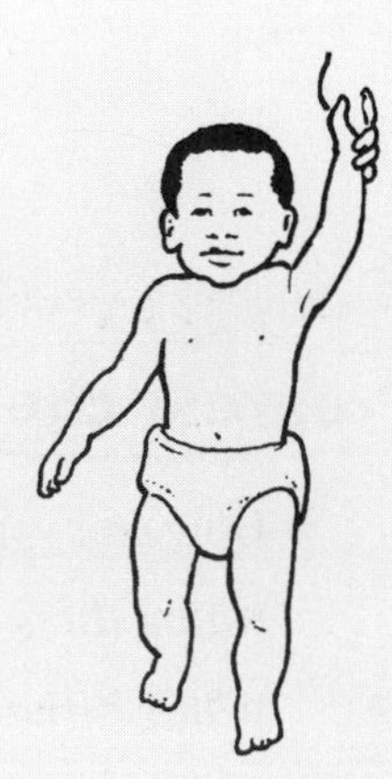

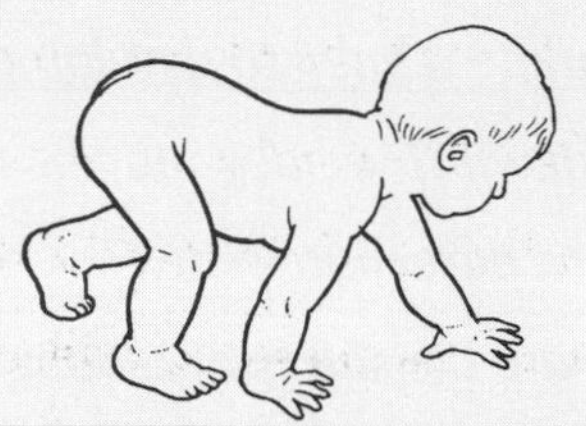

12 months

FINE MOTOR DEVELOPMENT

- The baby looks for objects hidden and out of sight.

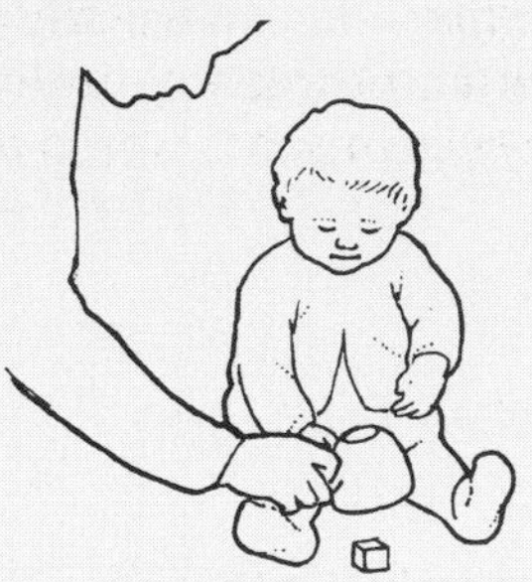
 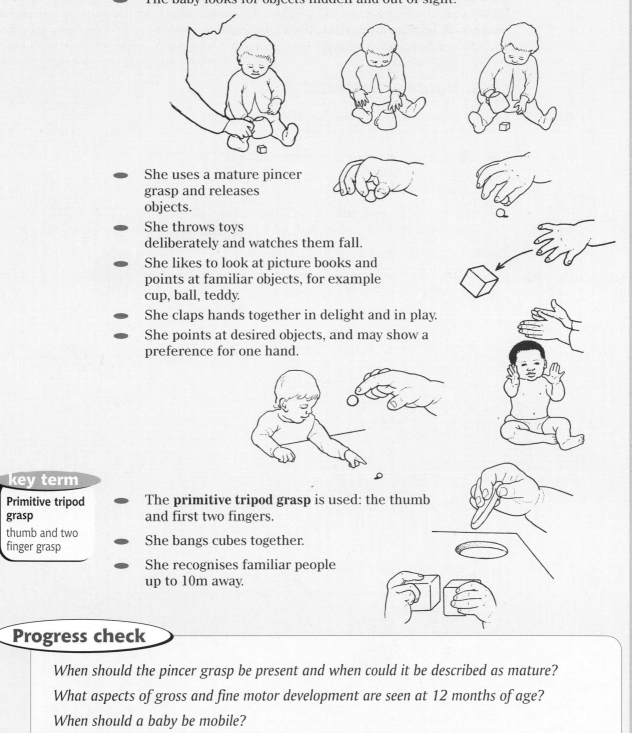

- She uses a mature pincer grasp and releases objects.
- She throws toys deliberately and watches them fall.
- She likes to look at picture books and points at familiar objects, for example cup, ball, teddy.
- She claps hands together in delight and in play.
- She points at desired objects, and may show a preference for one hand.

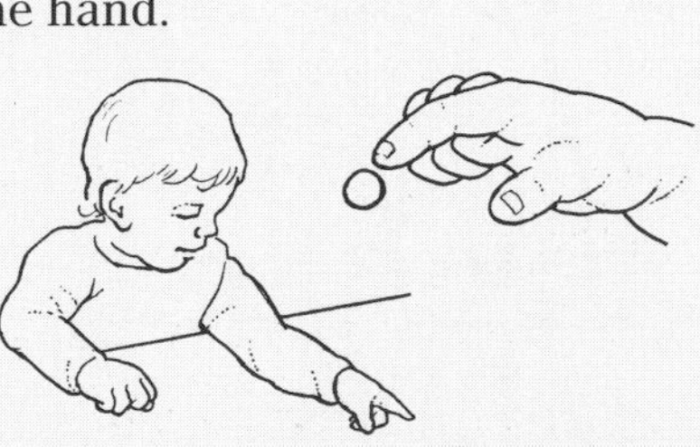
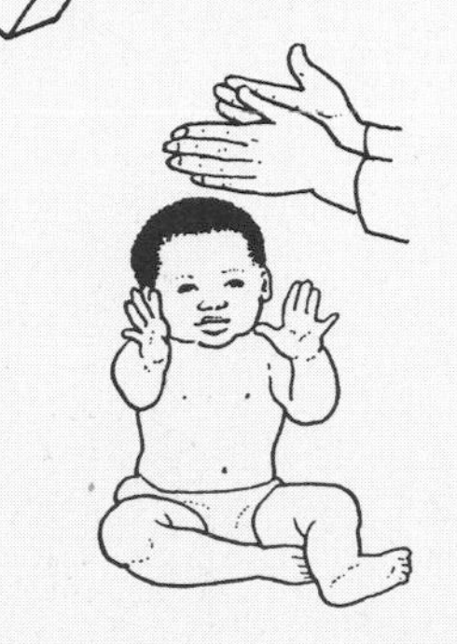

key term

Primitive tripod grasp
thumb and two finger grasp

- The **primitive tripod grasp** is used: the thumb and first two fingers.
- She bangs cubes together.
- She recognises familiar people up to 10m away.

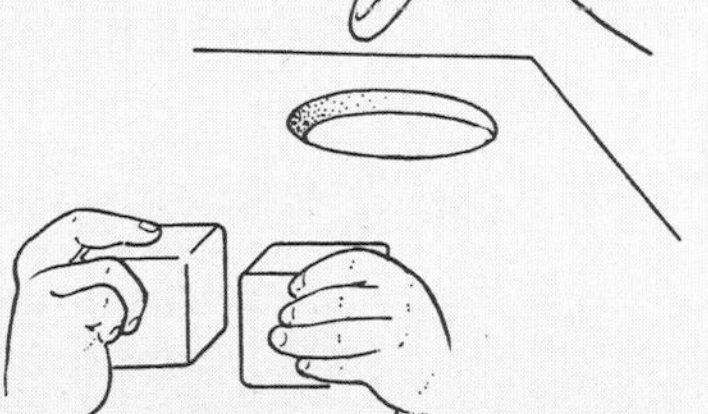

Progress check

When should the pincer grasp be present and when could it be described as mature?

What aspects of gross and fine motor development are seen at 12 months of age?

When should a baby be mobile?

Note five elements of physical skills at 12 months of age.

By what age should all the primitive reflexes have faded?

15 months

The baby at 15 months is usually walking unaided, but has limited control of stopping and starting, and falls over a lot. Supervision with steps and stairs is vital to prevent accidents. The desire to be independent is increasing at this age and feeding skills are improving. The child can usually try to use a spoon with some success. Throwing, trying to catch and throwing back balls, and pushing toys and trolleys are popular activities.

GROSS MOTOR DEVELOPMENT

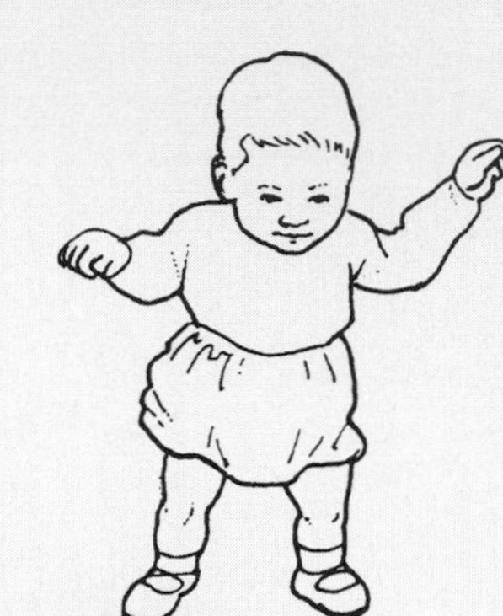

- The baby walks alone, feet wide apart with arms raised to keep balance.
- He falls easily, sometimes after just a few paces, and usually on stopping; he cannot avoid obstacles on the floor.
- He can sit from standing by falling backwards on to the bottom or forwards on to the arms.
- He gets to standing without help from people or furniture.
- She can climb the stairs on all fours.

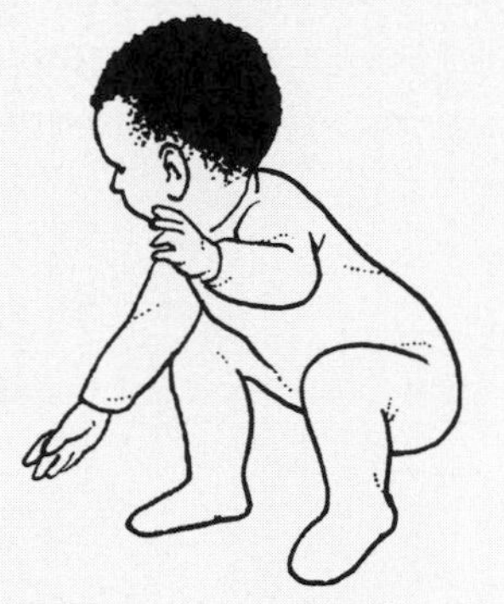

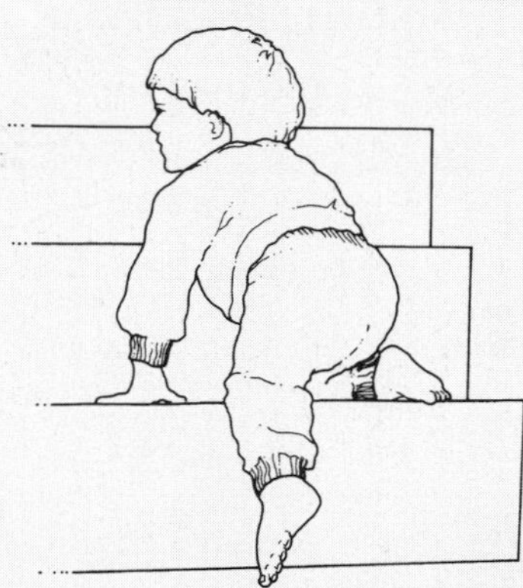

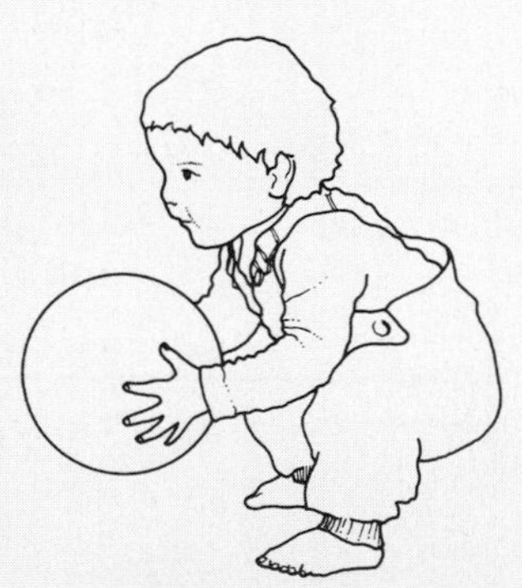

- She can throw back a ball, but often falls over.
- He kneels without support.
- He may climb forwards into a small chair and turn to sit.

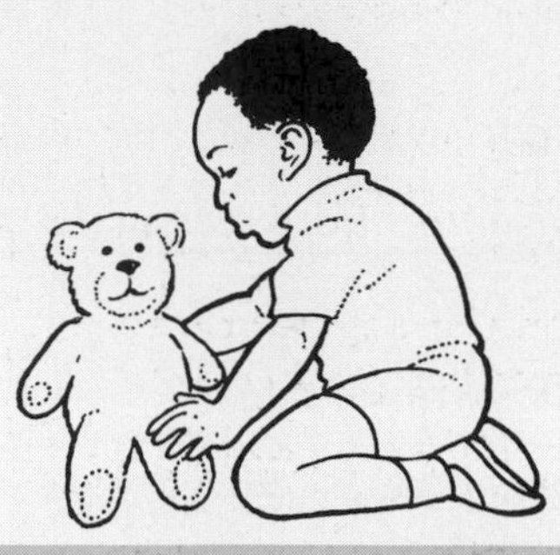

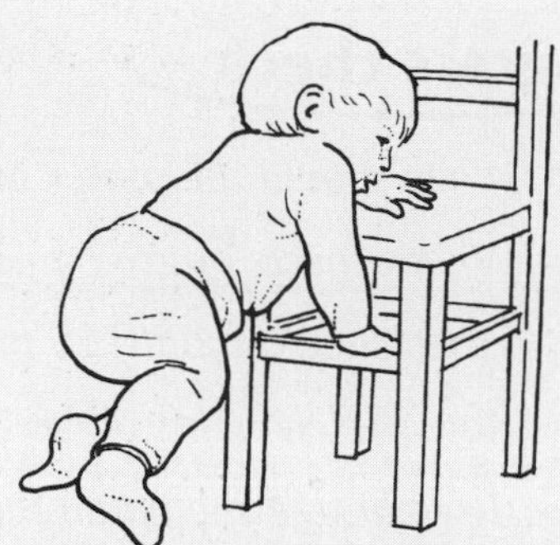

15 months

FINE MOTOR DEVELOPMENT

- The baby enjoys playing with small bricks.

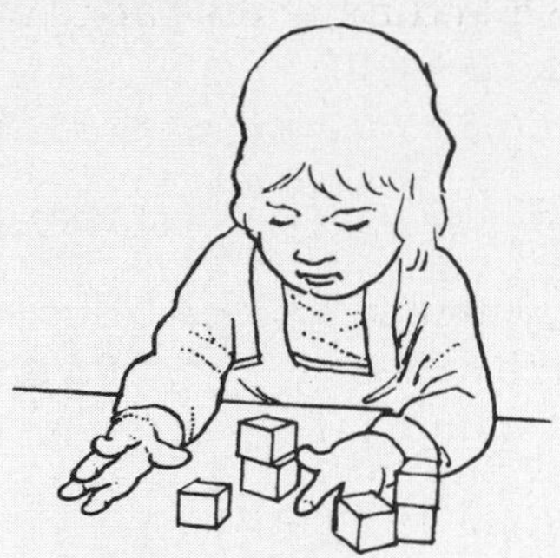

- She builds a two-brick tower.

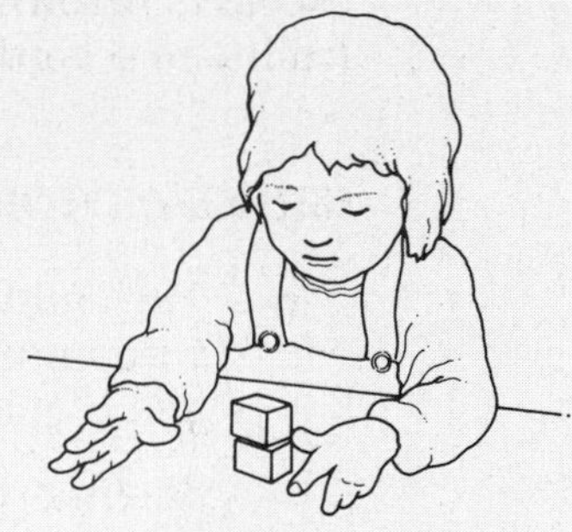

- She can put a button into the neck of a bottle.

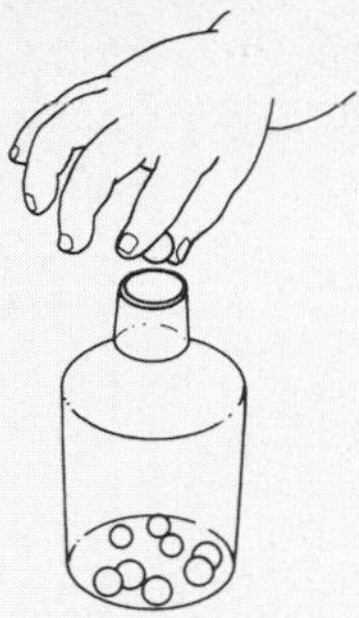

- He can hold a spoon, but puts it in the mouth upside down.

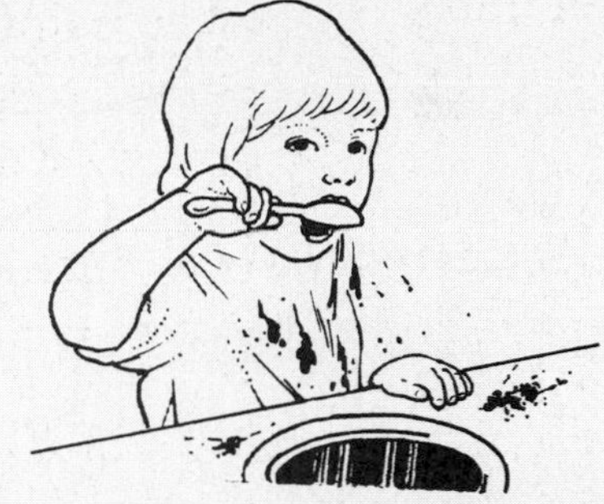

- He enjoys brightly coloured picture books and turns several pages at once.

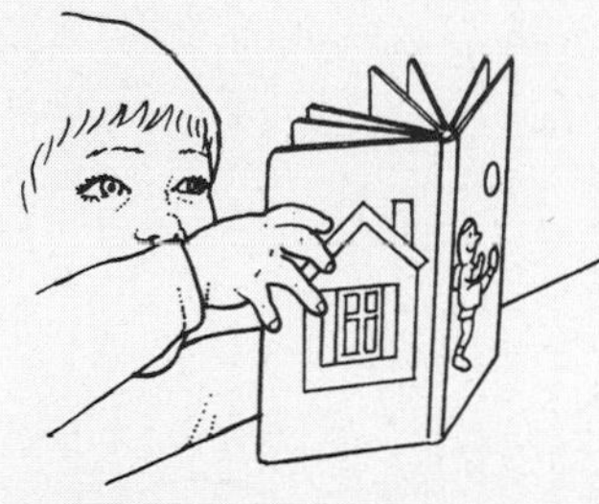

- He points at familiar objects in the book and pats the page.

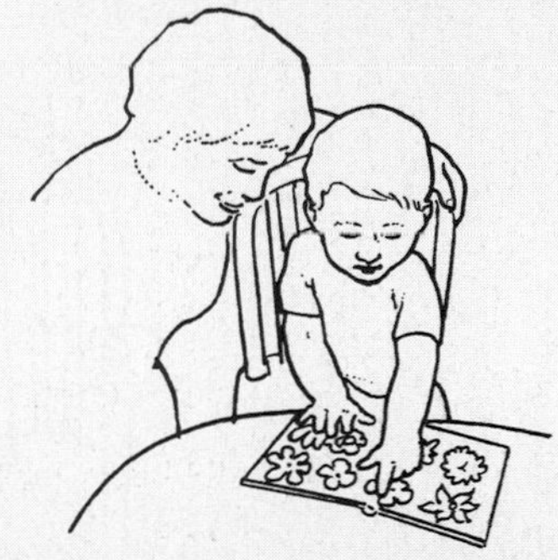

- He uses the index finger constantly to demand drinks, food and toys out of reach.
- He often stares out of the window for long periods watching and pointing at the activities outside with interest.
- He holds a crayon in a palmar grasp, scribbles backwards and forwards over the paper.
- He uses either hand but shows a preference for one.

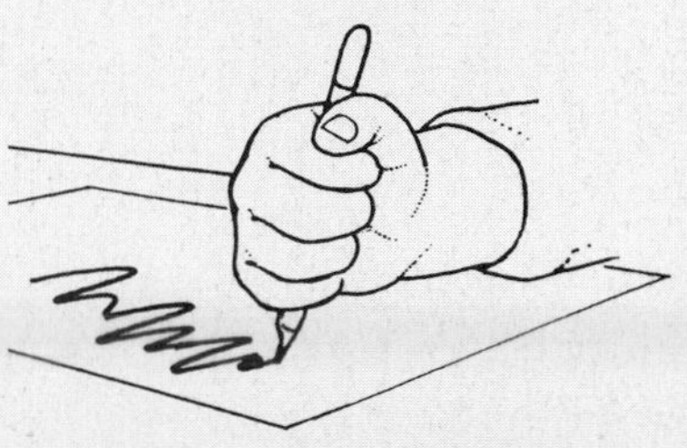

18 months

The 18-month-old child is extremely active, racing around at high speed to explore the environment. The child runs, with arms and legs apart, investigating corners and hurrying upstairs. Stopping and starting well, the child finds corners more difficult, but pulls large toys around and plays ball with whole-arm movements. Her world is one of 'here and now'. The child is self-willed and has yet to develop the ability to see others as people like herself.

GROSS MOTOR DEVELOPMENT

- The child walks confidently now, without using the arms for balance and is able to stop without falling
- She may carry large toys.

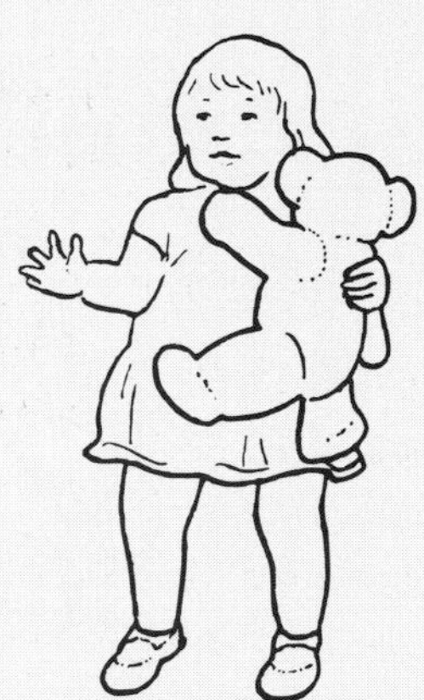

- She squats to the floor to pick up toys

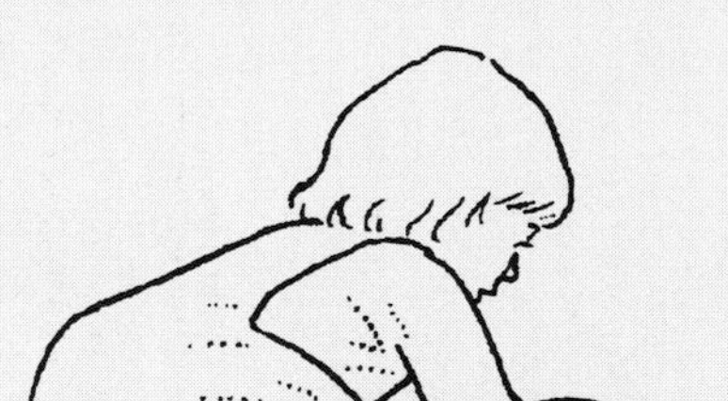

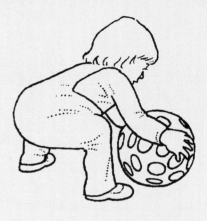

- He climbs into an adult-sized chair forwards and then turns round to sit down.

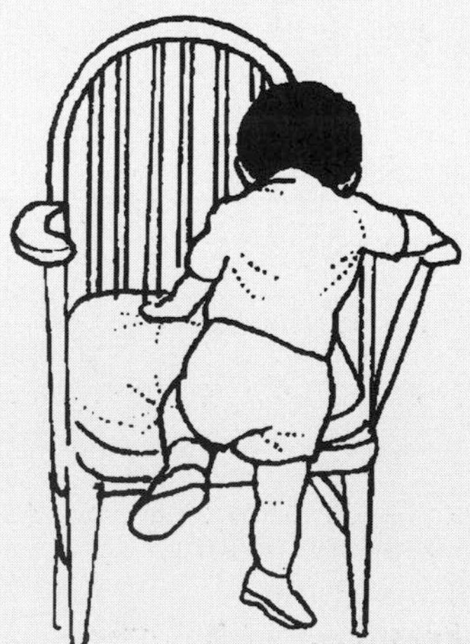

- He tries to kick a ball, often with success.

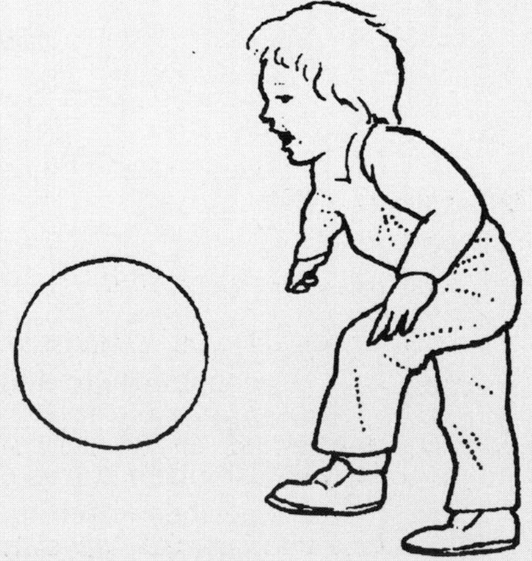

18 months (continued)

- He runs but often falls as he is unable to co-ordinate movements to get around objects in the way.

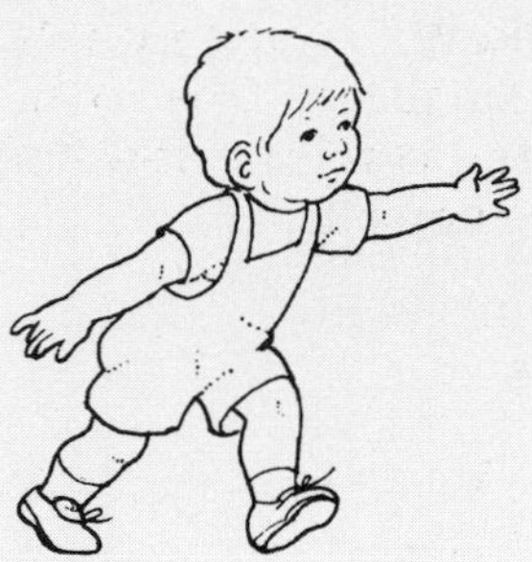

- He likes pushing a brick trolley or similar wheeled toy

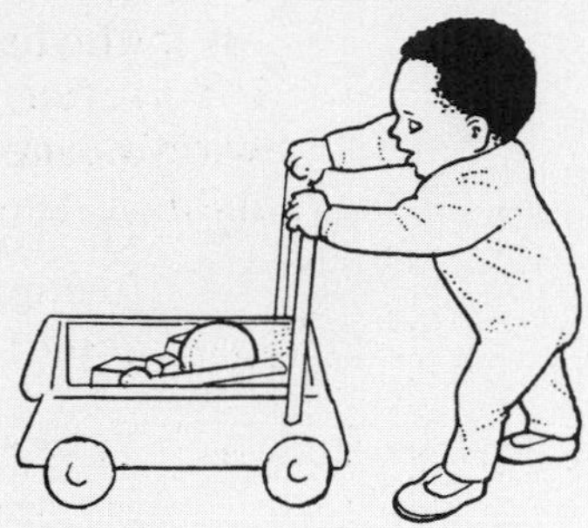

- She walks upstairs with hand(s) held.

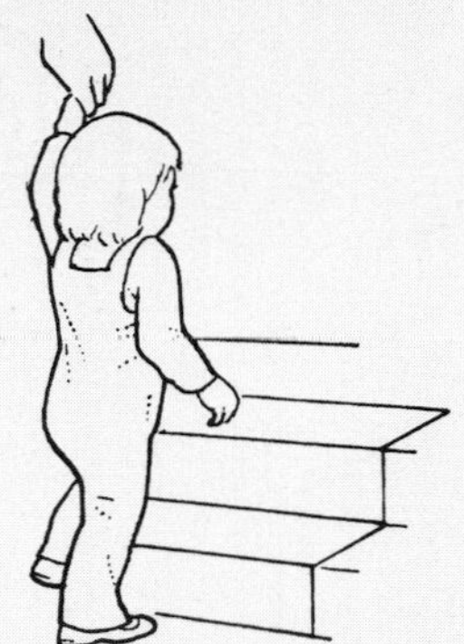

- She comes downstairs safely, either forwards on the bottom (one step at a time) or backwards crawling or sliding on the tummy.
- She may walk downstairs with a hand held or holding on to the rail.

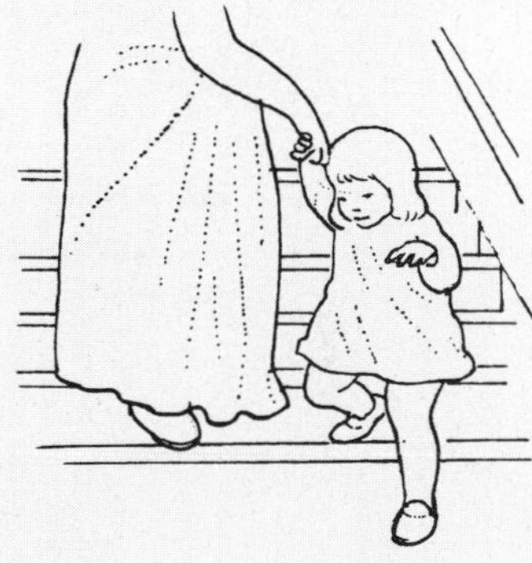

Progress check

List four gross motor skills that are typical at 18 months.

Explain why small bricks are a valuable tool to enable young children to develop fine motor skills.

How could an adult ensure the safety of young children who need assistance to go up and down stairs?

How does an 18-month-old child usually get into a large chair?

18 months

FINE MOTOR DEVELOPMENT

- The baby can now use a delicate, refined pincer grasp to put small objects through small spaces.
- The tripod grasp of crayon and pencil (using the thumb and two fingers in adult fashion) is developing.

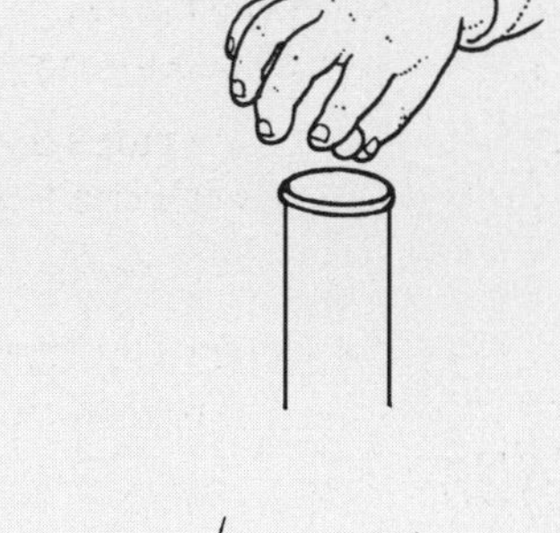

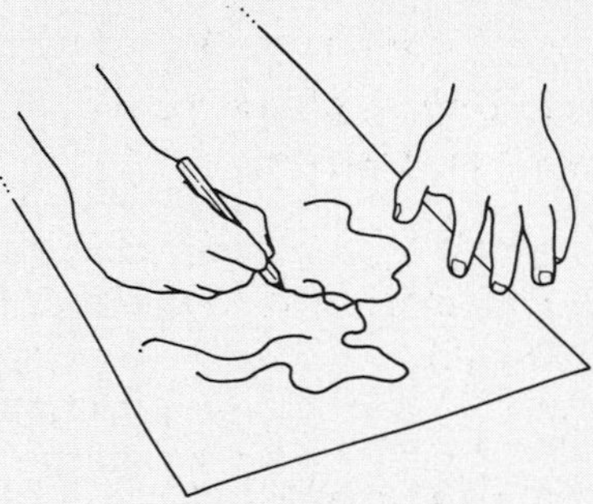

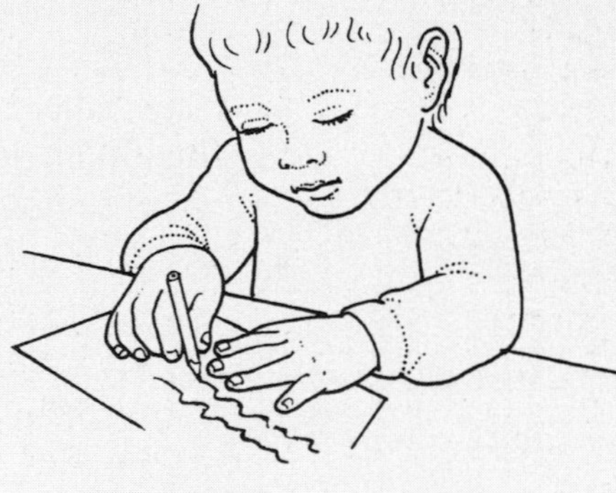

- She scribbles on paper to and fro and with random dots.

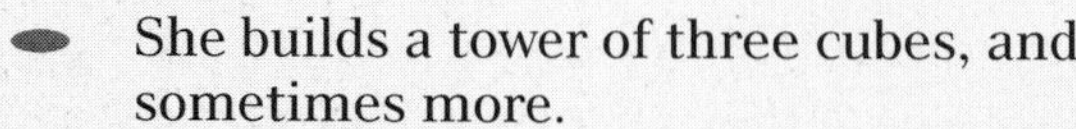

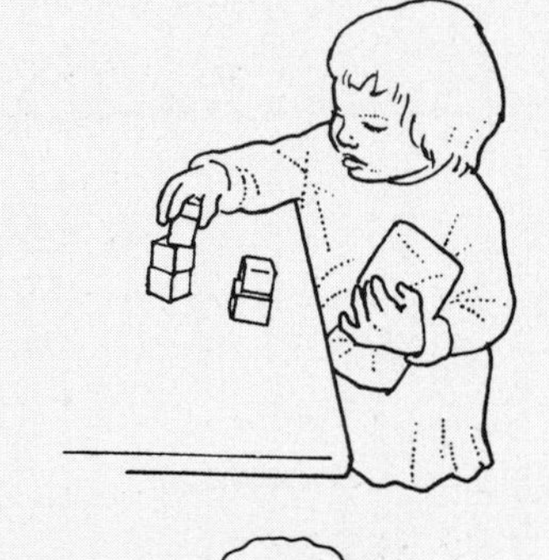

- She builds a tower of three cubes, and sometimes more.

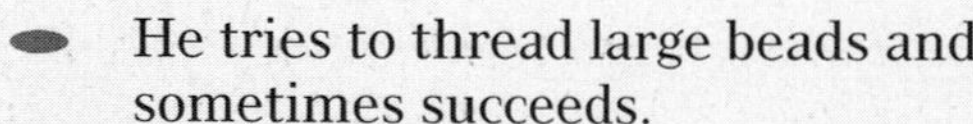

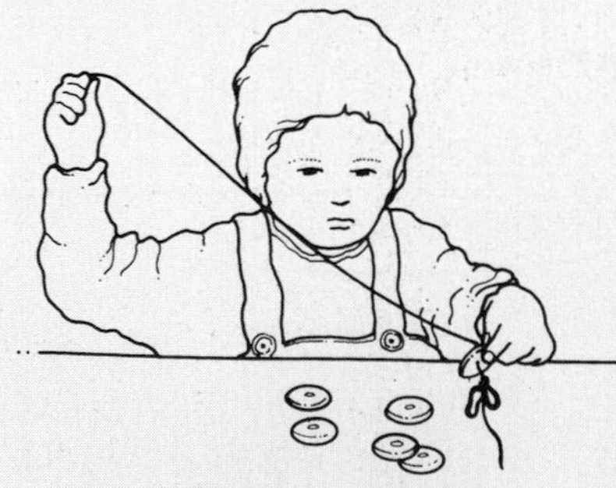

- He tries to thread large beads and sometimes succeeds.

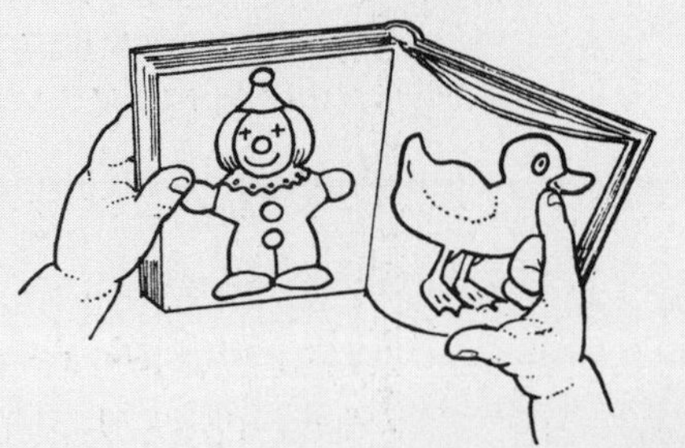

- She continues to enjoy picture books and points at known objects.

2 years

GROSS MOTOR DEVELOPMENT

key term

Locomotion
the developing ability to move from one place to another, usually by crawling, walking or running

key terms

Spatial awareness
a developing knowledge of how things move and the effects of movement

At 2 years children are very mobile and love exploring their surroundings. Their developing skills of **locomotion** and balance enable them to explore the environment by walking, running and climbing.

- He rides a small tricycle by pushing it along with the feet; he does not use the pedals.
- She tries to kick a ball but usually walks into it.
- He can climb up on to the furniture, usually to reach something or to see out of the window.
- She is beginning to show awareness of how she relates to other objects (**spatial awareness**).
- The child runs safely.
- She walks up and down the stairs holding on; she puts two feet on every step.
- He stops and starts easily.
- She pushes and pulls large wheeled toys; can pull along a small wheeled toy by the string and goes in the right direction.
- He squats down steadily to play with or pick up a toy, and gets up again without using the hands.

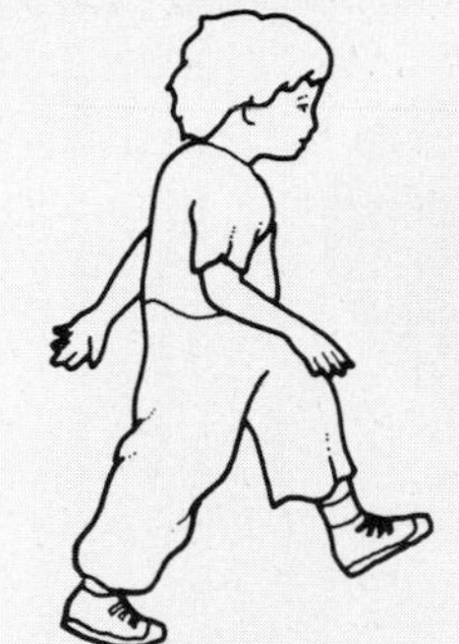

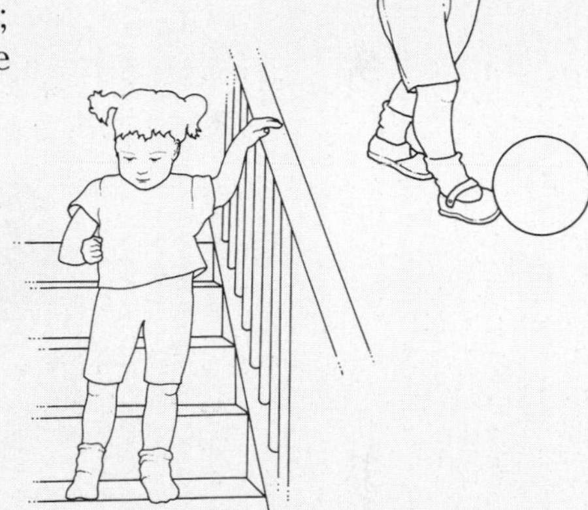

Case study . . .

. . . supporting the development of physical skills

Aaron is 2 years 3 months old and comes to the nursery every day. He has settled in well and enjoys playing outside. Although he is confident when riding the wheeled toys, he has not yet attempted to climb up the ladder and go down the slide. He has watched the other children with interest and on one occasion started to go up the ladder.

Today, Aaron approaches the slide as usual. Urmala, the nursery nurse, is nearby and encourages him, standing close to the ladder, helping him to place his feet and hands as he climbs. When he succeeds in climbing to the top, she praises him, helps him to sit on the slide and holds his hand as he slides down. When he arrives at the bottom, Aaron and Urmala clap their hands. Aaron immediately runs round to have another go and Urmala stands ready to support him.

1. *Why does Aaron spend time watching the other children?*
2. *How did Urmala help Aaron to achieve his goal?*
3. *What did Aaron do after he successfully went down the slide?*
4. *Why is this important?*

2 years

FINE MOTOR DEVELOPMENT

At 2 years children enjoy pulling things apart, fitting things together, pushing in, pulling out, filling and emptying. They will still often test by touch and taste. The use of the fine pincer grip is well established. By now, a 2-year-old child will use a preferred hand to hold a pencil, but both hands are used to perform complicated tasks.

- The child usually uses a preferred hand to hold a pencil; he draws circles, lines and dots.
- He can use a fine pincer grasp to pick up and put down tiny things.
- He can manipulate toys.
- She holds a pencil and draws circles, lines and dots.

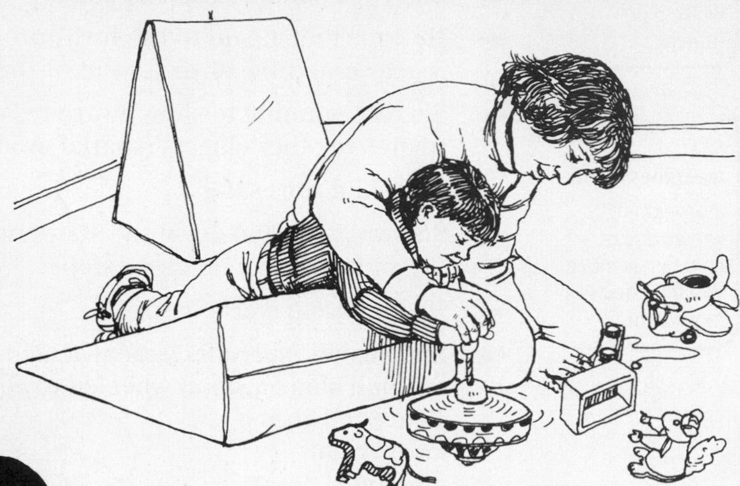

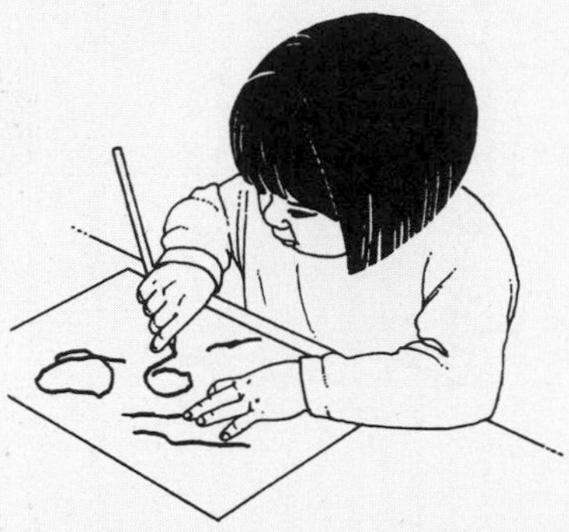

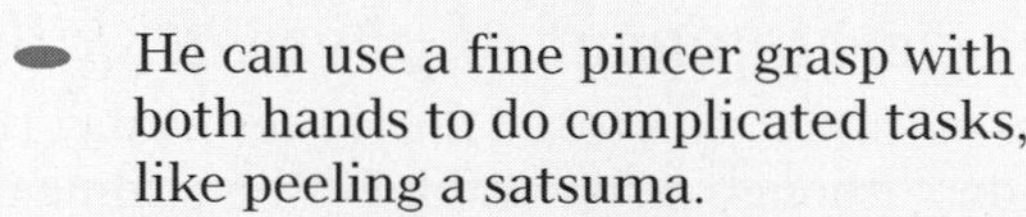

- He can use a fine pincer grasp with both hands to do complicated tasks, like peeling a satsuma.

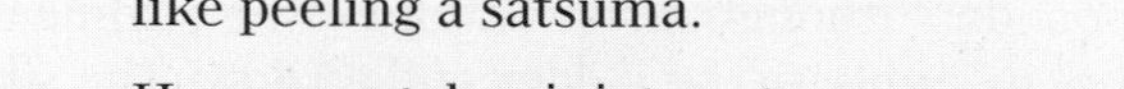

- He can match miniature toys on request.
- He carefully builds a tower of six or seven bricks.
- He likes picture books, enjoys recognising things in favourite pictures. He now turns the pages one at a time.

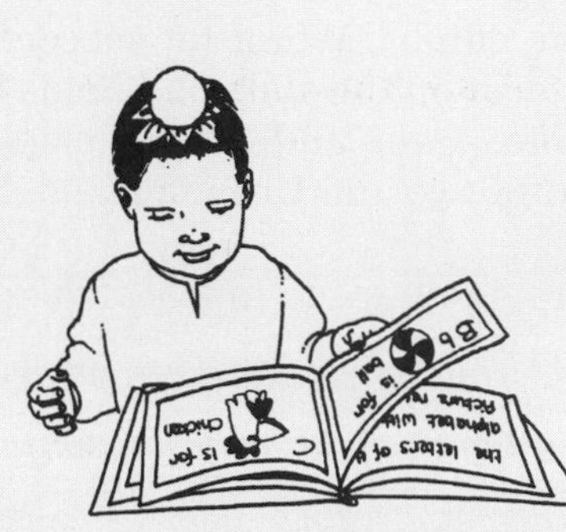

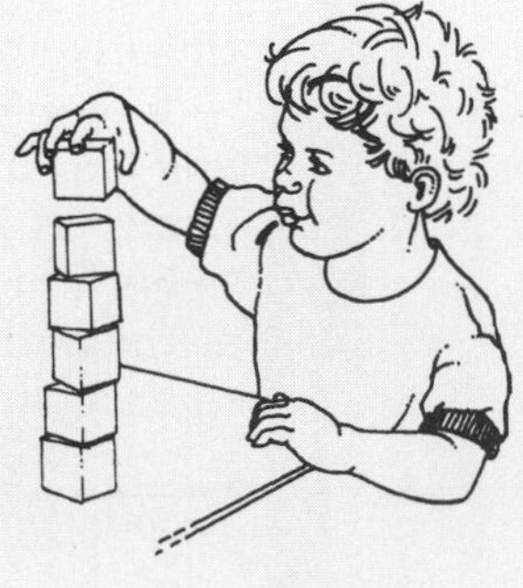

3 years

GROSS MOTOR DEVELOPMENT

At 3 years children's gross motor skills are developing well. They walk and run confidently, moving forwards, sideways and backwards, managing stairs easily. They use wheeled toys with skill and with an awareness of obstacles around them.

- The child can stand and walk on tiptoe.
- She walks forwards, sideways and backwards.
- She can kick a ball hard.

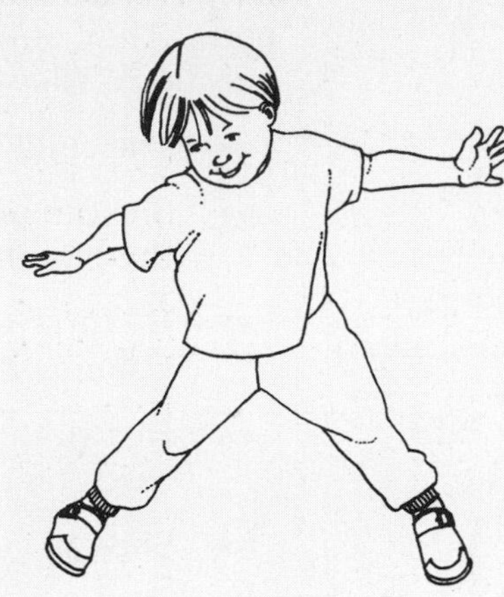

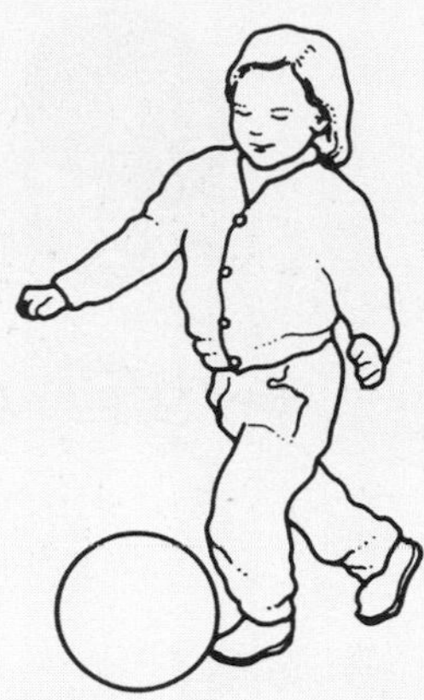

- She walks upstairs with one foot on each step.
- She walks downstairs with two feet on each step.

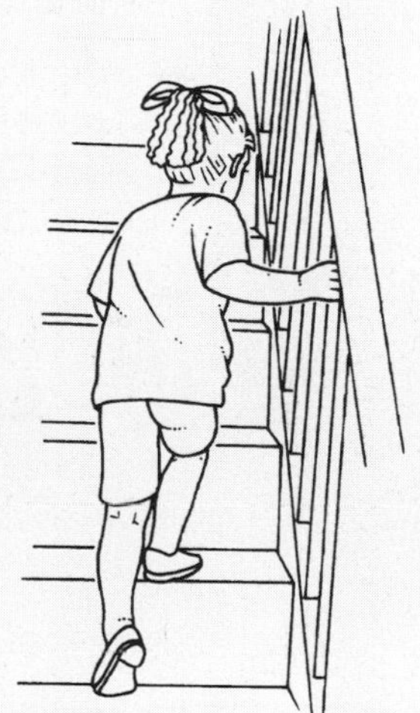

- She is now well aware of her own size in relation to things around her.
- She rides a tricycle using the pedals.

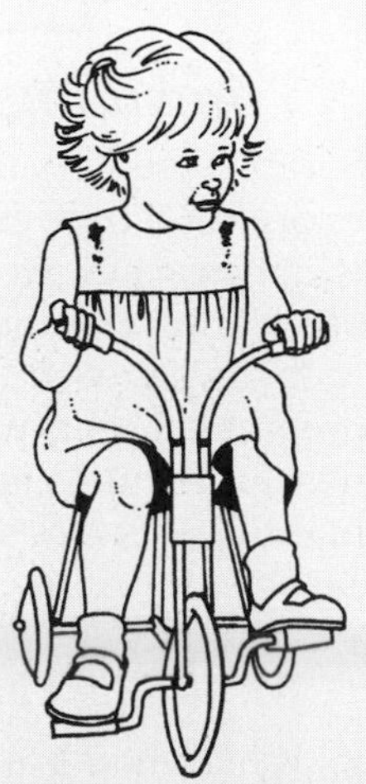

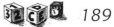

3 years

FINE MOTOR DEVELOPMENT

At 3 years old children's hand–eye co-ordination is good. They can pick up small objects, such as pieces of collage material and place them with some accuracy. Three year olds enjoy painting pictures with a large brush and usually name them when they are finished. Their drawings of people show the head and one or two other parts. They enjoy simple conversations about the current activity, asking many questions. They listen eagerly to stories and enjoy finger rhymes and action songs.

- The child can now build a tower of nine or ten bricks.
- She can pick up small pieces of collage material using the thumb and first finger.
- He can co-operate in simple vision tests by recognising toys.
- He can thread large wooden beads on to a lace.
- She can cut with scissors.
- She may know colours.
- She matches two or three primary colours.
- She controls a pencil in the preferred hand, between the thumb and first two fingers.
- She enjoys painting with a large brush.

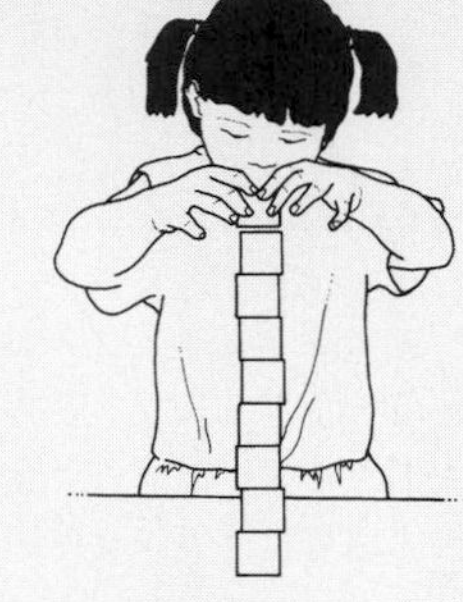

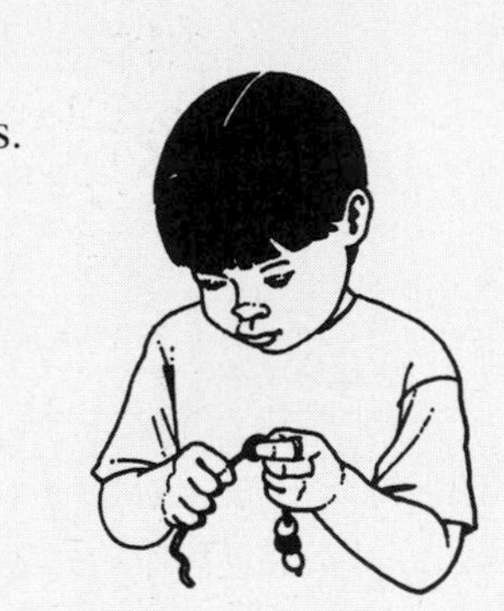

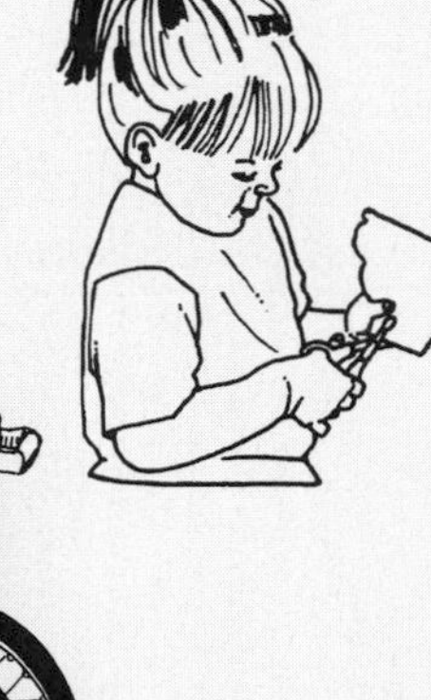

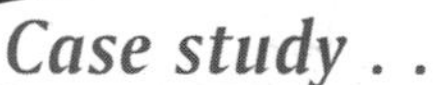

Case study . . .

. . . providing suitable equipment

Sarah, aged 3, is new to the nursery. She joins in many of the activities, and seems to prefer activities like collage and box modelling. Jason, the child-care worker who is Sarah's key worker, has noticed that she doesn't use scissors very easily and often tears collage material to get the shape and size she wants.

Jason sat with Sarah and showed her how to use the scissors and she made some progress. Later, when Sarah was using a pencil, Jason noticed that she was using her left hand. When Sarah wanted to do a collage activity, Jason made sure that left-handed scissors were available and sat with Sarah while she used them. With Jason's help and encouragement, Sarah was able to progress with her cutting skills.

1. *Why did the child-care worker intervene here?*
2. *What good practice enabled Jason to help Sarah effectively?*

4 years

GROSS MOTOR DEVELOPMENT

At 4 years children have developed good muscle control. This helps with energetic climbing, jumping, hopping and tricycle riding. They are adept runners and climbers, and enjoy any games that involve running and jumping. Four year olds are adding the skills of running on tiptoe. They are confident climbing over apparatus and, if they get the chance, up trees.

- The child can stand, walk and run on tiptoe.

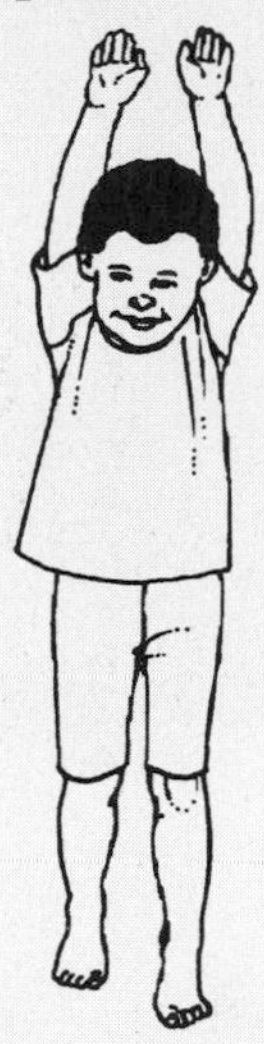

- Keeping the legs straight, he can bend at the waist to pick up things from the floor.

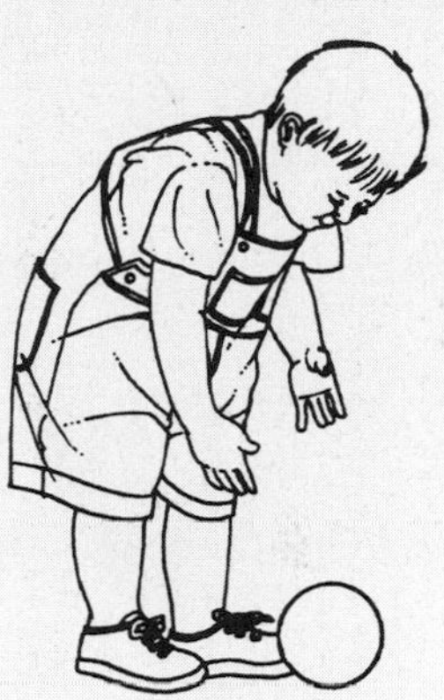

- He climbs trees, ladders, play equipment.
- She walks or runs up and down stairs, putting one foot on each step.
- He can catch, kick, throw and bounce a ball and hit it with a bat.
- Rides a tricycle well, able to make sharp turns.
- Children are confident at climbing over and through apparatus.

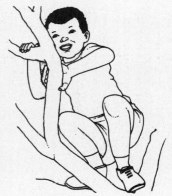

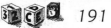

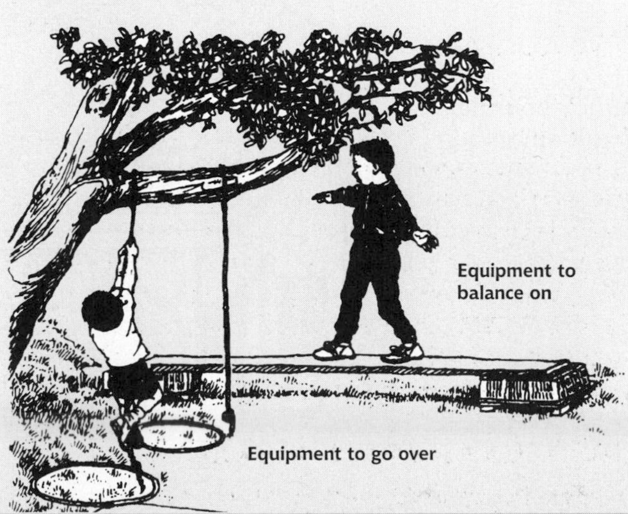

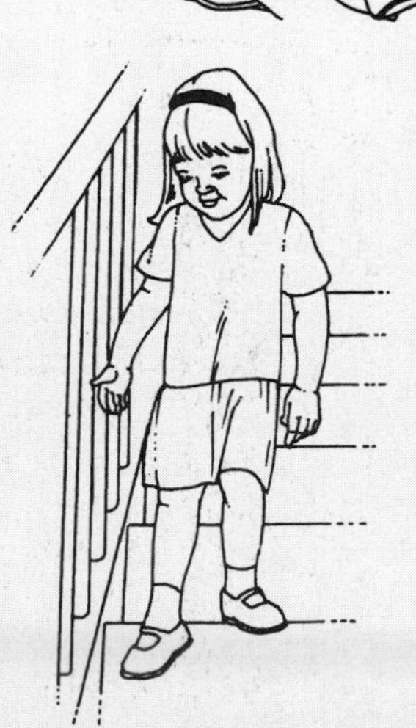

4 years

FINE MOTOR DEVELOPMENT

At 4 years old children are becoming adept at tasks needing careful hand–eye control. They are not so confident or accurate in their skills of catching and hitting as they are in games of running and jumping. They enjoy building with small- and large-scale construction materials and are learning to be more skilful in using scissors. They learn the combination of visual and fine manipulative skills that are required to complete jigsaws.

- He can build three steps with six bricks, after being shown how.

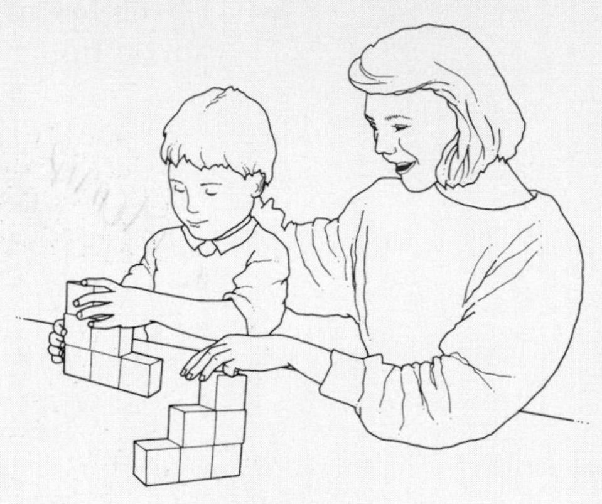

- The child is able to build a tower of ten or more bricks.

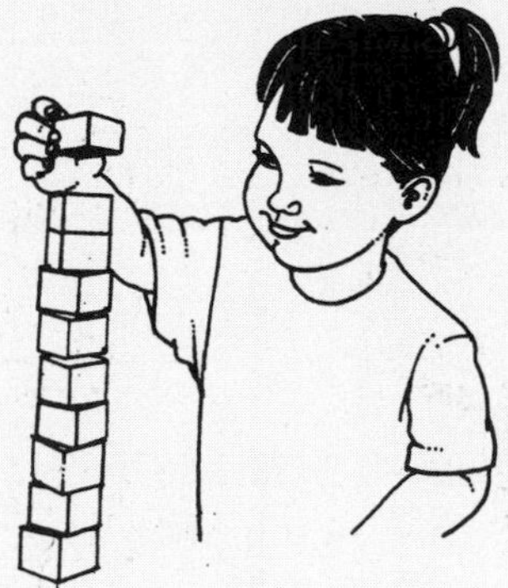

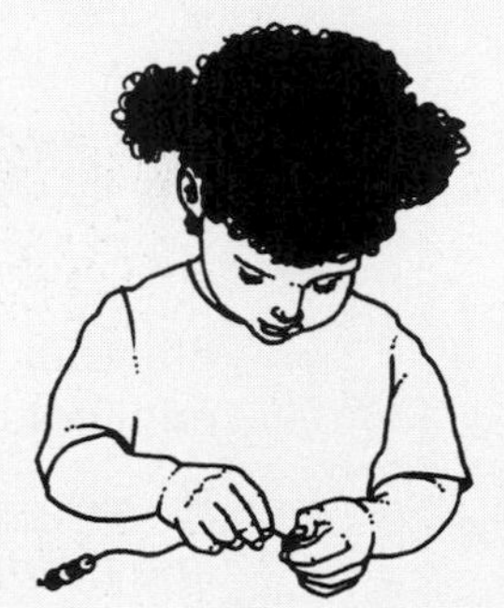

- She can thread smaller beads than at 3 years.

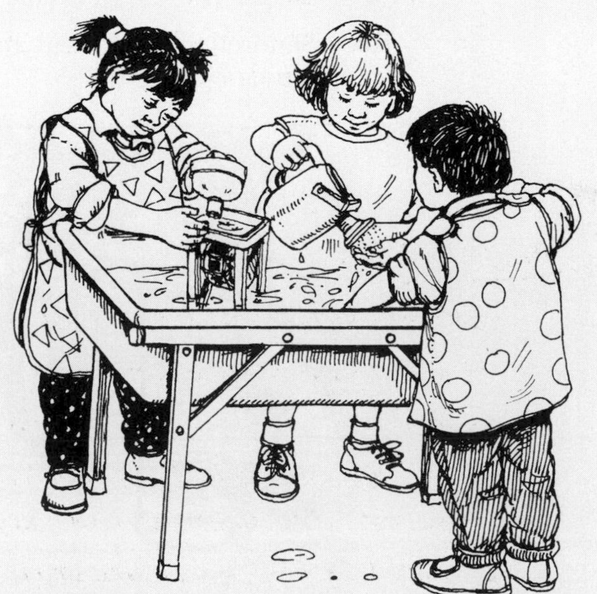

- They enjoy pouring, filling and emptying containers.

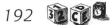

4 years

FINE MOTOR DEVELOPMENT

- He grasps a pencil maturely and has good control.
- He draws a person on request, showing head, legs and trunk.

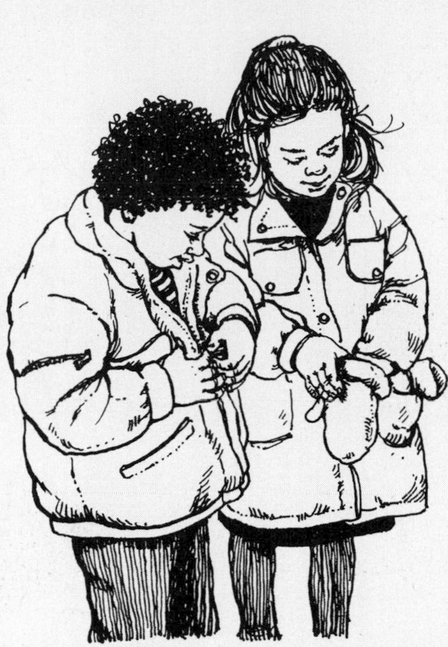

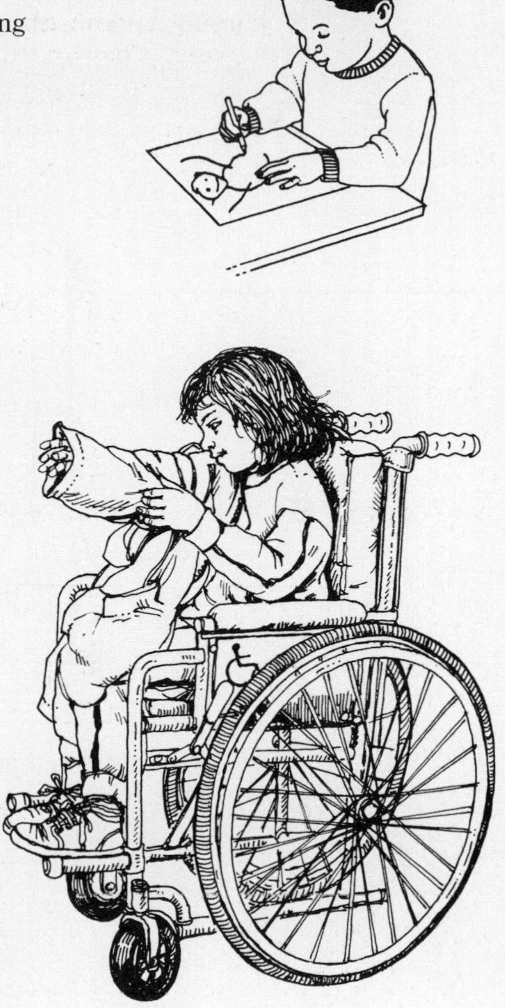

- They practise skills like buttoning clothes and fastening zips.
- They enjoy pouring, filling and emptying containers.

Progress check

At what age would you expect a child to be able to do the following:

(a) walk upstairs with one foot on each step, and down with two feet on each step?

(b) walk up and down stairs with one foot on each step?

(c) ride a small tricycle, pushing it along with the feet?

(d) be aware of their own size in relation to things around them?

(e) bend at the waist to pick things up from the floor?

5 years

GROSS MOTOR DEVELOPMENT

At 5 years children cope with most daily personal duties and are ready for the wider world of school. They run, climb, dance and jump about. Some children combine all this into some imaginative 'stunts'. Most children will use these skills in hiding and chasing games with each other, often involving any willing adults!

- She plays a variety of ball games quite well.

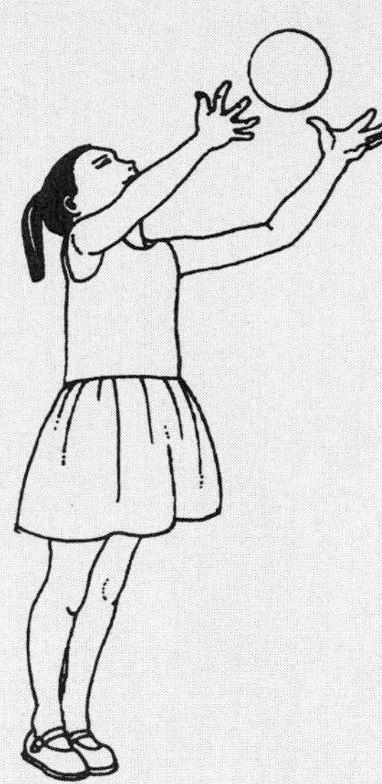

- The child moves rhythmically to music.

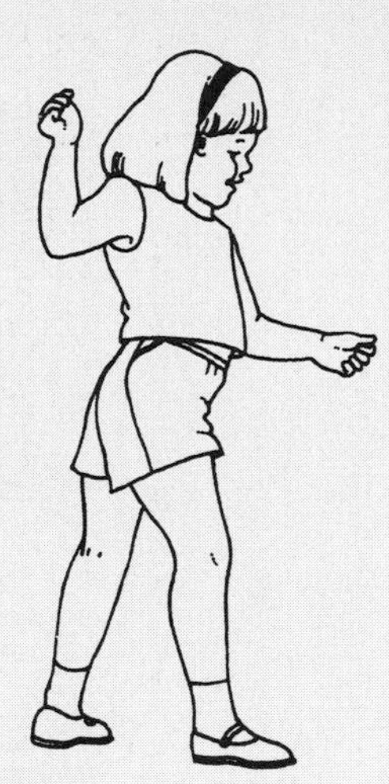

- He can hop and run lightly on the toes.

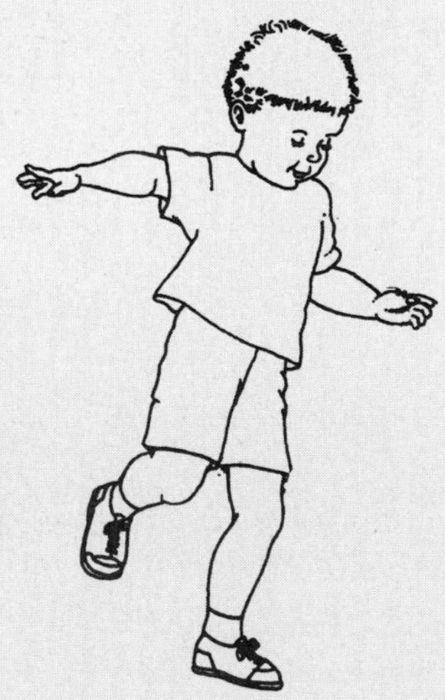

- He can walk along a thin line, climb, dig, and use slides and swings.

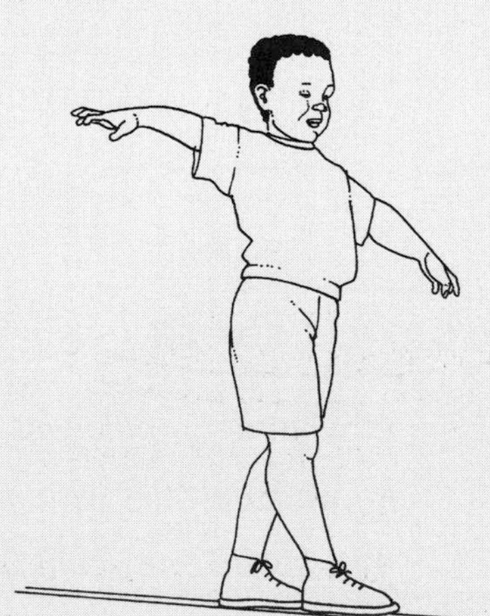

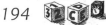

5 years

FINE MOTOR DEVELOPMENT

At 5 years fine skills are well co-ordinated and children can play games needing appropriate placing of objects. Five year olds will be able to manage most of the fastenings on their clothes, although they find tying laces difficult.

- He can draw a person with head, trunk, legs and eyes, nose and mouth

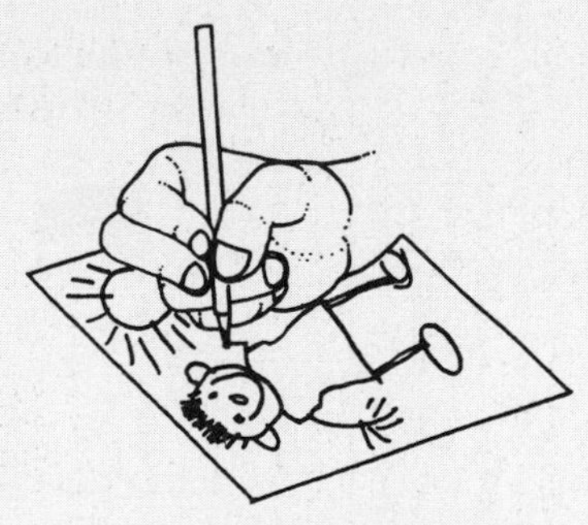

- He matches 10 to 12 colours.
- He can sew large stitches.
- He may be able to thread a needle.
- She builds three to four steps with bricks from a model.

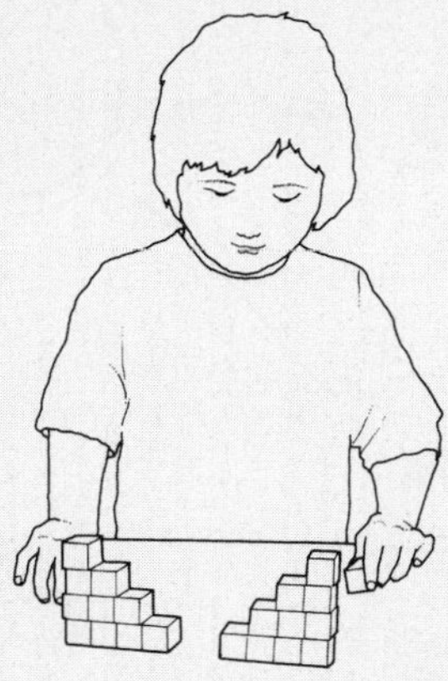

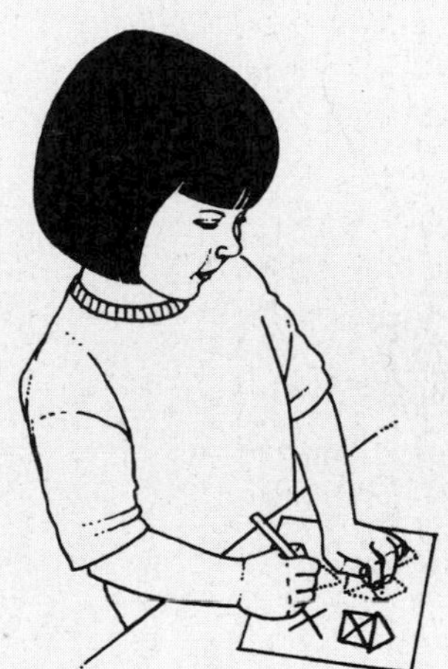

- There is good control of pencils and paintbrushes.

Progress check

Which combination of equipment will best stimulate fine manipulative skills when used by a 5 year old?

(a) water, dry sand, dough

(b) jigsaws, collage, sewing

(c) hats, dolls, pushchairs

(d) bicycles, trucks, tyres

6 years

GROSS MOTOR DEVELOPMENT

At 6 years the children have developed agility and strength. Six year olds become increasingly adept in climbing and jumping. They enjoy experimenting with their movements on the large apparatus, beginning to learn to suspend themselves by the arms and knees.

- He kicks a football a distance of 3–6 m.

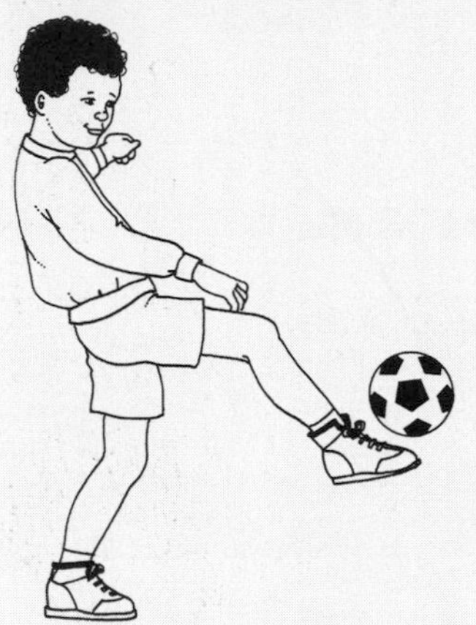

- He rides a two-wheeled bicycle.

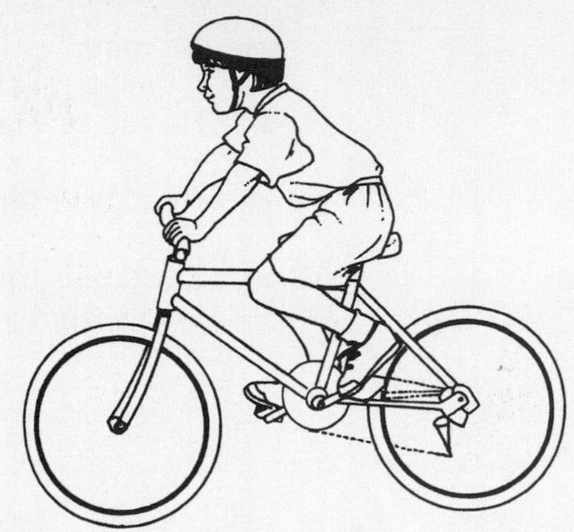

- He makes a running jump of approximately 100 cm.
- She can make a vertical jump of about 10 cm.

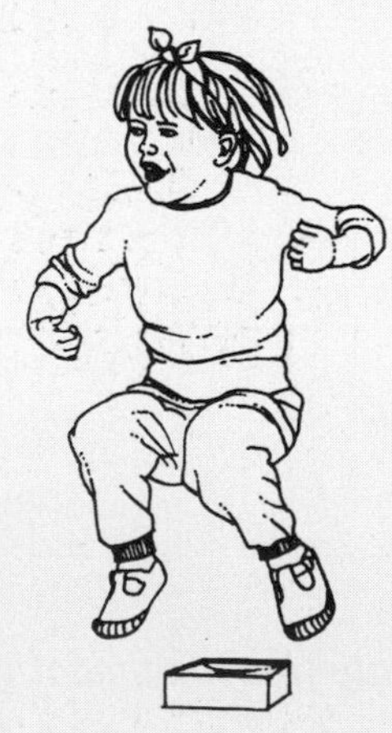

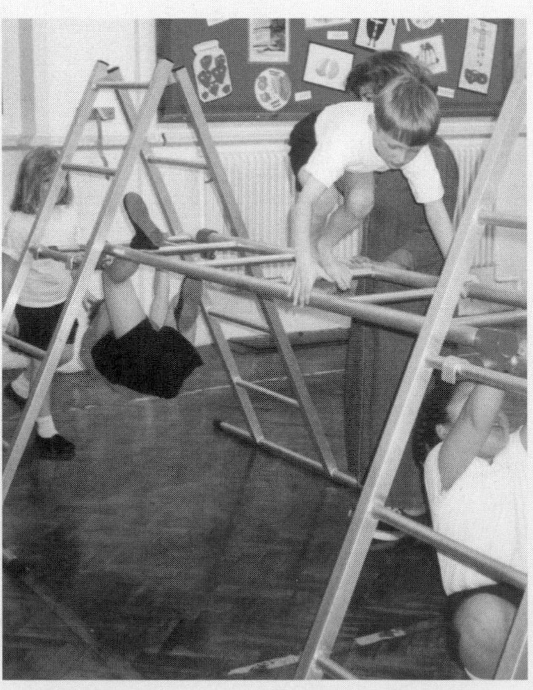

Children enjoy experimenting with movement on large apparatus

6 years

FINE MOTOR DEVELOPMENT

At 6 years old children can use a pencil, crayon or brush to produce drawings of people and buildings with much more detail. In order to write, children need to move from a whole-hand grip to a finer hold involving the thumb and fingers holding the pencil nearer the point. Six year olds are adjusting their grip on the pencil, forming letters and getting their writing to flow.

- The child can carefully align cubes to build a virtually straight tower.

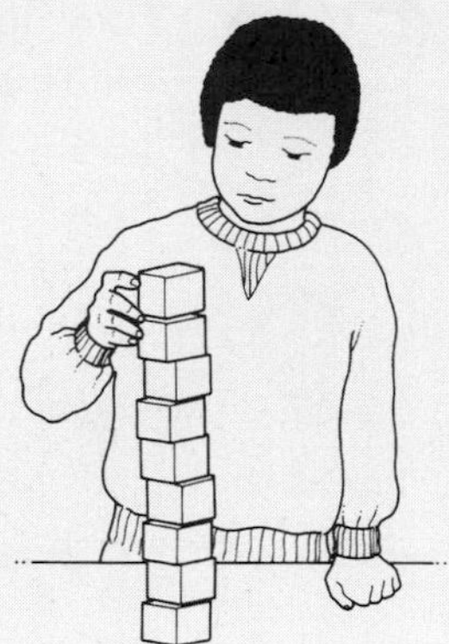

- He can catch a ball thrown from 1 m with one hand.

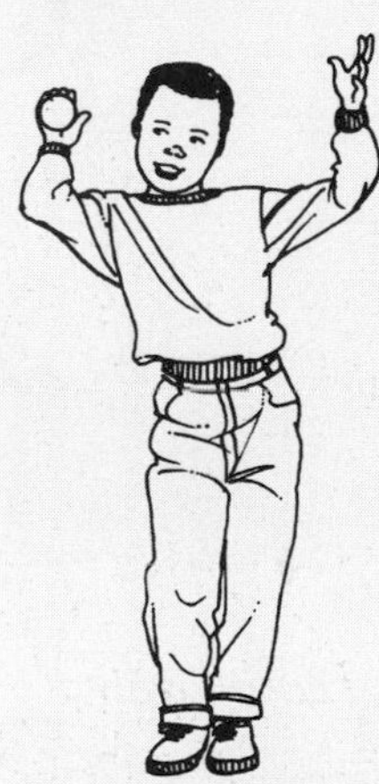

- She grasps and adjusts the pencil as at 5 years.
- The writing hold is similar to that of an adult.
- Writing is confined to a small area of the paper.
- He draws recognisable pictures.

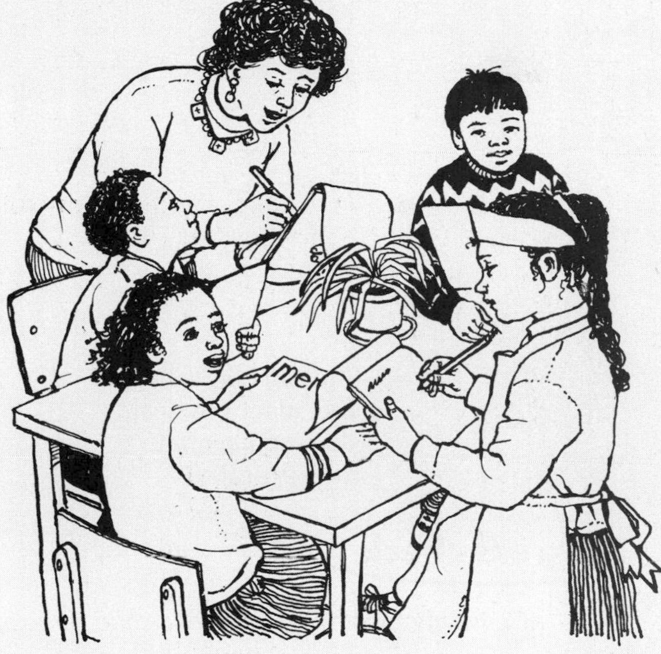

Progress check

Which combination of skills best describes the fine motor skills of a 6 year old?

(a) build three steps with six bricks; thread small beads; copy a square

(b) build a tower of nine or ten small bricks; cut with scissors; copy a circle

(c) catch a ball; draw recognisable pictures; adult writing hold

(d) draw a diamond; sew neatly with a needle and thread; tie shoelaces.

7 years

GROSS MOTOR SKILLS

At 7 years children's physical progress is consistently improving; they can balance and climb the apparatus with ease. Seven year olds become more able to experiment with the movements that they make and can deliberately vary their speed. These skills can be used in expressive movements, and children of this age enjoy dancing to music in various forms.

- The child can now ride a two-wheeled bicycle expertly.
- She can jump off the apparatus from about four steps high.
- He hops easily, keeping well balanced.
- They enjoy games and sports, and run around energetically.

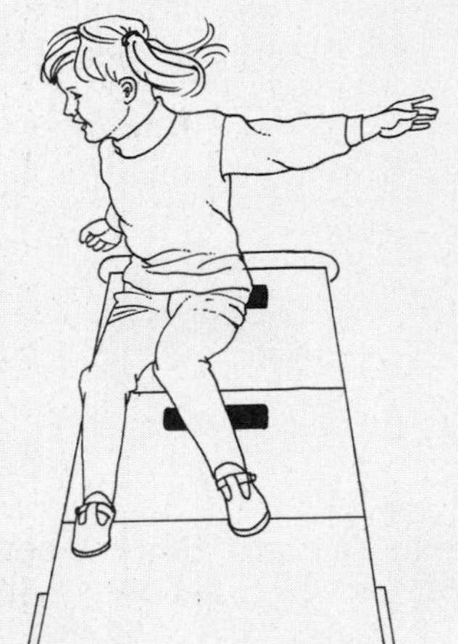

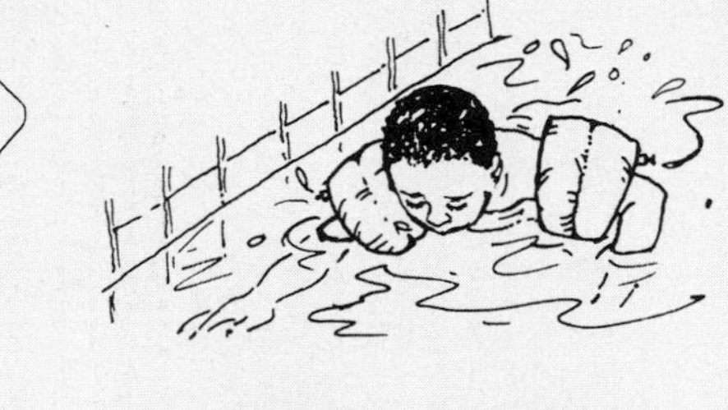

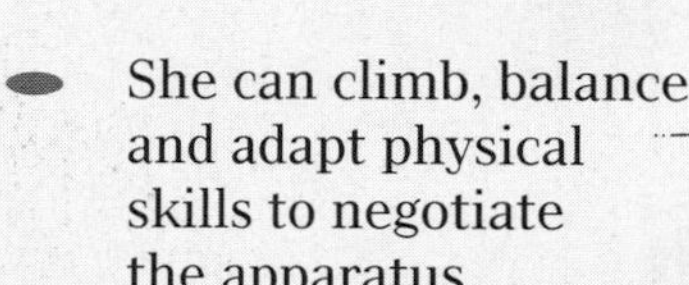

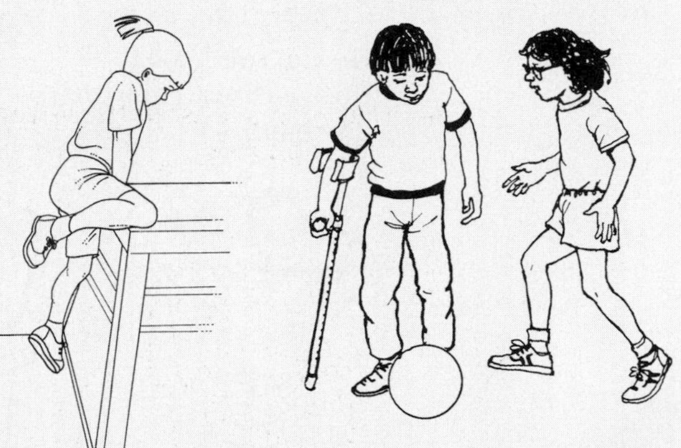

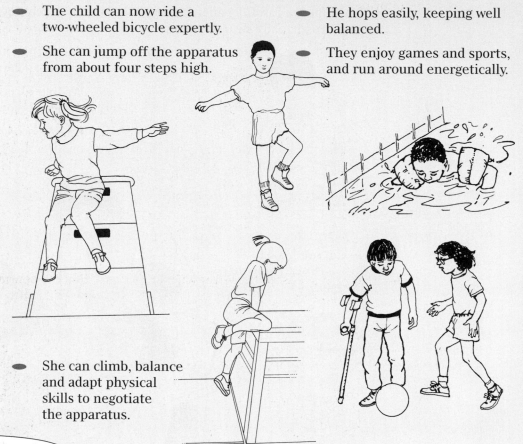

- She can climb, balance and adapt physical skills to negotiate the apparatus.

Progress check

At what age would you expect a child to be able to do the following:

(a) ride a tricycle using the pedals?
(b) walk upstairs and downstairs holding on and putting two feet on every step?
(c) balance on the apparatus beam?
(d) walk upstairs with one foot on each step, but downstairs with two feet on each step?
(e) draw a recognisable person with head, body, arms, legs and possibly eyes, nose, mouth?
(f) build a tower of ten bricks?
(g) build a tower of six or seven bricks?
(h) hold a pencil in the preferred hand?
(i) stand, walk and run on tiptoe?
(j) match and name four primary colours?

7 years

FINE MOTOR DEVELOPMENT

At 7 years children are generally learning to write. The skills of writing, forming and joining letters will only improve with a lot of practice. Children are beginning to get their writing to flow. Some children may also be aware that there are different scripts and different directions of writing. As with gross motor development, there will be differences in skill and confidence between individual children.

- She can build a tall straight tower with bricks.

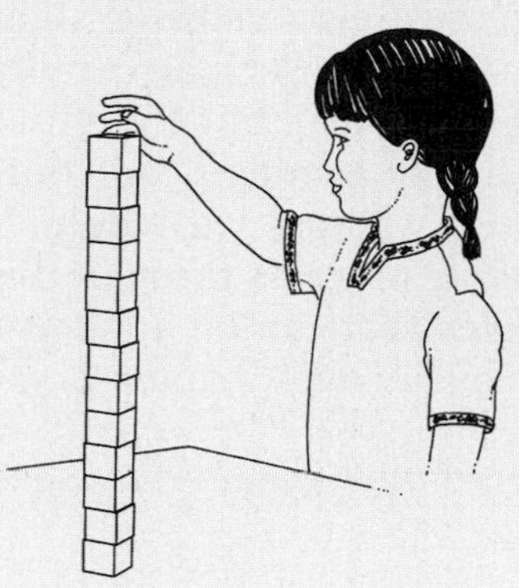

- She can draw a diamond neatly.

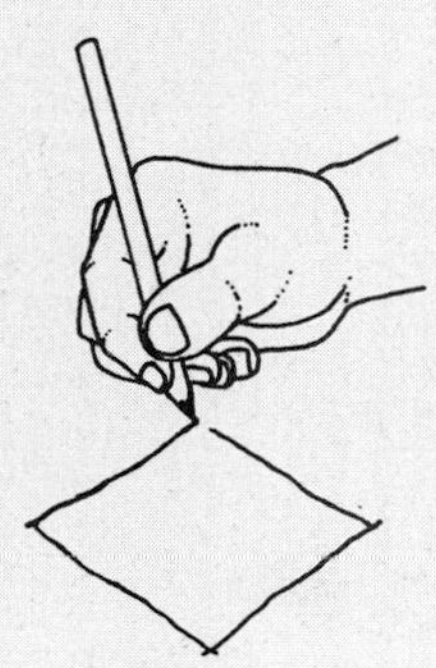

- He writes most of the letters of the alphabet.

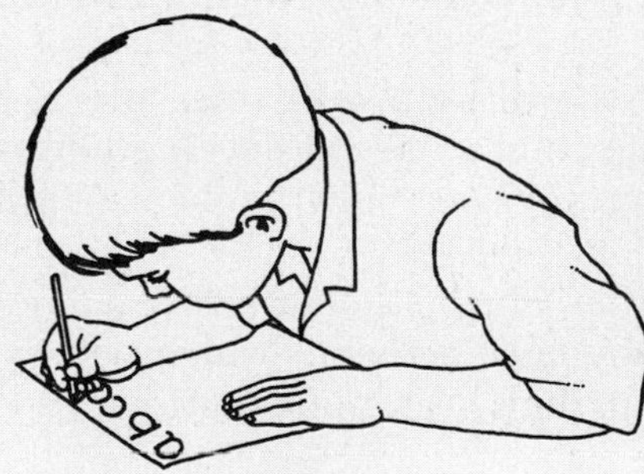

- She can sew neatly with a large needle.

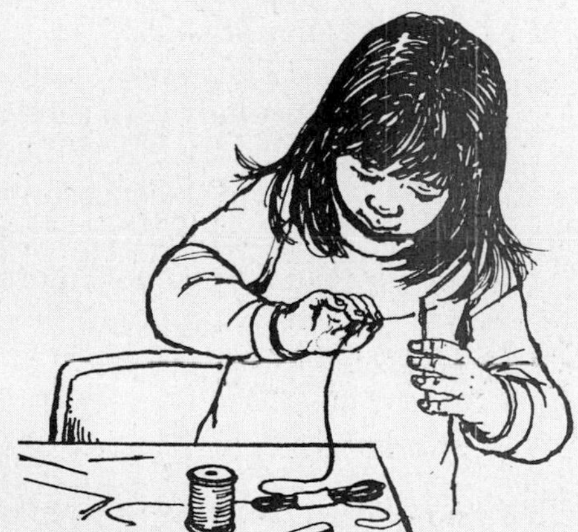

- He draws a person with originality, for example clothed and seated.

Progress check

At what age would you expect a child to be able to do the following:

(a) thread large beads?

(b) match two or three primary colours?

(c) draw a person showing head, legs and trunk?

(d) build three or four steps after a demonstration?

(e) draw a diamond?

Variations in developmental progress

The development of a child is a progression through stages. Very often an age is attached to a stage of development, such as children walking at 15 months. In reality some children walk as early as 9 months and others as late as 18 months. This is perfectly normal. Development is not a line but an area or range. Although you need a working knowledge of the *average* age at which children achieve their developmental milestones, you will always need to remember the *range* of achievement.

Children progress through the stages of development at their own pace. There may be many reasons why some children do this more quickly or more slowly. Factors may include race: African and Caribbean children often achieve the stages of gross motor more quickly than the average, sitting, standing and walking early in the range. Children who have a condition such as cerebral palsy may achieve the stages more slowly. Progress is individual, but the child will move through the stages in the same order, for example gaining head control, sitting with support, sitting unaided, pulling to stand, walking with help, walking alone. What is important is that the child is making progress through the stages.

There are other broad principles that can be applied to physical development and these are more thoroughly explained in Chapter 8.

The role of the adult

The adult needs to provide a safe environment for babies and children to extend their physical skills. Children need room to move around freely and the opportunity to extend their range of movements in both gross motor and fine motor skills.

There are many toys that will help with this, and it is important to choose carefully with safety and the child's stage of development in mind. Many toys will be labelled as suitable for certain age groups, but bear in mind the stage the child is at and select accordingly.

Providing toys and activities which stimulate development needs to be carefully undertaken. Children usually need activities which will extend their abilities, but not so difficult or easy that they lose interest. However much children enjoy a

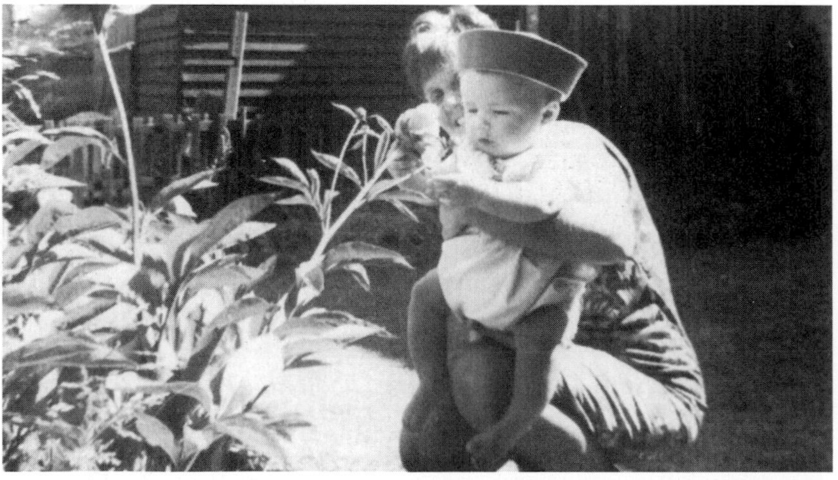

Exploring in the garden

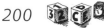

challenge, they will always enjoy their favourite toys. Children will work at achieving a skill, practise it and then enjoy themselves using their new-found achievement.

Although bought toys can be good, there are plenty of things around the home, garden and park that can be used by adults to stimulate children's physical development: boxes to climb in and out of, saucepans and cupboards to explore, wooden spoons, buttons, cotton bobbins to sort, hideaways under the table with a long cloth. Outside in the garden or park there is room to move around; there are plants, insects, animals, mud and water to explore. All these things can be observed, experienced and explored with imaginative, sensitive, adult encouragement and supervision. It is up to the adult to recognise the stage of development the child has reached and to provide the encouragement needed to help the child move forward at the pace each one needs. This pace may well vary with each child and should reflect individual needs.

Now try these questions

What are the stages in the development of locomotion?

Describe the stages in the development of fine manipulative skills.

What important points should adults be aware of when supporting children's physical development?

Discuss 'normal' and 'norms' in the context of development.

Describe the primitive reflexes present in the 'normal' neonate.

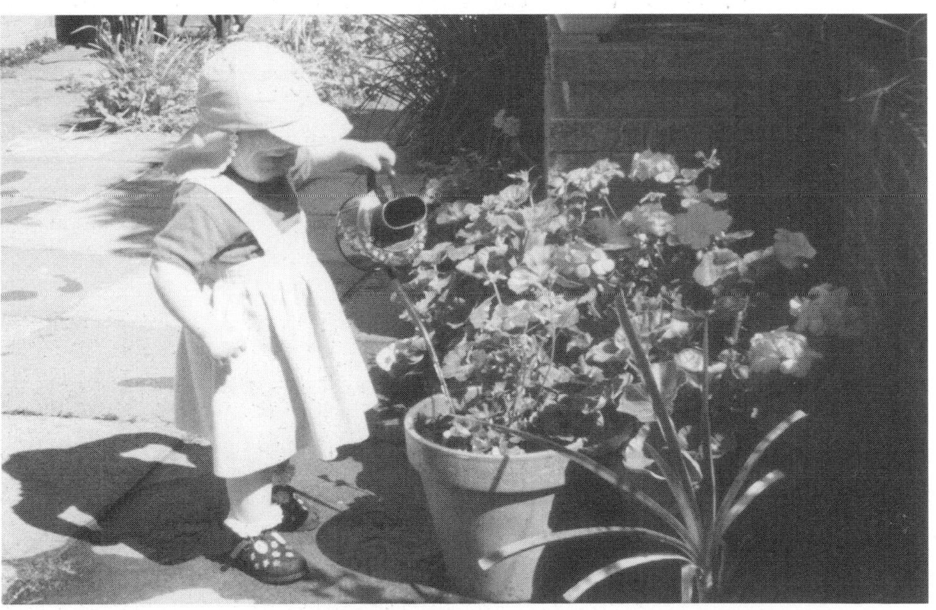

Refining and co-ordinating physical skills

key terms

You need to know what the key terms and phrases in this chapter mean. Go back through the chapter and find out.

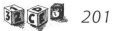

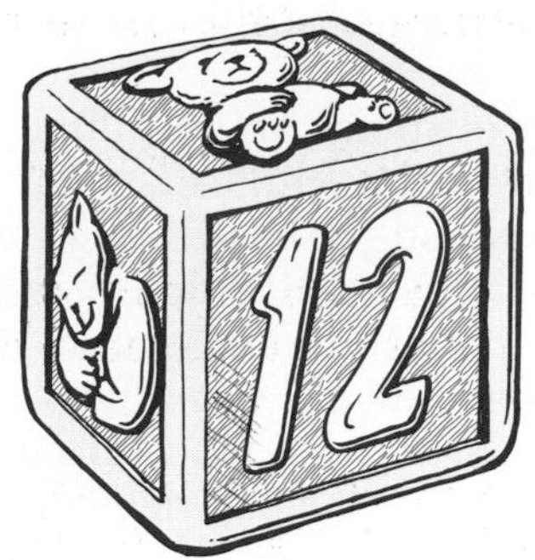

EMOTIONAL AND SOCIAL DEVELOPMENT

Emotional development is the growth of a child's ability to feel and express an increasing range of emotions appropriately. It includes the development of feelings about and for other people, and the ability to express them appropriately and with self-control.

Social development is the growth of a child's ability to relate to others appropriately, and become independent, within a social framework. It includes the development of social skills and independence.

An important strand in emotional and social development is the development of self-concept and self-image. This is the picture we have of ourselves and the way we think other people see us. Self-identity includes the characteristics that make us separate and different from others. It could also be referred to as our personality.

This chapter will cover the following topics:

- *general principles of social and emotional development*
- *the stages and sequence of emotional and social development, 0–1 year*
- *the stages and sequence of emotional and social development, 1–3 years 11 months*
- *the stages and sequence of emotional and social development, 4 years to 7 years 11 months*
- *factors that affect social and emotional development.*

General principles of social and emotional development

There are important things to remember when studying social and emotional development:

- Development is a whole process; all areas of development are integrated and interact with each other; they mix together and are affected by each other.
- The interaction of different areas results in an individual pattern of development that varies from one child to another.
- Development is usually made up of a period of rapid growth followed by a period of relative calm. During this period of calm, the previous growth is

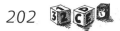

consolidated. This means that it becomes a definite and practised part of the child's being. One developmental area may be relatively calm while there is more rapid growth in another.

- The path of development moves from complete immaturity and dependence towards social and emotional maturity.
- Children do not develop in isolation; they develop within family systems. Families have individual characteristics that influence each child differently.
- A child's family exists within a larger cultural system. The experience of this cultural environment has a profound effect on both the family and a child's behaviour.
- Family and cultural environments interact with and affect children's developing skills, their awareness of themselves and their relationships with others.

In this chapter the stages of social and emotional development are outlined separately from physical, language and cognitive development. This is because it is simpler and easier to understand children's developmental progress by examining one area of development at a time.

The following sections of this chapter describe the path of emotional and social development of a newborn baby until the age of 8. The path moves from complete immaturity and dependence towards social and emotional maturity, and includes the development of social skills and independence. The main aspects of development covered are:

- *emotional* – children's ability to feel and express emotions
- *social* – children's relationships with other people
- *social skills* – the development of skills that lead to independence
- *self-image and identity* – children's view and awareness of themselves.

A child's self-concept and self-image is established gradually over the first few years of their life. By recognising and understanding the stages in this development, child-care workers can encourage the process and also enable children to feel worth while and valued. This is vital to their emotional well-being. Children's self-image and self-concept will influence their relationships through to adulthood.

The stages and sequence of emotional and social development, 0–1 year

BIRTH

At birth and for the first month or so of life, a baby's behaviour is largely governed by in-built reflexes and reactions. These reflexes govern the way the infant listens, looks around, explores and relates to others. However, even at this stage carers become aware of characteristics that they see as individual to the child, which seem to be the product of nature.

New-born infants begin to learn as soon as they are born, but at this stage their behaviour and communication with adults is limited. In general they cry to make their needs known and are peaceful when those needs are met.

Self -image

New-born infants do not realise that people and things exist apart and separate from them. It is thought that carers are perceived only as 'relievers of their distress', whether this is hunger, pain or loneliness.

Development

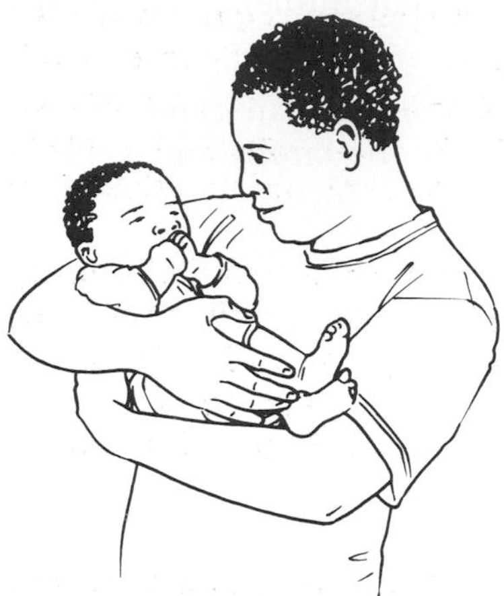

The newborn is usually content in close contact with the carer

At this stage babies:

- are utterly dependent on others
- have rooting, sucking and swallowing reflexes
- sleep most of the time
- prefer to be left undisturbed
- startle to noise, and turn to the light, providing it is not too bright
- cry when hungry, in pain or unattended to
- are usually content in close contact with carer
- are not aware of themselves as separate beings.

1 MONTH

Babies are observed to smile spontaneously from birth; but when they are 4–8 weeks old they begin to smile in response to happenings outside themselves. The baby learns to smile at a voice and a face; they are also attracted to the movement of faces.

key terms

Differentiate
to distinguish and classify as different

Personal identity
one's own individuality, the characteristics that make us different and separate from others, our personality

Self-image

Children learn to **differentiate** between themselves and other people or things through interaction with their carers and by exploration using their five senses. They gradually come to a realisation of who they are – their **personal identity** – and what they think and feel about themselves – their self-image and self-concept.

Development

Around this age babies:

- sleep most of the time when not being handled or fed
- cry for their needs to be attended to (different cries are evident for hunger, pain, panic and discomfort)
- will turn to the breast
- look briefly at a human face
- will quieten in response to a human voice and smile in response to the main carer's voice
- develop a social smile and respond with vocalisations to the sight and sound of a person (at around 6 weeks); the baby's response to a person separate from themselves
- grasp a finger if the baby's hand is opened and the palm is touched
- gradually learn to recognise themselves as separate individuals.

2 MONTHS

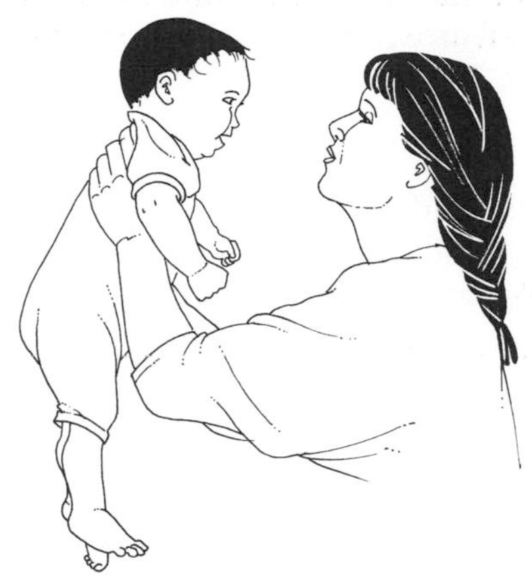

The baby smiles in response

From 2 months babies have fewer primitive reactions and gradually learn a range of responses and behaviour. These are the result both of physical maturation and of the baby beginning to explore the environment.

At 2 months the baby is capable of having 'conversations' with the carer. These are a mixture of gestures and noises, but follow the pattern of a conversation in that one person is quiet while the other speaks. Children start to recognise their carer's face, hands and voice. They may stop crying if they sense (i.e. hear, see or feel) their carer. This implies that they are beginning to be aware of their separateness, of the carer existing independently of themselves.

During this stage, early recognition of a child's **sensory impairment** will enable carers to adapt their approach to meet the child's needs, for example by using sign language with a deaf child. Carers who themselves have a sensory impairment are often skilled in adapting to accommodate the needs of their children.

key term

Sensory impairment hearing or sight loss

Self-image

Babies learn that touching a toy feels completely different to touching their own hand. In feeling the difference, they learn that the moving thing they see is their own hand, a part of them.

When they are held during feeding, changing and cuddling, babies learn that there are two kinds of feeling: one that comes from outside themselves; and the other, for example when they touch their own hand or chew on their own toes, that does not. These exploratory experiences start the process of differentiation between themselves and other people or things.

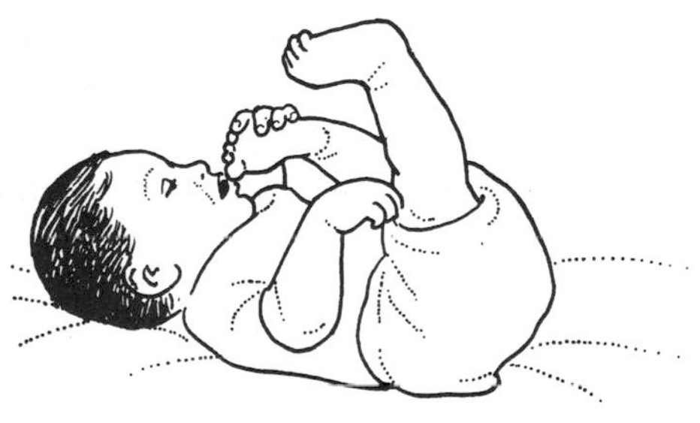

Is this part of me?

Development

Around this age babies usually:

- stop crying when they are picked up
- sleep less during the day and more during the night
- explore, using their five senses
- differentiate between objects, and begin to tell one face from another
- follow a human face when it moves
- smile and become more responsive to others.

3 MONTHS

Babies take a lot of interest in their environment at this stage. Physical maturation continues rapidly. Babies turn their heads in response to different sounds and to see what people are doing. They are rapidly beginning to learn a range of social skills from the people around them. Even during this early period, it is essential for babies that someone takes the time to communicate and be with them. Babies appear to have a natural capacity to communicate, but this does not develop without contact and interaction with other people. They need to be handled and talked to. By 3 months babies have learned to respond with pleasure to friendly handling. An infant and carer gradually build up a complex pattern of responses.

Self-image

Once children have distinguished themselves as separate, they will start to build a picture or image of themselves. Gradually they discover what kind of person they are and what they can do. This picture of themselves can be either:

- a **positive self-image** – the child feels they are valuable and worth while
- a **negative self-image** – the child feels worthless and useless.

Children measure their own worth by the responses of adults and children who are significant to them. They need to experience the approval and acceptance of these people to develop feelings of **self-approval** and **self-acceptance**.

At this stage, infants still react to the world as if they alone make things exist or disappear. If they are looking at something, it exists; if they don't see it, it doesn't exist. If something or someone disappears from their view, babies will keep looking at the place where they were before they disappeared, as if waiting for them to come back. If they do not return, the baby will probably forget about them. If it is a person who is important to them, they will probably cry.

key terms

Positive self-image
a view of oneself as worth while and valuable

Negative self-image
the child feels they are not worth while or valuable

Self-approval
being pleased with oneself

Self-acceptance
approving of oneself, not constantly striving to change oneself

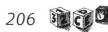

Development

Around this age infants usually:

- respond to friendly handling and smile at most people
- use sounds to interact socially and reach out to the human face
- become more oriented to their mother and other main carers, and look at their carer's face when feeding
- begin to connect what they hear with what they see
- are able to show an increasingly wide range of feelings and responses, including pleasure, fear, excitement, contentment, unhappiness
- have some awareness of the feelings and emotions of others
- still react to the world as if they alone make things exist or disappear.

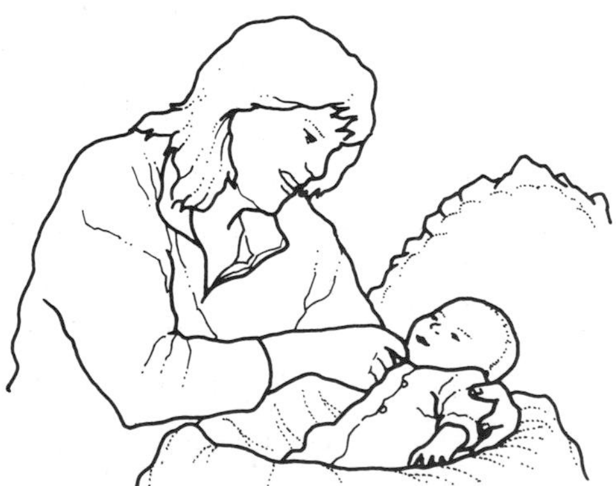

At 3 months babies respond to friendly handling and smile at most people

6 MONTHS

Development during the first 6 months is very rapid. Infants are awake for much longer periods by 6 months of age. If they have been stimulated by the presence of other people during this period, they will show great interest in their environment and respond happily to positive attention. Babies of 6 months laugh, show excitement and delight, and will also show likes and dislikes strongly.

Self-image

key terms

Stranger anxiety
fear of strangers

Separation distress
infants becoming upset when separated from the person to whom they are attached

This period may see the beginning of **stranger anxiety** and **separation distress**. This implies that babies recognise their separateness, and feel vulnerable without the support of the attachment relationship. If carers meet babies' needs at this stage, they will help to reinforce the babies' view of themselves as separate, but worth while.

Object permanence

During this stage, children are learning that people and things have a permanent existence. Even if they cannot see them, people and things still exist. This awareness is reinforced through games such as peek-a-boo: the infants are discovering that people and things that disappear temporarily are still there, but have to be looked for.

The importance of play in social and emotional development

Children from around 6 months are more able to join in play activities because of their developing physical skills. They may play alongside other infants in parallel play. Infants will develop a positive self-image if they are encouraged and enabled to learn by experience, especially through play. Play, at this stage, can be enhanced by the involvement of an interested adult. Their responses to the child, both positive and negative, will influence the child's self-image. Infants are aware of the feelings and emotions of other people. They experience all these emotions as reactions to themselves. They do not have the knowledge that would help them to see that anger and disappointment are not always caused by them. Infants start to feel towards themselves what they sense in others around them.

Development

Around this age infants:

- become more aware of themselves in relation to other people and things
- show a marked preference for their main carer(s)
- reach out for familiar people and show a desire to be picked up and held
- begin to be more reserved with, or afraid of, strangers
- smile at their own image in a mirror
- may like to play peek-a-boo
- show eagerness, anger and pleasure by body movements, facial expression and vocally
- play alone with contentment
- stop crying when communicated with.

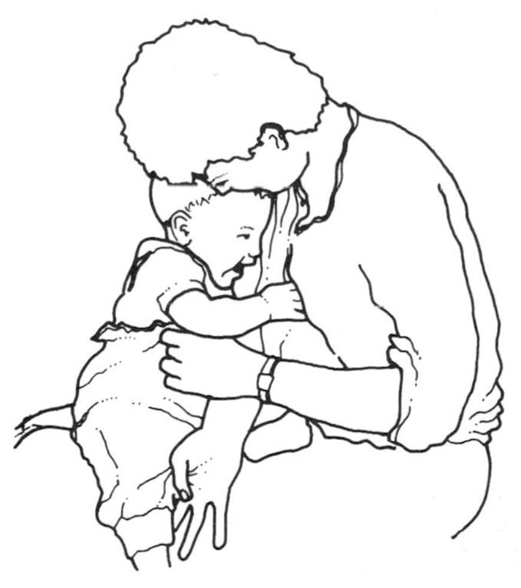

At 6 months babies show a preference for their main carer and begin to be more reserved with strangers

They may have the following skills:

- look at their hands and feet with interest
- use of their hands to hold things
- drink from a cup that is held for them.

9 MONTHS

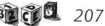

Given the right opportunities, babies of 9 months will have formed strong attachments with their main carer(s). They will also usually have begun to move around independently. These developments require new adaptations to be made by both infants and carers. Infants take great pleasure in playing with their carers and learn a great deal from this interaction. They can be a delight to be with. The development of infants who do not experience this positive interaction could be adversely affected.

Self-image

By this age, infants have become aware of themselves as separate from others, and have formed a definite image of other people who are significant to them.

Development

Around this age infants usually:

- clearly distinguish familiar people and show a marked preference for them
- show a fear of strangers and need reassurance when in their company, often clinging to the known adult and hiding their face in them
- play peek-a-boo, copy hand clapping and pat a mirror image
- still cry for attention to their needs, but also use their voice to attract people to themselves
- show some signs of willingness to wait for attention
- show pleasure and interest at familiar words
- understand 'No'
- try to copy sounds
- offer objects to others but do not release them.

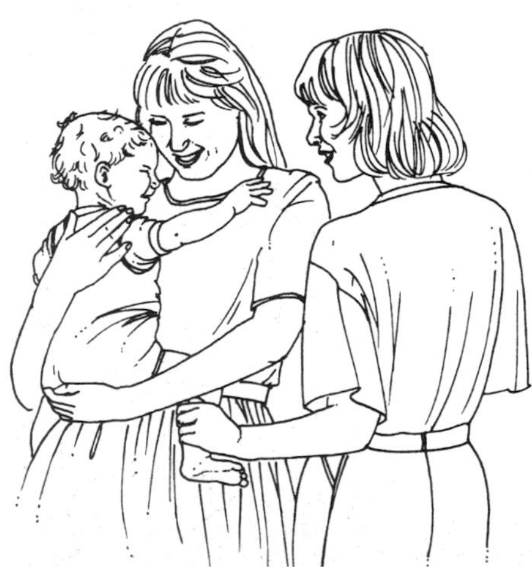

At 9 months babies show a fear of strangers, need reassurance, cling to known adults and hide their faces in them

They may have the following skills:

- put their hands around a cup or bottle when feeding
- awareness of self.

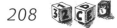

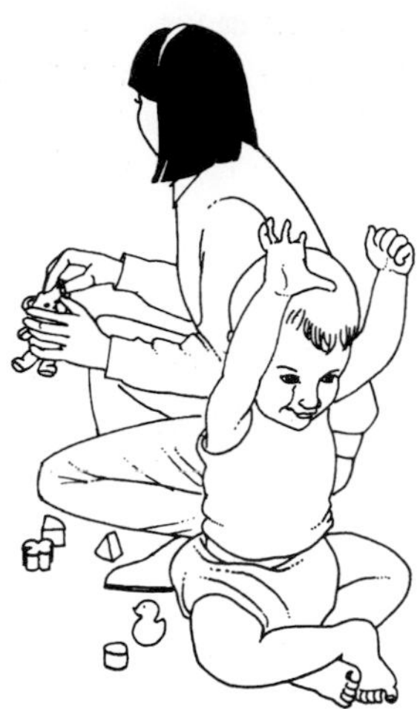

At 12 months infants like to be within sight and hearing of a familiar adult and will wave goodbye

12 MONTHS

Many infants have started to stand independently and possibly walk. They therefore gain a very different view of the world around them. Their physical skills enable them to pick up small objects, and to explore the environment. In a secure environment children can experience rich and varied interaction with adults. Their development will be adversely affected if they are not spoken to or played with at this age.

Self-image

By this stage, babies are aware of themselves as persons in relation to other people.

Development

Around this age infants usually:

- enjoy looking at themselves and things around them in a mirror
- know their name and respond to it
- like to be within sight and hearing of a familiar adult
- can distinguish between different members of the family and act socially with them
- will wave goodbye

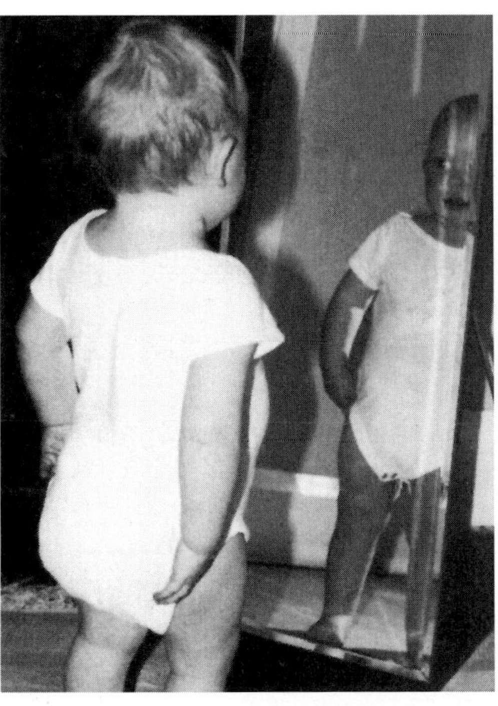

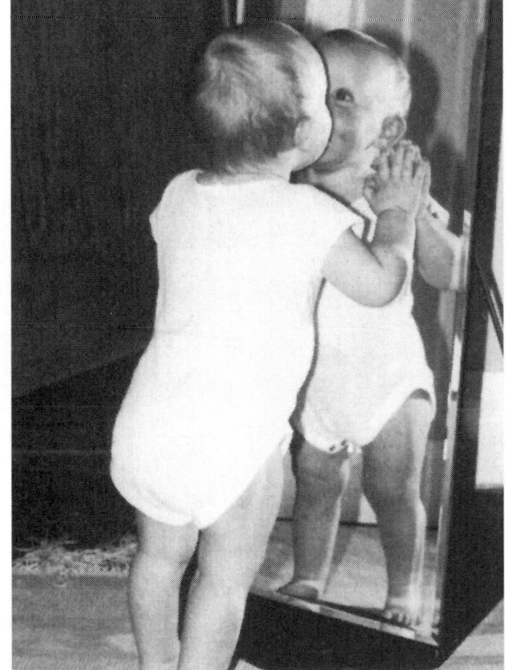

Is that me?

- appreciate an audience, repeating something that produced a laugh before
- begin to imitate actions they have seen others do
- respond affectionately to certain people
- may be shy with strangers

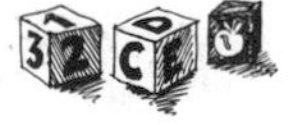

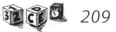

- are capable of a variety of emotional responses including fear, anger, happiness and humour
- show rage when thwarted
- actively seek attention by vocalising rather than by crying
- will obey simple instructions
- recognise other people's emotions and moods and express their own
- learn to show love to others, if they have been shown love themselves.

They may have the following skills:

- assist with feeding themselves by holding a spoon and may drink from a cup by themselves
- help with dressing by holding out their arms or legs.

Progress check

(up to 1 year)

What is a newborn baby's behaviour largely determined by?

At about what age do babies develop a social smile?

In order to develop communication skills what is it essential for babies to experience in their early life?

By what age do babies show a preference to be with their main carers?

How do 9-month-old babies often respond to strangers?

What range of emotional responses are babies capable of at 1 year?

The stages and sequence of emotional and social development, 1 year to 3 years 11 months

1–2 YEARS

From 1 to 2 years children become aware of themselves as people in their own right and begin to exert their will, sometimes in defiant and negative ways. At this stage children are very **egocentric**. Their defiant and resistant behaviour can be seen as an attempt to protect themselves and their individuality.

> **key term**
> **Egocentric**
> self-centred, from the words ego, meaning 'self' and centric, meaning centred on; seeing things only from one's own viewpoint

Factors that affect emotional and social development

The influence of cognitive development

Children's memory skills for objects and people are improving. By the end of their second year, they can remember whole situations and ideas, as well as concrete things. They could, for example, demonstrate their memory of a trip to the park with grandma. They could demonstrate that they remember the things in the park (the slide, swings, etc.), the fact that they went with grandma and that they enjoyed coming down the slide.

This growing intellectual ability enables them to know people by what they do, for example the person who dresses them, the one who smokes a pipe and so on, and it also enables them to define people outside themselves and remember them.

Children's developing language skills

Children's developing language skills enable them to express their needs more specifically and to express their will. Their growing understanding of language can have a positive or negative effect on their emerging self-image and self-concept. What is expressed to a child and how it is expressed are both significant. Between 18 months and 2 years children begin to call themselves by their name and talk about things as 'mine'. They recognise that some things belong to them and they can distinguish between 'mine' and 'yours'. They think of themselves as separate individuals and are learning to understand themselves in relation to others.

The role of the adult in promoting social and emotional development

Adult acceptance and approval

Infants learn to feel towards themselves what they sense in the responses of others. This applies both to them and their activities and efforts. Children begin to feel unworthy, incompetent, afraid and useless if:

- adults are impatient with their attempts to do things for themselves
- they are not allowed to explore and make new discoveries for themselves
- they always sense fear when they attempt new physical skills.

Infants' self-image is fragile at this stage. Even if adults are generally encouraging and approving, their feelings about themselves can swing dramatically. One moment a child may feel very powerful and successful, having learnt a new skill. The next moment they may feel small and weak when they find they cannot do what they have tried or seen another person do.

The importance of praise and encouragement

Appropriate encouragement and praise from adults for the effort children make at this stage is vital. Encouragement and praise for effort is more likely to develop a positive self-image than praise for achievement. This is especially true for children with learning difficulties, who may not be able to achieve in certain areas.

Children need to be encouraged to feel proud of any new accomplishments or independence skills, in effect to feel proud of themselves. Their feelings about themselves will have a significant effect on their relationships with other people.

The importance of play – parallel play

Towards the end of this period a child may be involved in playing alongside other children. They may form strong attachments to other children of the same age or older, although peers have not yet become very significant to their developing self-image.

15 MONTHS

By this age toddlers use their main carer as a safe base from which to explore the world. They are anxious and apprehensive about being physically separated from them, and tend to be very much 'under the feet' of their carers. They are very curious about their environment and their exploration of it can lead to conflicts with their carers.

Development

Around this age children:

- have a sense of 'me' and 'mine' and begin to express themselves defiantly
- begin to distinguish between 'you' and 'me', but do not understand that others are individuals just like themselves
- can point to members of the family in answer to questions like 'Where's granny?'
- tend to show off
- are not dissuaded from undesirable behaviour by verbal reasoning, react poorly to the sound of sharp discipline (the most useful disciplinary technique in this period is to distract a child and change the environment)
- have an interest in strangers, but can be fearful or wary of them
- show interest in other children
- show jealousy of the attention given by adults to other children
- throw toys when angry
- are emotionally changeable and unstable
- resist changes in routine or sudden transitions
- swing from dependence to wanting to be independent.

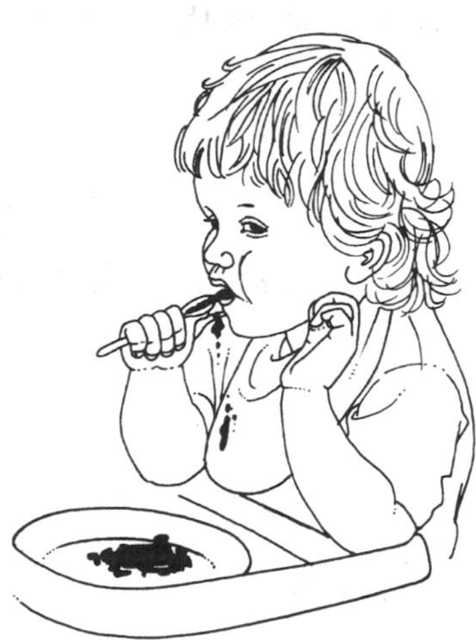

At 15 months toddlers will hold a spoon and bring it to the mouth, probably spilling some food in the process

They may have the following skills:

- hold a cup and drink without assistance
- hold a spoon and bring it to the mouth, spilling some food in the process
- help with dressing and undressing.

key terms

Internalise to understand the things that adults think are important and begin to believe and behave similarly

Reinforcement responding to an action or behaviour so that a particular consequence – a reward or punishment – is associated with the action and it is repeated (positive reinforcement) or not (negative reinforcement)

18 MONTHS

Development

At this age children usually:

- try to establish themselves as members of the social group
- begin to **internalise** the values of the people around them
- respond by stopping doing something when the word 'No' is used, but this usually needs **reinforcement**
- are still very dependent on a familiar carer and also often return to a fear of strangers
- tend to follow their carer around, be sociable and imitate them by helping with small household tasks
- are conscious of their family group
- imitate and mimic others during their play; engage in solitary or parallel play but like to do this near a familiar adult or sibling

- show intense curiosity
- show some social emotions, for example sympathy for someone who is hurt
- cannot tolerate frustration
- have intense mood swings, from dependence to independence, eagerness to irritation, co-operation to resistance.

They may have the following skills:

- use a cup and spoon well, and successfully get food into their mouth
- take off a piece of clothing and help with dressing themselves
- although still in nappies, they can make their carers aware of their toileting needs through words or by restless behaviour.

key terms

Social emotions
empathy with the feelings of others; the ability to understand how others feel

Empathy
an understanding of how other people feel

Self-awareness
a knowledge and understanding of oneself

Self-image

By the age of 2, some children have become sensitive to the feelings of others and display **social emotions**, such as sympathy if a person is hurt. This implies that children understand how such experiences make them feel (**empathy**), and is an indication of their growing **self-awareness**.

Progress check

How do babies learn to recognise themselves as separate individuals and differentiate between themselves and other people?

At what stage will babies first:

(a) exhibit stranger anxiety and separation distress?

(b) understand object permanence?

(c) usually know their name and respond to it?

(d) imitate something they have seen others do?

(e) call themselves by their name?

(f) engage in parallel play?

(g) demonstrate social emotions?

2 YEARS TO 2 YEARS 11 MONTHS

At this age children can be very self-contained; at other times very dependent. Children are capable of a wide range of feelings and are able to empathise with the feelings of those close to them. For example, if their carer is upset, they are capable of trying to comfort them.

Children are still emotionally and socially very dependent on familiar adult carers, although they are capable of self-directed behaviour. During this period extremes of mood are common. Children can change between aggressive and withdrawn behaviour, awkwardness and helpfulness very rapidly. They are also beginning to develop an understanding of those around them, enabling them to make friends with other children and play games based on shared interests.

Factors that affect emotional and social development

Children's developing language skills

By this stage, children are able to use symbols in language and these newly acquired linguistic skills promote their social development. Growing self-awareness depends on the development of a child's memory, the experiences they encounter and also on the development of language. Children who are encouraged to use language will develop more confidence in their own ability. This is because language enables children to explain how they feel, express more complex emotions than they could by non-verbal communication, receive reassurance and explanation, and handle problem situations.

The role of the adult in promoting social and emotional development

Role models

Adult role models with whom a child can identify are important. Disabled children and those from minority groups need to be able to model themselves on adults who are like them, rather than always seeing themselves as different from the significant adults in their world.

Self-image

Children at this stage are developing personal independence and taking important steps towards **self-reliance**; with improved motor development, children learn self-help skills. They will respond well if adults encourage this. Their developing competence confirms their **self-worth**. Adults can confirm children's separateness and individuality by, for example, setting certain things apart as belonging to the child – their own coat hook with their name and picture on.

Tasks that present children with a manageable challenge will give the opportunity for success and consequent enhancement of self-esteem. Too much frustration and consequent failure may produce a negative self-image and low self-esteem. This is one reason why disabled children, or those with learning difficulties, are more likely to have low self-esteem and a negative self-image.

> **key terms**
>
> **Self-reliance** the ability to depend on oneself to manage
>
> **Self-worth** thinking of oneself as having value and worth

Managing negative behaviour

Children's behaviour in the middle of this stage may seem rigid and inflexible. They do not like change, cannot wait and will not give in, often doing the opposite of what they are told. In fact, there may be a good reason for these behaviours. Children are just beginning to understand themselves and the world they live in. They are discovering that they have a will of their own and may practise exerting it!

The responses and reactions of adults at this time are vital to the child's emerging self-concept. Children need to be given clear guidelines for acceptable behaviour, but should not be 'put down' in a way that has a negative effect on their self-image. Carers have to limit their children's behaviour and impulses at this stage however, both for their future social development and the child's own survival.

The importance of play – role play

Between 2 and 3 years, children continue to develop their understanding of who they are and what they are like. They do this largely by observing and imitating the behaviour of people around them, particularly those who are significant to them.

This is shown in role play and imitation of actions and behaviours they have observed in others, such as feeding a doll or talking on the telephone. Pretending they are someone else helps children to take the point of view of others, to observe others and to generalise about the important aspects of other people's behaviour.

Such behaviour implies that children have developed a self-image and a view of other people separate from themselves. It may demonstrate something of what children think and feel about themselves in relation to other people.

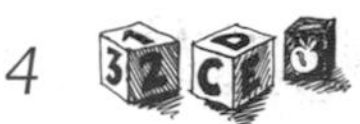

2 YEARS

Development

Around this age children:

- demand their carer's attention and want their needs to be met immediately they make demands
- can however respond to a reasonable demand to wait for attention or for the satisfaction of their needs
- will ask for food
- sometimes have tantrums if crossed or frustrated, or if they have to share the attention of their carer with another person
- are capable of being loving and responsive
- will try to be independent
- are possessive of their own toys and objects, and have little idea of sharing
- tend to play parallel to other children, and engage in role play, but begin to play interactive games
- tend to be easily distracted by an adult if they are frustrated or angry
- join in when an adult sings or tells a simple story
- can point to parts of the body and other features when asked.

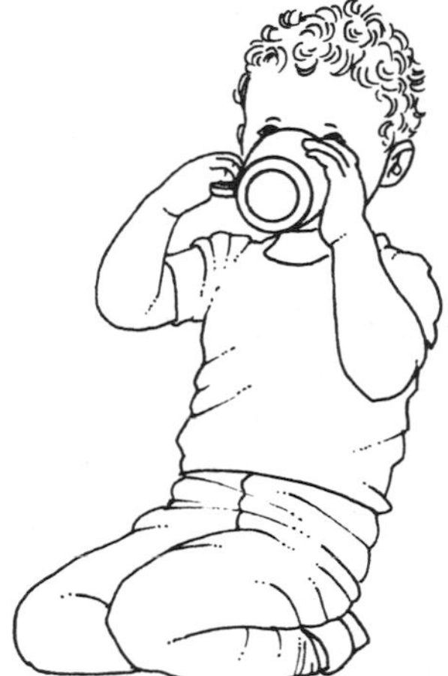

At 2 years children can lift up a mug and put it down again

They may have the following skills:

- feed themselves without spilling
- lift a cup up and put it down
- put some clothes on with supervision
- say when they need the toilet; become dry in the daytime.

2 YEARS 6 MONTHS

Development

Around this age children:

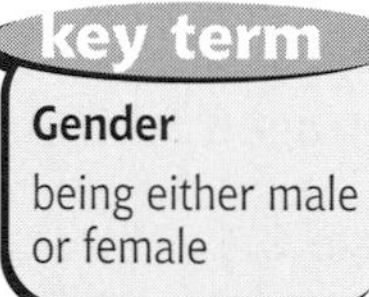

Gender
being either male or female

- develop their sense of self-identity – they know their name, their position in the family, and their **gender**
- play with other children – among other things this tends to reinforce their developing concept of gender roles. They also learn that different toys are intended for girls and boys
- may engage in pretend play including role or make-believe play
- behave impulsively, wanting to have anything they see, and do anything that occurs to them
- throw tantrums when thwarted and are not so easy to distract
- are often in conflict with their carers.

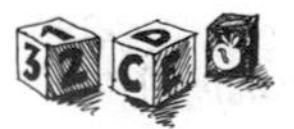

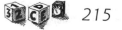

They may have the following skills:

- awareness of and ability to avoid certain hazards (like stairs and hot stoves)
- the ability to use a spoon well, and possibly a fork or chopsticks
- the ability to pour from one container to another and therefore to get themselves a drink
- dress with supervision, unzip zips, unbuckle and buckle, and unbutton and button clothing
- are toilet-trained during the day, and can be dry at night, especially if 'lifted' (taken to the toilet at night).

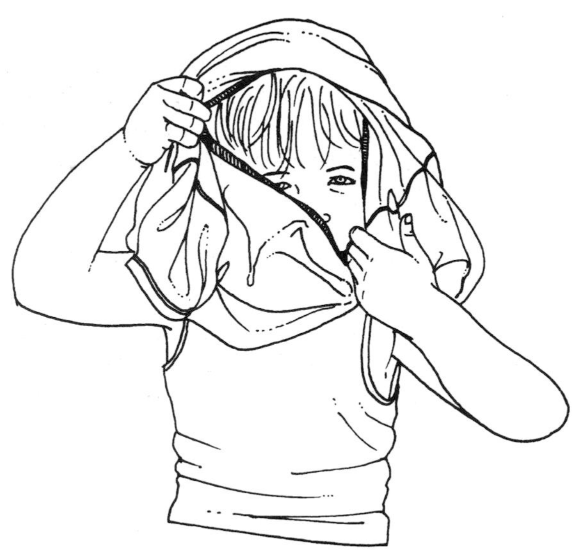

At 2 years 6 months children can dress with supervision

3 YEARS TO 3 YEARS 11 MONTHS

By this age children are usually happier and more contented than during the previous year. They have gained a certain amount of physical and emotional control. This can lead to more settled feelings and more balance in the way they express them. They are generally friendly and helpful in their manner to others. They are beginning to understand that other people have feelings, just as they do. They learn to sympathise with other children, and can be encouraged to think about their own and other people's feelings.

Factors that affect emotional and social development

Self-image

Between the ages of 3 and 5, the foundation of a child's self-concept is established. By 3 years, children call themselves 'I' and have a set of feelings about themselves. Their self-concept at this stage will influence how they respond to relationships and experiences now and in the future. It is still affected by the attitudes and behaviour of those around them. They see themselves as they think others see them.

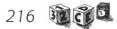

Peer group influences

At 3 to 4 years, children are more conscious of and concerned about others. They usually enjoy being with other children, and they begin to make strong attachments to individual children.

During this period, children test themselves out in different roles, for example as leader or as follower. Through this process they learn more about who they are and what they are like.

At this stage the reactions and responses of peers are very important and they will affect a child's self-concept. Comments like 'Here comes that dummy' and 'Oh no, it's that stupid boy again' will have a negative effect on a child's self-esteem and confidence. Adults can gain insight into children's views of themselves from observing if and how they join in group activities.

Adults are likely to find that a child with a positive self-image is easier to manage in a group situation.

Cultural background

In this period, children are beginning to learn the way of life of their cultural group. Learning to value and be proud of their own cultural background develops self-worth and self-confidence. Children should never be made to feel that what they learn in their own cultural setting is less valuable than what they learn in other cultural settings.

The role of the adult in promoting social and emotional development

Role models

All children will model themselves on the adults around them. Disabled children need to identify with disabled role models to construct their self-concept. It is not unknown for disabled children to think that they will grow out of their disability!

Avoiding gender stereotypes

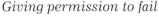

From 3 years most children know their own gender (that they are male or female) and start to learn society's ideas about appropriate attitudes and activities for each gender. To construct their self-concept, a child needs to identify with an adult role model of the same gender, but models of either gender should present children with choices of behaviours, activities and goals, not with **stereotyped roles**, such as men going out to work and women taking care of the home. Seeing men and women adopting non-stereotypical roles allows children of either gender to see that they can do and be anything they want. They do not have to be restricted by their gender.

key term

Stereotyped roles
pre-determined, fixed ideas to which individuals are expected to conform

Giving permission to fail

Children's feelings of confidence and self-worth will be strengthened if adults encourage them to develop independence skills and let them try to do things by and for themselves. Children need support to learn to accept their mistakes and not let them affect their feelings of self-worth. They need to be given permission to fail, with the message that it is perfectly acceptable to make mistakes.

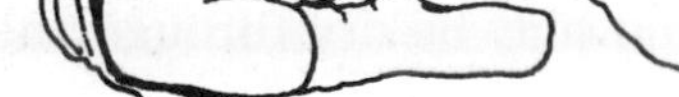

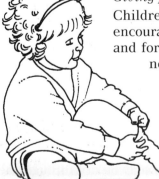

I can do this myself

Managing negative behaviour

By this stage, fear of punishment should be less important to children than their own internal set of standards – the standards by which they judge themselves and that guide their behaviour. Adults should explain rules so that children can understand them. Praising children for trying to do what they feel is right is more effective than punishing

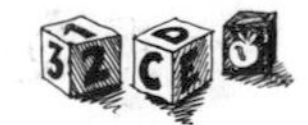

key term

Conscience the faculty by which we know right from wrong

them for doing wrong. If children misbehave, they should be given a chance to explain why they did so. This shows respect for the development of their inner **conscience**. They need to feel that while some actions are unacceptable, their participation in such activities does not make them bad people.

The importance of play – role play

Children continue to test out their self-image and explore that of others through role play. They also use role play to express their understanding of themselves and others' roles, behaviour and attitudes. Children can be involved in simple drama and take on characters and feelings. Role play can be used to help children understand other people's thoughts and feelings.

3 YEARS

Development

Around this age children:

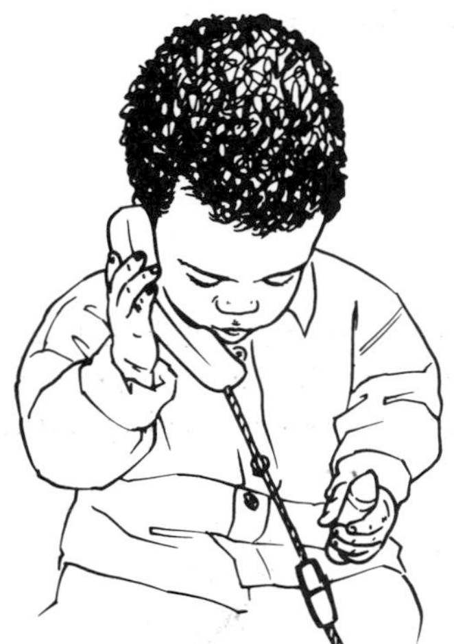
Is anyone there?

- can feel secure when in a strange place away from their main carers, as long as they are with people with whom they became familiar when they were with their carer
- can wait for their needs to be met
- are less rebellious and use language rather than physical outbursts to express themselves
- still respond to distraction as a method of controlling their behaviour – they are, however, also ready to respond to reasoning and bargaining
- are beginning to learn the appropriate behaviour for a range of different social settings – for example they can understand when it is necessary to be quiet or when they can be noisy
- adopt the attitudes and moods of adults
- want the approval of loved adults
- can show affection for younger siblings
- have an ability to share things and to take turns
- enjoy make-believe play, both alone and with other children
- project their own experiences on to dolls and toys
- may have imaginary fears and anxieties
- towards the end of this year may show some insecurity, expressed as shyness, irritability and self-consciousness.

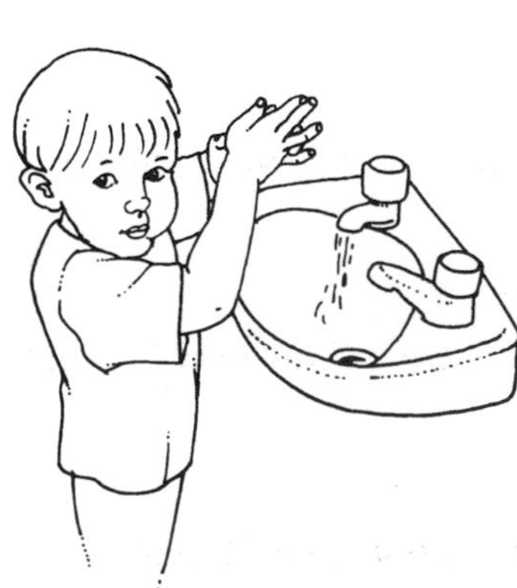
At 3 years children can toilet themselves and wash their hands

They may have the following skills:

- ability to use a fork and spoon to eat (in some cultures it will be more appropriate to use hands to eat some food) and can be proficient with chopsticks
- toilet themselves during the day, and may be dry through the night – will wash their hands but may have difficulty drying them
- learning to dress without supervision.

Case study . . .

. . . separation

Tom is 3 years old. His parents recently moved to another part of the UK, but they had to stay in temporary accommodation for some weeks before their house was ready. Tom is the eldest of two boys born 16 months apart. Tom happily attended a playgroup for a few months before they moved, and sometimes went to play next door.

Shortly after the family eventually moved into their new home, Tom was invited to a 4-year-old's birthday party at a neighbour's house. His mother left him, as she had to take his brother to the doctor. When she returned she was upset to find Tom asleep. Apparently he had cried so much when she left that he had exhausted himself. Following this Tom would not be left anywhere for several months and then only if his younger brother remained with him.

1. *Would you have expected Tom to have been staying on his own quite happily at playgroup at his age and why?*
2. *Why do you think Tom was so upset when his mother left him at the party?*
3. *Why was Tom not happy to be left for a few months after this, and what difference did his brother staying make?*
4. *How would you assess Tom's behaviour?*

3 YEARS 11 MONTHS

By this age children are constantly trying to understand and make sense of their experiences and of the world around them. Although they can be very sociable at this age, they often return to a more stubborn phase. This may involve using some physically and/or verbally aggressive behaviour at times.

Development

By this age children:

- are capable of being very sociable with, and talkative to, both adults and children, and enjoy 'silly' talk
- may have one particular friend
- can be confident and self-assured
- may be afraid of the dark and have other fears
- have adopted the standards of behaviour of the adults to whom they are closest
- turn to adults for comfort when overtired, ill or hurt
- play with groups of children – groups tend to centre around an activity, then disperse and re-form
- can take turns but are not consistent about this
- are often very dramatic in their play – engage in elaborate and prolonged imaginative play
- are developing a strong sense of past and future
- are able to cope with delay in having their needs met

- show purpose and persistence and some control over their emotions
- can be dogmatic and argumentative – may blame others when they misbehave, and may even behave badly in order to arouse a reaction
- may swear and use bad language.

They may have the following skills:

- feed themselves proficiently
- dress and undress, but may have difficulty with back buttons, ties and laces
- wash and dry hands and face and clean teeth.

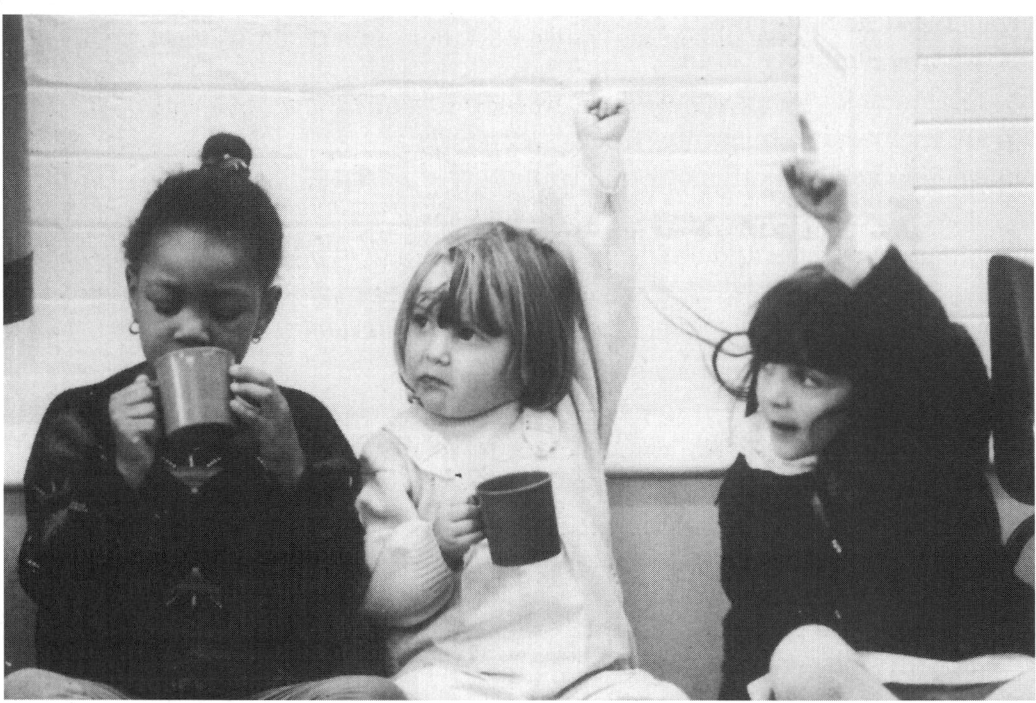

Between 3 and 4 years children can feel secure away from their main carers, are learning appropriate behaviour, are able to take turns and play in a group of children

Progress check

Name some of the emotions children can express at 1 year old.

At what age is a child most likely to begin to say 'It's mine'?

Children begin to 'internalise' the values of the people around them at around 18 months old. What does this mean?

At what age do children tend to begin to have tantrums?

When are children able to feel secure even if taken and left in a strange place? What does this depend on?

Use six words to describe a typical 4-year-old child.

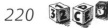

Case study . . .

. . . self-concept and behaviour

Elisha, aged 3 years 11 months, is of mixed parentage. Her adoptive parents are white and Elisha has no contact with her birth parents. The family live in a predominantly white, suburban area. Elisha was referred 6 months previously to a family centre, run by the social services department. Her rigid and inflexible behaviour had become difficult for her adoptive parents to manage. Elisha refuses to co-operate in day-to-day tasks such as washing, dressing, toileting, etc. She has severe temper tantrums and is deemed to be beyond her parents' control. Her adoptive mother explained that in the past she always did everything for Elisha, her 'little pet', but since becoming pregnant, she needs Elisha to 'grow up'.

The family centre is in the city centre and includes children from a variety of cultural backgrounds.

1. *Why may Elisha's behaviour pattern have developed?*
2. *How could the staff in the family centre manage Elisha's difficult behaviour?*
3. *Devise a play plan to include a range of activities to develop Elisha's self-esteem.*
4. *How can staff in the family centre work with Elisha's adoptive parents to prepare for and support them through the arrival of a new baby?*

The stages and sequence of emotional and social development, 4 years to 7 years 11 months

4–5 YEARS

Between 4 and 5 years children achieve a level of balance, self-containment and independence. They are usually friendly, willing to talk to anyone and are able to be polite. Most children have developed a stable self-concept (i.e. a view of themselves that remains constant and fixed). This is likely to be based on their own inner understanding and knowledge about who they are. If it is based only on other people's views, it will not be stable, but will change according to other people's ideas of them. Children at this stage who see themselves as likeable will not change this view of themselves when, from time to time, other children say that they do not like them.

Factors that affect social and emotional development

Internalising social rules

At this stage, social rules (for example not taking other people's things without their agreement) have been internalised by children. They do not have to be told what is right and wrong all the time. This does not mean, however, that they will always obey these internalised rules.

Children start to rely on their own judgement of their behaviour. They are beginning to understand the words 'good' and 'bad' in terms of consequences. They learn best if things are explained in terms of themselves as well as others, for example 'If you share your toys with Zaida, she will share hers with you'. Although children may not be able fully to put themselves into someone else's situation they can understand if the explanation is given in terms of themselves.

Development

By this age children usually:

- enjoy brief separations from home and carers
- show good overall control of emotions
- have a stable self-concept, are increasingly aware of a range of differences between themselves and other people, including gender and status differences
- want the approval of adults, show sensitivity to the needs of others and a desire for acceptance by other children
- are developing internalised social rules, an inner conscience and a sense of shame (an important development that affects the adult's ability to discipline and control the child)
- argue with parents when they request something
- still respond to discipline based on bargaining
- are not so easily distracted from their own anger as when they were younger
- often show the stress of conflict by being overactive – may regain their balance by having 'time-out'
- prefer games of rivalry to team games
- enjoy co-operative group play, but often need an adult to arbitrate
- boast, show off and threaten
- are able to see a task through to completion for their own self-satisfaction, show a desire to excel, and can be purposeful and persistent, which increases their own feelings of competence and self-worth.

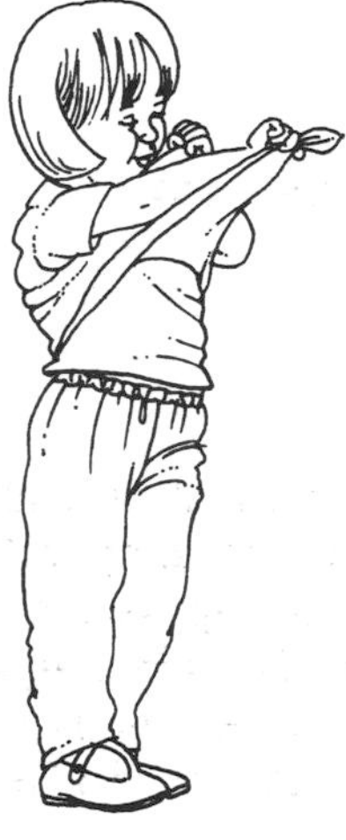

At 5 years children can undress and dress themselves

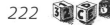

They may have the following skills:

- use a knife and fork well
- are able to dress and undress
- may be able to lace shoes and tie ties
- wash and dry face and hands, but need supervision to complete other washing.

Progress check

Why is role play important for children at this stage of development?

Why is it important that the tasks given to children are a manageable challenge?

Explain the importance of a child's involvement with their peer group at this stage?

Why is it important for a child to feel cared for, worthy and acceptable to their carers?

How do children develop an inner conscience?

Case study . . .

. . . a typical 5 year old

Christopher is 5 years old. He responds well to his parents, and smiles and enjoys it when they praise his efforts. He enjoys going to school. He especially likes playing in the playground with his two friends, Joel and James. Although he has a happy disposition, his parents are sometimes frustrated when he argues about going to bed, and other domestic routines. However, he usually responds well once his parents point out that they will be doing something enjoyable the next day or at the weekend, providing he gets enough sleep. He sometimes plays outside his home, as he lives on a safe cul-de-sac. He likes having races with his friends on their bikes. Sometimes they play imaginative games involving space travel and monsters, but they also argue and a parent sometimes has to come out and sort things out before they will continue playing. On occasions Christopher has to come indoors to calm down a little.

1. *How does Christopher relate to his peers?*
2. *How does he respond to his parents?*
3. *How does he like to play?*
4. *In what ways is Christopher's behaviour typical of a 5 year old?*
5. *Do you think he is at an appropriate developmental stage emotionally and socially?*

6–7 YEARS

Throughout these years children grow steadily more independent and truly sociable. They are generally self-confident and friendly; they are able to co-operate in quite sophisticated ways with adults and children. Their peer group becomes increasingly significant to them. Children's all-round development is increasingly sophisticated. This sophistication, coupled with skills of perseverance, opens up opportunities for success in many varied activities of increasing complexity, for example sewing, painting, playing a musical instrument and so on.

Development

By 6 years of age children:

- have progressed a long way along the path to independence and maturity
- have developed a wide range of appropriate emotional responses
- are able to behave appropriately in a variety of social situations
- have learned all the basic skills needed for independence in eating, hygiene and toileting routines
- are often irritable and possessive about their own things
- may have spells of being rebellious and aggressive.

At 7 years children:

- become very self-critical about their work
- may be miserable and sulky, and give up trying for short periods
- may be so enthusiastic for life that carers have to guard against them becoming overtired

- are more aware of gender characteristics – friendship groups are often separated by gender
- are influenced by the peer group, which becomes increasingly important to children over these years – peer group opinion is increasingly influential and will be used and quoted by children to carers as either their own ideas or to justify what they want to do. 'Hero' figures become influential and are used as role models by children at this stage.

7 YEARS TO 7 YEARS 11 MONTHS

The saying 'Give me a child until he is 7 and I will give you the man' sums up the fact that much of the child's personality is established by the end of this period. By the time they are 8 years old, children's experiences in their families and in their social and cultural environments will have led to the establishment of their:

- personal identity
- social and cultural identity
- gender role
- attitudes to life.

Disabled children

It is often at this stage that the differences of disabled children become more apparent. The development of sophisticated skills is the norm for children at this age; because of this the carers of a child who has a disability may be faced more starkly with their child's difference. They may struggle between:

- a concern to see their child treated as 'normal'
- acceptance of their child's disability and a recognition of the need for support.

The role of the adult in promoting social and emotional development

It is obvious that in this area of development children are fundamentally affected by the thoughts and actions of others. The following guidelines summarise, in a practical way, some of the principles involved in encouraging a positive self-image and self-concept, and healthy social and emotional development.

Twenty golden rules:

- From the earliest age, demonstrate love and give children affection, as well as meeting their all-round developmental needs.
- Provide babies with opportunities to explore using their five senses.
- Encourage children to be self-dependent and responsible.
- Explain why rules exist and why children should do what you are asking. Use 'do' rather than 'don't' and emphasise what you want the child to do rather than what is not acceptable. When children misbehave, explain to them why it is wrong.
- Encourage children to value their own cultural background.
- Encourage children to do as much for themselves as they can, to be responsible and to follow through activities to completion.
- Do not use put-downs or sarcasm.

- Give children activities that are a manageable challenge. If a child is doing nothing, ask questions to find out why. Remember that they may need time alone to work things out.
- Give appropriate praise for effort, more than achievement.
- Demonstrate that you value children's work.
- Provide opportunities for children to develop their memory skills.
- Encourage children to use language to express their own feelings and thoughts and how they think others feel.
- Provide children with their own things, labelled with their name.
- Provide opportunities for role play.
- Give children the opportunity to experiment with different roles, for example leader, follower.
- Provide good flexible role models with regard to gender, ethnicity and disability.
- Stay on the child's side! Assume they mean to do right rather than wrong. Do not presume on your authority with instructions such as 'You must do this because I'm the teacher and I tell you to', unless the child is in danger.
- Be interested in what children say; be an active listener. Give complete attention when you can and do not laugh at a child's response, unless it is really funny.
- Avoid having favourites and victims.
- Stimulate children with interesting questions that make them think.

Progress check

What aspect of development can make it easier for an adult to control a child of 5 years?

What are some of the more positive aspects of a typical 5-year-old child?

What difficulties can 5 year olds experience?

Describe the basic personal skills that most 6 year olds have developed.

What is the significance of the peer group to 7 year olds?

What is established by the time a child is 8 years old?

Factors that affect social and emotional development

Social development includes the growth of the child's relationships with others, **socialisation** and the development of social skills. **Emotional development** includes the growth of the child's feelings and awareness of themselves, the development of feelings towards other people, the development of self-image and self-identity, and therefore their intellectual development.

These two areas of development are closely linked and strongly affect one another. There are a number of theories about how and why emotional and social development happens.

key terms

Social development
the growth of the ability to relate to others appropriately and become independent, within a social framework

Socialisation
the process by which children learn the culture (or way of life) of the society into which they are born

Emotional development
the growth of the ability to feel and express an increasing range of emotions appropriately, including those about oneself

AN OUTLINE OF SOME OF THE THEORIES OF SOCIAL AND EMOTIONAL DEVELOPMENT

Biological theories

A biological or genetic explanation of how social behaviour and personality develop includes the ideas that:

- we are born with a definite personality and this determines how we respond and behave
- our temperament, sociability, emotional responses and intelligence are determined by what we inherit from our biological parents
- the way we behave and the pattern our development takes is programmed in our genes, and is sometimes affected by chemical changes in our bodies
- the way we mature and change follows a pre-set programmed pattern.

Support for the biological theory can be illustrated by the observation of parents who have more than one child. They comment that their children develop very different personalities and social skills, even though they have grown up in the same environment.

Learning theories

Learning theories hold that children develop as they do because they have contact with other people and learn from them. With regard to social and emotional development, learning theories hold that:

- children develop by learning from their experiences
- the only things babies are born with are some primitive reflexes – they do not have any social behaviour that is instinctive, or occurs automatically
- the environment, rather than inherited characteristics, is of the greatest importance in determining how children develop emotionally.

There is much evidence that points to nurture, or learning, being a very important factor in determining how children develop socially and emotionally.

key term

Psychoanalytical theory
a mixture of biological and learning theories, involving the idea that a child's development can be badly affected if at any stage their needs are not met appropriately

Psychoanalytical theories

Sigmund Freud, working at the beginning of the twentieth century, was the founder of modern **psychoanalytical theory**. Many others have since used his ideas.

Psychoanalytical theories are in some respects a mixture of biological and learning theories. They hold that:

- children are born with a set of needs (Mia Kellmer Pringle described these social and emotional needs as the need for love and affection, security, consistent care and reasonable guidelines, praise, encouragement and recognition and to be given appropriate responsibility)
- particular needs appear at different ages and stages through childhood
- children develop healthily only if these needs are met
- a child's future development can be badly affected if at any stage the appropriate needs are not met.

key term

Process
a continuous series of events, leading to an outcome

THEORETICAL PERSPECTIVES OF SOCIAL AND EMOTIONAL DEVELOPMENT – THE PROCESS OF SOCIALISATION

The sociologist Talcott Parsons used the term socialisation to describe the **process** through which children learn the way of life, the language and the behaviour that is acceptable and appropriate to the society in which they live – in other words their **culture**. The process of socialisation includes the combination of environmental influences that contribute to children's social and emotional development. It includes children learning from and being shaped by the experiences and relationships they have during childhood. This happens primarily within the family when they are very young and secondarily, as they grow older, through other influences such as their peer group and at school.

> **key term**
> **Culture**
> the way of life, the language and the behaviour that is acceptable and appropriate to the society in which a person lives

The process enables children to learn the behaviour that is expected and appropriate to their society and to become adult members of their society. During the process, children learn how to behave appropriately in a large number of **social roles** – positions in society that are associated with a particular set of expected behaviours.

> **key term**
> **Social role**
> a position in society that is associated with a particular group of expected behaviours

INFLUENCES ON SOCIAL AND EMOTIONAL DEVELOPMENT – HOW BEHAVIOUR IS LEARNED

There are several different ways that encourage children to learn the behaviour that is expected of them.

Rewards and punishments

Adults encourage acceptable behaviour in children by rewarding it. A reward can be a very simple thing like a smile, saying thank you, giving praise or a hug; it also includes giving children things such as toys, food or a treat. Children can also feel rewarded by the good feeling they get when they please an adult. Children want rewards to be repeated, and this encourages them to repeat the behaviour that brought the reward.

Adults discourage behaviour by punishing or ignoring it. Punishments, like rewards, can take a variety of forms: they include telling children they are wrong, physically or emotionally hurting them, depriving them of something they want, ignoring or isolating them. Children usually enjoy adults' attention and do not like to be ignored.

There are many different views about the relative effectiveness of rewards and punishments in changing behaviour.

Copying and imitating adults

Children learn how to behave by copying people in different roles. They use people as **role models**. For example, children copy what their mothers or fathers do and learn a lot about the roles of men and women. The idea that children develop partly by copying behaviour has implications for child-care workers, since children will also use them as role models.

> **key term**
> **Role model**
> a person whose behaviour is used as an example by someone else as the right way to behave

Role play

Children enjoy pretending to be someone else. In their play they sometimes act as if they are another person; this is called **role play**. They often copy the adults who are close to them, or the ones they see on the television. When they do this, they may not be able to tell whether or not the adult's behaviour is socially acceptable. This may happen, for example, when children copy violent parents in their play or general behaviour.

> **key term**
> **Role play**
> acting out a role as someone else

Peer group pressure

Peers (other children) can exert very strong pressure on children to behave in certain ways. Children change their behaviour when they are with their peer group, and may sometimes behave in ways that they know are unacceptable to adults. A peer group can punish a child who does not conform to their expectations by excluding the child from the group or by making the child feel different. The fear of exclusion from the group can be stronger to some children than fear of adult punishment. This peer group pressure can become a form of bullying. There is an increasing awareness of the different forms that bullying can take, and a greater commitment by many schools to introduce policies to try to prevent it.

Case study . . .

. . . promoting healthy development – using praise

Jo attends a nursery school. She is a lively and responsive 4-year-old child who uses the nursery resources enthusiastically. One morning Jo is sitting in the book area looking at different books, she asks a child-care and education worker who is standing near the area if she can read a book to the worker. The worker knows that Jo can read very few words, but willingly agrees, knowing that the policy of the school is to encourage free reading in this way. Jo turns the pages of the book and mainly uses the pictures to tell the story; she also reads a few words correctly and the worker helps her with a few others. The worker says 'I think you are very clever, well done! Would you like to read another book to me?'

1. *Why would this response encourage Jo to want to go on reading books?*
2. *If the worker had said to Jo, 'That wasn't very good, you didn't know many words', what effect could this have on the child's behaviour in future?*
3. *What knowledge about children's social and emotional development and their behaviour is the worker basing her responses on?*
4. *List some other rewards that can be used in a school to foster healthy social and emotional development and encourage acceptable behaviour.*

STRATEGIES TO HELP CHILDREN TO RELATE TO OTHERS

The importance of play

Play is recognised as stimulating and encouraging growth in every area. Child-care workers have an important role in using play to promote children's social and emotional development, particularly in helping children to relate to other children and adults.

By the time they are 3 many children are capable of taking account of other people's actions and needs, and to co-operate with them by taking on a role in a group. Workers should therefore be aware of the range of activities that could positively encourage children to play and do things co-operatively both indoors and outdoors. These will include imaginative play experiences, games that involve sharing and taking turns, and activities that include using resources co-operatively. Adults should also provide opportunities for children to talk and listen to each other, to share their experiences, and to explore and investigate objects and events together. By doing this adults help children to develop and to learn socially acceptable behaviour.

Children sometimes need help to express themselves and what they are feeling. Play can form an important part of this. Expressive play can be encouraged through the provision of malleable materials and sensory experiences with water and sand. Small world play and imaginative play areas will also help a child to act out what they are feeling in a safe environment.

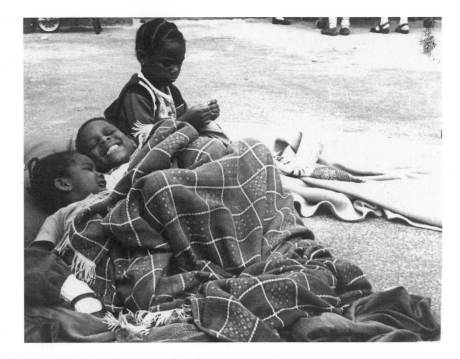

Play helps children to relate to each other

Dealing with conflict

Sometimes children behave in ways that produce conflict between them and other children. Children should be encouraged to resolve minor conflicts themselves through developing the skills of negotiation and compromise. Adult intervention is however sometimes essential, particularly if children are being physically or verbally aggressive. In this case the adult should stop the child who is being aggressive, tell them that what they have done is wrong, comfort the child who has been hurt, and discuss why the action was wrong with the aggressor. Workers can use the discussion to extend their understanding and to reinforce the difference between right and wrong.

This is particularly so if children are aggressive to a child because they are of a different race or they are disabled. Further strategies within a nursery or school to promote tolerance can be to celebrate differences, provide positive images of different groups of people in society, and provide activities and resources to encourage familiarity with and acceptance of difference. Play and learning experiences can be used effectively to develop mutual understanding and respect between those from various social and cultural backgrounds.

Progress check

What are the main things that children learn during the socialisation process?

What are the main things that influence children's behaviour?

What rewards can encourage positive behaviour?

What is role play?

What do children fear their peer group might do?

What is a role model?

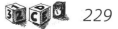

THE INFLUENCE OF THE FAMILY AND OTHERS ON SOCIAL AND EMOTIONAL DEVELOPMENT

There are two identifiable periods in the process of a child becoming a social being:

- the social development that occurs in the early years of life – *that is primary socialisation*
- the social development that takes place as children grow older – *that is secondary socialisation.*

These two periods overlap in a child's life. A child does not leave one and go into the other; the first merges into the second. Any adult working with children may be involved in either or both of these processes.

Primary socialisation

Primary socialisation is the name given to the early social development that takes place within the child's close family and also in a day-care setting. It is a very important period, as during this time the child is learning the basic patterns of behaviour, skills and responses that are appropriate and acceptable both within the family and also in society. This lays the foundation for the later social development of the child.

The main influences during this early period are the people closest to the child. These people are usually the child's parent(s) and other close family members, together with any substitute carers, for example a childminder, a nanny or a day-nursery officer or a foster carer.

Research shows that it is better for children to have close contact with a small number of main carers during this early period. This enables them to experience continuity and consistency in the way they are handled. It also helps them to build up a pattern of acceptable behaviour: they learn what is right and wrong from the adults around them. If children receive conflicting messages about appropriate behaviour during this early period, they may not establish a consistent pattern of behaviour. Healthy emotional development is best promoted by the stability and consistency of care that comes from having a limited number of carers.

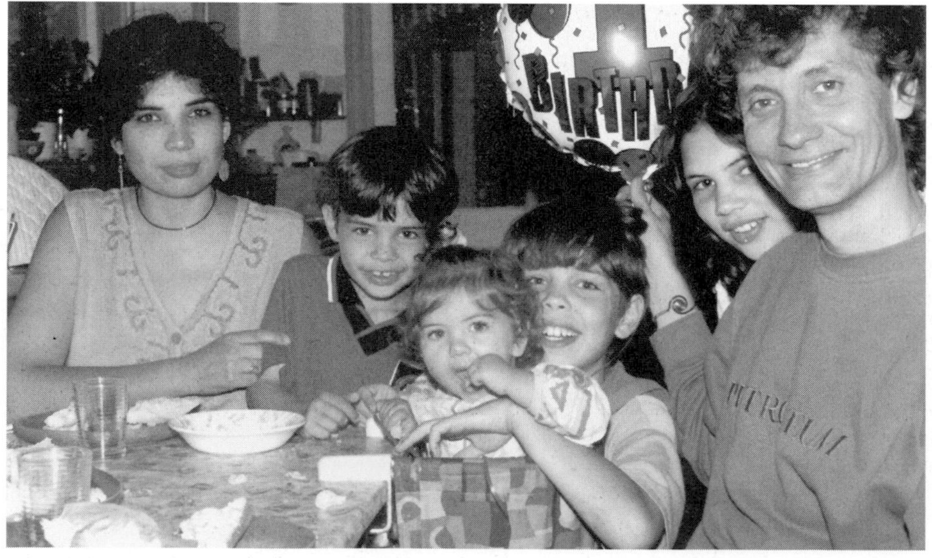

Primary socialisation takes place in the early years of life, mainly within the child's close family

This knowledge has been reflected in recent legislation and child-care practice. The Children Act 1989 has clear guidelines about the ratios of staff to children required in day-care settings; the younger the children the higher the ratio of staff required. The Children Act also gives guidelines about a suitable environment and accommodation for children. It is partly for this reason that many child-care settings have introduced a key worker system to enable a worker to form a special relationship with a child, and gain a thorough knowledge and understanding of them. This enables them to meet the individual needs of the child and also to work more effectively in partnership with parents.

Secondary socialisation

As children get older they are also exposed to influences outside the family and their close environment. They develop friendships, mix with their peers, go to school, watch the television, read books and magazines, join clubs and begin to learn the rules for behaviour in the wider society. These activities lay the foundation for children becoming adult members of that society. Growing children need to be encouraged and enabled to develop a range of relationships and interests. Workers who help to extend the child's experiences beyond the immediate family and close social group can do this. Through this children develop the ability to adapt to a variety of situations. They therefore become increasingly independent and socially mature. Children develop differences in values and ways of behaving that in part reflect differences in their environment. Adults need to encourage children to be sensitive to other people who may have different **customs**.

key term

Customs
special guidelines for behaviour, which are followed by particular groups of people

Progress check

What is primary socialisation and where does it mainly take place?

What is secondary socialisation and what are the main influences during this period?

List some advantages of a key worker system in a day-care setting.

CULTURAL INFUENCES ON SOCIAL AND EMOTIONAL DEVELOPMENT

What is culture?

An important aspect of social development involves children learning the culture of their society. Culture is the learned, shared behaviour of people in a society. It includes a shared language, **values**, **norms** and customs. Values are beliefs that certain things are important and to be valued, for example a person's right to personal freedom or to own their belongings. Norms are the rules and guidelines that turn values into action. A custom is another word used to describe particular norms. Customs are special guidelines for ritual behaviour, which are followed by particular groups of people.

Values and norms guide people and inform them about how to behave or do something. The value that children are precious and should be protected from harm leads to the norm that children should learn how to cross the road. The origins of customs often go back a long way into the past. An example of a custom is the celebration of birthdays.

key terms

Values
beliefs that certain things are important and to be valued, for example a person's right to their own belongings

Norms
the rules and guidelines that turn values into actions

The role of the adult in promoting children's cultural and moral development

In the early stages of their social development children learn language, values, norms, customs and acceptable behaviour from the people who are very close to them. This is usually their close family, but also includes any substitute carers.

Part of the carer's role is to teach children appropriate behaviour and a moral code. Such teaching has to be repeated until children behave automatically in certain situations, for example being considerate of the needs of others, taking turns to speak, remaining on the pavement and not running into the road, or how to greet familiar people. Sometimes it is sufficient to reinforce rules and customs by rewarding children. It may also help to explain to them the reasons that certain customs exist or behaviour is expected. In this way carers are also helping children to understand the underlying values.

Schools, playgroups and nurseries also have particular values, norms and customs. It is important, in any group, that rules are kept by everyone and that the norms for behaviour are shared. Social contact would be uncontrolled and unpredictable without this, as we would have no way of knowing how people are likely to behave.

key term

Multi-cultural society
a society whose members have a variety of cultural and ethnic backgrounds

SOCIAL AND EMOTIONAL DEVELOPMENT IN A MULTI-CULTURAL SOCIETY

A **multi-cultural society** is one whose members have a variety of cultural backgrounds. Britain can be described as a multi-cultural society that is committed to promoting equality of opportunity for all its members. It is essential that anyone caring for children examines the particular rules and customs of the establishment in which they work. They need to distinguish between rules that are essential for everyone to follow (for example, rules concerning safety and mutual respect) and those that can be varied (for example, those connected to dress, food and religious customs). Establishments sometimes have rules that are both unessential and culturally biased.

The Children Act 1989 requires establishments to have a multi-cultural approach to caring, and most establishments encourage understanding and respect for the customs of all children and their families. Many have examined their rules to ensure that they promote equal opportunities and avoid discriminatory practices.

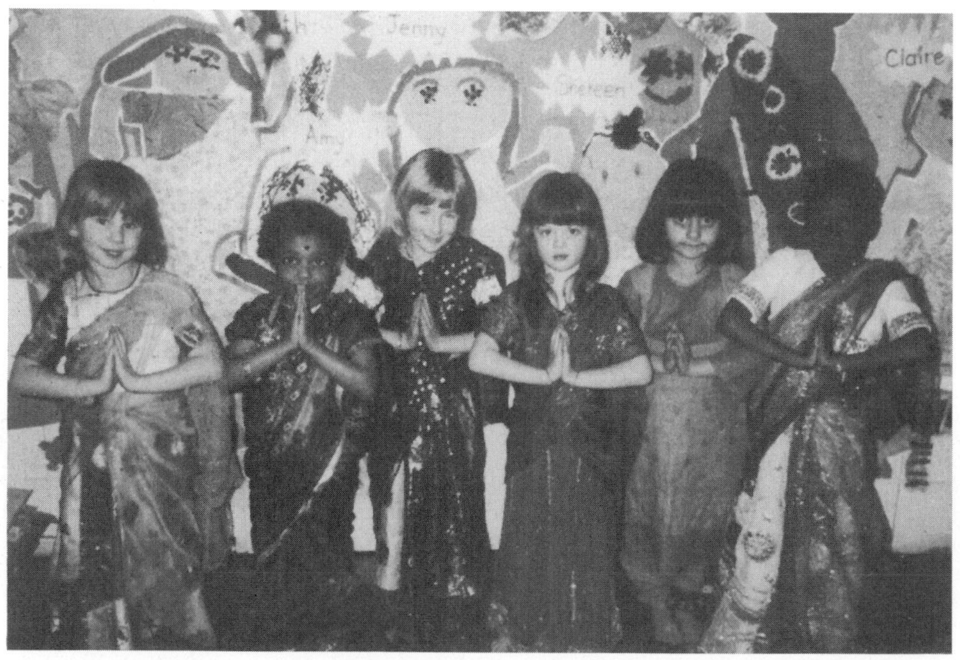

Many establishments now encourage understanding and respect for the customs of all children and their families

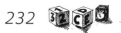

The role of the adult in promoting children's positive self-image in a multi-cultural society

> **key term**
>
> **Positive images**
> the representation of a cross-section of a whole variety of roles and everyday situations, to challenge stereotypes and to extend and increase expectations

Children build up pictures of themselves and images of how others see them through the process of socialisation. All children need to develop a positive identity. One of the things that help them to do this is if they see **positive images** of themselves in everyday life and in special roles in their environment. A positive image in this context is a balanced representation of a cross-section of people in the objects, pictures and books that surround children, showing them in different roles and everyday situations.

It is important, for example, that classroom displays show a representative range of people of different races so that black people are not invisible and by implication unimportant. Doctors, for example, are valued in society, so showing a black doctor in a book or on television will help a black child's positive self-identity, as the child can identify with a black person in a valued role. The positive visual portrayal of people of differing racial origins also enables white children and adults to build up positive images of all members of society.

When children are not of the dominant ethnic group in a society, they may find it more difficult to see positive visual images of themselves. Their teachers, people on the television, children and adults in books are more likely to be of the majority ethnic group, which in the case of the UK is white. The need for a positive identity has been recognised in the Children Act 1989. This legislation recognises for the first time every child's right to be part of a community that is free from racial discrimination and a society that values different backgrounds and encourages a sense of identity. The importance of this principle, and its relevance to every aspect of children's care, is emphasised throughout the guidance to the Children Act 1989. As a result when people provide day care for children they are required to:

- take account of their religious persuasion, racial origin and cultural background
- have a commitment to treat all children as individuals and with equal concern
- enable children to develop positive attitudes to differences of race, culture and language.

The role of the adult in promoting positive self-images for children with disabilities

Similarly, as well as adopting a multi-cultural approach in an early years setting, it is important that workers provide images of people with disabilities participating fully in all areas of life. Children with disabilities need to identify with disabled role models in their environment in order to develop a positive self-image.

> **Progress check**
>
> *What is culture?*
>
> *What is a multi-cultural society?*
>
> *What is a value?*
>
> *What is a norm?*
>
> *What does the Children Act 1989 recognise about culture?*

CULTURAL INFLUENCES ON CHILDREN'S SOCIAL DEVELOPMENT – THE LEARNING OF SOCIAL ROLES

An important aspect of social development is that children learn an increasing number of social roles. This means that they learn the appropriate behaviour associated with different social positions. This learning may include the behaviour appropriate to being a daughter or a son, a sibling, a grandchild, a school pupil, a friend or a member of a club.

The learning of social roles helps children to:

- know how to behave in a wide range of social situations
- know how they can expect other people to behave
- understand that people will respond differently to them according to that person's role, for example, that a teacher will behave differently towards them than a grandparent. Children also learn to cope with this difference
- perceive their social world as structured and predictable, and therefore have a feeling of security
- be aware that they have a place and belong in a social system.

The role of the adult in helping children to learn social roles

Adult carers can help children to learn varied social roles by:

- giving them opportunities for imaginative play where they can explore their social world in a safe manner
- providing a good role model themselves
- making clear to the child the behaviour that is appropriate and expected
- supporting them at times of potential stress as they learn social roles
- providing activities that help them to relate to others and co-operate with them.

The table below shows the potential stress associated with the learning of social roles.

Potential stress associated with the learning of social roles and the adult's role in supporting a child

Causes of stress	Definition	Example	Adult role
Role transition	Children move from one role to another	Change from pre-school to school child	Provide preparation and support
Role loss	Lose one role completely	From an only child to having a sibling	Give special attention, understanding, make allowances
Role conflict	Meeting the demands of one role clashes with meeting another's demands	Peer group encourages behaviour not approved by carer	Show understanding, provide firm boundaries

THE INFLUENCE OF GENDER ON CHILDREN'S SELF-IMAGE AND SOCIAL AND EMOTIONAL DEVELOPMENT

key term

Stereotyping when people think that all the members of a group have the same characteristics as each other; often applied on the basis of race, gender or disability

Sex-role **stereotyping** is still present in society. Stereotyping occurs when people think that all the members of a group have the same characteristics as each other, for example boys are tough and active, girls are soft and passive.

Sex stereotypes develop in children's minds when they learn what behaviour is expected of them as a boy or a girl. Although the process may be less pronounced than in the past, by the time children are 5 or 6, they appear to have a clear awareness of gender differences and the behaviour that goes with them. These ideas are firmly held by the time they are 7 or 8.

Children learn rules about how boys and girls behave from a variety of sources. They learn from their adult carers, other children, and from television and the mass media in general.

Children are disadvantaged by sex-role stereotyping if it limits the opportunities available to them. This happens when children believe they cannot do something because of their gender, or when those around them believe this. Developing an awareness of stereotyping and how to avoid it is vital for those who care for children.

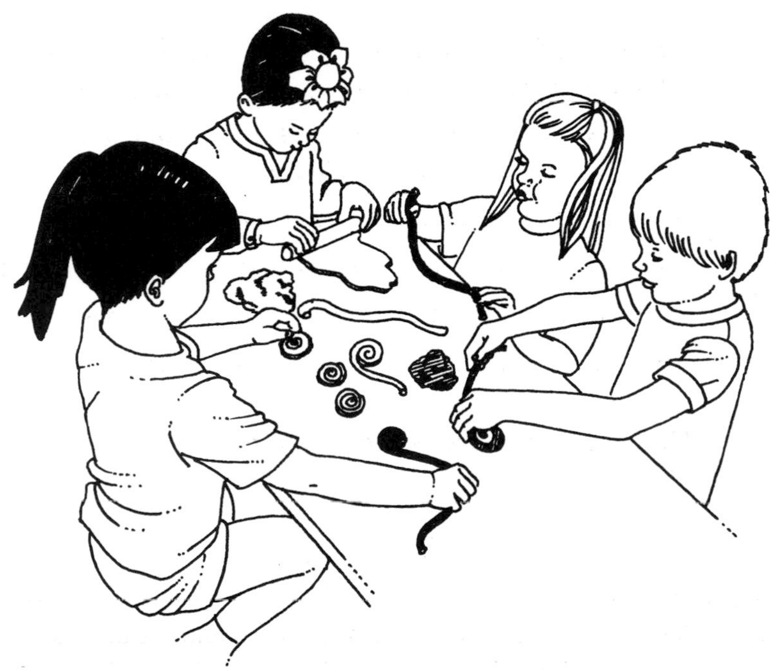

It is preferable to concentrate on the many similarities between girls and boys

The role of the adult in counteracting sex-role stereotyping

No one can argue with the fact that there are physical differences between girls and boys. However, workers must aim to provide an environment for children that avoids gender bias. To do this it is preferable to ignore gender differences and to concentrate on the many similarities between girls and boys. It is also preferable to avoid dividing children into groups according to their gender as this draws attention to gender unnecessarily.

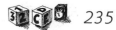

Dividing children into gender groups increases the likelihood of differences being emphasised. When this happens, children are seen in terms of their gender first and as individuals second. One of the problems created by stereotyping is that children (and adults) begin to believe the picture others have of them and start to behave in ways that are expected of them. If a girl repeatedly hears a teacher asking for 'a nice strong boy' to carry something and 'a nice tidy girl' to clear up, she may begin to believe she is not strong and that her role is to clear up after others.

Children sometimes see differences between gender emphasised in books and other visual images. Girls have traditionally been portrayed as passive and domesticated, boys as active and dominant. Schools and nurseries are increasingly aware of this bias and avoid using such books. Good practice is to present positive images of both genders through the staff, range of activities, books, displays, visitors and any other means that can be used.

Workers who avoid making any divisions between children on the basis of their gender will be more likely to provide an environment in which all children reach their full potential.

Progress check

What is a social role?

What does stereotyping mean?

What practices reinforce gender stereotyping?

What good practices can prevent gender stereotyping?

THE INFLUENCE OF THE ECONOMIC AND SOCIAL CIRCUMSTANCES ON SOCIAL AND EMOTIONAL DEVELOPMENT

The link between social status, the 'openness' of a society and success

key term

Social status the value that a society puts on people in particular roles

Child-care and education workers need to have some awareness of the potential influence of a family's economic and social circumstances (or **social status**) on a child's self-image and social and emotional development. They should understand that these circumstances might influence the child's potential to be successful. Social status is the value that a society puts on people in particular roles in society.

In all societies there are some people who are more successful than others. Success is usually measured in terms of the 'power' that a person has. In most societies, people who have power and influence also have higher social status. What constitutes or makes up high social status varies between societies: in some societies, religious leaders have the most power and highest status; in others it may be military leaders, business people, politicians, people with inherited wealth and status, or those who achieve wealth and success.

Power includes:

- having easy access to things that are valued (for example, wealth, education and health)
- the potential to influence directly what happens to other people (for example, religious, military or political power).

Some societies, such as the UK, are considered to be 'open societies'. The structures of such societies (for example, the education system, job opportunities) enable a child to change their position within their lifetime. We have seen in recent years how the daughter of a grocer and the son of a circus performer became prime ministers in the UK.

A closed society is one in which it is impossible for a child to move beyond the social status of their birth family, as for example in the Hindu caste system in parts of India.

Through education, people in the UK and other European countries can achieve high social and economic status. The introduction of comprehensive education in the 1950s aimed to make educational success for all children possible. Previously a system of selection to grammar or secondary modern schools existed throughout England and Wales.

Despite this, however, a large body of research shows that others factors must be influencing success in education and in society in the UK, and that they are not linked to children's ability alone. League tables and research shows that children from families who are poorer economically and have lower social status are less likely to achieve success in the education system. Whatever the intentions, children from different social backgrounds do not appear to experience equality of opportunity.

THE INFLUENCE OF THE FAMILY ON DEVELOPMENT AND EDUCATIONAL SUCCESS

Children from families with fewer economic resources are *statistically less likely* to do well at school. It is important to recognise and understand this fact when we aim to promote equality of opportunity for all children. While avoiding the possibility of generalising and stereotyping a group of people, it is only by finding out the causes of this unequal achievement that we can begin to support and compensate children who are less successful.

Children who are successful at school are more likely to be:

- brought up in a secure and loving environment
- have parents or carers who see the value of educational achievement
- experiencing a language-rich environment with opportunities for play.

Families have different abilities to provide the above.

Families who provide a secure and loving environment

Families from all social backgrounds can provide security and love for their children. Children brought up in a secure and loving environment are more likely to be responsive, confident, to behave in a socially acceptable way, to have high self-esteem, to be more willing to learn and therefore be more successful.

The life experience of some families, however, prevents them from putting the needs of their children first and providing security during the crucial period of primary socialisation. This inability may be because of difficult relationships within the family and these can exist within any social group. However, relationship difficulties may also be linked to the stress caused by living in long-term poverty, poor housing or a run-down environment, and people in lower social groups more commonly experience these. Many people, however, continue to achieve a happy secure home for their children in these difficult circumstances.

Parents and carers who support educational achievement

Parents and carers who recognise the value of educational achievement are more likely to encourage their children's intellectual and social development. They recognise the value of encouraging socially acceptable behaviour, and realise that this is more likely to lead to success at school. Such parents visit the school and show interest in their children's progress. Any family, regardless of social status, can to do this.

However, carers who have themselves achieved success through the education system inevitably have a greater understanding and knowledge of how to succeed than those who have not. They are more likely to feel at ease with teachers because

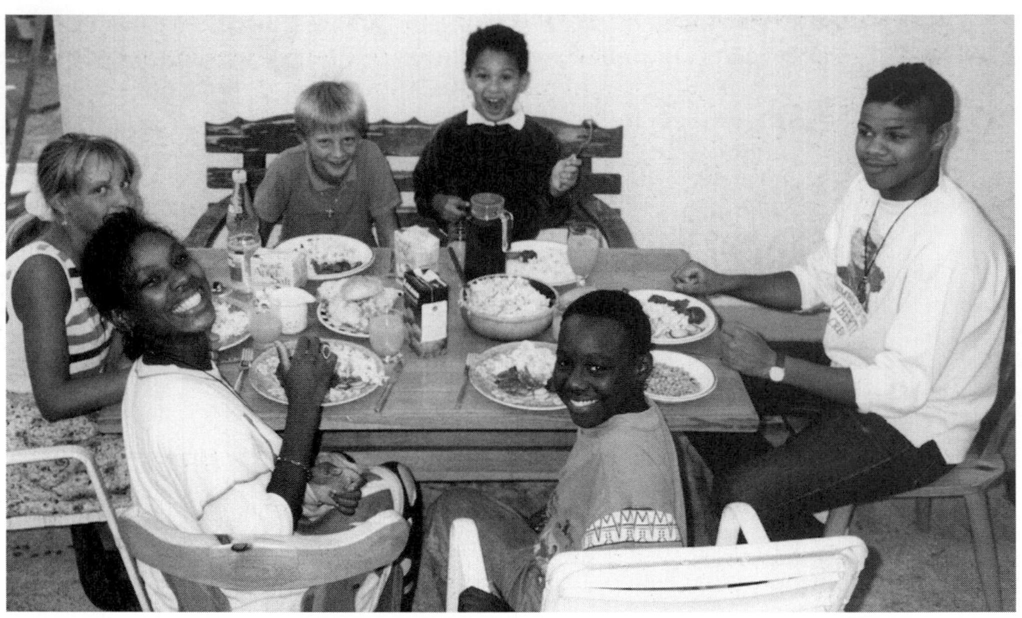

Carers who have a close and loving relationship with their children are more likely to spend time with them and establish language-rich communication patterns

they are similar to them. There is less to prevent them, both practically and psychologically (in their mind), from going into school to see how their child is progressing or from helping in the classroom.

Parents and carers who provide an environment rich in language

Children who experience a language-rich environment, with good opportunities for play, establish the early speech and thought patterns that are essential to the development of literacy skills (reading and writing) when they go to school. A good experience of play is essential to their future intellectual development.

Carers who have a close and loving relationship with their children are more likely to spend time with them, establish language-rich communication patterns and encourage play. Children from any social background can be deprived of this if their parents' attention is directed elsewhere. Parents may be distracted from close contact with their children by the demands of their jobs and careers, by their own physical or mental health, or by their personal, social or economic circumstances.

Parents who have money, power and higher social status are more likely to be able to pay for care and education for their children to complement the time they spend with their children. This care may be by a nanny or in a nursery. The disadvantages experienced by some children from families with low social status, whose carers cannot pay for substitute care, has long been recognised by some local authorities who provided nursery education in areas of high social deprivation. In the late 1990s it became an increasingly central feature of government policy to provide subsidised child care and education at the foundation stage to provide all young children with early play experiences and language stimulation. This aims to enable all children to achieve early learning goals and be more prepared when entering statutory education.

Children have very different experiences during their early years. Some of these directly affect their social development and their potential to be socially successful. Some of these differences are common to all social groups; others, notably those who are affected by economic status, are more likely to occur within a high or lower social and economic group.

Case study . . .

. . . success at school

Winston is an only child and lives with his mother in a small house on a private housing estate. His parents are separated. He sees his father occasionally and his extended family regularly. He and his mother have a warm, close relationship. His mother visits his school for regular parents evenings and knows that he is a bright child. If she ever feels that Winston is experiencing any particular difficulties, she makes an appointment to see his teacher. His mother and he eat together each evening, they discuss what they have done that day and often laugh and joke about things that have happened. Each day his mother listens to him read and they look at books together.

1. *How would you describe Winston and his mother's relationship?*
2. *Why do you think it is likely that Winston will do well at school?*
3. *Write a description of a child, and their family, who might be less likely to succeed at school.*

OVERVIEW OF THE VARIED EXTERNAL INFLUENCES ON THE DEVELOPMENT OF A CHILD'S SELF-IMAGE AND THEIR SOCIAL AND EMOTIONAL DEVELOPMENT

- Infants and young children become truly human through contact with other people. This is one of the reasons that working with and caring for young children is important and responsible work.
- Children need close contact with carers during their early years.
- The learning process is continuous.
- Caring adults help children to develop social skills, relationships, rules for behaviour, social maturity and independence.
- It is essential that workers base their professional good practice on a knowledge of the social and cultural backgrounds of children in their care.
- Families provide differing social environments for children and these affect children's social and emotional development, and their self-image and can strongly influence a child's eventual position in society.

Progress check

What does the term social status refer to?

What are the advantages of having high social status?

What should the introduction of comprehensive schools have ensured?

In what ways can the family influence children's educational success?

Now try these questions

What are the main aspects of emotional and social development?

What relationship do all the different areas of development have to each other?

Why is it important for a child to value their own cultural background?

How can child-care workers encourage children to be independent and self-reliant when they are developing self-help skills?

How does cognitive and language development affect the development of self-concept and self-image?

key terms

You need to know what the key terms and phrases in this chapter mean. Go back through the chapter and find out.

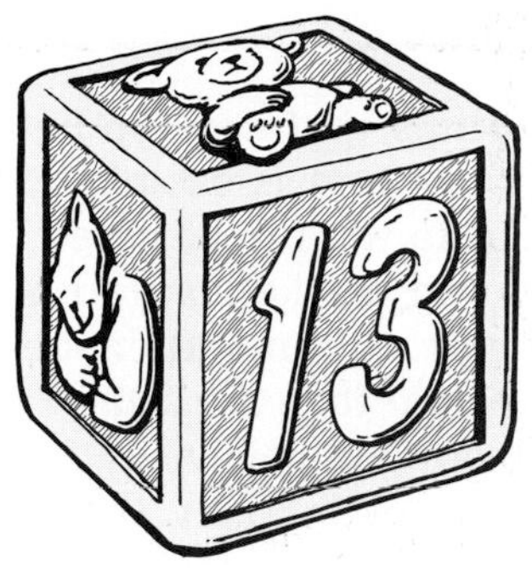

ATTACHMENT, SEPARATION AND LOSS

The quality and character of children's early close relationships is now believed to be of central importance to their social and emotional development. Pioneering research into the nature and effect of early relationships, particularly concerning the development of attachments between infants and their main carers, was carried out in the 1940s and 1950s. During this period John Bowlby, an influential British child psychiatrist, studied the long-term developmental effects on children who had been separated from their parents when they were orphaned or evacuated during the Second World War. He observed that many of these children suffered a range of behavioural, emotional and mental health problems.

The experience of secure attachments is very important to children's all-round development. Child-care workers are usually looking after children who are separated from their primary carers and need to understand:

- *the possible long-term consequences for children who have insecure attachments*
- *the possible effects of an 'interruption' to an attachment caused by the separation, or loss, of the child from their main carer(s), either temporarily or permanently.*

The preparation for separation and loss and the quality of substitute care provided are of great significance to the short and long-term emotional and social development of the child. The child-care worker has a significant role to play in minimising the negative effects of separation and loss, and also in caring for children who are experiencing grief.

This chapter will cover the following topics:

- *what are attachments?*
- *how attachments are established*
- *the implications of disability*
- *attachment behaviour patterns*
- *the importance to children's development of the experience of attachment*
- *the effects on children and their families of separation and loss*
- *strategies for minimising the adverse effects of separation*
- *transitions*
- *loss and grief.*

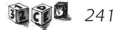

What are attachments?

key term
Attachment
an affectionate two-way relationship that develops between an infant and an adult

key term
Instincts
patterns of behaviour that are not learned

Attachments are the affectionate two-way relationships that develop between infants and their close carers. When a secure attachment is established the infant will try to stay close to that adult and will appear to want to be cared for by them. By the end of their first year the infant will show a marked preference for that person and may show anxiety towards strangers. Infants then become distressed if they are separated from those adults to whom they are attached and try to regain contact with them. Bowlby called this 'attachment behaviour'.

Bowlby concluded that babies have a biological need, or **instinct**, to form an attachment to the person who feeds and cares for them. He maintained that this was a survival instinct without which the helpless infant would be exposed to danger and might die.

Together with Bowlby, James and Joyce Robertson, Mary Ainsworth and other researchers went on to study the nature and effects of early parent–child relationships. Bowlby was the first person to link together the biological, psychological, social and cultural influences on children's development and from this he developed the 'theory of attachment'. He and others discovered that the experience of an attachment is crucial to children's healthy social and emotional development. This 'relationship-based' theory of personality development is now accepted as fundamentally important to an understanding of the path of children's social and emotional development.

Child-care workers need to understand why and how these attachments develop, why they are so important and what happens if they are broken by separation.

THEORIES ABOUT WHY ATTACHMENTS OCCUR

Maternal instincts

The notion that mothers have 'maternal instincts' that motivate them to love and care for their children is widely confirmed from observations. However, such instincts do not appear to occur in *all mothers* immediately, or ever in a few cases. Nevertheless, research shows that most mothers seem highly alert and sensitive to their baby's physical and emotional states immediately after birth. Babies in their turn appear to be ready to interact and relate with their carers from birth.

Affection or contact comfort

John Bowlby found that 'contact comfort', or affection, is very important to the formation of a bond of attachment and that the adult's demonstration of physical affection is crucial to this. The experiments of Margaret and Harry Harlow with rhesus monkeys during the 1960s and 1970s also demonstrated the theory that contact comfort was more important than feeding in nurturing emotional development.

Sensitive responsiveness theory

Many psychologists now believe that human infants are born with skills that allow them to attract and keep adult's attention. They appear to be programmed to become aware of and to respond to the people around them. They seem to prefer things that are human, like voices and faces. From an early age babies give out strong signals that draw adults to them and make them respond, for example crying, smiling, gazing, grasping.

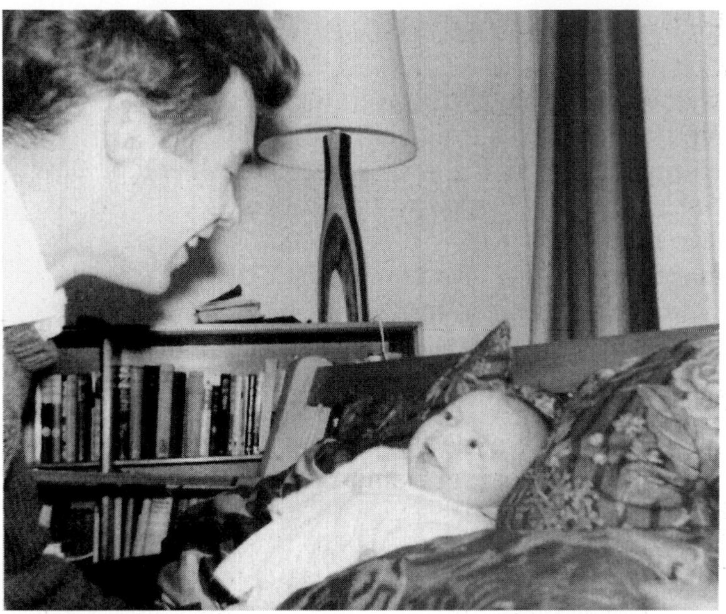

Infants seem to prefer things that are human

The carer's role in forming attachments

An adult must want both to become emotionally involved and to spend time with a child. An attachment is not formed immediately. Carers who are sensitive to the signals given by the infant and respond to them encourage the bond to develop over a period of time.

Making multiple attachments

John Bowlby maintained that babies need to attach to their mothers and that mother is best. However, it is now recognised that a child is capable of multiple attachments, for example with father, grandparents, other family members and substitute carers. Babies who attach to several adults can be deeply attached to each.

In 1964, Rudi Schaffer and Peggy Emerson undertook a study of 60 Glasgow children from birth to 18 months. They concluded that when several adults took an interest in a baby, the baby could attach to them all. Schaffer and Emerson found that each attachment was much the same in quality. The infants responded in the same way to each attached adult. They seemed to use different adults for different things; if they were frightened they usually preferred their mother; if they wanted to play they usually preferred their father.

Schaffer and Emerson concluded that attachments are more likely to be formed with those people who are most sensitive to the baby's needs. They do not necessarily attach to those people who spend most time with them.

Progress check

Explain what causes attachments to develop.

What do babies do to attract and keep an adult's attention?

What response is necessary from the adult if healthy attachments are to develop?

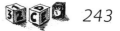

How attachments are established

In order to develop an attachment, babies need to experience a warm, continuous, loving relationship with a small and relatively permanent group of carers who respond sensitively to them.

Certain conditions are thought necessary to the formation of attachments:

- interaction needs to occur between the baby and carer(s) who want to spend time and get involved with them
- relationships need to develop with a few people who will stay with the baby most of the time (continuous care), not deserting them
- communication needs to develop between the infant and carers who respond sensitively to them
- carers giving loving physical affection.

STAGES IN THE DEVELOPMENT OF ATTACHMENTS

Attachments are established over a period of time. Factors that affect their development include the responses of both infant and carers, and external or environmental factors such as birth experiences and financial security. Secure attachments are more likely to develop if many of the factors below occur. Insecure attachments can result if some of the factors below are experienced negatively and lead to a mother being insensitive to her infant's needs. Four significant stages are:

1. *During pregnancy* A positive bond is encouraged by a planned, confirmed, wanted pregnancy that is welcomed by partners and the wider family; by partners being emotionally mature and having a stable and mutually supportive relationship; by a normal healthy pregnancy; feeling fetal movements; making full use of antenatal health care, which includes an understanding of the process of pregnancy and preparation for delivery; by security in material things such as finances and housing; by making physical preparations for the baby's arrival.
2. *During delivery* A secure attachment is encouraged by a planned and expected delivery; a delivery with minimal medical intervention that fulfils parents' expectations, during which the mother remains reasonably alert and in control; the attendance of health-care staff who are known and caring; a friendly, non-medical setting; the support of a partner or relative or friend; giving birth to a healthy 'normal' baby of the desired gender, whose appearance fulfils parents' expectations; if the baby is given immediately to parents and placed in contact with their skin or put to the breast; a period of undisturbed contact between baby and parents in the first few hours of life.
3. *The period shortly after birth* This can be a very **sensitive** period. Mothers who recognise their baby's needs and respond appropriately to their signals are regarded as 'sensitive'. 'Insensitive' mothers fail to read their infant's signals and interact with them according to their own needs. Research has shown that attachments are encouraged by the baby staying physically close to the parents, rather than being separated for long periods of time; health-care staff being supportive but not intrusive; mother feeling well; being

key term

Sensitive (or critical) period
a period of time vital for the achievement of a particular skill

emotionally stable and mature, having experienced a strong bond with their own parent or carer; mother sharing the parenting role with a chosen adult; a healthy, thriving baby, who feeds and sleeps well; siblings and the wider family welcoming the baby.

4. *The first 6 months of life* By the end of this stage, infants and their main carer(s) will usually have established a strong attachment. Experiences during this period are crucial. Many of the factors already described will continue to influence the development of attachments, the interaction between carers and baby is very significant during these months. This interaction often focuses on carers meeting the child's needs, but positive feedback from baby to carer also strengthens the bond. For example, the baby expresses needs by crying, smiling, babbling, clinging or raising her arms and the carer meets the baby's needs by feeding, talking and cuddling the infant. The infant gradually learns to trust that the carer will meet their needs and in this way the attachment is established. The carer, for their part, may initiate positive interaction, for example talking to the baby. The baby responds positively by perhaps cooing or smiling. The carer is then motivated to initiate further positive interaction and the cycle begins again. This leads to feelings of self-esteem and self-worth on the part of the carer and strengthens the attachment.

The quality of care

The meeting of children's needs encourages attachments to develop. The success and the intensity of the attachment do not, however, depend on the *amount of time* the carer spends with the infant, but on the *quality* of that involvement. Infants can develop attachments with people who spend relatively short periods of time with them, if that time is spent in certain ways that are of good quality; these include the carer playing with the baby, cuddling them, providing them with individual attention, entering into 'conversations' with them, and generally creating a situation in which both of them are enjoying each other's company. The baby forms a stronger attachment with this person than with someone who cares for them physically for a longer period of time, but does not play or interact with them.

This aspect of bonding has implications for those providing substitute care for a child. In the absence of their primary carers, for example in day-care settings, it is essential that all carers interact closely and meaningfully with an infant. A key worker system is one way to ensure that one member of staff forms a special relationship with particular children.

The implications of disability

The media often portray disability in a negative way. Society tends to view disability as a condition to be pitied rather than a difference to be celebrated. Consequently, parents of disabled children may feel a sense of disappointment and failure when they discover their child has a disability. This may lead to difficulty or delay in the formation of a bond of attachment.

RECOGNISING THE DIFFERENCES

The formation of a bond of attachment may be encouraged in a different way by disabled carers and/or children. While recognising that all disabled people are individuals, it is important to think about the possible implications of particular disabilities on the bonding process.

Disabled children and carers have the same needs as other people, but the methods of meeting these needs may vary according to the nature of the disability. Children and carers with sensory impairment, sight or hearing loss in particular, will need to have alternative or additional ways of responding to one another.

RESPONDING APPROPRIATELY

Blind babies or carers may not be able to join in communication games that rely on visual clues such as facial expression or body posture. They will not recognise the carers'/baby's face by sight and respond to this. If sight loss has not been diagnosed, babies may be considered unresponsive by their carers. For example, when the carer of a blind baby enters the room, the baby 'freezes' so they can listen very hard. Some carers may interpret this as the baby not welcoming them. Strategies need to be worked out to encourage alternative patterns of interaction.

Carers and/or children with hearing loss also need to use alternative methods of responding to one another. This is vital to the development of the bond, which in turn affects all-round development.

THE IMPORTANCE OF LANGUAGE

Many of the difficulties disabled children and adults face are related to the responses of other people to them, rather than to the disability itself.

For example, children with hearing loss often experience difficulty in developing an understanding of language. The development of language relies on communication between children and others. This communication must be accessible and meaningful to children. Recent research indicates that early use of sign language develops deaf children's understanding and does not delay the acquisition of spoken language.

Relatively few deaf children are exposed to sign language early enough. The exception to this is deaf children with deaf carers. Research by Susan Gregory and Susan Barlow (1989) highlighted the skills deaf parents show in interaction with their deaf children. This research confirmed subjective observations that deaf children with deaf carers tend to be more advanced in all-round development than other deaf children.

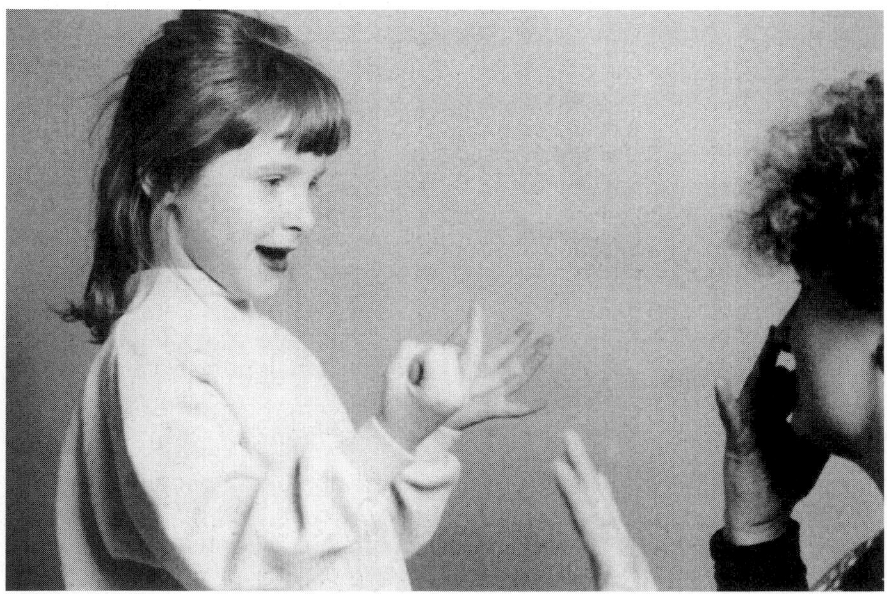

Early use of sign language develops deaf children's understanding and does not delay the acquisition of spoken language

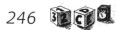

Attachment behaviour patterns

The following attachment behaviour has been observed at these ages:

- *0–2 months* At this age babies are not usually selective, neither do they show a preference for their main carers. However, they do exhibit social behaviour by showing a preference from birth for the human face and voice and enjoying social interaction.
- *3–6 months* Babies begin to recognise particular people and their faces. Babies generally do not mind who is with them; they will often smile at strangers, but respond with more smiling and noises to familiar faces. They develop a growing interest in and preference for the main carer, and their interaction becomes increasingly attuned. Babies start to decide whom they feel safe with. They may 'freeze' if approached by a stranger.
- *6–8 months* If contact has been sufficient, most babies will be firmly attached to their primary caregivers. Evidence for this can be observed in two ways. First, a baby with a firm attachment at this stage will show stranger anxiety (fear of strangers); second, they will show separation distress, that is, they become upset when they are separated from the person to whom they are attached. Babies express their preference clearly and behave in ways that are designed to bring about a response in the carer such as following, clinging, crying. Stranger anxiety is more likely if the baby is not being held by the person they are attached to and they are in a strange place. The way the stranger approaches the baby is also significant. If the stranger approaches slowly, does not get too close, does not try to pick up the baby, and does not talk too loudly, the baby will show less fear.
- *8–18 months* Babies start to make additional attachments if other adults are willing and responsive to the child's needs. With increasing mobility and later with the development of language the child becomes more active in searching for and keeping contact with the person to whom they are attached.
- *2 years onwards* Stranger anxiety and separation distress slowly disappear in well-attached children, so long as the separation is not for too long. Well-attached children will be increasingly independent and willing to explore new situations. Less well-attached children are less adventurous and less independent.
- *3–5 years* By this age there is less need to be within sight of primary carers and children are becoming steadily less clingy too. The child needs to develop a sense of independence and begins to separate and be willing to act alone. Just knowing that through experience the parent is going to be available enables them to feel secure. Peer group relationships become important.

Progress check

What conditions are necessary to the formation of a bond of attachment?

What periods are important to the development of a bond of attachment?

Explain how meeting a baby's needs helps to develop attachments in infants.

Why may blind babies be considered unresponsive by their carers?

At what age may stranger anxiety occur?

The importance to children's development of the experience of attachment

Attachments are important because they affect all aspects of children's development; insecure attachments have far-reaching implications for a child and the effects may extend into the next generation. This section looks at the importance of secure attachments to each aspect of children's development.

PHYSICAL DEVELOPMENT

Secure attachments motivate carers to meet children's physical needs. In a young baby this can be a very demanding task. If a baby is responsive, the carers' self-esteem will be increased and the attachment will provide them with the motivation to put the needs of the baby before their own, for example getting up in the night, sacrificing their own sleep to meet the baby's need for food.

Failure to meet children's physical needs may lead to neglect and **failure to thrive**.

> **key term**
>
> **Failure to thrive**
> failing to grow normally for no organic reason

COGNITIVE DEVELOPMENT

Children with secure attachments will have the confidence to explore and make discoveries. Attachment and dependency are not the same thing. The researcher Mary Ainsworth concluded that 'the anxious, insecure child may *appear* more strongly attached to his mother than the secure child who can explore fairly freely in a strange situation, using his mother as a safe base', but it is the securely attached child who is the more confident and freer to leave their carer. This child is more likely to explore the environment and learn from new experiences.

During the first year of life, children learn consequences and they learn cause and effect. For example, they learn that being fed stops the discomfort of hunger; they learn that crying brings adult attention. Cognitive development is built on this foundation. Studies in the US show that children in the care system (who are therefore more likely to have had erratic parenting and insecure attachments) are four or five times more likely to have learning difficulties.

LANGUAGE DEVELOPMENT

Attachments develop through interaction between carers and babies. Long before babies can talk or understand words, carers and babies hold 'conversations'. These conversations are a mixture of words and gestures from the carer and noises and movement from the baby, patterned like adult conversations. Early signs of pre-speech are evident even in newborn babies; babies appear to be born with a natural drive towards communication. Strong attachments motivate carer and baby to engage in early conversations that encourage the development of language.

EMOTIONAL DEVELOPMENT

Attachment experiences affect many aspects of emotional development, as follows:

Coping with frustration

If babies have their emotional needs met through secure attachment relationships, they will be more able to cope with stress and frustration. This is true both in

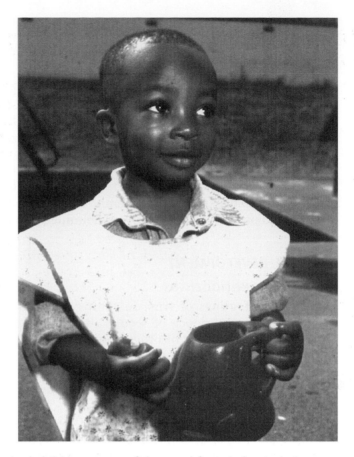

A securely attached child is more confident and freer to leave their carer

childhood and later in life. From her research, Mary Ainsworth concludes that 'an infant whose mother has responded promptly to his cries in the past, develops both trust in her responsiveness and confidence in his increased ability to control what happens to him'. Ainsworth used the term 'sensitive mother' to refer to one who is quick to respond to her baby's needs. These babies, she says, feel loved and secure, which helps them become more independent later on. Babies whose needs are not dealt with sensitively and consistently tend to demonstrate attachment behaviour by becoming more demanding and clingy.

Developing a positive self-image

Children with secure attachments develop a positive self-image. They understand themselves through the responses and reactions of those close to them. They believe the messages that are repeatedly given to them. When these messages are positive, they help to build self-esteem and a positive self-image.

Responding to control and discipline

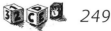

Children with a positive self-image, who think they are worthwhile, valuable human beings, will be able to tolerate frustration more easily; they will also be easier for adults to manage, control or discipline. Effective methods of control and discipline rely on children wanting to be remain attached to their carer. The carer can discipline the child by distancing themselves physically and emotionally, for example with disapproving looks or perhaps sending the child to their room. *They rely on children wanting to re-establish closeness.* This process will only work with children who are securely attached and who modify their behaviour to re-establish closeness.

Children who feel worth while and valued expect good things to happen to them. They believe that they are worthy of rewards and they trust the carer to give them if they behave appropriately. They will modify their behaviour appropriately to obtain the reward.

Coping with fears and worries

Children with secure attachments are better able to cope with fears and worries. Their experience of life leads them to feel safe and to trust that people will care for them and protect them from overwhelming fears and anxieties.

SOCIAL DEVELOPMENT

Making relationships

Children's feelings of trust in their carer and their sense of security develop through the experience of secure attachments. This experience makes children feel safe and trusting of other people, and this provides the foundation of later relationships, influencing their desire and ability to relate to others throughout life. Through the experience of secure attachment relationships, children learn how to take their part in other, reciprocal (give-and-take) relationships.

The development of social emotions

Around the age of 18 months, children with secure attachments demonstrate social emotions. Toddlers are able to display some empathy or understanding of how other people feel in particular situations. They can demonstrate care for others, sympathy (feeling sorry for others), pride and embarrassment. Children whose own needs have been met by the attachment relationship are freer to care for others.

The development of conscience

Through experiencing embarrassment children can be made to feel shame and guilt. In the right balance, these feelings are healthy. They lead to the development of a conscience. A conscience relies on the ability to know right from wrong and is important to the development of relationships. Without conscience, children's behaviour is self-centred. Self-centred children have difficulty forming and maintaining relationships.

Case study . . .

. . . failure to thrive

Philippa had always assumed she would have a second child but had not planned to get pregnant. She and her partner John, both used to their way of life in the Services, were not surprised when John was posted abroad for 6 months during the pregnancy.

Philippa did, however, feel let down and unsupported when John was unable to return for the delivery. After a long and difficult labour, James was born by Caesarean section. Slow to start breathing, he was placed in the Special Care Baby Unit for the first few weeks of his life. A few days after delivery, Philippa, still feeling very tired, was relieved to leave hospital without James. She was anxious to return to caring for Thomas, her eldest child, who was only 2. Finally, James was allowed home.

The health visitor visited Philippa when James was 3 months old because she had not attended any of the baby clinics. The health visitor found Philippa and Thomas playing together in the lounge. James was in his cot in the bedroom. There were no baby things visible and Philippa seemed surprised at the health visitor's interest in James.

After careful monitoring by the health visitor, James was deemed to be failing to thrive and was re-admitted to hospital. Once in hospital, he gained weight. James was subsequently accommodated away from home by the local authority social services department.

1. *What factors may have led to the weak bond of attachment between Philippa and James?*
2. *Why did James put on weight in hospital?*
3. *Why was James accommodated away from home by the social services department?*
4. *Why was his brother Thomas not accommodated away from home by the social services department?*
5. *How could James be reintegrated into the family?*

Progress check

Why is it important for a baby's physical well-being that they are responsive?

How is cognitive development encouraged through the experience of secure attachments?

What are the qualities of a 'sensitive mother'?

Why are children with secure attachments better able to cope with fears and worries?

What are social emotions?

The effects on children and their families of separation and loss

key term

Maternal deprivation
'the prolonged deprivation of young children of maternal care' (Bowlby)

During the 1940s, John Bowlby, whose work on attachment was mentioned above, studied young people who persistently broke the law. In his work *Maternal Care and Mental Health* (1951), he explained their delinquency by their 'prolonged deprivation of maternal care'. This lack of maternal care was referred to as '**maternal deprivation**', then defined as the loss by a child of their mother's love.

During the 1950s and 1960s, James and Joyce Robertson, colleagues of John Bowlby, undertook observations of children who were admitted to hospitals or residential nurseries. They were convinced that separating young children from their parents was harmful. At this time the idea was not accepted by the medical profession. The Robertsons used a cine-camera to film children during these periods of separation. (These films or videos are still available.) They noted that during periods of separation, many of the children went through a similar sequence of behaviour. This process appeared to occur if children were separated from the

key term

Distress syndrome the pattern of behaviour shown by the children who experience loss of a familiar carer with no one to take their place

people to whom they were attached but did not then receive appropriate care. They called it **distress syndrome**.

When the Robertsons cared for a 2-year-old in their own home and filmed her responses, they did not observe the distress syndrome because, as they explain in the film, the child Kate was well prepared, took many familiar objects with her which gave her reassurance and a sense of security, and was given appropriate one-to-one care that took the place of the most important aspects of her parents' love and care. That is, she received good substitute care.

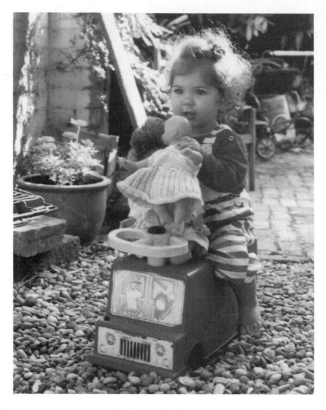

Familiar objects give reassurance and a sense of security

THE DISTRESS SYNDROME

The distress syndrome is the name given to the following pattern of behaviour shown by children who are not prepared for separation and who do not receive appropriate substitute care:

- It starts with a period of *distress* or protest, shown by crying, screaming, and other expressions of anger at being left.
- This gives way to a period of *despair* when children, fearing their carer might not return, become listless, need more rest, are dull, disinterested and refuse to play.
- Finally, there is a period of *detachment* when the children, believing their carer will not return, appear to try to separate themselves from any memory of the past. They lack concentration, their behaviour is erratic; they seem sometimes dull and lifeless, at others highly active and excitable. If children reach this stage it appears that long-term damage is done to their future emotional security.

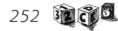

The Robertsons also noted the difficulty children experienced in linking up and relating to their parents when the separation ended. They studied some of the children after separation and noted that they cried more than previously, had tantrums and did not show as much affection as before the separation. They concluded that these negative separation experiences might have long-term effects.

Fortunately, as a result of their research fewer children are now exposed to such trauma.

Case study . . .

. . . hospital admission

Jill was born in 1948. She had a happy childhood and had never been apart from her parents. When she was 4, after periods of prolonged illness, it was decided that she needed to have her tonsils removed, for which she would be in hospital for 10 days. The hospital was in the country many miles outside her town and her family had no car so travel was a problem. Her parents were told that, although there was a visiting hour each afternoon, it was better not to visit because 'it might upset her'. Her parents therefore did not visit her for the whole time and she was taken and brought home in a hospital car.

When Jill first arrived at the hospital, she was cheerful and interested, but was quickly frightened when she was made to drink some medicine and change into a hospital gown. Nobody in particular looked after her; the nurses took their duties in turns. The preparation for the operation was bewildering for her and she started to cry for her mother. After the operation she was very uncomfortable and cried even more. No one was actually unkind to her, but little notice was taken. She gradually became quiet and subdued and took little notice of anyone.

When she was taken home, Jill was cold and distant from her parents. She did not respond to their attempts to cuddle her. She became a tense and nervous child, and when she started school at 5 years old she was very distressed and took a long time to settle.

1. *What pattern of behaviour do Jill's responses illustrate?*
2. *Why do you think she responded in this way?*
3. *Why did her parents not visit her?*
4. *What long-term effects did the experience appear to have?*
5. *In what ways are the admission of children to hospital different today?*

Strategies for minimising the adverse effects of separation

CURRENT GOOD PRACTICE

Michael Rutter in his book, *Maternal Deprivation Reassessed*, concluded that the needs of children can be met satisfactorily by good substitute care, organised in a sensitive way, and that the children observed by the Robertsons missed the individual caring behaviour that they were used to as much as their parents. Children are less likely to be so profoundly affected by separation if an environment provides good substitute care.

Bowlby's findings, together with those of the Robertsons and other researchers, have resulted in far-reaching changes to child-care practice. Many professions concerned with children have now changed their practices to avoid the unnecessary separation of children from their parents, for example hospital admissions, and to prepare children when separation is unavoidable, such as going to school.

These changes include:

- new babies being kept beside their mothers on maternity wards
- parents of babies in Special Care Baby Units being encouraged to be involved in the care of their ill or tiny babies
- parents being encouraged to remain with their children in hospital, and the provision of facilities for them to stay overnight
- many social workers being taught to regard the separation of children from their primary carers as the worst possible solution to a family's problems
- preparation for starting school and for hospital admission.

GOOD SUBSTITUTE CARE

> **key term**
> **Substitute care** the care given to children during periods of separation from their main carers

The Robertsons' observations highlighted the importance of good replacement or **substitute care** (now often known as 'short-term breaks') for children during periods of separation. Substitute care is good when it is organised in a way that meets the emotional needs of children.

Substitute care is unlikely to meet children's needs if children are:

- cared for by constantly changing caregivers, with limited time to provide individual attention
- given little opportunity to form an attachment with any one caregiver
- poorly prepared for separation or for being reunited
- not encouraged to keep in contact with the people they were attached to.

The research of the Robertsons and others has had an effect on the provision of care for all children in the many settings in which they are separated from the carers with whom they have developed attachments. In the past, children were often cared for in large institutions. The staff had responsibility for many children and were not encouraged to develop special relationships with individual children

> **key term**
> **Key worker** works with, and is concerned with the care and assessment of, particular children

RESIDENTIAL CARE

Today, children who cannot remain with their parents are cared for, if possible, by members of their extended family or by people they know. Those who are cared for by the local authority social services department are now placed in foster homes or small group homes. Residential nurseries are now rare.

The emphasis now is on substitute care that is as much like family care as possible. Substitute carers are encouraged to develop a bond with the children. Children in small children's homes will have a limited number of carers, one of whom will be their **key worker** or special carer. In addition, many children in the long-term care of the social services department are now adopted. Disabled children, previously cared for in residential institutions, may also be placed with adopters.

> **key term**
> **Day care** the provision of care during the day in a variety of settings outside a child's own home with people other than close relatives, either full-time or part-time

DAY CARE

Day care means care for children who are looked after for the whole or part of the day, but who return to their main carers at night. This may be with childminders, in day nurseries, nursery schools and primary schools. Children looked after by nannies usually remain in their own home and may or may not have their parent(s) present for some of the time; they may still experience some loss.

Under the Children Act 1989, local authorities are encouraged to provide a range of services to enable 'children in need' to remain in their own homes and to be cared for by their own families. This avoids the emotional damage that can be caused by separation. These services include:

- day nurseries or family centres
- respite care, for disabled children – this provides short-term care that enables families to have a break and hopefully prevents family breakdown
- liaison with voluntary agencies who also provide services to children and their families.

Progress check

What is 'maternal deprivation'?

Describe the distress syndrome and when it might occur.

What are the measures laid down in the Children Act to enable 'children in need' to remain in their own homes?

Transitions

key term

Transition
the movement of a child from one care situation to another

A **transition**, in the context of child care, refers to the movement of a child from one care situation to another. This usually involves a change of physical environment and a change of carer(s) for part or all of the day.

Transitions are experienced across a range of situations. These include a child going to a childminder, day nursery, family centre, crèche, nursery school or infant school.

Transitions involve change and loss of attachment figures, both of which are potentially threatening to children's feelings of security and trust.

STRATEGIES TO HELP CHILDREN AND FAMILIES COPE WITH TRANSITIONS

Young children need stability and security in their environment and because of this they need help to cope with any transitions they make. Significantly they need preparation, good substitute care and help with being reunited.

key term

Residential care
the provision of care both during the day and the night outside a child's home with people other than close relatives

The research that has been carried out into the effects of separation and loss has had a direct effect on the way that children are both prepared for transitions and cared for when separated from their carers both in day care, **residential care** and in hospital.

Preparation

Children's reactions to separation can be affected by the way they are prepared for change. In the past, there was little or no awareness of the value of preparation. Children were taken to school or hospital and left to cope with the experience. Good preparation is now accepted as beneficial to all children when moving to any setting. Preparation has become part of the policy of most institutions, including nurseries, schools, hospitals, childminders and long-term foster care.

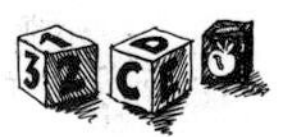

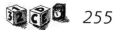

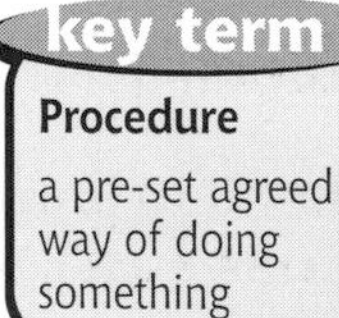

Procedure
a pre-set agreed way of doing something

Preparation is often built into the **procedures** of a day-care setting or school. (A procedure is a pre-set agreed way of doing something.) People dealing with children at times of change need to understand and be sensitive to children's needs.

The following guidelines for preparation can be applied to a variety of settings including schools and hospitals. Before a transition, prepare children by:

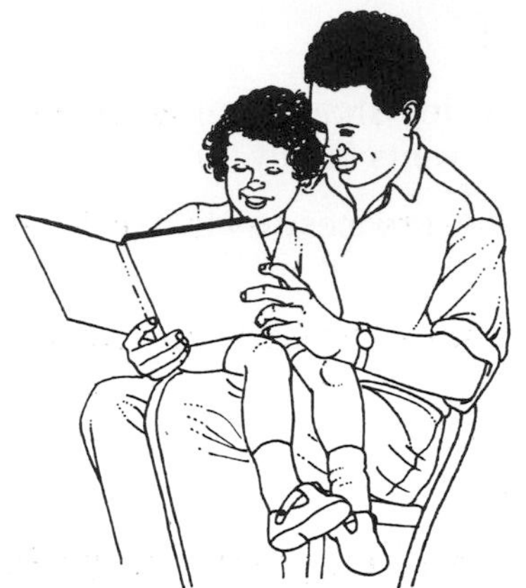

Reading relevant books can help to prepare a child for change

- talking to them and explaining honestly what is about to happen
- listening to and reassuring them
- reading books and watching relevant videos with them
- providing experiences for imaginative and expressive play, which will help children to express their feelings
- arranging introductory visits for them and their carers, when information and experiences can be given both at their own and an adult's level
- making sure that any relevant personal details about a child, including their likes and dislikes and cultural background, are available to the substitute carer.

CARING FOR CHILDREN DURING SEPARATION AND TRANSITION

Workers should assess children's behaviour during separation, recognise if there is any cause for concern and give appropriate attention. As shown in the table below, the Children Act 1989 recognises that younger children have a need for close contact with a familiar carer. It therefore provides guidance for the ratios of children to carers: the younger the child, the higher the ratio. Many day-care settings have key workers who are concerned with the care and assessment of particular children.

When caring for children the following points are relevant:

- Children under 3 years benefit from a one-to-one relationship with a specific person.

Suggested adult-to-children ratios (Children Act 1989)

Setting	Age	Children:carer ratio
Day care	Under 2	3:1
	Over 2 but under 3	4:1
	Over 3 but under 5	8:1
	Over 5 but under 8	8:1
Childminders	Under 5	3:1
	Over 5 but under 8	6:1
	Under 8 (of whom no more than three are under 5)	6:1

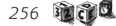

- The particular needs and background of children need to be known.
- Children's comfort objects should be readily available to them.
- Children should be provided with activities appropriate to their developmental age and stage, especially play that encourages the expression of feelings.
- Honest reassurance should be given.
- Children's parents should have access to them if appropriate, whenever possible.
- Children should have reminders of their parents or carers, such as photographs, when they are apart.
- Positive images of parents, reminders of home culture should be promoted.

REUNITING CHILDREN WITH THEIR MAIN CARERS

Children who have been prepared for separation and cared for appropriately will find it easier to be reunited with their carers and to readjust to their home environment. This can apply as much to children starting school as to children who are returning home from full-time care. Children can be helped with being reunited if carers remember to:

- be honest about when they will be reunited
- allow them to talk and express their feelings through play
- advise the parent(s) to expect and accept some disturbance in their child's feelings and possibly some *regressive* (going back to an earlier developmental stage) behaviour.

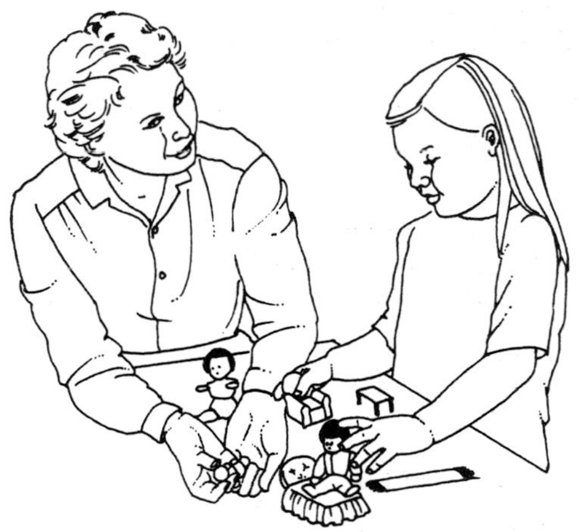

Allow the child to talk and express feelings through play

TRANSITIONS TO NURSERY OR SCHOOL

Most children go to school. Some may start by attending a nursery school, others start when they are the statutory school age of 5. Whatever their age, children may experience anxiety and stress when they start school.

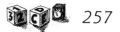

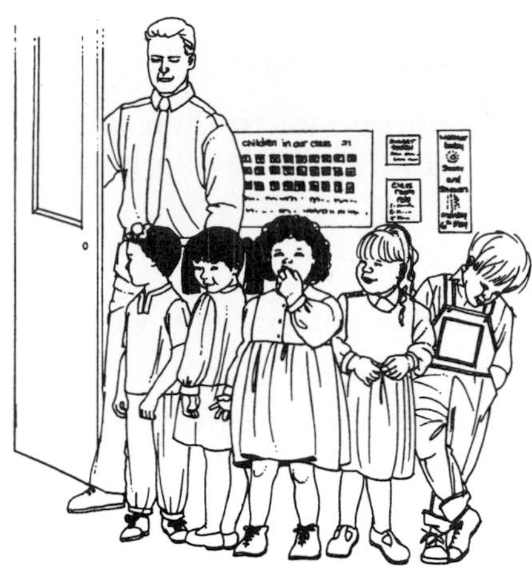

The routines may be unfamiliar and they may have a fear of doing something wrong

Possible sources of anxiety when starting nursery or school are:

- separation from their carer
- being among a large unfamiliar group of children who may already be established in friendship groups
- the day may seem very long
- they may be unfamiliar with the predominant culture and language of the school
- the routines will be unfamiliar and they may have a fear of doing something wrong
- different activities such as PE, playtime, milk and dinner time can feel strange to them
- the scale and unfamiliarity of the buildings may be frightening
- being directed and having to concentrate for longer than they are used to.

Easing the transition from home to school

Possible sources of help for children when they start school are shown in the figure on page 259. These sources include the policies of the school to admissions and to parents, the staff of the school and the child's parents or family.

Case study . . .

. . . starting school

Marcus started in the reception class at his local infants school the week after his 5th birthday. This was the school policy for all admissions. Previously, he went to a private day nursery full-time for 4 years while his mother and father worked. His parents were given a helpful information brochure about the school and attended a meeting held for parents of all new children. Marcus attended pre-school sessions with other new children during the term before he started. These were held in one of the school classrooms on one afternoon a week, with the reception teacher.

1. *How was Marcus prepared for the reception class?*
2. *How could Marcus's parents use the information they were given about school?*
3. *How well do you think Marcus settled into school and why do you think this?*
4. *Why might Marcus not have settled without this preparation?*

FREQUENT TRANSITIONS

key term

Respite care
short-term care for a child to receive training and assessment and/or to allow their family to have a break

Children, whose admission to school is handled sensitively with attention to the points above, usually learn to cope with attending school each day. Children can also be helped to adjust to frequent hospital admissions if necessary. Some children also have to cope with movement between their family home and residential accommodation or foster care. This may be because of family difficulties; parents may be unable to care for them because they are experiencing problems. Sometimes, if a child has a disability, a period of **respite care** in a community children's home enables the child to receive training or assessment. It also gives their families a rest. If it is handled well, a child can adjust to periodic changes of residence of this kind.

POLICIES

School policies can include:
- an appropriate admission programme
- an admission policy that staggers the intake of children
- a helpful and informative brochure, provided in the home languages of parents and children
- appropriate classrooms and staff
- good liaison with parents
- a welcoming environment.

Strategies to help children when starting school

STAFF

Staff (teachers, nursery nurses, classroom assistants, etc.) can provide:
- a relaxed classroom routine
- appropriate activities and expectations
- individual attention
- observation and monitoring of new children
- an awareness of cultural and language differences
- a welcome to parents to participate.

PARENTS

Parents and carers can help by:
- encouraging independence skills, e.g. dressing, washing, eating
- giving children some experience of separation before they start school
- being there for the child when they need reassurance
- having a positive attitude towards school
- reading books about starting school and encouraging realistic expectations
- establishing routines (e.g. bedtime) that will fit in with school
- providing the appropriate equipment (e.g. lunch box, PE kit).

Strategies to help children when starting school

MULTIPLE TRANSITIONS

Some children, however, experience frequent moves. This may be because of constant and unpredictable family breakdowns. Such children become increasingly distrustful of adults. They become accustomed to change, but become increasingly unable to relate closely to any carers. Their emotional and social development is disturbed and this makes them difficult to care for. It is for this reason that frequent changes of environment for young children are avoided if at all possible. Social workers try to make long-term permanent plans for children. These may involve placing children with adopters or long-term foster parents.

Progress check

What is a key worker?

What is a transition?

When might children experience separation from their main carers?

What can significantly affect children's reactions to a transition?

What are the main sources of anxiety for children when starting nursery or school?

Loss and grief

key term

Grief
feelings of deep sorrow at the loss, through death, of a loved person

We have a limited number of very close attachments in our lives. Amongst the closest relationships are those between grandparents, parents and children, between siblings, and between life partners.

The term **grief** is usually reserved for feelings of deep sorrow at the loss, through death, of a loved person. The term also applies to the feelings and reactions of children to the long-term loss in other circumstances of a person with whom they have formed an attachment. This long-term loss may occur when a carer:

- separates or divorces from their partner and loses contact with the child
- is in prison for a long period
- is seriously ill and unable to communicate (for example, in a coma)
- goes away, including to another country, leaving the child behind.

If any of the above happens, the child may experience feelings of grief. Research has shown that grief felt by both children and adults follows a recognisable path or pattern. It is essential to have an awareness of this pattern when working with children who are experiencing grief. This awareness will enable you to:

- understand the child's feelings and behaviour
- be sensitive to the child's needs
- be able to provide and care for the child in the most appropriate way.

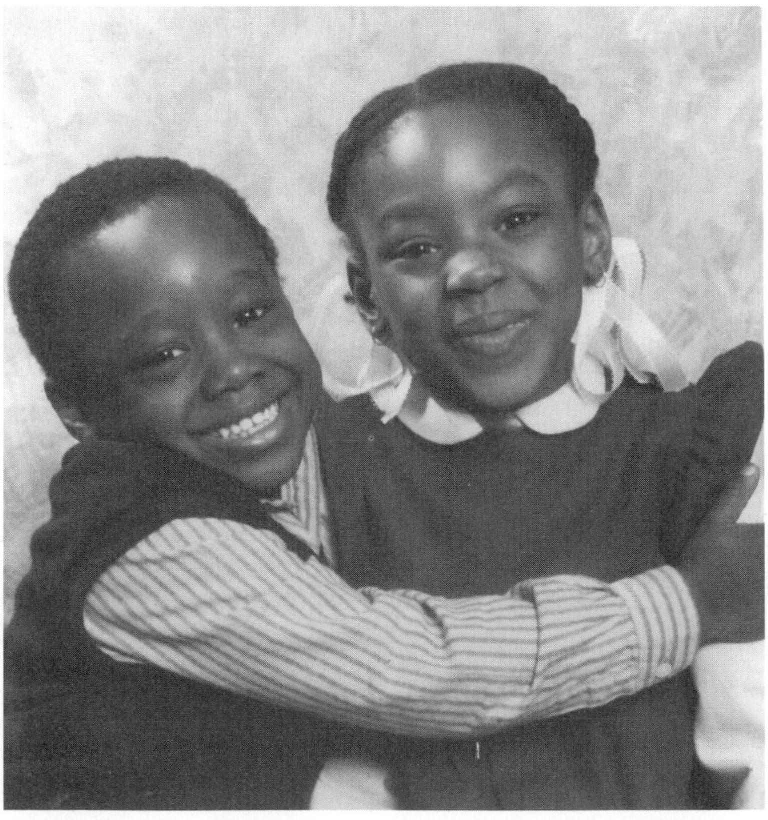

We have a limited number of very close attachments in our lives. Amongst the closest of these is the attachment between siblings

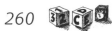

THE STAGES OF GRIEF

This section will concentrate on the child whose carer has died; however a child may feel *as if* a carer has died in any of the other circumstances listed above. People usually experience very powerful feelings of grief when they lose a person with whom they have a close attachment. In any person's life, the number of people with whom they have such attachments is quite limited.

The process of grief can be understood as a number of stages that people pass through. Each stage involves experiencing feelings and behaving in certain ways. One stage has to be worked through, at least in part, before a person can move on to the next. Although it is useful to look at stages in this way, it can make the process appear orderly and systematic. In practice the stages tend to merge into one another. Children (and adults) may return to the feelings of a previous stage at any time during the process of grieving.

The strength of feeling people have when they lose someone or something is directly linked to the strength of feeling they have for the person or to the value they place on the object. The length of time the feelings last vary with the importance of the loss. Children may work through the main stages of grief for a person within a year. Adults may take considerably longer; 3 years can be quite normal. It is usually necessary for the dates of special anniversaries associated with the lost person, for example their birthday, to pass at least once before both children and adults can begin fully to adjust to the loss.

The table below summarises the possible feelings and behaviour of a child during stages of grief. The stages of grief that a child (or an adult) goes through when they lose a person can be divided into early grief, acute grief and subsiding grief.

DEALING WITH GRIEF

Children are immature and very vulnerable at times of loss. They need special consideration and care. However, it is possible that the adults who are closest to them could also be suffering the same loss. This means that the child's needs may not always be given the highest priority. It is very common in white British culture, unlike perhaps in Asian families, for children to be excluded during the period of

The stages of grief

Stage of grief	Possible feelings of the child	Possible behaviour of the child
Early grief Immediately after the loss or death	Shock, numbness, disbelief, denial, panic, alarm	Listlessness, or hyperactivity, dislike of being alone, prone to illness
Acute grief Follows the acceptance of the loss	Extreme sadness, anger, guilt, shame, yearning, despair	Pining, searching, restlessness, crying, compulsive and irrational acts, lack of concentration, prone to illness
Subsiding grief When acute feelings have been worked through	Less absorbed by grief, calmer, less preoccupied, shows interest in other things, higher self-esteem	Shows interest in life, forms other attachments, involved in activities, better concentration

mourning for the death of a relative for example. They may not be informed of a death until later, they may not be allowed to attend a funeral even if they want to, or they may be sent away to stay with people who are not directly involved. This exclusion is probably the result of adults believing it is better not to upset the child, and also feeling that they do not have the emotional energy to cope with the child's grief as well as their own. Whatever the reasons, all available research shows that excluding a child at this time can create problems for the child later on. In the long term their unexpressed and unresolved feelings can return and complicate their adult mental health.

Adults who are not themselves involved in the grief of a child, for example child-care workers and teachers, can be of great help to a child. They can give the child uncomplicated attention and consideration. Despite this, many adults find such involvement difficult. This may be because they:

- themselves have unresolved grief. Perhaps they were denied a period of mourning when they were young. Any contact with a grieving child can therefore activate painful memories
- do not understand the process of grief, or the time that it takes, or the appropriate way to respond
- have, along with many people, a fear of death, and an unconscious wish to avoid any contact with death.

It should be a part of any child-care worker's training that they examine their own feelings and attitudes, and learn as much as possible about the process of grief. Avoidance is not helpful to a child.

THE ROLE OF THE ADULT WHEN WORKING WITH A GRIEVING CHILD

Adults should give as much warning to a child as possible and tell them honestly if they are about to experience loss through separation or death. They should encourage children to accept that the loss has happened and allow them to share their sorrow with others, attending a funeral if appropriate. They should provide a quiet environment and give physical comfort to the child. In the stages of acute grief children need time and attention, patience and reassurance from adults. Allowances may need to be made for regressive behaviour and appropriate play provided so that a child can express their feelings safely. Adults should be less demanding and help the child to reorganise gradually, helping the child to participate in activities when ready. They should give time throughout to listen to the child, care for them and promote their welfare.

THE EFFECTS OF GRIEF ON GROWTH AND DEVELOPMENT

Grief can be such a powerful experience that the developmental growth of a child may be affected in every area (see the table on page 263).

GRIEF AND MOURNING IN A MULTI-CULTURAL SOCIETY

People have differing cultural practices for dealing with death and mourning. The mourning period is the time when people show conventional signs of grief, such as wearing black, or wearing white, weeping together, closing curtains. A knowledge of and respect for different customs and beliefs is vital when you are working with children whose cultural and religious background is different from yours. Without this knowledge, a child-care worker might respond unsuitably, or offer words of comfort that are inappropriate and even offensive.

The effects of grief on development

Area of development	Possible effect of grief on development
Physical	Child may not want to eat or run around
Cognitive	Child may be unable to concentrate or be too sad to play
Language	Child may be self-absorbed and unwilling to communicate
Emotional	Child may feel insecure, lose trust in adults, have low self-esteem
Social	Child may not want to be with friends or relatives

Progress check

What are the main stages of grief?

How can an adult best provide for a child who is experiencing grief?

How may grief affect a child developmentally?

Now try these questions

Why do attachments develop?

What behaviour encourages attachments during the first 6 months of a baby's life?

How do we know if attachment has occurred?

Why are secure attachments important?

What may result from poor or weak attachments?

Describe the possible consequences of long-term separation of an infant from their parent/carer.

Describe the characteristics of good substitute care.

What are the advantages for young children of foster care, rather than care in a residential establishment?

Why is it that adults who work with children might find it difficult to respond appropriately to a grieving child?

key terms

You need to know what the key terms and phrases in this chapter mean. Go back through the chapter and find out.

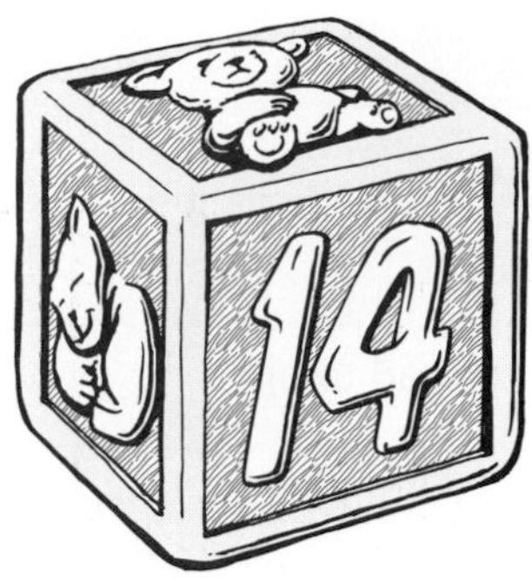

MANAGING BEHAVIOUR

In this chapter you will learn about managing children's behaviour effectively. You will learn how to encourage children to behave in an acceptable way and how to respond to unacceptable behaviour. You will begin to understand why some children exhibit unacceptable behaviour and learn some ways in which to manage and mould this behaviour so that it becomes more acceptable.

This chapter will cover the following topics:

- *what is behaviour?*
- *how is behaviour learned?*
- *young children's behaviour*
- *managing children's behaviour*
- *behaviour modification.*

What is behaviour?

key term

Behaviour
acting or reacting in a specific way, both unacceptably and acceptably

Behaviour is acting or reacting in a specific way. It is what we exhibit to others. It includes all that we do and say, both acceptable and unacceptable.

Patterns of behaviour are learned from the people with whom we have contact, both direct and indirect. This includes such influences as television, books and magazines. However, our earliest and most powerful influences are parents or carers and other influential adults in the immediate community.

Behaviour is therefore socially and culturally defined. We learn our behaviour from the social and cultural groups in which we grow up. There are, of course, many similarities between societies and cultures. There are also many differences in expectations and what is regarded as acceptable behaviour. This is important – do not assume that because someone's behaviour is unusual to you it is necessarily unacceptable.

Ideas of what are acceptable patterns of behaviour are acquired from a number of sources:

- immediate and extended family
- local community

 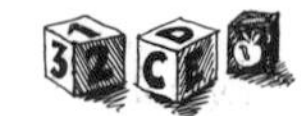

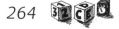

- peer group
- national government
- history, culture and/or national heritage.

At different times in an individual's life, different influences will predominate. For young children, the family is the most powerful influence. As children get older, peers and the wider community become increasingly important.

Progress check

Who and what are patterns of behaviour learned from?

Who are the most powerful influences in a young child's learning?

From what other sources are patterns of acceptable behaviour learned?

How is behaviour learned?

key terms

Sanction
a negative outcome attached to a specific behaviour

Subconscious
thoughts and feelings that a person is not fully aware of

Behaviour is learned through a complex process of imitation of role models, expectation expressed verbally and non-verbally, and rewards and **sanctions** that mould behaviour. Much of this process is **subconscious**: we are not aware that it is happening. It is a constant, life-long process. Both acceptable and unacceptable behaviour is learned in this way.

The patterns of behaviour that are established in childhood influence our behaviour throughout our lives. It is essential therefore that young children are given the opportunity to develop acceptable patterns of behaviour from an early age. To enable them to achieve this, children need:

- positive role models
- loving adults who have realistic expectations of young children's behaviour
- clear and consistent expectations expressed verbally and non-verbally
- fair and consistent boundaries of acceptable behaviour, rewarded when appropriate.

Where these conditions exist most children will develop acceptable patterns of behaviour with a minimum of conflict.

key terms

Prejudice
an opinion, usually unfavourable, about someone or something, based on incomplete facts

Discrimination
behaviour based on prejudice, which results in someone being treated unfairly

Behaviours that children learn are more complex merely than what is either acceptable or unacceptable. They also learn different roles. Children pick up the different expectations that society has of different groups of people. For example, how does society expect a female to behave? How is a male expected to behave?

Many people feel that the expectations of society are unfair to some groups of people, for example, the expectation that females should be responsible for all the domestic work in a home, or the expectation that males do not cry when upset. These roles are perceived to be restrictive because they do not reflect what individual people are really like. The learning processes described above, however, are so powerful that many people conform to the expectations.

Children also learn the value placed upon each role by society. They learn that the behaviour of some groups is more highly valued than others. This leads to **prejudice** and **discrimination** against some groups of people. Prejudice and discrimination are not acceptable. People who have contact with young children

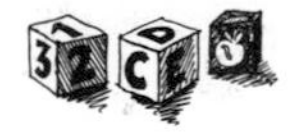

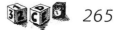

have a unique opportunity to work towards changing this through the powerful influence they have on children's expectations of what is acceptable and what is unacceptable behaviour.

Young children's behaviour

key term

Labelling
giving a reputation (or label) to someone based upon a small part of their behaviour. For example, a child who is very noisy may be labelled as disruptive. This creates a prejudiced view of the child

It is important to have realistic expectations of young children's behaviour. If expectations are unrealistic, the possibility for conflict and **labelling** arises. Acceptable behaviour causes little concern.

Unacceptable behaviour needs more careful consideration and is therefore the focus of the rest of this chapter. The following points are important in the discussion.

- The vast majority of children want to be approved by adults and others, and therefore wish to behave in an appropriate way. With positive role models, loving adults who are fair and consistent in their expectations and who set clear boundaries, most children will develop acceptable patterns of behaviour.
- Behaviour is not 'naughty' just because it does not conform to adult standards of behaviour. Children need to learn which behaviour is acceptable and which is unacceptable.
- There is often a reason why a behaviour occurs. This reason may be hidden, unconscious or in the past.
- Behaviour can often be attributed to how a child is feeling. The feelings that a child has do exist and cannot be changed. It is the behaviour that results from the feeling that is either acceptable or not acceptable. You must never reject a child's feelings, only their behaviour.
- Similar feelings in children can lead to very different behaviours. For example, the feeling of anger may result in one child being physically or verbally aggressive, but another child may well become withdrawn.
- Some behaviours are well established and it is difficult to understand why they occur.

Most young children will consistently exhibit acceptable behaviours as they grow and learn what is expected of them. However, while they are still in the process of learning, it is important that adults have appropriate expectations of what is common behaviour for young children. This will reduce the possibility of conflict and labelling. If the child is in an environment that promotes positive behaviour unacceptable behaviours will diminish with time as the child learns and grows.

SOME COMMON BEHAVIOURS IN YOUNG CHILDREN

Some common behaviours include:

- physical aggression
- use of aggressive language
- temper tantrums
- defiance
- withdrawing
- jealousy.

WHY DO THESE BEHAVIOURS OCCUR?

There are many reasons for a behaviour occurring. Listed below are some suggested answers to this question. However, the reasons are not always straightforward; simple solutions are not easy to find, and the feelings and reasons that influence the behaviours are not always obvious.

> **key term**
> **Curiosity**
> an inquisitive interest

Curiosity

A child learns by being active and interacting with their environment, and by being curious about their environment. There may be a clash between the child's curiosity and need to be active, and the adult's wish for the child to be safe and/or to establish boundaries of what is acceptable.

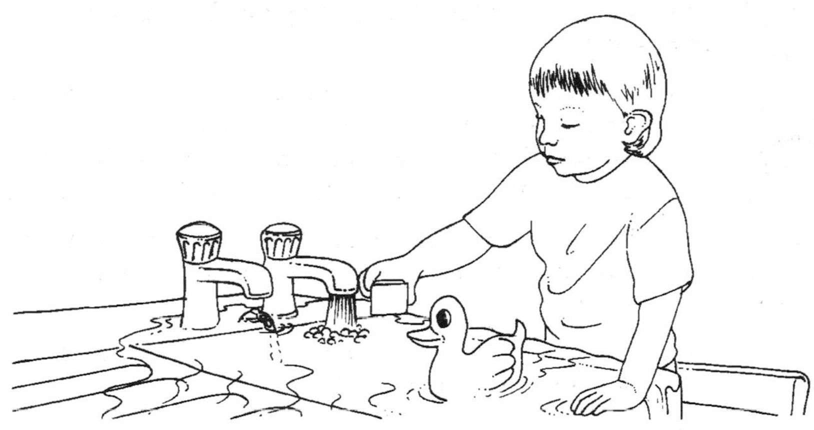

There may be a clash between the child's need to be active and the adult's wish for the child to be safe

> **key term**
> **Imitate**
> to copy closely, take as a model

Imitation

Children will **imitate** what they see others doing. This may at times be acceptable behaviour for an adult or older child, but not for a young child. Who or what are the child's role models?

> **key term**
> **Egocentric**
> seeing things only from one's own viewpoint

Egocentricism

Being **egocentric** means seeing things only from one's own viewpoint. It is not the same as being selfish, when both sides can be seen and the selfish one is chosen. Some psychologists believe that young children are incapable of seeing things from another person's viewpoint. It is a skill that children need to acquire over a period of time.

Developing independence

Children need to find ways of exhibiting their growing independence, and this may result in them trying to influence others in unacceptable ways.

Attention-seeking

Human beings need and want attention from other people. Children's behaviour can be a way of attention-seeking, that is attracting the attention of other people. For some children negative attention is better than none at all.

Anger and/or frustration

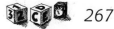

A lack of experience of the world sometimes means that children have unrealistic expectations of what is and what is not possible. This may result in anger or frustration, which is shown in their behaviour. For example, a child may have a tantrum when told that mummy cannot stop it raining so they can go to the park.

Anxiety or fear

A lack of experience and understanding of the world may lead to an unrealistic interpretation of events. For example, a child who experiences anxiety at being left in child care may be aggressive towards a parent who picks them up at the end of the session. This is often an expression of relief that the parent has returned.

Children may also become anxious and/or fearful when changes in familiar patterns and/or routines occur. This is likely to be reflected in their behaviour. Examples might be a change in child care, starting school, changes in friendships, lack of sleep. The feelings associated with these changes and the resulting behaviour is often short term and behaviour usually settles down once new or different routines are established.

EMOTIONAL NEEDS

Children have many emotional needs, for example:

- **affection** – the feeling of being loved by parents, carers, family, friends and the wider social community
- **belonging** – the feeling of being wanted by a group
- **consistency** – the feeling that things are predictable
- **independence** – the feeling of managing and directing your own life
- **achievement** – the feeling of satisfaction gained from success
- **social approval** – the feeling that others approve of your conduct and efforts
- **self-esteem** – the feeling of liking and valuing oneself.

The absence of any of the above may lead to unacceptable behaviour as children struggle to get what they need. There are likely to be times in all children's lives where they experience short-term stress because some of their emotional needs are not being met, for example, moving house, a new baby in the family or a short period of hospitalisation. If these situations are handled sensitively any behavioural difficulties are not likely to be long term.

However, when children's emotional needs are not met for a sustained period of time their behaviour can be severely affected. For example when children experience separation, loss and/or grief (see Chapter 13) or children are abused (see Unit Nine), their distress is likely to be evident in their behaviour. This may be anything from extreme withdrawal to violent behaviour. It is important to remember that all children are individuals and that the same feelings or events can result in different behaviours in different children. These can be long-term problems, which require long-term strategies to mould behaviour so that it becomes acceptable. Specialist help and guidance will probably be required.

There are a number of different ways of accessing help and guidance. It will depend upon the situation that you are in. In education help is usually accessed through the Special Educational Needs co-ordinator who will be a named member of staff. Once the child's needs have been identified an individual education plan (IEP) will be drawn up, which may eventually involve an educational psychologist (see Chapter 42).

Other help can be accessed through health professionals (e.g. health visitors, GPs), or through social services (e.g. staff in nursery/family centres, social workers). All these people can be contacted directly by parents or family members seeking help, by concerned friends or neighbours, or by professionals and others

key terms

Affection
the emotional need to feel loved by parents, carers, family, friends and the wider social community

Belonging
the emotional need to feel wanted by a group

Consistency
the emotional need to feel that things are predictable

Independence
the emotional need to feel you are managing and directing your own life

Achievement
the emotional need for the satisfaction gained from success

Social approval
when a person's conduct and efforts are approved of by others

Self-esteem
liking and valuing oneself

 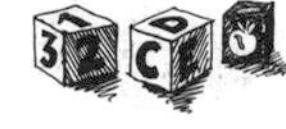

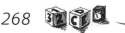

from statutory or voluntary agencies. The aim of all these professionals is to address the child and family needs through the development of strategies to manage behaviour (see Chapter 33).

Progress check

Why is it important to have realistic expectations of young children's behaviour?

List some common behaviours for young children.

Suggest some reasons why these behaviours occur.

What are children's emotional needs?

What may happen when children's emotional needs are not met and how can you help?

How can you access specialist help and guidance if it is required?

Managing children's behaviour

Behaviour is learned. People who work with children need therefore to be aware of effective ways of managing and moulding children's behaviour. The same techniques can be applied during the child's initial learning and when it is necessary to alter existing unacceptable behaviour.

Work settings will have policies and procedures for managing behaviour, and it is important that all staff are familiar with them. This will ensure consistency in approach, which is vital to good behaviour management. It is important to note that physical punishment is not allowed in most establishments. This is for many reasons but perhaps most importantly because we know which techniques are most effective. Behaviour management that communicates which behaviours are acceptable, rather than punishes unacceptable behaviour, is a more effective way of managing and moulding behaviour.

The situation regarding guidelines and procedures in other settings, for example working as a childminder or nanny is less clear. It is therefore vital that issues of behaviour management are discussed and clear guidelines established at the outset.

key term

ABC of behaviour
the pattern of all behaviour: Antecedent – what happens before the behaviour occurs; Behaviour – the resulting behaviour, acceptable or unacceptable; Consequence – the result of the behaviour, positive or negative

THE ABC OF BEHAVIOUR

All behaviours that occur, both acceptable and unacceptable, follow a similar pattern, known as the **ABC of behaviour**:

- *the Antecedent* – what happens before the behaviour occurs
- *the Behaviour* – the resulting behaviour, either acceptable or unacceptable
- *the Consequence* – the results that occur because of the behaviour, either positive or negative.

The most effective way of managing young children's behaviour is by controlling the antecedent. By being aware of what leads up to a particular behaviour, it is possible to have some influence on the behaviour that follows. Careful observation of situations is required for the antecedent to be identified before changes can be made. By anticipating the antecedents to behaviour, carers can encourage children to behave in an acceptable way and the possibility for conflict is minimised. This can be done, for example, in the following ways.

- In a nursery or school setting, remind children of the behaviour that is expected, e.g. 'I'm going to read the story now. Please be quiet until I have finished the story so that we can all listen and enjoy it.'
- Give children clear instructions about what you want them to do, e.g. 'We are going outside. It is cold. Get your coat and put it on. If you need help ask me.'
- Set up systems for children to have jobs in the setting, e.g. collecting the register, setting out some activities, checking everything is tidy, setting the table for snacks or lunch. All these activities allow children to feel independent and to have a sense of ownership and belonging to the setting.
- Welcome children by name to the establishment; this is likely to produce a feeling of being part of the group, and can exert a powerful influence on behaviour.
- Be careful about grouping children where there are some within the group who do not work well together.
- Provide enough space and equipment to reduce the likelihood of problems occurring.
- Praise effort; this is likely to encourage a child to continue trying this and other activities.

Changing the antecedent of unacceptable behaviour is one way of beginning to manage children's behaviour effectively so that it becomes more acceptable. Again, careful observation of situations is necessary to establish the antecedent. Here are some examples.

- *Temper tantrums* – When do they occur? What leads up to them? Can this be altered?
- *Physical aggression* – Who is involved? When does it occur? What leads up to it? Who or what are the child's role models?
- *Verbal aggression* – Who is involved? Who or what are their role models? When does it occur? What leads up to the behaviour?

Children's behaviour can also be managed by altering the consequence of a behaviour. This may mean rewarding acceptable behaviour, or attaching a negative outcome to a behaviour. For this to be effective, it is important that the child is aware of the consequence of the behaviour, both positive and negative. It is also important that the resulting outcome is applied consistently. Where possible all the adults who have close contact with the child need to be applying the same consequences to behaviours.

Case study . . .

. . . managing behaviour effectively

Tom, aged 3, who was normally quite a placid child, often became upset and difficult when activity time ended and the children came together for a story. He wouldn't put his toys away and shouted at the staff that he didn't want to have a story. This was clearly upsetting to Tom and disruptive to the group.

The staff decided to observe Tom over a period of a week to try and establish the pattern of events that led up to this behaviour.

The staff noted many things:

- that Tom often became engrossed in the activities, especially construction activities
- that he produced quite complex structures with the equipment
- that when the children were asked to clear up, he became agitated, he quickly tried to finish his construction and became anxious that the other children were going to break it up
- this behaviour only occurred when he was part-way through an activity at story time.

The staff implemented the following plan.

- Tom was told, 10 minutes before story time, that the session was ending soon to give him time to complete what he was doing.
- Completed models were kept until the following day.
- If Tom didn't finish what he was doing, his partly finished model would be saved until the following day when he could choose either to finish it or to break it up himself.

1. *What were the antecedents to Tom's behaviour?*
2. *What unacceptable behaviour was evident?*
3. *What consequences did this behaviour have?*
4. *How did the staff establish what was causing this behaviour?*
5. *How did they plan to manage Tom's behaviour?*

Progress check

What is the ABC of behaviour? Explain each element.

What is the most effective way of managing children's behaviour?

Give some examples of changing the antecedent.

How else can children's behaviour be managed?

What are the important features of managing behaviour by altering the consequence?

Behaviour modification

key term

Behaviour modification
techniques used to bring about changes in unacceptable behaviour so that it becomes acceptable

Behaviour modification is the term used for techniques that bring about changes in children's behaviour so that it becomes acceptable. It is based on the work of B.F. Skinner and his theory of operant conditioning. It works on the basis that:

- children will repeat behaviour that receives a positive response
- children will not repeat behaviour that receives no response or a negative response.

Behaviour is therefore moulded by manipulating the outcomes of a behaviour. This may be done by attaching a positive outcome to a behaviour so that the child is encouraged to repeat it. It may be done by ignoring a behaviour. It may also be done by attaching a negative outcome to a behaviour, so that the child is discouraged from repeating it. (This is the same as altering the consequence of a behaviour in the ABC of behaviour outlined above.)

This way of modifying children's behaviour is a long-term strategy. The rewards and/or sanctions need to be applied over a substantial period of time for them to be effective, especially if the unacceptable behaviour has been evident for some time.

For behaviour modification to be successful an assessment of how a child behaves is essential. This can be done using the ABC of behaviour. Patterns within a child's behaviour can be established through observation. Their needs can then be assessed and decisions made about a suitable behaviour-modification programme.

ATTACHING POSITIVE OUTCOMES TO CHILDREN'S BEHAVIOUR

The following outcomes may be attached to behaviours to encourage repetition:

- adult attention, which can be verbal or non-verbal (nods, smiles, winks)
- adult praise directed solely at the child
- peer group attention, where the group's attention is drawn to the child and the behaviour
- attention from other groups within the establishment
- responsibilities within the group
- extended privileges
- choice of activity
- tokens to exchange for privileges/activities/extended time at an activity
- positive reports to the parent or carer.

ATTACHING NEGATIVE OUTCOMES TO CHILDREN'S BEHAVIOUR

The following outcomes may be attached to behaviours to discourage children from copying or repeating them:

- ignoring the behaviour
- adult attention directed towards a child who is behaving acceptably
- removal from a positive situation to a neutral or negative situation, for example 'time out'
- adult disapproval, verbal or non-verbal, directed solely at the child
- peer group disapproval, which must come from the other children, not as a result of humiliating comments from the adult
- loss of responsibility or privileges.

APPLYING SANCTIONS TO UNACCEPTABLE BEHAVIOUR

Where a sanction is applied, wherever possible it should follow a pattern of natural justice; for example helping to rebuild models that were broken in anger; not being allowed on the apparatus if the child has consistently misbehaved when on it; clearing up mess created through misbehaviour, i.e. water tipped on to floors.

For behaviour modification to work effectively, it must meet the following criteria:

- Rules must be established and the children must be aware of them.
- The children must be aware of the outcomes attached to behaviours, whether they are positive or negative.
- The outcomes must be appropriate to the children's age and/or stage of development and understanding.
- The outcomes must be applied each time the behaviour occurs.
- The outcomes must be applied immediately.
- Outcomes must take individual likes and dislikes into account. What an adult sees as a negative outcome may be positive for a child. For example, removing a child from a group for being disruptive: the child may not want to remain in the group as they feel their lack of knowledge or competence is going to be shown up and by removing them the adult has actually rewarded the unacceptable behaviour.
- Behaviour modification needs to involve all adults who have close contact with the child or children. This means that the rules are consistently reinforced within an establishment and at home.

MAKING CONTRACTS

key term

Contract
an agreement between an adult and child – the child agrees to behave in a particular way and the adult agrees to reward that behaviour when it occurs

To encourage a child to behave in an acceptable way over a period of time, a **contract** may be drawn up between the child and an adult. The child agrees to behave in a particular way over the period of time and the adult agrees to reward the acceptable behaviour.

For young children this can be done by filling in a chart. Each time a child behaves in an appropriate way a section of the chart is filled in. When the chart is completed an agreed reward is received. Examples of such charts are shown below.

The benefit of this is to encourage the child to be behave consistently in an acceptable way, as the reward is not received until the child has maintained the behaviour over a period of time.

Managing behaviour effectively is an essential part of working with children. Adults who work with them need to know how to manage and mould behaviour so that it is, or becomes, acceptable.

Effective behaviour management should have the following features:

- *Confident* – adults need to know how to manage behaviour, where possible in a positive way, and how to modify unacceptable behaviour, with help where necessary.
- *Clear* – rules and expectations should be clear to the adults and the childen in the group.
- *Consistent* – rules and expectations should be fair and applied every time a behaviour occurs.
- *Caring* – most children want to please and will respond to a fair system of behaviour management. Children who consistently exhibit unacceptable behaviour are often children in need.
- *Catch children being good* – positive behaviour management is the most effective way of managing behaviour.

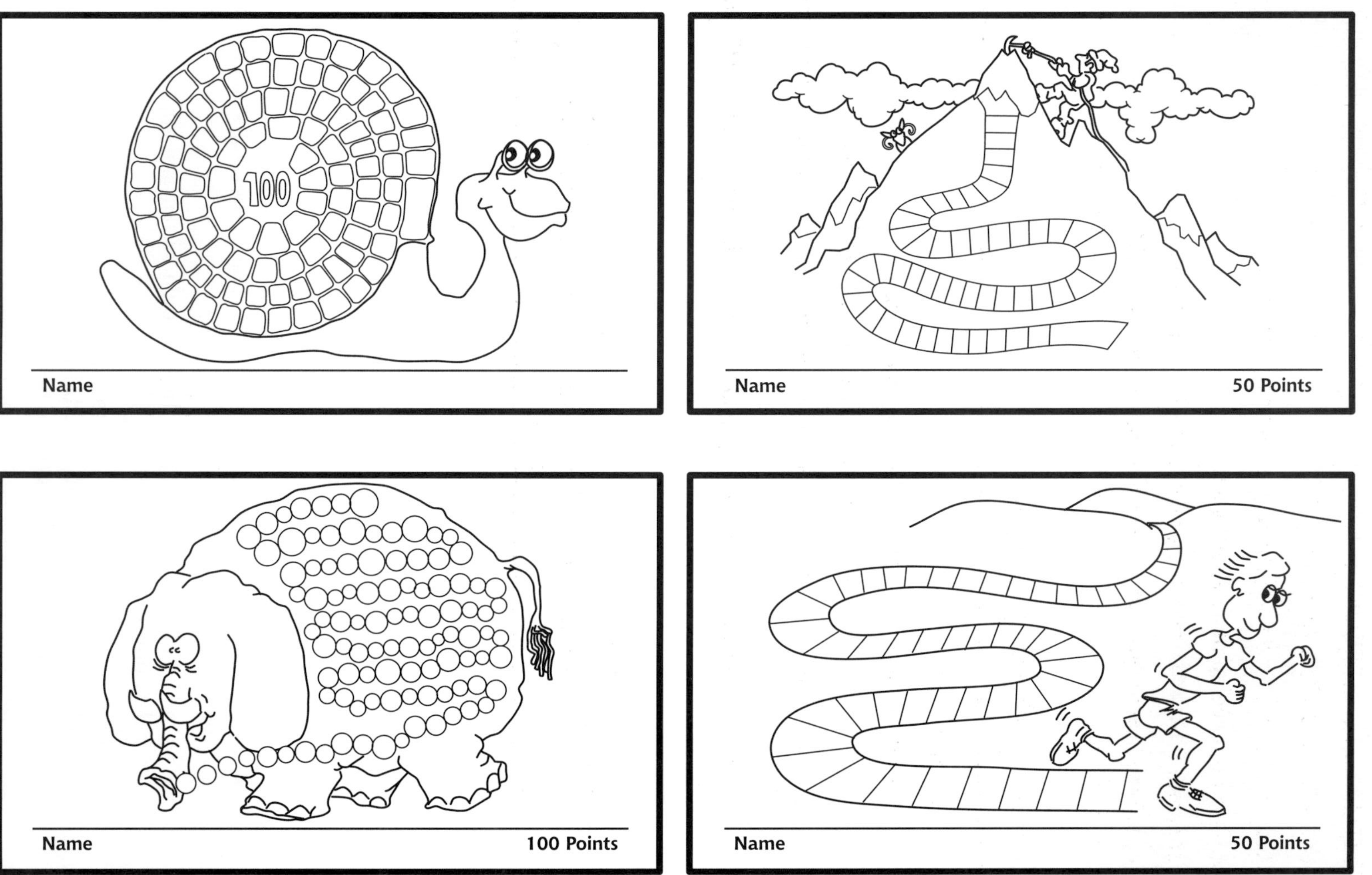

Examples of behaviour charts to be filled in by the child

Progress check

What is behaviour modification?

What are the underlying principles?

What is meant by 'attaching a positive outcome to behaviour'?

Give some examples of positive outcomes.

What is meant by 'attaching a negative outcome to behaviour'?

What are the benefits of making behaviour contracts with children?

Now try these questions

What is behaviour?

How do humans learn their patterns of behaviour?

What does a child need to develop positive patterns of behaviour?

Describe some common behaviours in young children and outline why they may occur.

Describe the ways in which unacceptable patterns of behaviour can be effectively managed.

key terms

You need to know what the key terms and phrases in this chapter mean. Go back through the chapter and find out.

Unit 5: Health and Community Care

In this unit you will learn about the promotion and maintenance of health, including surveillance programmes, childhood illnesses, the care of the sick child and a child with a life threatening or terminal illness. This unit will provide you with the basic knowledge required to work in most early years care and education settings, and an introduction to working in a hospital setting.

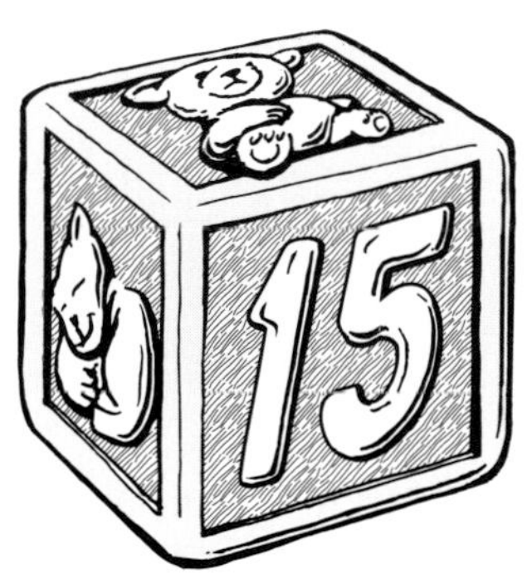

THE PROMOTION AND MAINTENANCE OF HEALTH

Promoting a healthy lifestyle can encourage positive aspects of improving and maintaining health. An important part of health promotion includes a health surveillance programme to monitor children's health, and to detect and prevent illness.

This chapter will cover the following topics:

- *defining health*
- *the role of the child-care worker in health promotion and education*
- *child health surveillance*

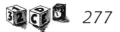

- *screening for hearing impairment*
- *screening for visual impairment*
- *Guthrie test*
- *hip test.*

Defining health

Health is a difficult word to define because it means different things to different people. Some may consider themselves to be healthy because they do not smoke; others because they have not been ill recently. Being healthy involves more than the physical condition and may include being fit, not being ill and living to a very old age.

The World Health Organisation defines health as 'a state of complete physical, mental and social well-being and not merely the absence of disease or infirmity'.

This definition recognises that there are three aspects to health, physical, mental and social, that will affect overall health. However, this definition has been criticised for being too idealistic as it makes healthy status out of reach of a large proportion of the world's population. Poverty or disability may affect health, but need not imply that poor health is inevitable.

The World Health Organisation also states that 'The enjoyment of the highest attainable standard of health is one of the fundamental rights of every human being without distinction of race, religion, political belief, economic or social condition . . .'.

One of the main issues in health is the person's capacity to make their own choices. These choices may be based on:

- traditions of the cultural group
- the family
- self-awareness
- knowledge.

Adults make choices for themselves and also for their children. Examples include when to wean their babies, which foods to give to children, whether to immunise and raising awareness of safety. Choices made by parents and child-care workers should be informed choices. The Health Education Authority and health professionals seek to inform the population in the UK so that they can make their own informed choices.

HEALTH EDUCATION

The main objective of health education is to improve the general health of the population, and to enable people to take responsibility for their own and their children's health by:

- changing behaviour or attitude
- providing knowledge and raising awareness

- empowering people to choose their own lifestyle and to be aware of the implications of their choices
- promoting the interest of a particular group
- meeting local and national targets in health, e.g. promoting self-examination to detect breast cancer.

The role of the child-care worker in health promotion and education

There are many important factors involved in maintaining children's health and keeping them safe from illness. Child-care workers can have an impact on the health of the children in their care by providing routines, activities and education that increase adults' and children's awareness of the importance of good health and ways of keeping healthy.

It is important that health topics and activities are part of the planned programme for children. It is often possible to link these successfully with other areas of the curriculum. For example, topic work about 'Ourselves' will cover aspects of 'Knowledge and Understanding of the World' as part of the Early Learning goals, while helping children to understand how their bodies work.

Health issues should be part of the daily routines and reminders, and explanations about health and hygiene will reinforce healthy life skills. Child-care workers should work in ways that will promote children's self-esteem so that they can feel good about themselves, develop independence and form positive relationships. This will have a positive effect on their health and well-being.

Child-care workers should provide children with positive role models. For example, children who see their carers smoke are more likely to go on to smoke themselves. Smoking should be positively discouraged in child-care settings.

The child-care environment should be safe. Both staff and children should be aware of safety issues at all times, and child-care workers should use all available opportunities to raise children's awareness and understanding of safety and keeping themselves safe.

Providing healthy choices at mealtimes and discussing food with children will enhance their understanding of the importance of a healthy diet and its influences on good health.

HEALTH-RELATED ACTIVITIES

Many activities can be offered to children to raise their awareness of and promote good health. They must be appropriate for the developmental stage of the child and be interesting and stimulating. They may also be successfully linked with children's learning in other areas of the curriculum.

Activities could include:

- *imaginative play* – setting up the imaginative play area as a health centre, dental surgery, hospital, shop, cafe
- *visits to places of interest* – to food shops, farms and gardens where vegetables and fruit are grown
- *visitors* – the **health visitor**, school nurse, road crossing patrol, dentist
- *daily routines* – hygiene routines, safety routines

key term

Health visitor
a trained nurse who specialises in child health promotion

- *books and stories* – books in child-care settings should present health issues positively; story and group time can be used for discussion
- *games* – board games created with a health aspect in mind
- *displays and interest tables* – displays can be created to convey particular health messages. Children's work can contribute to displays, for example, their writing, drawing and paintings about health topics
- *demonstrations* – of hand washing, hairbrushing, crossing the road safely.

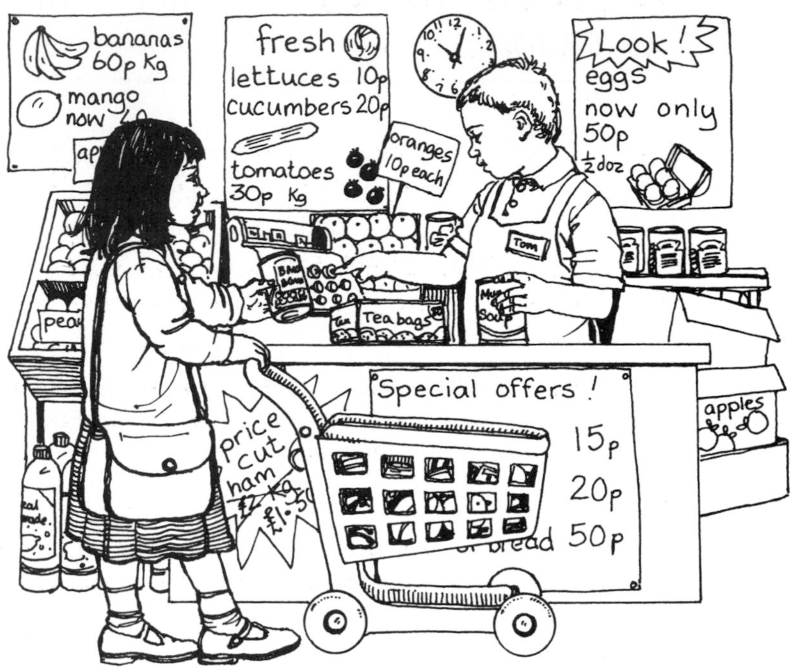

Activities such as this can be related to health promotion and to other areas of the curriculum (healthy eating, mathematics and communication, language and literacy)

Progress check

Define health.

List five activities related to health topics that would be suitable for each of the following age groups:

(a) 1–3 years *(b) 3–5 years* *(c) 5–7 years.*

Child health surveillance

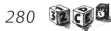

Child health surveillance is a system of reviewing a child's progress. These reviews are carried out at certain ages in the child's life. Programmes with regular reviews at fixed ages safeguard children from slipping through the net, especially when families move home frequently and change doctors and health visitors. In many areas of the UK the child health record is held by the main carer of the child in the form of a book. This book, the child health record, has spaces that can be filled in by the parent or carer and other people who care for the child. These may be:

- health visitors
- family doctors
- child health clinic staff
- hospital emergency department staff
- hospital outpatient staff
- school health team
- dentists.

In this way information can be shared and is easily available to all those caring for the child. Parents or carers have an ongoing record to which they can refer.

PRINCIPLES OF CHILD HEALTH SURVEILLANCE

There are certain principles that underpin the effective use of a child health surveillance programme. Child health surveillance should be:

- carried out in partnership with the parents or carers – they are the experts and the best people to identify health, developmental and behavioural problems in their own children
- a positive experience for parents or carers
- a learning experience for the parents or carers, the child and the health professional – it should involve exchanging information
- an opportunity to provide guidance on child health topics and health promotion
- a continuous and flexible process – as well as fixed assessments there should be opportunities for other reviews as required by each child
- carried out by observation and talking with the parents or carers – tests and examinations should complement the process
- based on good communication and teamwork.

The professionals involved

Most child health surveillance is carried out in the child's own home or at the child health clinic. Clinics are held in health centres, GPs' premises or in other convenient places, like church halls. The professionals most concerned with child health surveillance are health visitors and doctors. Health visitors are trained nurses who have undertaken further training in midwifery and health visiting. The doctors have a special interest in child health and could be the child's GP. Each of these professionals is responsible for part of the child health surveillance programme; they work as a team with the parents or carers. The general practitioner and the health visitor are part of the **primary health-care team** and are involved with **primary health care.**

key terms

Primary health-care team
a group of professionals who are concerned with the delivery of first-line health care and health promotion

Primary health care
first-line health care and health promotion

THE CHILD HEALTH SURVEILLANCE PROGRAMME

Assessment of the developmental progress of the child and discussion about relevant health promotion topics are part of each review.

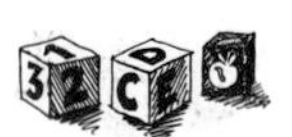

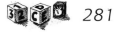

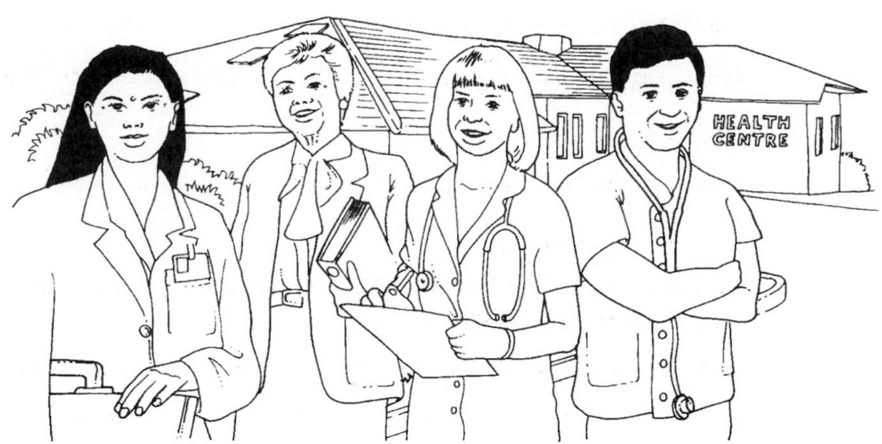

The primary health-care team

Birth review

The birth review is normally carried out before discharge from hospital, or by the family doctor if the birth is at home. The birth review includes:

- measurements – weight and head circumference are recorded on a **percentile chart**
- Guthrie test to exclude phenylketonuria (see page 289)
- hip examination to detect any congenital dislocation or instability of the hip (see pages 289–90)
- general examination to exclude congenital conditions or acquired disease.

> **key term**
>
> **Percentile chart**
> Specially prepared charts that are used to record measurements of a child's progress in growth or development. There are percentile charts to measure weight, height, head circumference and development

Health promotion topics covered at this review include advice on feeding, safety and car transport.

10–14 days review

The 10–14 days review is usually carried out by the health visitor at the child's home and includes:

- review, with the parent or carer, of progress and development since the birth
- general examination
- hip examination repeat
- measurements – head circumference and weight are recorded on the percentile chart.

Health promotion topics covered at this review include immunisations, feeding, further health reviews and safety.

6-week review

The 6-week review is usually carried out by the doctor at the child health clinic and includes:

- review, with carer, of progress and development from 2 weeks
- physical examination
- measurements – weight and head circumference are recorded on the percentile chart

 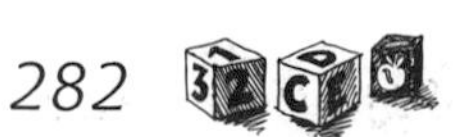

- hip examination repeat.

Health promotion topics covered at this review include feeding and safety.

3–4 months review

There is another hip examination for any signs of disability or instability.

6–9 months review

The review at 6–9 months is usually carried out by the health visitor at home or at the clinic and includes:

- review, with parent or carer, of progress and development from 6 weeks
- measurements – weight and head circumference are recorded on the percentile chart
- hip examination
- hearing test, using a distraction test (see pages 285–6)
- observation of visual behaviour
- check for **undescended testicles** – in males the testes, which are in the body before birth, should come down into the scrotum.

> **key term**
> **Undescended testicles**
> when the testes remain located in the body, instead of coming down into the scrotum

Health promotion topics covered at this review include safety, use of fireguards, stairgates, car seats and the dangers of glass doors.

18–24 months review

The review at 18–24 months includes:

- review, with parent or carer, of development and progress from 9 months
- measurements – weight is recorded on the percentile chart
- language development is checked (see Chapter 10)
- vision test.

Health promotion topics covered at this review include accident prevention, water safety (for example, ponds), safe storage of medicines and other dangerous fluids, and kitchen safety.

Heart check

Between 1 and 3 years, all children should have a heart check by the doctor.

Testicular examination

Between 1 and 3 years all males should have their testes checked again, to make sure both of them have come down into the scrotum.

3 years to 3 years 6 months review

The review at 3 years includes:

- review of progress and development with parent or carer, especially of language development
- measurements – height is recorded on the percentile chart.

Health promotion topics covered at this review include road and car safety. At this stage the doctor and health visitor will review the records with the parents or carers and discuss the need for further regular reviews.

School entry review

The school entry review is undertaken by the school nurse and doctor. The review involves:

- review, with parent or carer, of progress and development
- measurement of height and weight
- vision test
- hearing test
- immunisation booster (for more on the immunisation programme see Chapter 16).

Health promotion topics covered at this review include road safety and 'stranger danger'.

8 years appraisal

This appraisal is carried out by the school nurse and involves:

- review of progress and development
- measurement of height and weight
- vision test.

Health promotion topics covered at this review include road safety, 'stranger danger', dental health, diet and exercise.

Progress check

Who writes in the child health record?

Who are the best people to identify health and developmental problems?

How are reviews carried out?

Which professionals are most involved in child health surveillance?

What measurements are recorded in the first year?

Where are the measurements recorded?

What is the starting point of each review?

What does the hip examination detect?

What is the testicular examination for?

When should all children have a heart check?

Screening for hearing impairment

Parents or carers will often recognise that their child has a hearing loss. Child-care workers should listen carefully to these concerns and refer the child for further investigation. There are special tests that are done as part of the child health surveillance programme, but tests can, and should, be done at any time if a hearing problem is suspected. There is more information about deafness in Chapter 21.

NEONATAL SCREENING

Parents or carers will know whether their child is responding to sounds. Responses to loud sounds at this age include:

- stiffening
- blinking
- the Moro (startle) reflex (described in Chapter 11)
- crying.

key term

Neonate
a newborn baby

The baby may respond to quieter, prolonged sounds by becoming still and quiet. There are methods of testing the hearing of **neonates**, but these are not tests that are done routinely on every newborn baby. Tests include:

- auditory response cradle (ARC)
- otoacoustic emissions (OAE)
- brainstem evoked response audiometry (BSERA).

These are complex tests. They are usually used if there is some reason to suspect a hearing problem.

DISTRACTION TEST

key term

Distraction test
a hearing test carried out at about 7 months

key term

Localising
searching for and locating the source of a sound

The best age for screening hearing in the first year of life is at about 7 months old. All babies should have their hearing tested at this age. Developmentally, the baby must be able to sit and have good head control. The **distraction test** needs two people as well as the carer: one to observe and one to test.

The baby sits on the carer's lap facing the observer. The observer holds the baby's attention with a soundless toy. When the observer has engaged the baby's attention, the toy is withdrawn and the tester makes the stimulus sound at ear level. The baby should turn, search for and find the source of the sound. This is called **localising**. Both ears must be tested with a range of quiet sounds, both high-pitched and low-pitched.

Stimulus sounds include:

- rattles – there are specialised rattles, such as Manchester and Nuffield rattles
- voice – low-pitched sound such as *oo*, high-pitched sound such as *ss*, quiet conversation using the baby's name.

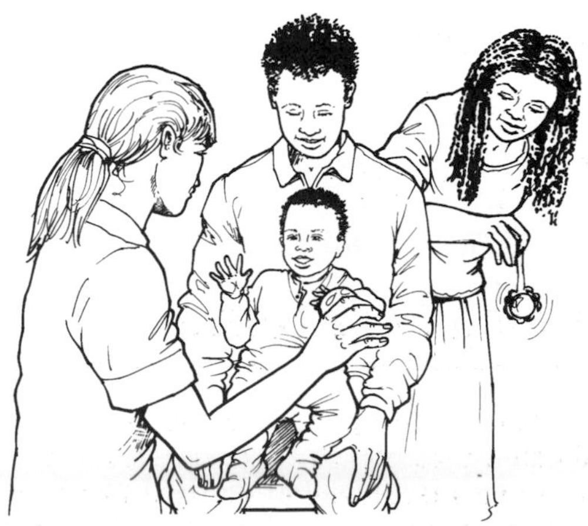

The sounds are made very quietly

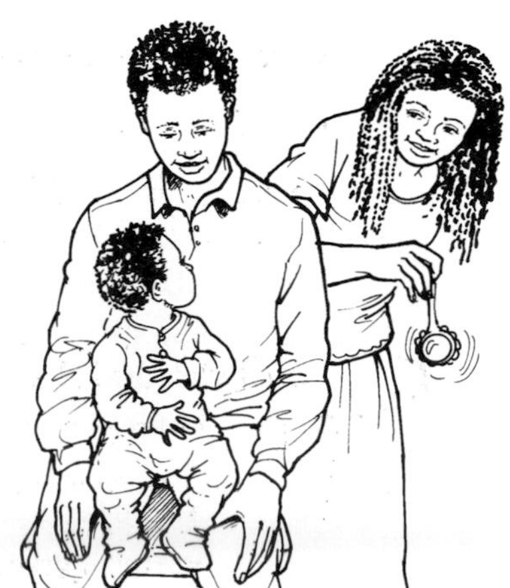

The baby locates the sound

A distraction hearing test

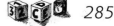

There are many reasons, such as illness or tiredness, why a baby might not respond to a hearing test. If the baby does not respond at all to the test, it is repeated after 2 to 4 weeks. Further failure to respond needs referral for a full audiological assessment.

TESTS FOR OLDER CHILDREN: 2–5 YEARS

As children develop, it becomes possible to use tests that need the child's co-operation. Examples of these are the Go game and the speech discrimination test.

Go game

In this game test, the child is asked to post a brick into a box when they hear the word 'Go'. An experienced tester can vary the pitch and sound level of the voice and each ear can be tested separately.

Speech discrimination test

This test is more difficult than the Go game and the child's co-operation and understanding are needed. The child is presented with a selection of toys. These toys are specially selected to test the child's ability to hear different consonants, for example *p*, *g*, *d*, hard *c*, *s*, *m*, *f*, *b*. After naming the toys in a normal voice with the tester, the child is asked in a quiet voice to identify each of the toys, for example 'Show me the duck'; 'Give the brick to Mummy'. Again, each ear is tested though the range.

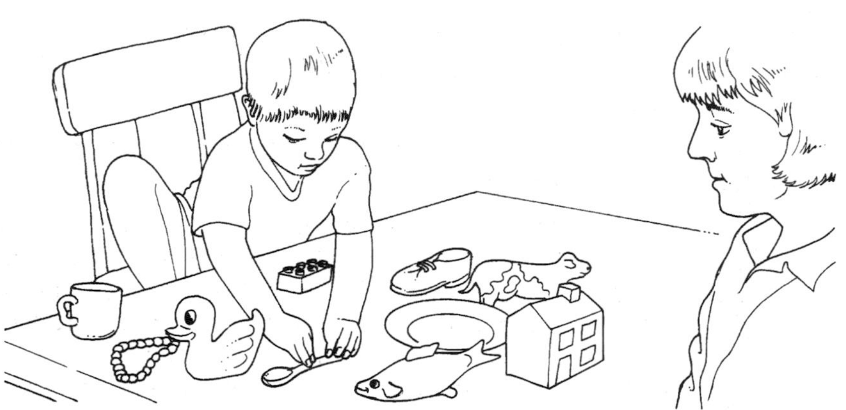

The speech discrimination test

PURE TONE AUDIOMETRY (FROM 5 YEARS)

For pure tone **audiometry**, the child puts on earphones and listens for the tone produced by the audiometer. The tones are given at different pitch and intensity. Each ear is tested separately. This is a lengthy and complicated test.

Sweep audiometry

Sweep audiometry is a less complicated method of pure tone audiometry, where a range of selected frequencies is tested. This test is usually performed at around the time of school entry.

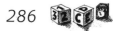

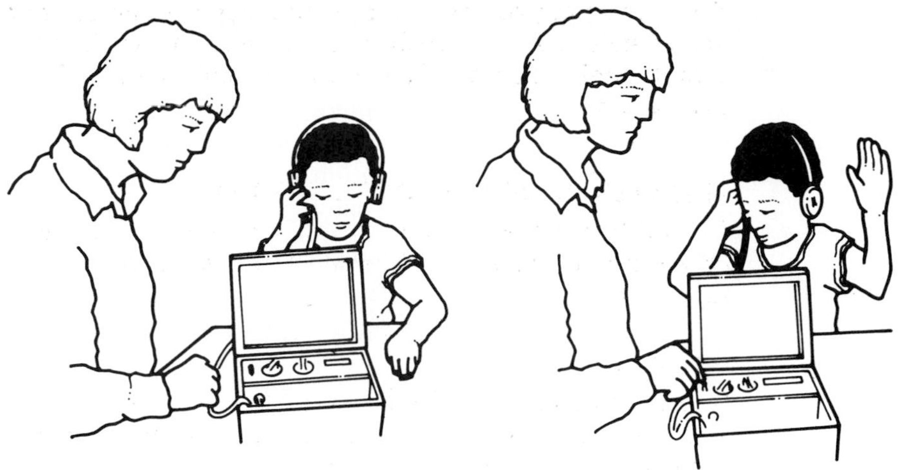

Audiometry using an audiometer to measure hearing

Progress check

What is the best age to test a child's hearing using a distraction test?

Name two other tests that can be used to test hearing.

What does localising a sound mean?

What sort of sounds are used to test hearing?

Why is it important to have two people involved in the distraction hearing test?

Case study . . .

. . . a hearing test

Jade is 8 months old and has come to the health centre with Dulcie, her mother, for her routine hearing test. Ruth, her health visitor, talks to Dulcie about Jade's development and Dulcie tells her that Jade is vocalising and making sounds with two syllables. Ruth observes Jade and notes that she is sitting up unsupported and has good head control. Jade sits on her mother's knee and faces Colin, another health visitor, who is helping Ruth with the tests. Colin plays with Jade for a while and keeps her attention. Meanwhile, Ruth makes a very quiet sound, level with Jade's ear and about 1m away. Jade immediately turns to find the sound, sees Ruth and smiles broadly. Ruth praises her and then encourages her to return her attention to Colin. Ruth continues the test in this way using different sounds including high-pitched and low-pitched sounds. Jade quickly responds to all the sounds, Ruth is satisfied with the test and she tells Dulcie that Jade is hearing normally.

1. *Between what ages is it best to test the hearing of a baby under 1 year?*
2. *Why did Ruth check with Jade's mother about her development?*
3. *Why are two people needed for the hearing test?*
4. *Why did Ruth wait for Jade to turn to the sounds?*
5. *What is the term used to describe this?*
6. *If the test had not been conclusive what would Ruth's action have been?*

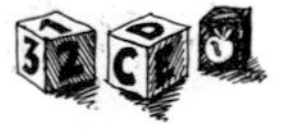

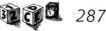

Screening for visual impairment

In many instances, visual defects are first detected by parents or carers. The child-care worker should be sure to listen carefully to any concerns expressed and refer the child for further investigation to the GP or health clinic. Some of the general signs that will indicate that a baby's vision is developing normally are as follows:

- *At birth*, the baby will look briefly at the mother's face.
- *At 1 month*, the baby will watch the carer's face intently while being fed and follow the carer's face as it moves from side to side.
- *At 3 months*, the baby will follow a dangling toy held in front of his face; he starts to look at his own fingers.
- *At 6 months*, the baby can see across a room and can see small objects like a Smartie.
- *At 9 months*, the baby can recognise toys across a room and see small crumbs on the floor and try to pick them up.

If a child does not seem to be doing these things, it is important that further tests on vision are carried out.

In addition to general observation of the child's progress, there are routine checks on children's vision that are part of the child health surveillance programme:

- *At birth and 6 weeks*, the doctor will examine the eyes for any signs of abnormality, in particular any evidence of cataract, a condition where the lens of the eye is not transparent.
- *Between 6 weeks and 6 months*, the doctor and health visitor will look for any sign of a squint, a condition where the eyes do not work together properly and the baby seems not to look straight at you. There are special tests used to identify a squint: the corneal reflection test and the cover test.
- *Between 2 and 5 years* – by this age children are able to co-operate with vision testing. Distance vision can be assessed using single letters with a letter matching chart. The child looks at the letter being held up by the tester, then points to the matching letter on her chart. Older children will be able to name the letters. Each eye must be tested separately from a distance of 3 m.

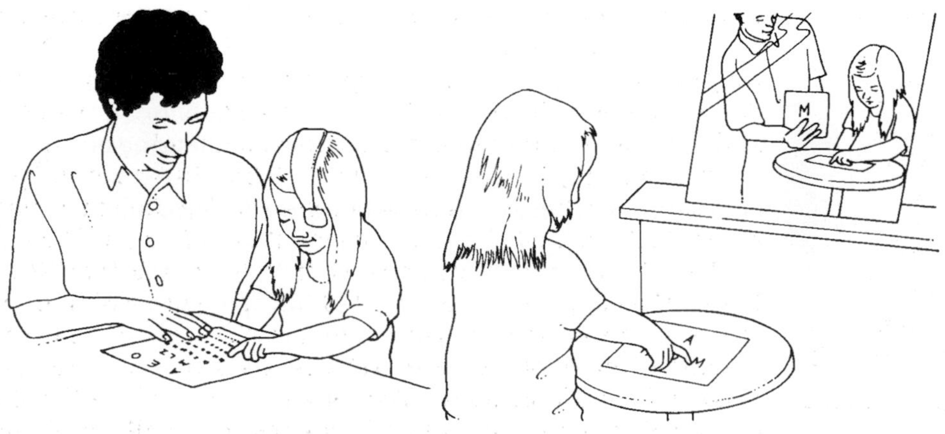

Vision testing, for close and distance vision

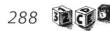

- *Pre-school* – routine screening of vision is usually carried out at school entry and at 3-yearly intervals.
- *Colour vision defects* – screening for colour vision impairment is usually recommended at the beginning of secondary school.

Progress check

What are the general signs that vision is developing normally at:

(a) birth? (b) 3 months? (c) 9 months?

What might lead you to suspect that a baby of 6 weeks was not able to see?

Guthrie test

The Guthrie test is a screening test to detect phenylketonuria (PKU is an inherited condition affecting the baby's ability to metabolise part of protein foods). Other conditions such as hypothyroidism (a condition in which the thyroid gland is not working properly) and cystic fibrosis (an inherited condition) may also be detected. The test is carried out when the baby is about 6 days old and has been taking milk feeds for several days. Blood is collected from a heel prick to cover four circles on a specially prepared card that is then sent to the laboratory. Early treatment of PKU gives the child a good chance of developing normally.

Progress check

When is the Guthrie test carried out?

What feeds must the baby have had before the test can be done?

What does the Guthrie test detect?

Hip test

key terms

Congenital
a disease or disorder that occurs during pregnancy and is present at birth

Femur
the long bone in the thigh

Pelvis
the bones that make up the hip girdle

CONGENITAL DISLOCATION OF THE HIP

Congenital means occurring at birth. The hip joint consists of the head of the **femur** (the long bone in the thigh) and the socket in the **pelvis** (hip girdle). In **congenital dislocation of the hip**, the hip joint is unstable because of failure to develop properly before birth; this may be associated with the position of the fetus in the uterus, but there may also be a genetic link.

When the hip is dislocated or unstable, the head of the femur may become displaced from the socket in the pelvis. One leg then appears to be shorter than the other. If left untreated the development of walking will be affected.

The baby's hips are tested soon after birth and then at regular intervals up to 1 year. The baby's legs are abducted (turned outwards) and the typical 'click' can be felt as the dislocated head of the femur slips back into the socket.

The treatment takes place in stages and is aimed at preventing dislocation and at making the hip joint stable. The baby's legs are held in the abducted position by the use of splints or a 'frog plaster'. Progress is usually good and normal walking can usually be achieved.

key term

Congenital disorders of the hip
the hip joint is unstable or dislocated because it fails to develop properly before birth

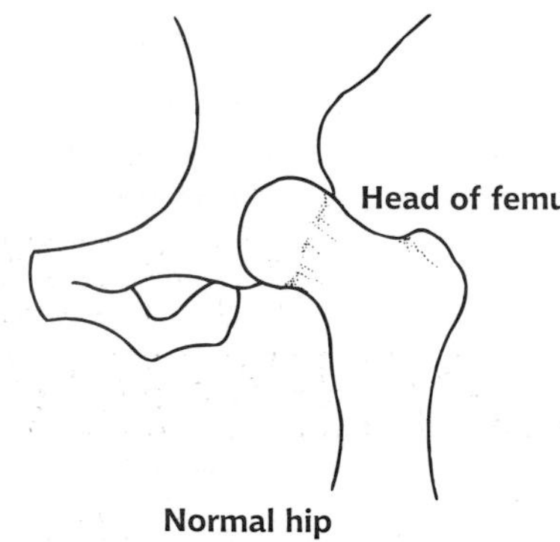

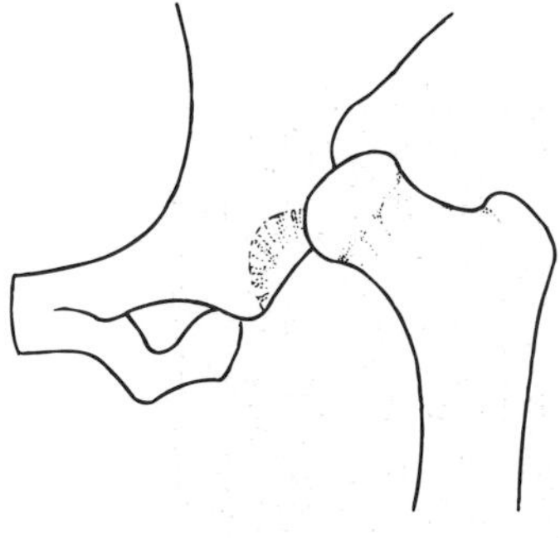

Congenital dislocation of the hip

Progress check

When is the hip test carried out?

Which bones are involved in the hip test?

Now try these questions

What factors may influence people's individual health choices?

Why is it important for parents and carers to be informed about health issues?

Why is it important to detect any hearing loss that a child might have as early as possible?

Why is health promotion an important part of the role of the child-care worker?

What is the contribution of the health surveillance programme to the ongoing health of the child?

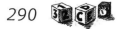

key terms

You need to know what the key terms and phrases in this chapter mean.
Go back through the chapter and find out.

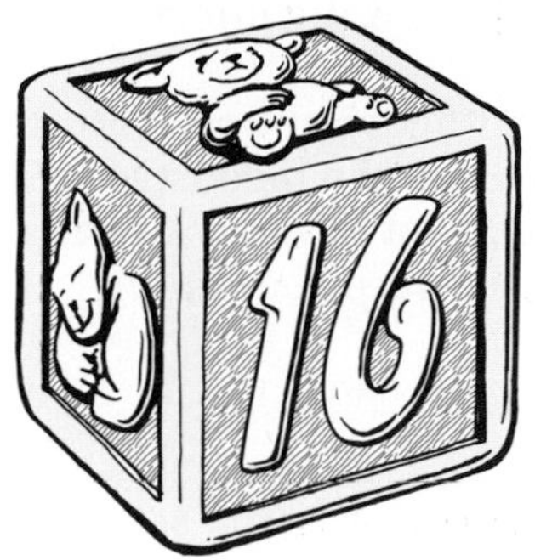

CAUSES AND PREVENTION OF ILL HEALTH

Children have illnesses and infections that are passed very easily from one child to another. Understanding how diseases are spread will help child-care workers to prevent children from becoming infected and from passing that infection on to others. Many children will develop their own natural immunity, but they will also benefit from a programme of immunisation.

This chapter will cover the following topics:

- *disease transmission*
- *immunity*
- *genetics*
- *immunisation.*

Disease transmission

Disease is a condition that arises when something goes wrong with the normal working of the body. As a result the child becomes ill. Signs that a child is ill and has a disease include:

- raised temperature (38°C or above)
- headache
- sore throat
- rashes on the skin
- diarrhoea.

Other possible signs of illness are a lot of crying, being irritable and behaviour that is unusual. Possible signs of illness are always more worrying and significant in a baby or very young child.

Organisms that cause disease are called **pathogens**. The most important pathogens are bacteria, viruses and some fungi. The everyday name for pathogens is *germs*. Pathogens get into the body mainly through the mouth and nose, and sometimes through cuts on the skin. Once they are inside the body, they multiply very rapidly. This is called the **incubation period** and can last for days or weeks,

key terms

Pathogens
germs such as bacteria and viruses

Incubation period
The time from when pathogens enter the body until the first signs of infection appear

depending on the type of pathogen. Although the person is infected during the incubation period, they only begin to feel ill and have signs of the infection towards the end of the incubation period.

Pathogens work in different ways when they infect the body. Some attack and destroy body cells; others produce poisonous substances in the bloodstream called **toxins**. The intense activity of the pathogens produces a lot of heat, so one of the signs of infection by pathogens is that the child's temperature goes up.

key term

Toxin
a poisonous substance produced by pathogens

HOW DISEASES SPREAD

Diseases are spread by:

- droplets of moisture in the air
- touch
- food and water
- animals
- cuts and scratches.

Droplets in the air

When you cough, sneeze, talk and sing, tiny droplets of moisture come out of your nose or mouth. If you have a disease, these droplets will be swarming with pathogens. If these infected droplets are breathed in by another person, the disease can be spread to them. Colds (caused by viruses) spread rapidly in this way.

Touch

It is possible to catch some infectious diseases by touching an infected person, or by touching towels or other things used by that person. The skin disease impetigo (caused by bacteria) is spread in this way. Another skin disease, athlete's foot (caused by a fungus), can be picked up from the floors of public changing rooms and showers.

Food and water

The urine and faeces of an infected person will contain pathogens. Drinking water may be contaminated if sewage gets into it. Food and drinks can be contaminated if they are prepared or handled by a person with dirty hands, or if the food preparation area is dirty. This is why washing hands after visiting the lavatory and before handling food is so important. Food poisoning (caused by bacteria) easily spreads in this way, especially in places where lots of children play and eat together, such as nurseries. For more information on food handling, see Chapter 7.

Animals

Pathogens are brought on to food by animals like flies, rats, mice and cockroaches. Animals that suck blood spread other diseases; an example of this is malaria, which is spread by mosquitoes.

Cuts and scratches

Pathogens can enter the body through a cut or other injuries to the skin. Examples of these are the tetanus bacteria and the hepatitis virus.

Progress check

What are the signs of disease?

What are pathogens?

Give some examples of pathogens.

Explain briefly the different ways that diseases are spread.

What are toxins?

Immunity

key terms

Antibody
a substance made by white cells to attack pathogens

Phagocytosis
the process by which white cells absorb pathogens and destroy them

When pathogens do enter, the body does not just sit back and let the pathogens take over. White blood cells work to try to destroy the invading bacteria or viruses. The white cells identify the invading pathogens as a foreign substance and begin to make **antibodies**. Antibodies make the pathogens clump together so that the white cells can destroy them by absorbing them – this process is called **phagocytosis**.

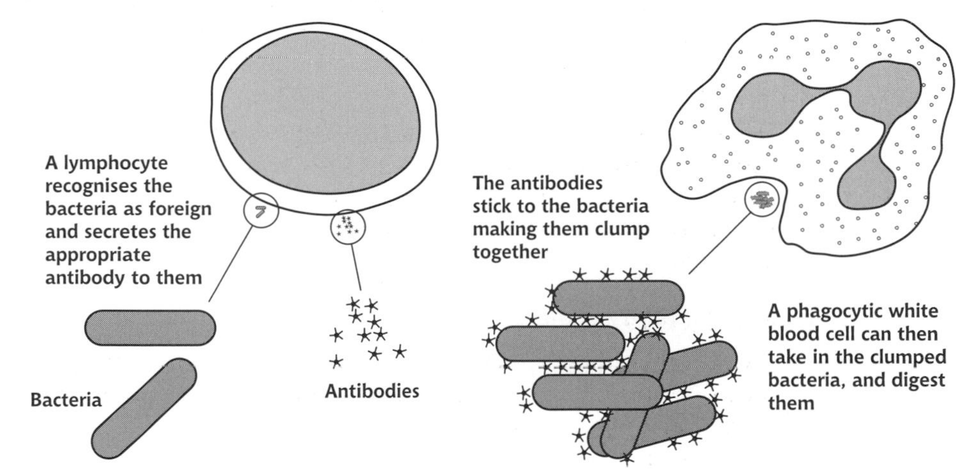
A lymphocyte recognises the bacteria as foreign and secretes the appropriate antibody to them
Bacteria
Antibodies
The antibodies stick to the bacteria making them clump together
A phagocytic white blood cell can then take in the clumped bacteria, and digest them

Phagocytosis: how white cells destroy bacteria

key term

Immunity
the presence of antibodies that protect the body against infectious disease

It will take some time for the white cells to make enough antibodies. This may give the pathogen enough time to multiply so that the child shows signs of having the disease. Eventually, however, the white cells make enough antibodies to destroy the pathogens and the child recovers from the illness. If the same pathogen attacks again some time later, the white cells recognise it and can quickly make large quantities of antibody so that the pathogen is destroyed before it has a chance to multiply – **immunity** has been created; the child is now immune to that pathogen and the disease it causes.

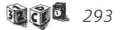

ACTIVE IMMUNITY

Having a disease and recovering from it is one way of becoming immune to it. This is called **active immunity**, because the white cells make the antibodies against the pathogens causing the disease. Active immunity is also acquired by having an immunisation with a **vaccine**. Vaccines contain killed or weakened forms of the pathogens that cause the particular disease. The BCG vaccine for tuberculosis, for example, contains bacteria that have been weakened. When they are injected into the body, they are too weak to multiply, but the white cells can identify them as foreign cells and begin to make antibodies to overcome them. Immunity to the disease is then acquired because the body has learnt to recognise that pathogen and can make the antibody required to combat it.

key terms

Active immunity
the body's ability to resist a disease that has been acquired by having the disease or by having a specific immunisation

Vaccine
a preparation used to stimulate the production of antibodies and provide immunity against one or several diseases

PASSIVE IMMUNITY

Another type of immunity is called **passive immunity,** where the antibody is put into the body ready-made. Passive immunisation can be given by injecting a serum that contains antibodies into the body, but this is not done very often. The most common example of passive immunity is when breast-fed babies acquire immunity to diseases because there are antibodies in breast milk that are passed to the baby from the mother. Passive immunity does not last indefinitely, because the antibodies gradually disappear from the blood. Active immunity lasts much longer because the white cells have learnt to make the antibody and can do this if the pathogen enters the body on future occasions.

Progress check

What is an antibody?

Which cells in the body destroy pathogens?

What is phagocytosis?

How is active immunity acquired?

How is passive immunity acquired?

Genetics

Some illnesses and conditions are inherited and are carried by the chromosomes and genes.

key term

Passive immunity
the body's ability to resist a disease, acquired from antibodies given directly into the body, for example the antibodies passed on in breast milk

RECESSIVE INHERITANCE

This is where both parents carry a defective gene for a particular condition or illness, e.g. cystic fibrosis or sickle cell disease. There is a one-in-four chance of the disorder being passed on with each pregnancy.

DOMINANT INHERITANCE

This is where one parent carries a dominant gene for a particular condition, e.g. Huntington's chorea. There is a one-in-two chance of this being passed on with each pregnancy.

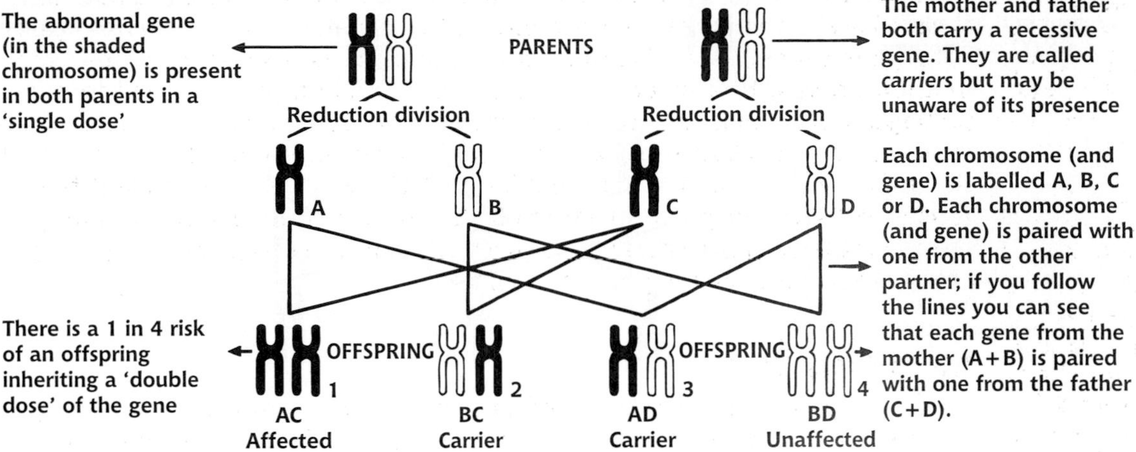
The abnormal gene (in the shaded chromosome) is present in both parents in a 'single dose'
PARENTS
The mother and father both carry a recessive gene. They are called carriers but may be unaware of its presence
Reduction division
Reduction division
A
B
C
D
Each chromosome (and gene) is labelled A, B, C or D. Each chromosome (and gene) is paired with one from the other partner; if you follow the lines you can see that each gene from the mother (A+B) is paired with one from the father (C+D).
There is a 1 in 4 risk of an offspring inheriting a 'double dose' of the gene
OFFSPRING
OFFSPRING
1
2
3
4
AC
Affected
BC
Carrier
AD
Carrier
BD
Unaffected

Recessive inheritance

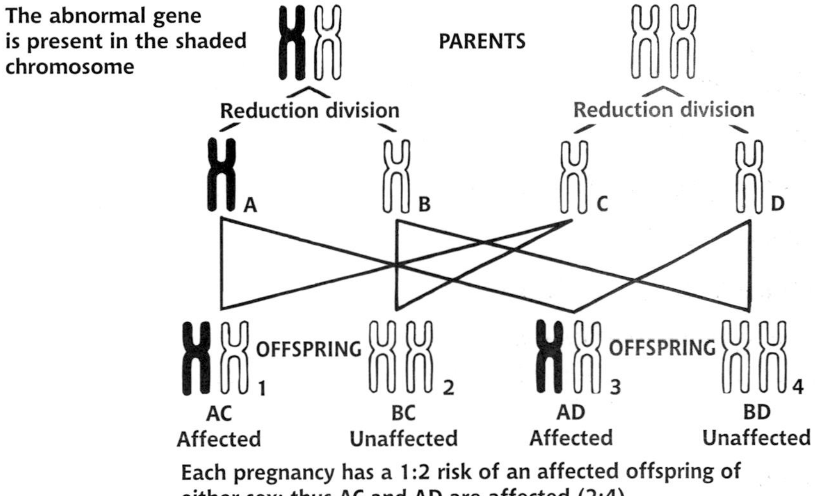
The abnormal gene is present in the shaded chromosome
PARENTS
Reduction division
Reduction division
A
B
C
D
OFFSPRING
OFFSPRING
1
2
3
4
AC
Affected
BC
Unaffected
AD
Affected
BD
Unaffected
Each pregnancy has a 1:2 risk of an affected offspring of either sex; thus AC and AD are affected (2:4)

Dominant inheritance

SEX-LINKED INHERITANCE

Sex-linked or X-linked conditions are passed from mothers to their sons, e.g. haemophilia and Duchenne muscular dystrophy. With each pregnancy, mothers who carry an affected gene on their X chromosome have a one-in-two chance of each boy being affected and a one-in-two chance of each girl being a carrier.

CHROMOSOMAL ABNORMALITIES

Conditions that result from defects in the chromosomes have a characteristic pattern. Down syndrome is a well-known chromosomal abnormality.

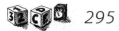

FEMALE

MALE

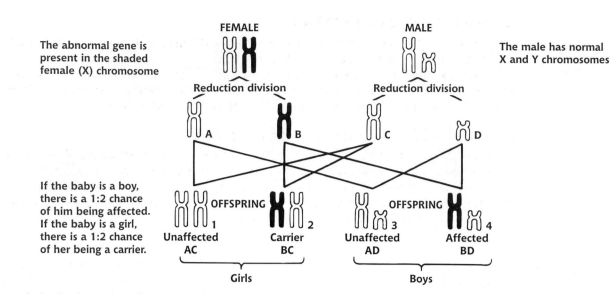

The abnormal gene is present in the shaded female (X) chromosome

The male has normal X and Y chromosomes

Reduction division

Reduction division

A B C D

If the baby is a boy, there is a 1:2 chance of him being affected. If the baby is a girl, there is a 1:2 chance of her being a carrier.

OFFSPRING

OFFSPRING

1 Unaffected AC

2 Carrier BC

3 Unaffected AD

4 Affected BD

Girls

Boys

Sex-linked inheritance: female parent carrier

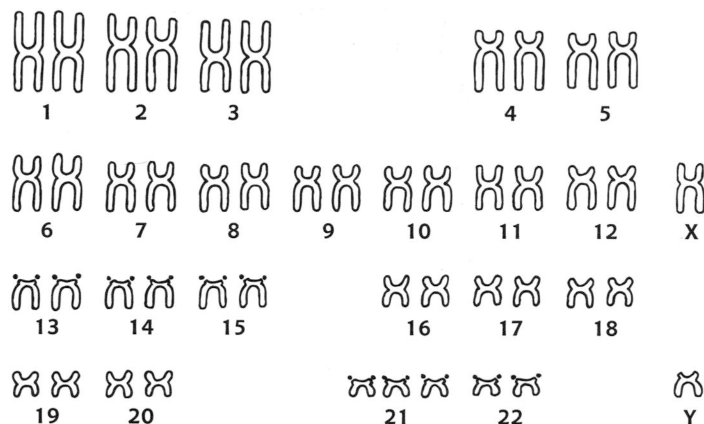

The chromosome pattern of a male infant with Down syndrome. Note the presence of the extra number 21 chromosome, Trisomy 21.

The chromosome pattern of a male infant with Down syndrome

Immunisation

key term

Booster

an additional dose of a vaccine, given after the initial dose

Immunisation is the use of vaccine to protect people from disease. Vaccines used in immunisations contain either small parts of the viruses or bacteria that cause the disease, or very small amounts of the chemicals (toxins) they produce. These have been treated to make sure that they do not cause the disease, but are still capable of stimulating the body to make antibodies. In this way, the body will be able to defend itself against future infections. Vaccines provide most children with effective and long-lasting protection. Some immunisations need topping up and **boosters** may be needed as the child gets older.

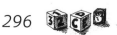

THE IMMUNISATION PROGRAMME

Immunisation protects children from serious diseases. It also protects other children by preventing diseases being passed on.

Advice and guidance on immunisation is part of the programme of child health promotion. Doctors and health visitors will advise parents or carers about immunisations and discuss any worries they may have about their child.

The booster MMR (measles, mumps and rubella)

Since October 1996 all children having their pre-school booster against diphtheria, tetanus and polio are also offered a booster dose of measles, mumps and rubella. A booster is needed because around 5 to 10 per cent of children remain unprotected after their first MMR immunisation. A second dose will offer protection to those children and boost the immunity of the others.

The immunisation programme

Age	Vaccine	Method
2 months	Hib (haemophilus influenzae type b meningitis) Diphtheria, tetanus, pertussis (whooping cough) (DTP) Polio	1 injection 1 injection By mouth
3 months	Hib DTP Polio	1 injection 1 injection By mouth
4 months	Hib DTP Polio	1 injection 1 injection By mouth
12–15 months	Measles, mumps and rubella (MMR)	1 injection
3–5 years (school entry)	Diphtheria, tetanus MMR Polio	1 injection 1 injection By mouth
Girls 10–14 years	Rubella	If not previously given at 12–15 months 1 injection
Girls/boys 10–14 years (sometimes shortly after birth)	Tuberculosis	1 injection (BCG)
School leavers 15–19 years	Diphtheria, tetanus Polio	1 injection Booster by mouth

SIDE-EFFECTS AFTER IMMUNISATION

After immunisation some children may be unwell, have a fever or be irritable for a while. Sometimes the skin becomes red and swollen around the place where the injection was given, or a small lump appears. If the child does develop a fever after being immunised, keep them cool and give plenty to drink. The doctor or health visitor may advise a dose of paracetamol syrup, but always check first to make sure the right dose is given. Any red or swollen area around the injection site should gradually disappear. If there are any other worrying symptoms such as a high temperature or a convulsion, consult the doctor immediately.

Side-effects of the DTP triple immunisation

Side-effects after having the DTP (diphtheria, tetanus, pertussis – whooping cough) immunisation are mild. The baby may become miserable, fretful and slightly feverish in the 24 hours after the injection. Some children may have a convulsion (fit) after the DTP immunisation. It is the whooping cough part of the triple vaccine that often worries parents and carers. There have been questions about the safety of the vaccine and the possibility of brain damage. New research has not found a link between the vaccine and permanent brain damage.

Side-effects of the Hib (haemophilus type b) immunisation

About one baby in ten will have some redness or swelling at the site of the injection. The swelling goes down very quickly and has usually disappeared after a day or so.

Side-effects of the MMR (measles, mumps and rubella) immunisation

Some children develop a mild fever and a rash about 7 to 10 days after the immunisation. This usually lasts for a day or two. A few children get a mild form of mumps about 3 weeks after their immunisation. These are all mild symptoms and are not infectious to other children or pregnant women. A few children may have more serious reactions such as a convulsion or encephalitis (inflammation of the brain), but this is very rare. Recently, the MMR vaccine has been linked to incidences of autism and bowel disorders in children, but research has *not* found conclusive evidence to support this.

Side-effects of the polio immunisation

The polio vaccine is a live virus given by mouth. The virus is passed through the digestive tract and into a dirty nappy. It is very important, therefore, for care workers to wash their hands carefully after changing nappies to avoid becoming infected. Child-care workers need to check that their own polio immunisation is up to date.

CHILD-CARE WORKERS AND IMMUNISATION

Immunisation protects children from serious diseases. It also protects other children by preventing diseases being passed on.

Child-care workers will benefit from keeping their own immunisations up to date. Immunisations requiring boosters are polio and tetanus. Child-care workers could also be protected against hepatitis.

Progress check

Give two reasons why it is important for children to be immunised.

Describe the most common mild reactions to an immunisation.

Describe the more serious side-effects.

Which vaccine is given by mouth?

If a baby has had the polio vaccine, what special precautions should the carer take?

What is contained in the triple vaccine?

Now try these questions

In what different ways are diseases spread?

Describe how immunity is acquired. What are the different types of immunity?

Why is it important for children to be immunised?

key terms

You need to know what the key terms and phrases in this chapter mean. Go back through the chapter and find out.

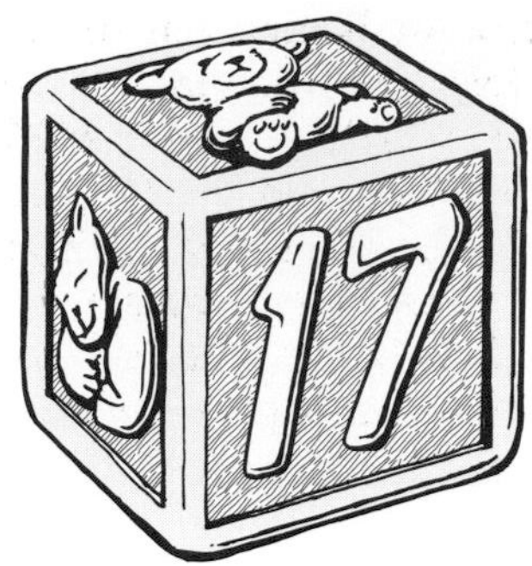

RESPONSES TO CHILDHOOD ILLNESSES

Childhood illnesses can be passed very easily from one child to another. Some illnesses are more common and are experienced by many children, when they will need loving care and some simple treatments. Other, more serious illnesses will require prompt action and referral on the part of the carer.

This chapter will cover the following topics:

- common childhood illnesses
- infectious diseases
- infestations.

Common childhood illnesses

COLDS

Viruses cause colds, and children get many colds because there are many different cold viruses and young children are infected with each virus for the first time. As they grow up they build up immunity, so they get fewer colds. Viruses, not bacteria, cause colds, so antibiotics will not help. There are things you can do to help the child breathe more easily: keep the nose clear and use a menthol rub or decongestant capsule, especially at night. Make sure the child has plenty to drink, and give light, easily swallowed food. Don't fuss if a child does not want to eat for a while, just give plenty to drink.

COUGHS

A virus causes most coughs, like colds. If a cough persists or the chest sounds congested, a doctor should be consulted. Most coughs are the body's way of clearing mucus from the back of the throat, or from the air passages in the lungs. The cough, therefore, serves a useful purpose and should be soothed rather than stopped. Honey and orange or lemon in warm water or a bought cough mixture will help. If you use a bought cough mixture, check that it is suitable for the age of the child and stick to the recommended dose. Do not combine cough mixtures with other medicines, such as paracetamol, without advice from a doctor.

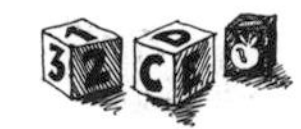

key term

Stools
faeces, the product of digested food

DIARRHOEA

Young babies' **stools** are normally soft and yellow, and some babies will soil nearly every nappy. If you notice the stools becoming very watery and frequent, with other signs of illness, consult the doctor. Young babies who get diarrhoea can lose a lot of fluid very quickly, especially if they are vomiting as well. This can be very serious. Call the doctor and, in the meantime, give as much cooled, boiled water as you can. Use a teaspoon if the baby is reluctant to suck and try to give some water every few minutes. Diarrhoea in older children is not so worrying, but maintain the fluid intake. If the diarrhoea persists for more than 2 or 3 days, consult the doctor.

EAR INFECTIONS

Ear infections often follow a cold. The child may be generally unwell, pull or rub the ears or there may be a discharge from the ear. There may be a raised temperature. The child may complain of pain, but small babies will just cry and seem unwell or uncomfortable. If you suspect an ear infection, it is important that it is treated promptly by the doctor to prevent any permanent damage to the hearing. Ear infections, especially of the middle ear (**otitis media**), are quite common. These infections will often temporarily affect the hearing of a child and this can then affect their ability to participate at nursery and school. Repeated infections of the middle ear where infected material builds up in the middle ear (sometimes called **glue ear**) can result in long-term problems with hearing.

key terms

Otitis media
an infection of the middle ear

Glue ear
where infected material builds up in the middle ear, following repeated ear infections

SORE THROAT

Like colds, sore throats are caused by viruses. The throat may be dry and sore a day or so before the cold starts. Sometimes a sore throat is caused by tonsillitis, and the throat is red and sore with white patches on the tonsils, which are enlarged. The child may find it hard to swallow and have a raised temperature with swollen glands under the jaw. If there is a raised temperature, consult the doctor who may suggest giving paracetamol. Meanwhile, give plenty of clear drinks, soft food to eat and keep the child warm and comfortable.

key term

Bronchitis
a chest infection caused by infection of the main airways

BRONCHITIS

Infection and inflammation of the main airways cause **bronchitis** (chest infection). The child will have a persistent chesty cough and may cough up green or yellow phlegm. There may be noisy breathing, a raised temperature and the child feels very unwell. Consult the doctor as soon as possible, who may give antibiotics. Meanwhile, allow the child to rest quietly. Sitting well propped up will help breathing. Give paracetamol to reduce the temperature and plenty of warm soothing drinks such as honey and lemon. It may help to moisten the atmosphere by putting a damp towel on a warm radiator. This could help to loosen phlegm in the airways so that coughing becomes easier. Some children are prone to repeated attacks of bronchitis.

TEMPERATURES

As we saw in Chapter 16, a raised temperature of 38°C or above, is a sign that pathogens have entered the body and are multiplying. Children, especially babies, can develop high temperatures very quickly. If a baby has a raised temperature and/or other signs of illness, always consult the doctor as soon as possible. With older children, contact the doctor if the temperature remains high or if the child has other signs of illness. It is important to bring the temperature down to avoid any complications. Do not wrap a baby up; take off a layer of clothing. Let older children wear light clothes. Keep the room cool and fan the child if possible. Give plenty of cool drinks, little and often. Give paracetamol to help lower the temperature, but consult the doctor first if the baby is less than 3 months old.

key term

Febrile convulsions a fit or seizure that occurs as a result of a raised body temperature

FEBRILE CONVULSIONS

Febrile convulsions are dealt with in more detail in Chapter 19. Briefly the signs to look out for are:

- loss of consciousness
- stiffness of the body
- twitching movements of the body
- the eyes may roll back
- child may wet or soil themselves.

It is important to act effectively and quickly:

- Stay with the child and protect them from injury or falling.
- Get medical aid.
- Put the child in the recovery position when the convulsions have stopped.
- When the child regains consciousness, continue to try to reduce the temperature.

THRUSH

Thrush is a fungal infection that forms white patches in the mouth, usually on the tongue and the inside of the cheeks and lips. If you try to rub off the fungus, it leaves a red sore patch. A baby may also have a sore bottom because the thrush has infected the skin in the nappy area. Consult the doctor who will give the specific anti-fungal treatment to clear up the infection. Thrush is often spread from one child to another because feeding equipment is not properly sterilised and handled. It can also be passed on from an infected adult. It is very important that all feeding equipment is thoroughly cleaned and properly sterilised before use. Effective hygiene practices in kitchens where feeds are prepared and good personal hygiene routines by child-care workers will prevent the spread of thrush.

VOMITING

All babies will bring up some milk from time to time. If the baby is vomiting often or violently and/or there are other signs of illness, contact the doctor. Babies can lose a lot of fluid if they vomit frequently. Maintain the fluid intake, but stop giving milk and give clear fluids as often as possible. Oral rehydration fluids may also be given and may be advised by a doctor.

Progress check

List all the signs you can think of that would indicate that a child has an infection.

Why is it important to act quickly if a baby has diarrhoea?

Why do children get repeated colds?

What does a raised temperature indicate?

How is thrush spread?

Infectious diseases

The table on pages 304–306 lists some of the diseases child-care workers are likely to meet. Note: Rashes look different on different people. The colour of the spots may vary and on black skin rashes can be less easy to see. If you are doubtful, check with the doctor, especially if the child is showing other signs of illness. Some infectious diseases can be prevented by immunisation.

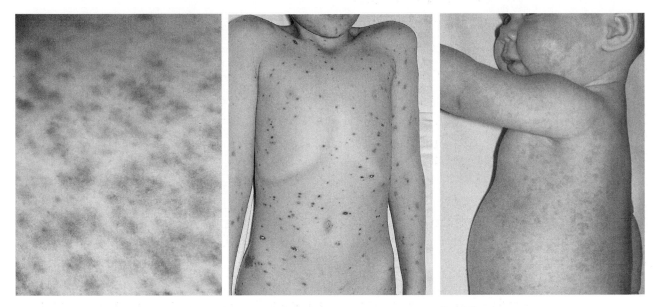

Measles

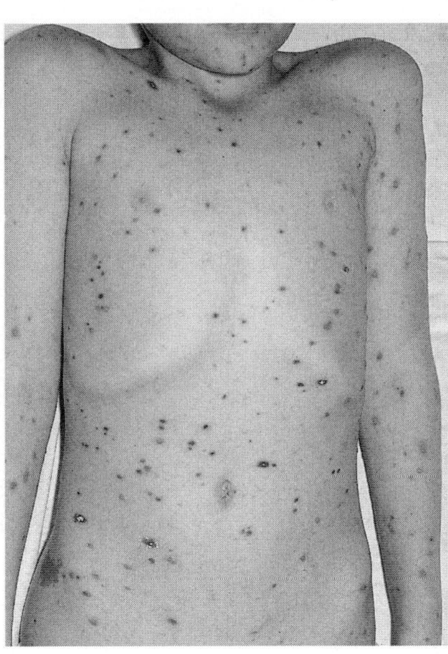

Chicken pox

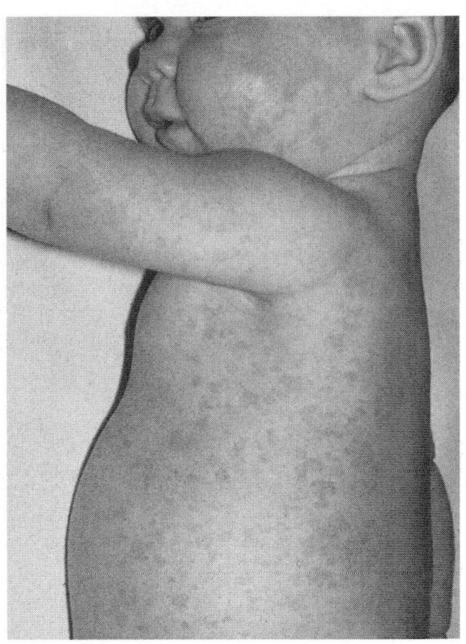

Rubella

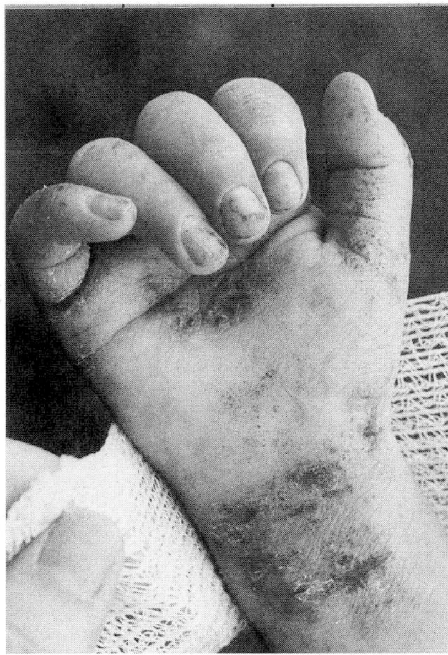

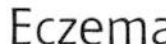

Eczema

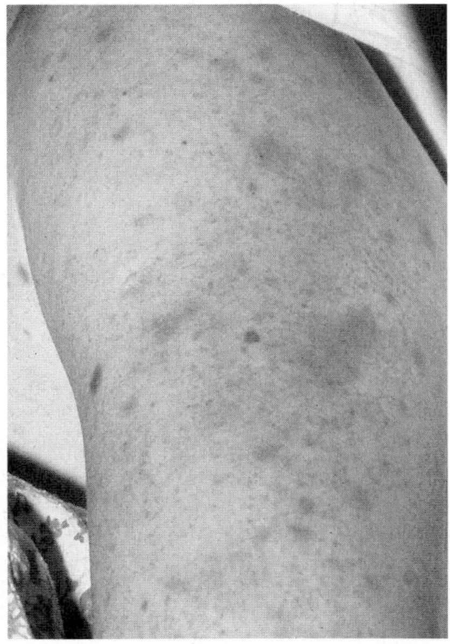

Meningococcal rash

Skin rashes and blemishes

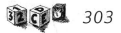

Infectious childhood diseases

Disease	Incubation period	Signs to look for	Care
Chicken pox: viral infection	14–16 days	Begins with general signs of feeling unwell, maybe a slight temperature; spots appear first on the chest and back and then spread; red at first but become fluid-filled blisters; they eventually dry off into scabs which drop off; spots come in successive crops and are very itchy	Give plenty to drink, keep the child as comfortable as possible, with baths, loose comfortable clothes and calamine lotion to ease the itching; prevent scratching as this may leave scars
Diphtheria: bacterial infection	2–6 days	General signs of being unwell, difficulty with breathing; classic sign of diphtheria is white membrane forming across the throat and restricting the airway; toxins produced by the bacteria can damage the heart and brain	Requires prompt medical treatment with antibiotics and admission to hospital
Gastroenteritis: bacterial or viral infection spread by direct contact or eating infected food or water	Very variable: 1–14 days; viruses affect more quickly	Child is generally unwell, with severe vomiting and diarrhoea; babies and young children quickly show signs of dehydration, with dry mouth and skin, decreased urine output; anterior fontanelle in small babies sinks down	Call the doctor, initial treatment in hospital may be necessary; keep the child cool and comfortable; give drinks of water very regularly; oral rehydration solutions may also be given
Measles: viral infection	7–12 days	Begins with signs of bad cold and cough; child gradually becomes more unwell and miserable with raised temperature and sore eyes; before rash appears on the skin white spots can be seen inside the mouth (Kopliks spots); when rash appears spots are red and rash is blotchy; rash usually starts behind the ears and quickly spreads downwards to rest of the body	Child may be very unwell; call the doctor; in addition to any medical treatment, give rest and plenty of fluids; eyes may need special attention and gentle bathing; keep mouth clean and moist; watch for signs of ear infection
Meningitis: inflammation of the membrane covering the brain; can be caused by bacterial or viral infection	2–10 days	Important to recognise meningitis early as it develops very rapidly; usually begins with high temperature, headache, vomiting, confusion, irritability; later signs may develop, pain and stiffness in the neck, dislike of the light	Get medical help early; treatment and care in hospital will be required (for more details see pages 307–8)

If meningitis is suspected, it is important to get medical help as quickly as possible

Infectious childhood diseases continued

Disease	Incubation period	Signs to look for	Care
Mumps: viral infection	14–21 days	Generally unwell; pain and tenderness around the ear and jaw, uncomfortable to chew; swelling starts under jaw and up by the ear, usually on one side of the face, followed (though not always) by the other	Keep the child comfortable and give plenty to drink; doctor may advise analgesic (such as paracetamol) to ease soreness; rest is necessary as rare complication in boys is inflammation of the testes
Poliomyelitis (polio): viral infection that attacks the nervous system causing muscle paralysis; a water-borne infection	5–21 days	Becoming suddenly unwell, with headache, stiffness in the neck and back, followed by loss of movement and paralysis; maybe difficulty with breathing	Initial hospital care, followed by rest and rehabilitation
Rubella (German measles): viral infection	14–21 days	Begins like a mild cold, but often child does not feel unwell; rash appears first on the face, then spreads to the body; spots are flat and only last for about 24 hours; glands in the back of the neck may be swollen	Children with rubella often do not feel unwell; give plenty to drink; if a pregnant woman gets rubella, there is a risk of damage to her baby; keep the child away from anyone who is pregnant or likely to be; if the child was with anyone who is pregnant before you knew about the illness let them know; any pregnant woman who has had any contact with rubella should see her doctor urgently
Scarlet fever: bacterial infection	2–6 days	Begins with child suddenly feeling unwell, with sore throat, temperature, feeling sick; tongue looks very red, cheeks are flushed, throat looks red and sore, with white patches; rash starts on the face and spreads to the body	Make sure child rests and drinks plenty; doctor may prescribe antibiotics; observe for complications, such as ear and kidney infections
Tetanus: bacterial infection; bacteria found in soil, dirt and dust, enter the body through cuts, scratches and other wounds	4–21 days	Tetanus attacks the nervous system, causing painful muscle spasms; muscles in the neck tighten and the jaw locks	Any cuts, etc. must be properly cleaned; immunisation kept up-to-date; immediate hospital treatment needed for suspected tetanus

Infectious childhood diseases continued

Disease	Incubation period	Signs to look for	Care
Tuberculosis (TB): bacterial infection	28–42 days	Persistent coughing, weight loss, further investigation shows lung damage	Initial period of treatment in hospital may be required; specific antibiotics given, rest and good quality diet essential
Whooping cough (pertussis): bacterial infection	7–14 days	Begins like cough and cold; cough usually gets worse; after about 2 weeks coughing bouts start; long bouts of coughing and choking are exhausting and frightening, as coughing can go on for so long that child finds it hard to breathe and may be sick; sometimes there is a whooping noise as child draws in breath after coughing; coughing bouts can continue for several weeks	Call doctor, who may prescribe antibiotics; child will need lots of support and reassurance, especially during coughing bouts; encourage child to drink plenty; may be necessary to give food and drink after coughing bouts, especially if child is being sick; possible complications: convulsions, bronchitis, hernias, ear infections, pneumonia and brain damage

Note Rashes look different on different people. The colour of the spots may vary and on black skin rashes can be less easy to see. If you are doubtful, check with the doctor, especially if the child is showing other signs of illness. Some infectious diseases can be prevented by immunisation (see Chapter 16).

MENINGITIS AND SEPTICAEMIA

Meningitis is an inflammation of the lining of the brain. It is a rare but very serious illness. There are two main types of bacterial meningitis in the UK. They are named after the pathogens (germs) that cause the infections.

The two types are:

- meningococcal
- pneumococcal.

Septicaemia is a form of blood poisoning that may be caused by the same pathogens (germs) that cause meningitis. Septicaemia is very serious and must be treated straight away; it is the more life-threatening consequence of meningococcal infection. The pathogen enters the body through the throat (droplet infection) and travels though the bloodstream. In some cases, the pathogens multiply in the bloodstream and cause blood poisoning.

Meningitis and septicaemia occur most commonly in:

- babies
- children
- teenagers.

In children under 4 the most common type of meningitis used to be *haemophilus influenzae* type b (Hib). This pathogen could also cause septicaemia. Immunisation against Hib infection is now part of the routine childhood immunisation programme and, as a result, Hib has virtually disappeared.

Recognising meningitis

Meningitis is not easy to recognise at first because the symptoms are similar to those of flu. Symptoms may not all appear at the same time, and they may be different in babies, children and adults.

Symptoms in babies

- a high-pitched, moaning cry
- difficult to wake
- refusing to feed
- vomiting
- pale or blotchy skin
- red or purple spots that do not fade under pressure – *do the glass test* (see overleaf).

Symptoms in older children and adults

- red or purple spots that do not fade under pressure – *do the glass test* (see overleaf)
- stiffness in the neck
- drowsiness or confusion

- severe headache
- vomiting
- high temperature
- dislike of bright light.

The glass test
Press the side of a glass firmly against the rash. You will be able to see if the rash fades and loses colour under the pressure. *If it doesn't change colour, contact the doctor immediately.*

Symptoms of septicaemia

These are:

- a rash that may be small spots or large, blotchy bruise-like spots
- pale, clammy skin
- joint and limb pains
- high temperature.

Note that the rash will be more difficult to see on a dark skin. The rash may develop very quickly in a matter of hours – the spots can grow to red or purple bruises.

If you suspect either meningitis or septicaemia, call the doctor immediately.

Treatment

Bacterial meningitis and septicaemia are treated with antibiotics, which are also given to the immediate family and any close contacts.

Case study . . .

. . . recognising early signs and symptoms of an illness

David had been playing happily all morning at playgroup. His dad had fetched him at lunchtime because this was the afternoon that his mum went to work. David ate all his lunch and went off to play in the garden with his friend, Andrew. David's dad took the paper into the garden to read so that he could keep an eye on the children. They had not been playing long before David came over and said he felt 'funny and his tummy hurt'. David's dad took him inside and made him sit in the cool, but he was immediately sick and said he felt much worse. David's dad put him to rest in bed and went to telephone Andrew's mum to ask her to come and take him home. When she arrived, they went in to look at David and they were alarmed to find that he was much worse – he looked hot and sweaty, his neck hurt and he had a purple rash on his tummy.

1. *What action should David's parents take now?*
2. *What illness could David's symptoms be a sign of?*
3. *Who else should consult the doctor?*

Progress check

Name two water-borne infections.

What are the signs of measles?

What are the complications of measles?

If a child in your care has rubella, what is the important thing you must do as well as caring for the child?

Describe a chickenpox rash.

Where is the tetanus bacteria found?

What are the possible complications of whooping cough?

What are the signs of meningitis in:

(a) a baby?

(b) an older child?

Describe the 'glass test' for meningitis.

What are the symptoms of septicaemia?

What are the two pathogens that cause meningitis and septicaemia?

Infestations

key term

Parasite
lives on and obtains its food from humans

Parasites obtain their food from humans and are likely to affect all children at some time. Common parasites that infest children include:

- fleas
- head lice
- ringworm
- scabies
- threadworms.

FLEAS

Fleas are small insects. They cannot fly, but jump from one person to another. The type of flea that feeds on human blood lives in clothing next to the skin. When it bites to suck blood, it leaves red marks that itch and swell up. Fleas lay their eggs in furniture and clothing to be near to humans, their source of food. The insect bites can be treated with antiseptics or calamine lotion to stop itching and swelling. To get rid of fleas, it is important to get rid of the eggs as well as the live insects. Insecticide powder can be applied to clothes and bedding. Cleanliness is very important; regular washing of clothes and bedding will get rid of the eggs. Sometimes children are sensitive to fleas that normally live on cats and dogs. Animals need to be treated regularly to prevent this problem.

HEAD LICE

Head lice are small insects that live in human hair, near to the scalp, where they can easily bite the skin and feed on blood. Many children get head lice; they catch them by coming into contact with someone who is already infested. When heads and hair touch, the lice simply walk from one head to another. Children are vulnerable because they work and play with their heads close together. The lice lay eggs, called nits, close to the scalp and cement the eggs firmly to the hair. Nits look like specks of dandruff, but when you try to remove them they are firmly attached to the hair. The first sign of head lice is usually an itchy scalp.

If a child has head lice, the condition must be treated straight away. Treatment is an insecticide lotion available from the chemist, clinic or doctor. Follow the instructions carefully and treat the whole household. The lotion kills the lice and nits, but the nits are not washed off. To remove dead nits you need to use a plastic tooth-comb, which is obtainable from the chemist. Some head lice are becoming resistant to these lotions and there has been concern about the safety of some lotions; so treatment is now relying more on natural methods.

Fine tooth-combing is the preferred natural method of treatment and should be done every 2 to 3 days. Wet the hair and apply a little conditioner, comb the hair from root to tip, over a piece of white paper, paying particular attention to the areas behind the ears and in the nape of the neck. Lice will fall out of the hair and will easily be seen on the paper.

Oils like tea-tree oil and eucalyptus oil have some effect when dealing with head lice.

The most effective way of preventing and discouraging head lice is to:

- inspect the hair regularly
- comb the hair thoroughly at least twice a day and always after school or nursery – this injures the lice so that they don't lay eggs
- wash brushes and combs regularly in hot, soapy water.

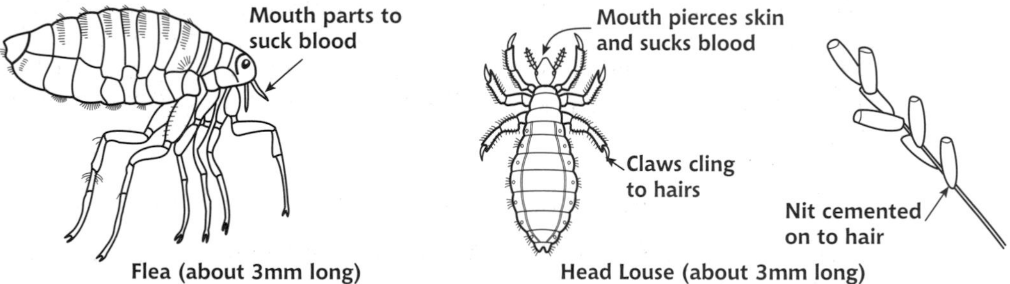

A head louse and nits

RINGWORM

Ringworm is a fungus that can be caught from animals. It is seen as a raised red circle with a white scaly centre. It is very itchy. Ringworm patches can occur on the body and on the scalp. Contact the doctor who will prescribe the specific treatment, usually an antibiotic cream.

SCABIES

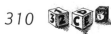

Scabies is caused by a tiny mite, *sarcoptes scabiei*, that burrows under the skin, causing intense itching. The mites spend their lives feeding on the skin and laying their eggs. It may be possible to see the burrows, or red raised spots, which are very itchy. Scratching may cause redness and infection. Scabies is mostly seen on the hands between the fingers, on the wrists and sometimes in the armpit and groin. Scratching and scratch marks may draw attention to the presence of scabies in a child. The mites crawl from one person to another and several family members may be affected. If there is severe itching and soreness the doctor may prescribe a specific treatment such as an antihistamine cream. Otherwise calamine lotion or a mild antiseptic cream will soothe the itching. The doctor will prescribe a lotion to kill the mites and eggs; it will be necessary to treat all the affected members of the family. All the bedding and clothing will need to be washed and all family members treated.

THREADWORMS

Threadworms are small white worms that look like pieces of cotton. They live in the bowel and can be seen in the stools. Threadworms come out of the bowel at night to lay their eggs around the bottom. This causes itching and, when the child scratches, the eggs are transferred to the fingers and under the nails. Later, the child will lick their fingers and eggs are swallowed, to hatch and develop in the bowel, perpetuating the cycle. Constant itching and scratching may cause a very sore bottom and disturb the child's sleep. The doctor will prescribe specific anti-worm treatment. Everyone in the household needs to be treated, keep their nails short and wash their hands well after using the lavatory and before eating. At night, close-fitting pyjamas may help to stop the child scratching. All bedding, nightclothes and pants need to be washed and changed regularly.

Case study . . .

. . . coping with head lice

Aaron is 5 years old and started at his local infant school a few months ago. The school has sent home a letter to parents and carers informing them that there are problems with infestations of head lice and that children in school have been affected. When Aaron returns home from school, his mother Marcia decides to look carefully at his hair. She finds a few live head lice. Marcia comes to you for advice.

1. *How would you advise Marcia to treat Aaron's hair now?*
2. *How would you advise her to care for Aaron's hair in the future to try to prevent further infestations?*

Progress check

How can you discourage head lice?

How is ringworm caught?

What signs might lead you to suspect that a child has scabies?

Where are threadworms seen?

What are nits?

Now try these questions

In what different ways are diseases spread?

Describe how immunity is acquired. What are the different types of immunity?

Describe meningitis and septicaemia. What are the signs and symptoms of meningitis and septicaemia?

key terms

You need to know what the key terms and phrases in this chapter mean. Go back through the chapter and find out.

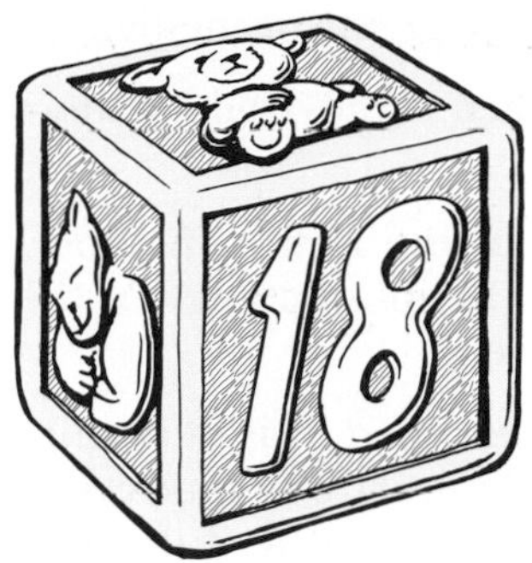

CARING FOR SICK CHILDREN

Babies and children require special care when they are ill, whether they are ill at home or become ill while they are being cared for outside their home environment.
This chapter will cover the following topics:

- *caring for sick children at home*
- *caring for sick children in the work setting.*

Caring for sick children at home

Babies and children need to be with their main carer when they are ill. Unless the doctor suggests that the child stays in bed, they may feel less isolated if they come downstairs. Here they can see and hear what is going on, and a bed could be made up, for rest, on the settee. Some children may need the quiet and comfort of bed, and in this case the carer and other adults should try to spend as much time as possible with them.

PHYSICAL CARE

The child should be kept clean and comfortable. Change their clothes frequently and make sure they are loose and made of absorbent material. If the child is staying in bed, give an all-over wash if a bath is not possible. Straighten up the bed, smooth the sheets and pillows, wash the hands and face and comb the hair at regular intervals.

FOOD AND DRINK

Drinking is important. Having plenty of fluids during illness will help recovery and prevent dehydration, especially if the temperature is raised, so it is vital to encourage a child to drink as much as possible. Offering a variety of drinks may encourage an unwilling child to drink more. Appetite may be affected by illness, so do not worry about food for the first day or so unless it is wanted; after this, try to find ways of making food tempting. Offering favourite foods and serving small appetising portions will help to encourage a reluctant child to eat.

ROOM TEMPERATURE

Make sure the room is kept warm and well ventilated (not too hot), day and night.

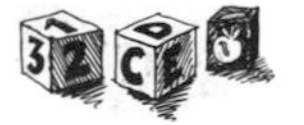

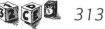

MEDICINES

The following points are important to note regarding the giving of medicines.

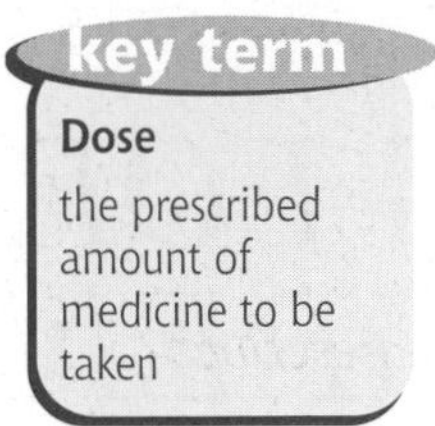

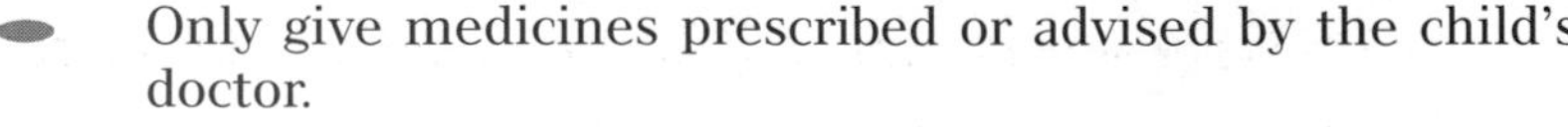

- Only give medicines prescribed or advised by the child's doctor.
- Medicines need to be given at the right time and in the right **dose** (quantity); check the instructions on the label each time the medicine is given.
- If a course of medicine is prescribed, it is very important to finish the full course. This must be done even if the child seems to be better, so that the full benefit is obtained.
- When a medicine is prescribed, ask about any possible side-effects. If you think the child is reacting badly to a medicine (for example, with a rash or diarrhoea), stop giving it and tell the doctor.

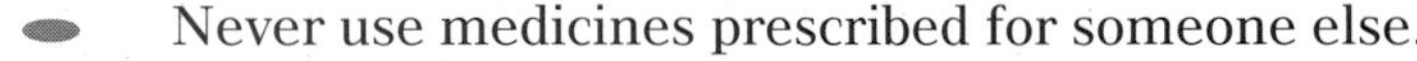

- Never use medicines prescribed for someone else.
- Aspirin should not be given to children. There is a risk of Reye's disease, which causes damage to the liver.
- Keep all medicines in a locked cupboard if possible.
- Do not keep prescribed or out-of-date medicines.

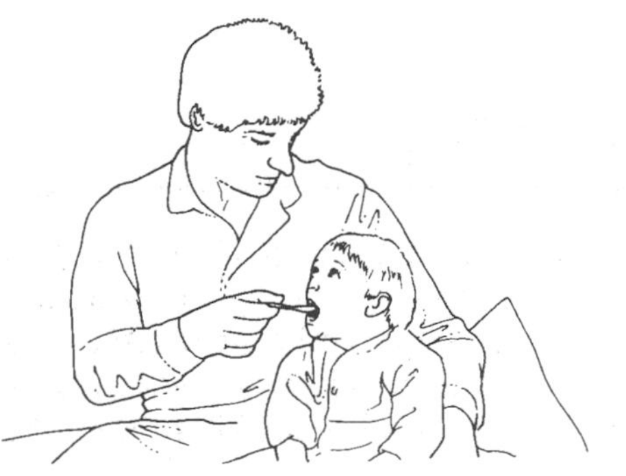

Giving medicine

TAKING A TEMPERATURE

Thermometers that you hold on the child's forehead show the skin temperature, not body temperature; to take an accurate temperature it is best to use a mercury thermometer.

First shake down the mercury in the thermometer. Hold the child on your knee and tuck the thermometer under the armpit next to the skin. Leave the thermometer there for about 3 minutes; it might help to read a story to the child while you do this.

A normal temperature taken under the tongue is 37°C; taken under the arm, it is 36.4°C.

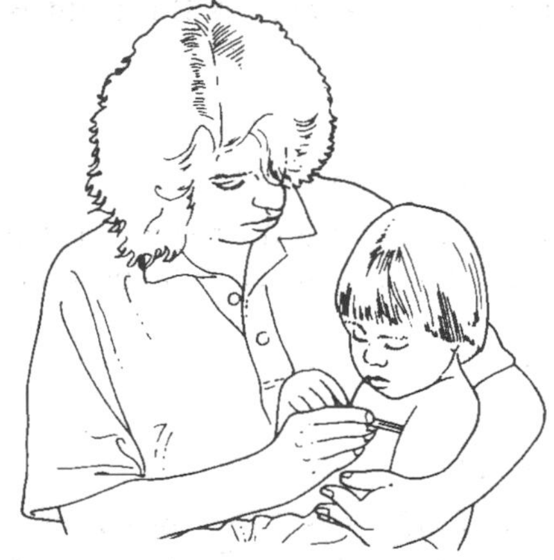

Taking a temperature under the arm

ACTIVITIES

A carer should allow time for games, stories, company and comforting the sick child. Children will need activities that are not too difficult or needing lots of concentration. They may like to return to activities and games that they enjoyed when they were younger.

Sick children are easily tired and need plenty of rest. They may not manage to concentrate for long and may want you to do things for them that they did quite capably when they were well.

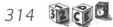

Progress check

When giving medicines to children, what two important things should be checked?

What is a normal temperature taken under the arm?

What is a normal temperature taken under the tongue?

Why is it important to finish the full course of a medicine that the doctor has prescribed?

If a sick child has no appetite, what is the best thing to do?

Caring for sick children in the work setting

When a child is taken ill outside the home environment, it is important to report any concerns to the appropriate people so that the illness can be properly diagnosed. At a nursery, school or playgroup, the illness should be reported to a senior staff member who will follow the workplace policy and decide whether to contact the child's parents/carers. A childminder or nanny should contact the parents direct.

It is important to keep a record of the symptoms, noting how they first appeared and how they have progressed, as this information may need to be passed on to a doctor and the parents. When caring for a child who is unwell at school or nursery you will need to:

- give practical help, for example take a temperature, help if the child is vomiting, provide a quiet place for them to lie down
- provide reassurance and stay with the child
- tell the child what you are doing, for example contacting a parent
- relax your normal expectations of the child – a child who is feeling ill will not be able to concentrate, and may be very miserable and distressed and want their parent or carer.

WHAT TO REPORT TO A DOCTOR IF A CHILD IS ILL

It is very important to have a clear history of the child's illness so that you can give accurate information to the child's parent/carer or to a doctor. These are the important things to record:

- when you first noticed that something was wrong and suspected that the child was ill
- what the symptoms were
- what action you took, for example taking a temperature, taking steps to cool the child, arranging for the child to rest
- how the symptoms have progressed since you first noticed them
- the child's behaviour and what they told you about how they were feeling.

WORKING WITH PARENTS

If a child is ill, parents will need information and reassurance. The child-care worker can help parents by:

- informing them promptly if there are concerns about a child
- remaining calm
- giving parents accurate information about their child
- reassuring parents that appropriate steps have been taken
- showing understanding of parents' concerns
- offering support and practical help where possible.

The parents of other children may need to know if another child in the setting has an infectious disease, so that they can take steps to ensure their child's health and well-being. This information will need to be given while ensuring confidentiality, so it is important not to name children in these circumstances.

INFORMATION NEEDED ABOUT EACH CHILD IN YOUR CARE

Child-care workers need to keep information about each child to enable contact to be made in the case of an emergency. Records should include:

- child's full name and date of birth
- child's full address and telephone number
- names and addresses of child's parents/carers
- emergency contact telephone numbers
- telephone numbers for the child's GP and health visitor and other agencies, if applicable, such as a social worker.

All the records should be regularly updated and child-care workers should stress the importance of parents/carers informing them of any changes.

PROVIDING AN HYGIENIC ENVIRONMENT

Children are very vulnerable to infection and diseases can spread very quickly in a child-care setting. Infection can be transmitted between adults and children, and also between the children themselves. Basic workplace routines can prevent diseases being spread if they are carried out efficiently, thoroughly and regularly. Three important areas of routine hygiene in child- care settings are:

- personal hygiene
- environmental hygiene
- disposing of waste materials.

Personal hygiene

Good personal hygiene routines involve thorough cleansing of the skin, hair, teeth and clothes.

Hands

Hand washing is especially important because it is the single most effective means of preventing the spread of infection. Child-care workers should ensure that they:

- wash their hands often throughout the day, especially after going to the toilet, cleaning up after accidents and *before* handling food

- keep nails short and free of nail varnish – bacteria grow where the varnish is chipped
- disinfect nail-brushes
- use disposable paper towels or hot air hand-dryers – if this is not possible towels should be washed at least daily and kept as dry as possible
- cover any cuts or abrasions with a waterproof plaster
- wear latex gloves when changing nappies, or dealing with blood or any other body fluids.

Hair

Hair should be kept clean, brushed often and tied back if long. Check regularly for head lice.

Environmental hygiene

A clean child-care setting is not only more welcoming but also less likely to contain harmful pathogenic organisms. Spread of infection can be prevented by good practice aimed at reducing the number of pathogenic organisms in the environment and preventing them spreading. Good practice includes:

- ensuring good ventilation
- supervising children when they use the lavatory and making sure that they wash and dry their hands properly afterwards
- avoiding overcrowding – the Children Act stipulates how much space is required
- providing separate rooms for babies and toddlers
- keeping laundry facilities separate from food preparation areas
- cleaning toys and play equipment regularly – toys should be cleaned daily if children are under 12 months old
- damp dusting daily
- using cloths and mops in their designated areas, e.g. separate floor mops for the toilet area and for the play room
- regular checking of the toilet/bathroom area
- using paper towels and tissues and using covered bins for disposal
- washing and sieving the sand regularly
- ensuring that any pets are kept clean and well cared for
- encouraging parents and carers to keep children at home if they are unwell – including this in the written policies may prevent misunderstandings
- observing strict hygiene procedures in the food preparation areas (see Chapter 7 for more information about this)
- checking the outside area for animal excrement or other hazards, like broken glass or refuse.

Disposing of waste materials

All child-care settings should have a health and safety policy that covers the disposal of hazardous waste. Care must be taken with all bodily waste (blood, faeces, urine, saliva) to prevent the transmission of diseases. Infections can be present without showing signs so the policy must be strictly maintained.

The following guidelines should be implemented when handling and disposing of waste materials:

- cover any skin abrasions with a waterproof dressing
- wear disposable latex gloves when dealing with bodily waste
- cover blood with a 1 per cent hypoclorite solution before wiping up
- wash hands with an antiseptic soap
- dispose of nappies, dressings and used gloves in a sealed bag and place in a sealed bin for incineration
- provide designated areas with covered bins for different types of waste.

GIVING MEDICINES IN THE WORK SETTING

There are occasions when children will be taking medicines and the child-care worker could be required to give these medicines. Each child-care establishment will have its own policy about giving medicines to children in its care. Child-care workers should always follow this policy.

These are the important points to remember when giving medicines to any child in your care:

- Follow the policy of your establishment.
- Get the parents'/carers' written consent.
- Only give medicines advised or prescribed by the child's GP or hospital doctor.
- Follow the instructions for dosage and frequency carefully.
- Store medicine safely in a locked cupboard.
- Keep a record of all the medicines given, include the date, time and dose.

Case study . . .

. . . feeling ill at nursery

Leroy is 3 years old and comes to the nursery on 3 days each week while his parents are working. He has been coming to nursery for 2 months now and has settled in happily. He is very sociable and loves to play with the staff and with the other children. Leroy came into nursery this morning his usual bright, cheerful self, but as the morning went on Sandra, the worker in charge of his group, noticed that he was sitting alone looking miserable. She tried to involve him in the activities, but he was reluctant to join in and became tearful. When Sandra went to comfort him, she noticed he was hot and decided to take his temperature. Leroy's temperature was raised and Sandra noticed that he had a flat, red rash on his face and body.

1. *What should Sandra do now?*
2. *What information should Sandra record?*
3. *What should Sandra tell Leroy's mother?*

Progress check

What important points should you check when giving medicines to children?

What facts should you report to a doctor about a child who is ill?

What information is needed about a child for emergency contact purposes?

How can you help parents when their child is ill?

Now try these questions

Describe how you would care for a child at home who is recovering from measles.

What important points need to be considered if medicines are being given to a child who is ill at home?

What action would you need to take if a child was taken ill in the child care setting?

How would you take a child's temperature using a mercury thermometer?

key terms

You need to know what the key terms and phrases in this chapter mean. Go back through the chapter and find out.

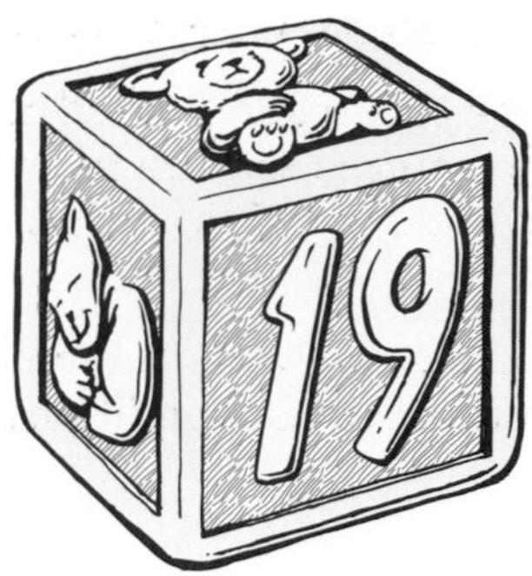

RESPONDING TO EMERGENCIES

This chapter provides an overview of emergency aid for children. Undertaking a recognised first aid course is recommended.

This chapter will cover the following topics:

- first aid in emergencies
- examining a casualty
- ABC of resuscitation
- recovery position
- first aid for minor injuries
- asthma
- diabetes
- febrile convulsions
- workplace policies and procedures.

First aid in emergencies

First aid is the assistance given to casualties before an ambulance arrives or the casualty arrives at a hospital. The principles are to:

- **p**reserve life
- **p**revent the worsening of the condition
- **p**romote recovery.

It is important to act logically and calmly in any emergency situation and remember the following four actions.

1. *Assess the situation* – If you are the first person to arrive at the scene of any accident, it is vital to assess quickly what happened and how it occurred. Find

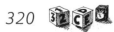

out how many children are injured and whether there is any continuing danger. Are there any other adults who can help? Is an ambulance required?

2. *Safety first* – Thinking of safety includes the safety of all children and adults, including yourself. You cannot help if you are injured too. Remove any dangerous hazards from the child and move the child only if it is absolutely essential. Try to make the area safe.
3. *Priorities* – Treat the serious injuries first. As a general rule, the quietest casualty is in most need of help – they may be unconscious. Conditions that are immediately life-threatening in children are:
   - severe bleeding
   - inability to breathe.
4. *Seek help* – Shout for help or ask others to get help, for example if a playground accident occurs, another child may be sent to fetch the first aider or another adult from the establishment. Call an ambulance and administer first aid. Move the child to safety if this is required.

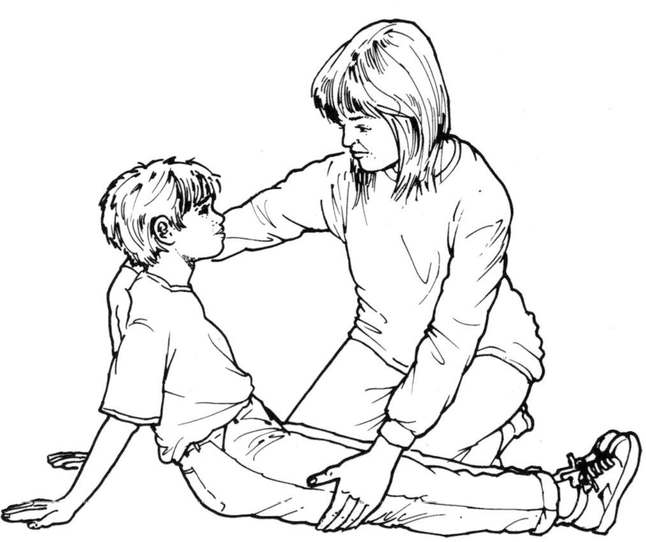

Assess the situation

Examining a casualty

> **key term**
> **Unconscious**
> showing no response to external stimulation

It is vital to find out if the child is conscious or **unconscious**. This can usually be done by gently talking to the child to assess their condition.

- Check for response – call the child's name, pinch the skin.
- Shout for help.
- Open the airway and check for breathing.
- Check the pulse.
- Act on your findings according to the chart below.

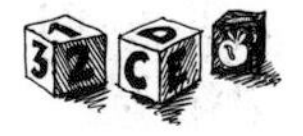

How to deal with an unconscious casualty

Unconscious **Breathing, pulse present**	**Unconscious** **Not breathing, pulse present**	**Unconscious** **Not breathing, no pulse**
1 Treat life-threatening injuries, e.g. bleeding, burns	1 Artificial ventilation – about 20 breaths of mouth-to-mouth ventilations for 1 minute	1 Cardiopulmonary resuscitation (CPR) – 5 chest compressions – 1 breath of mouth-to-mouth ventilations Repeat for 1 minute
2 Place in recovery position (see page 324)	2 Call an ambulance	2 Call an ambulance
3 Call an ambulance	3 Continue ventilations	3 Continue CPR until help arrives
	4 Check for pulse each minute	

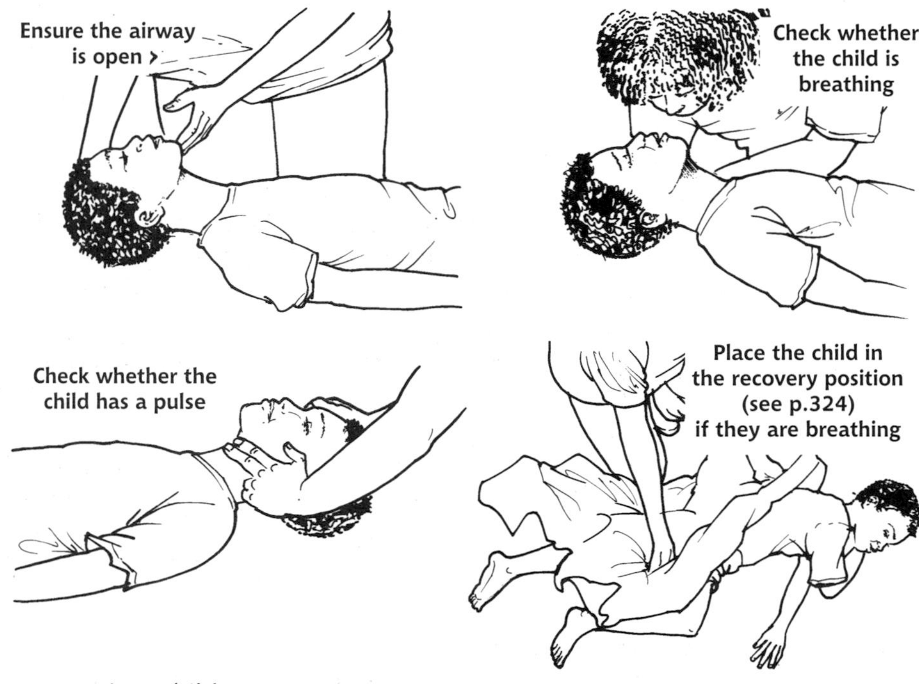
Ensure the airway is open
Check whether the child is breathing
Check whether the child has a pulse
Place the child in the recovery position (see p.324) if they are breathing

The unconscious child

Progress check

What are the principles of first aid?

Which four steps should the child-care worker remember if an accident occurs?

Explain why it is important to remain calm in the event of an accident.

How can you find out whether a child is conscious?

What steps should be taken for a child who is unconscious, breathing and with a pulse?

What is CPR?

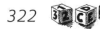

ABC of resuscitation

If a child stops breathing, they will quickly become unconscious because no oxygen can reach the brain. The heartbeat will slow down and eventually stop because of lack of oxygen.

The ABC of resuscitation

A is for airway

Is it clear?

Open the airway (mouth) and remove any obstructions. Lift the head and tilt the chin to bring the tongue away from the back of the throat.

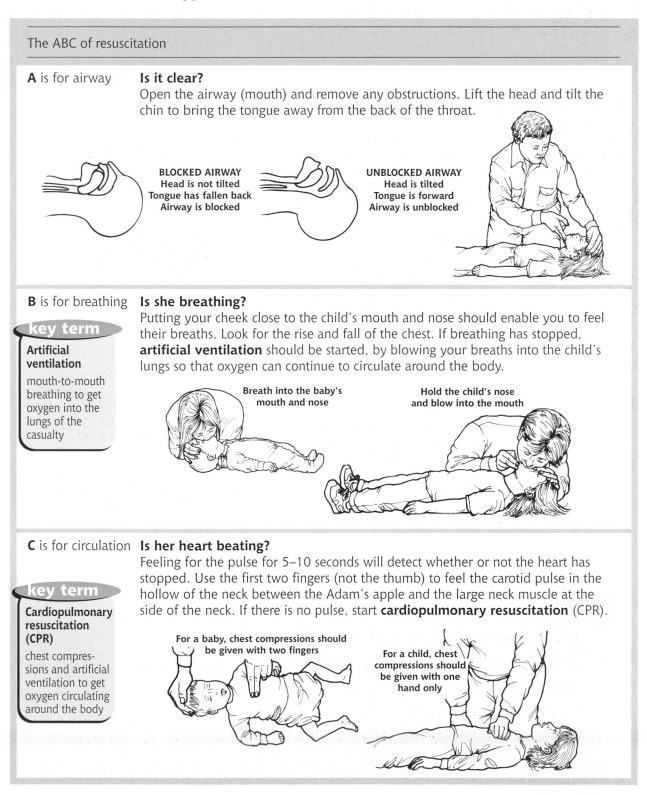

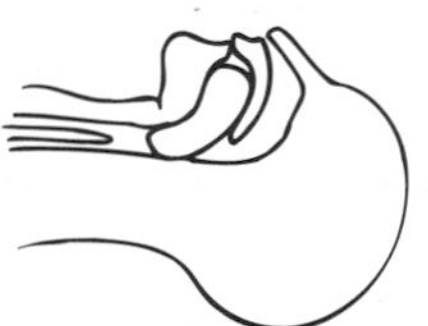

BLOCKED AIRWAY
Head is not tilted
Tongue has fallen back
Airway is blocked

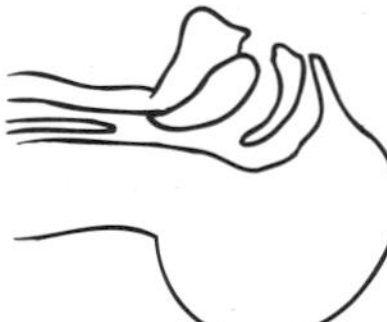

UNBLOCKED AIRWAY
Head is tilted
Tongue is forward
Airway is unblocked

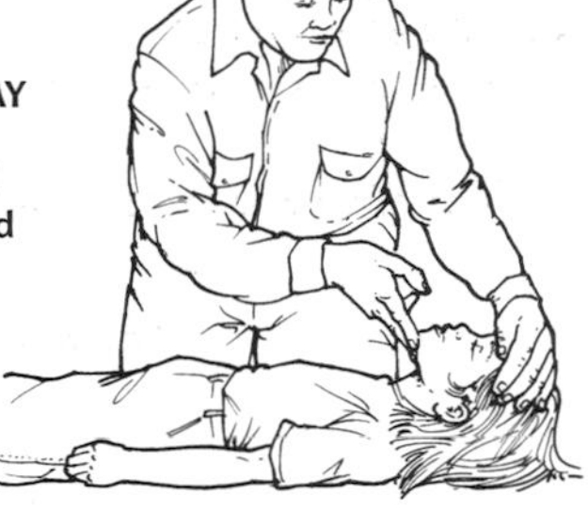

B is for breathing

Is she breathing?

Putting your cheek close to the child's mouth and nose should enable you to feel their breaths. Look for the rise and fall of the chest. If breathing has stopped, **artificial ventilation** should be started, by blowing your breaths into the child's lungs so that oxygen can continue to circulate around the body.

key term

Artificial ventilation mouth-to-mouth breathing to get oxygen into the lungs of the casualty

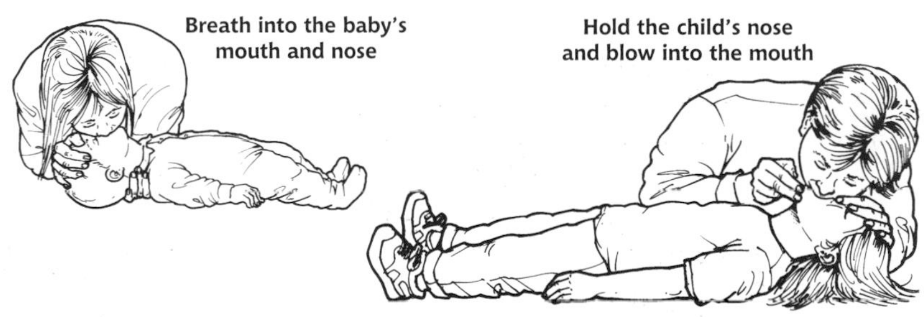

Breath into the baby's mouth and nose
Hold the child's nose and blow into the mouth

C is for circulation

Is her heart beating?

Feeling for the pulse for 5–10 seconds will detect whether or not the heart has stopped. Use the first two fingers (not the thumb) to feel the carotid pulse in the hollow of the neck between the Adam's apple and the large neck muscle at the side of the neck. If there is no pulse, start **cardiopulmonary resuscitation** (CPR).

key term

Cardiopulmonary resuscitation (CPR) chest compressions and artificial ventilation to get oxygen circulating around the body

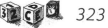

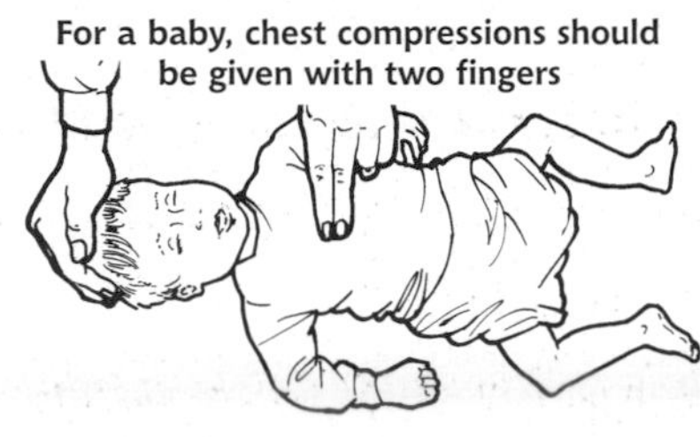

For a baby, chest compressions should be given with two fingers

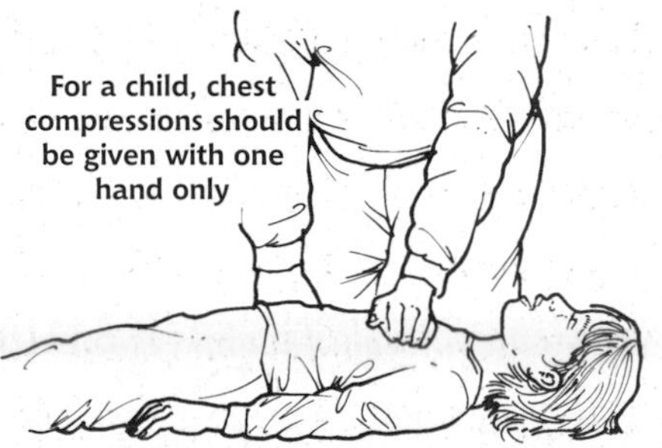

For a child, chest compressions should be given with one hand only

Recovery position

key term

Recovery position
safe position in which to place an unconscious casualty if they are breathing and have a pulse

An unconscious child who is breathing and has a pulse should be put into the **recovery position** to keep the airway clear by preventing choking on the tongue or vomit. Check for breathing and the pulse until medical help arrives.

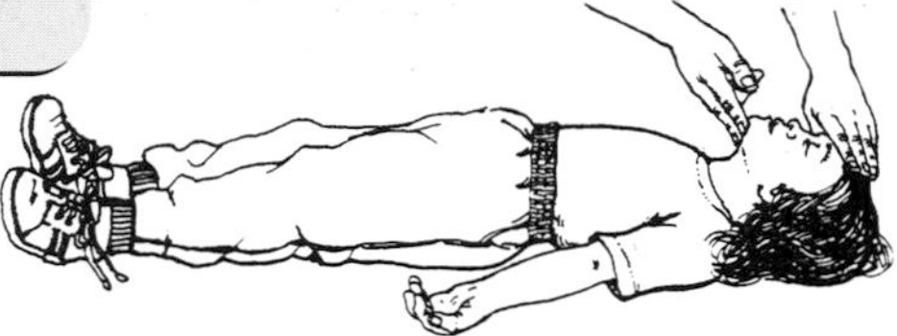

1 Lay the child on their back
Tilt the head back
Lift the chin forward
Ensure the airway is clear

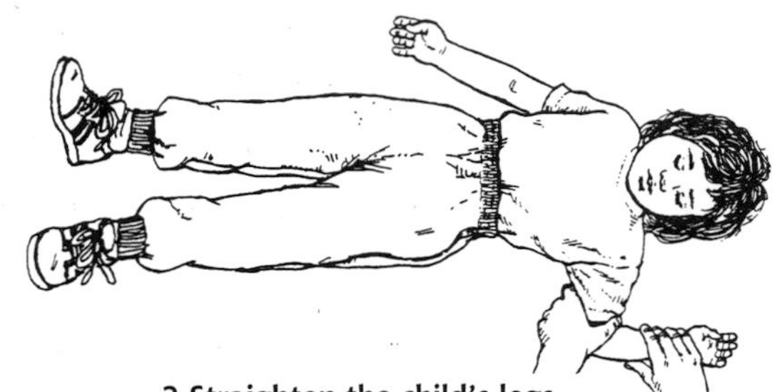

2 Straighten the child's legs
Bend the arm nearest to you at a right angle

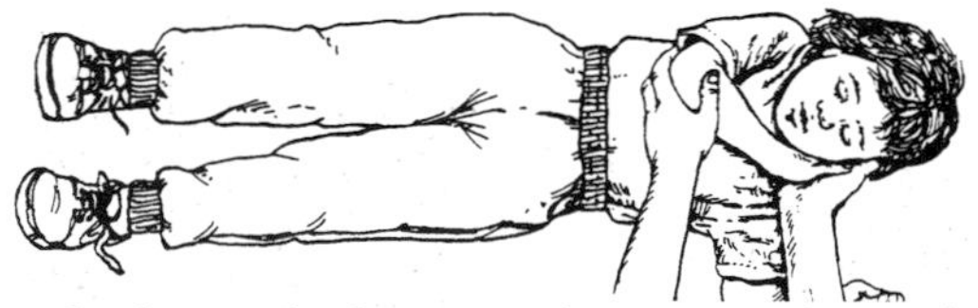

3 Take the arm furthest away from you and move it across the child's chest, bend it and place it on the cheek

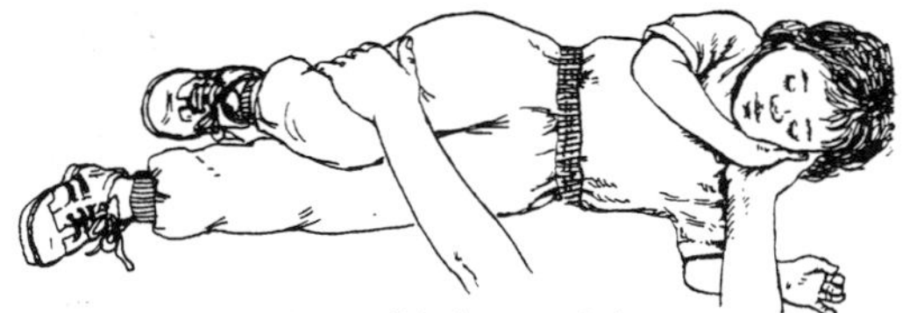

4 Keep this leg straight
Place foot flat on ground
Clasp under the thigh of the outside leg and bend it at the knee

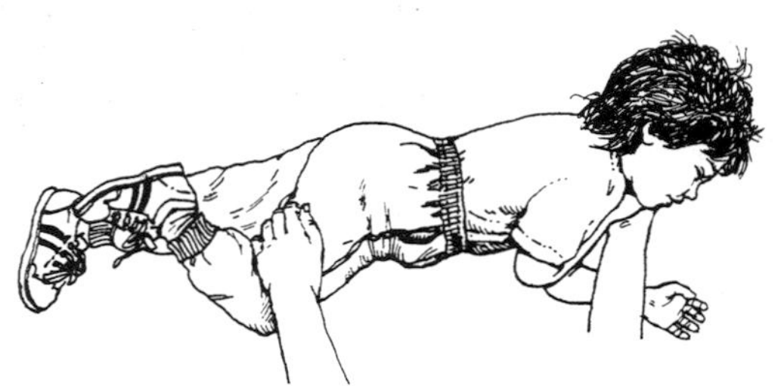

5 Pull the bent leg towards you to roll child on to their side
Use the knees to stop the child rolling on to their front
Keep hand against cheek

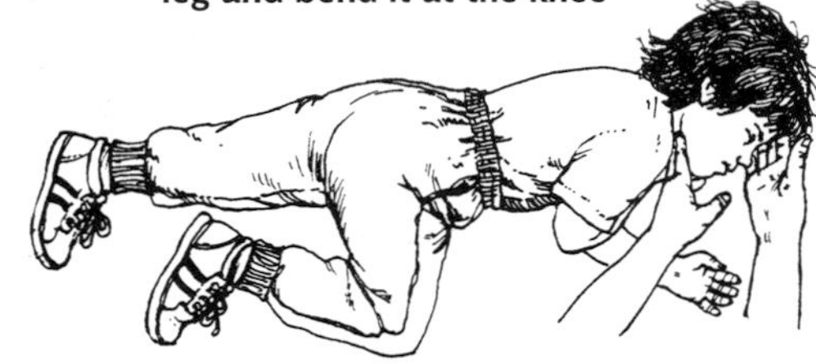

6 Bend top leg into a right angle to prevent child rolling forward
Tilt head back to keep airway open
Adjust hand under child's cheek

The recovery position

Progress check

Why does a child quickly become unconscious when they stop breathing?

What does ABC stand for?

How can you check the airway?

How can you tell if a child is breathing?

Where can the pulse most easily be felt in a child?

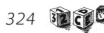

First aid for minor injuries

It is essential to remain calm when dealing with an injured child. They need to be reassured that they are in safe hands and everything will be all right.

BURNS AND SCALDS

- Do not remove any fabric that may be sticking to the affected area.
- Use cold water to cool the burn or scald for at least 10 minutes. (Use another cool liquid, such as milk, if cold water is unavailable.)
- Avoid touching the burn or blisters.
- Avoid immersing the child in cold water.

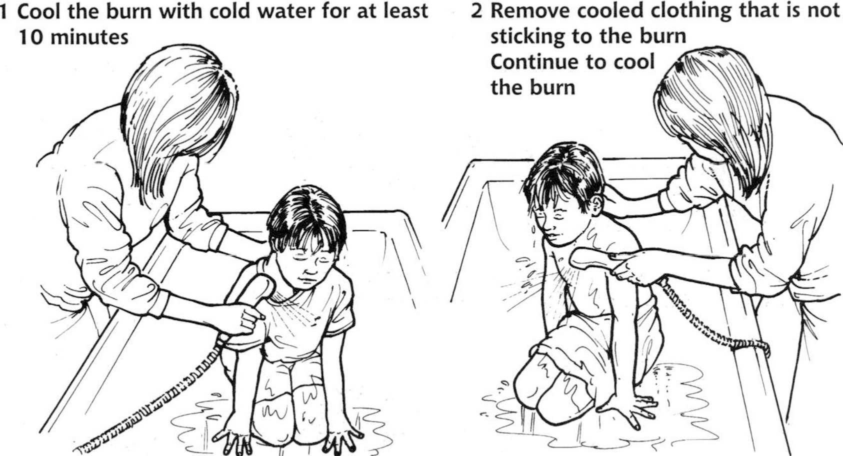
1 Cool the burn with cold water for at least 10 minutes
2 Remove cooled clothing that is not sticking to the burn
Continue to cool the burn

Dealing with burns and scalds

BLEEDING

- Minor bleeds must be cleaned and covered.
- Major bleeds must be stopped by direct pressure as quickly as possible:
  - if possible, keep the injured part raised
  - lay the child down to keep the head low
  - cover the wound with a firm, sterile dressing and a bandage.
- Remember that you should always wear gloves when dealing with blood or any other body fluids.

NOSEBLEEDS

- Sit the child leaning forwards and pinch the soft part of the nose above the nostrils for 10 minutes.
- Allow the child to spit or dribble into a bowl.

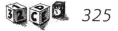

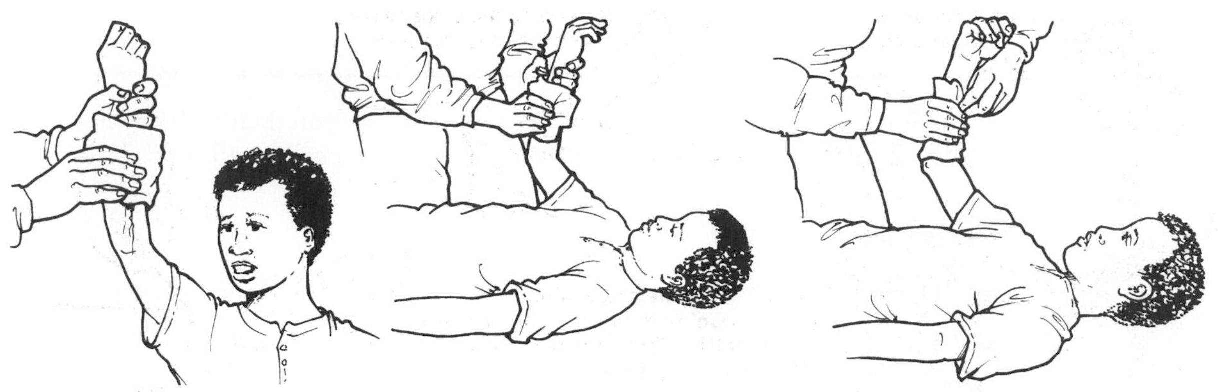

1 Apply pressure to the wound and raise the injured part

2 Lay the child down, while continuing to apply pressure and keep the injured part raised

3 Keeping the injured part raised cover the wound with a firm, sterile dressing and a bandage

Dealing with bleeding

- Continue to pinch the nose until the bleeding has stopped, checking after 10 minutes.
- Clean the child gently and tell them not to blow their nose, and breathe through their mouth.

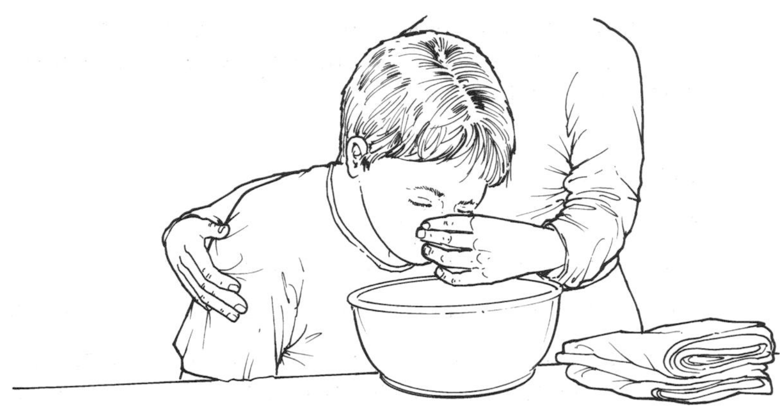

Dealing with a nosebleed

SPRAINS

- Raise and support the injured limb to minimise swelling. Remove shoe and sock if it is a sprained ankle.
- Apply a cold compress – a polythene bag of ice or a pack of frozen peas would do, if available.
- Wrap the limb in cotton wool padding and then bandage firmly.
- Keep the limb raised.

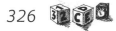

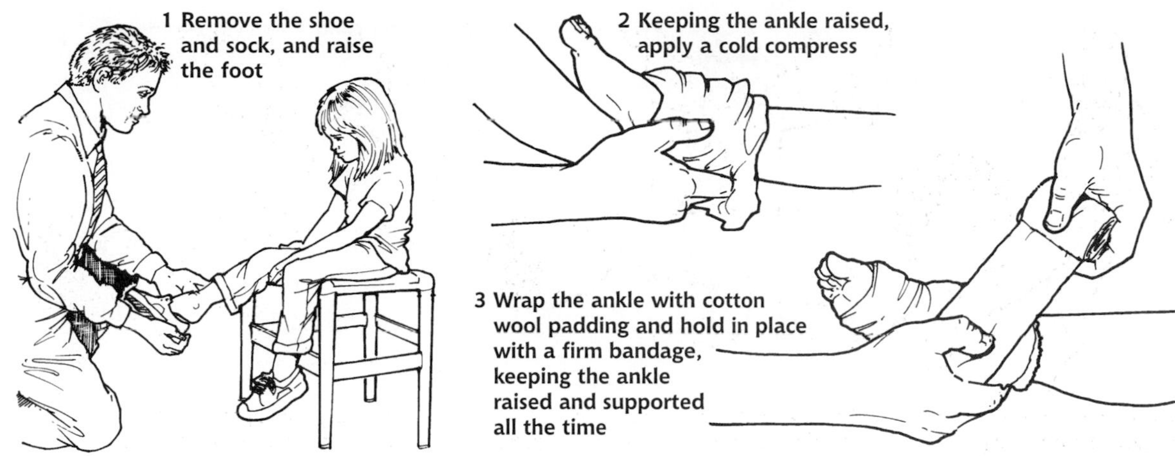

1 Remove the shoe and sock, and raise the foot
2 Keeping the ankle raised, apply a cold compress
3 Wrap the ankle with cotton wool padding and hold in place with a firm bandage, keeping the ankle raised and supported all the time

Dealing with a sprained ankle

RICE will help you remember what to do:
Rest
Ice
Compression
Elevation.

FOREIGN BODY

Children who have poked an object into their nose or ears should be taken to the nearest hospital Accident and Emergency Department, where the object can be safely removed.

CHOKING

If you are dealing with a young child:

- Put the child over your knee, head down.
- Slap sharply between the shoulder-blades up to five times.
- Turn the child over, and give five downward thrusts – place the heel of your hand on the child's lower breastbone (at the base of the sternum). Push sharply downwards five times.
- Check to see if the object has become dislodged and is in the mouth.
- If the object cannot be removed, give five upward thrusts – place the heel of your hand on the abdomen just below the rib-cage. Push firmly upwards five times. Then check the mouth again.
- Call for medical aid – take the child to the phone with you if you are alone.
- Check ABC.
- Repeat the process again until help arrives or the object can be removed.

If you are dealing with an older child, start by giving back slaps with the child standing and bent forwards. Then lie the child on the floor and continue as for the young child.

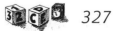

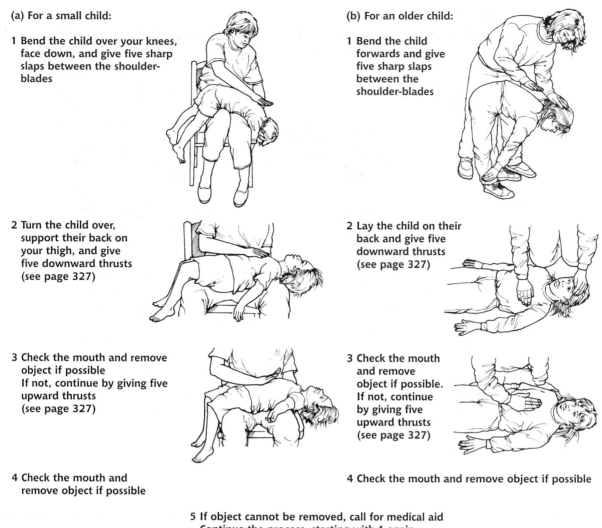

(a) For a small child:

1 Bend the child over your knees, face down, and give five sharp slaps between the shoulder-blades

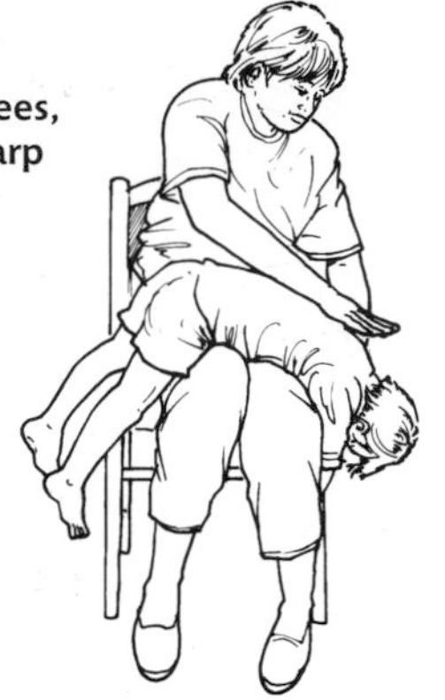

2 Turn the child over, support their back on your thigh, and give five downward thrusts (see page 327)

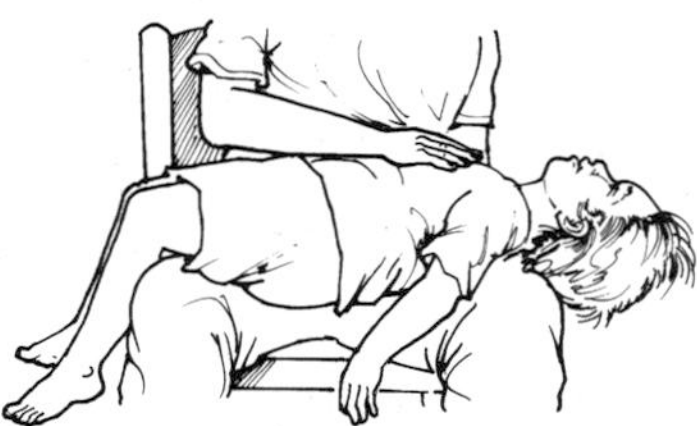

3 Check the mouth and remove object if possible
If not, continue by giving five upward thrusts (see page 327)

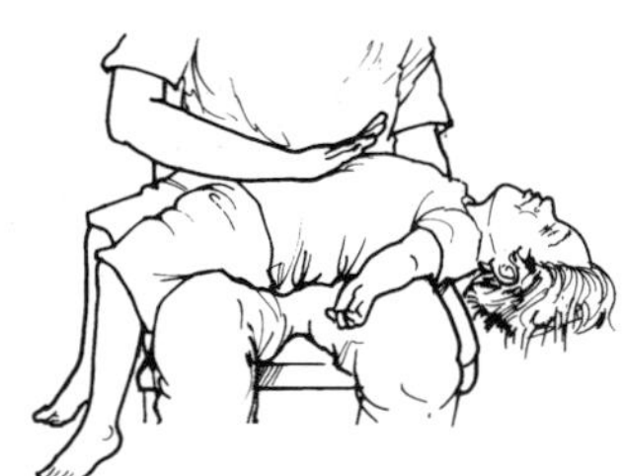

4 Check the mouth and remove object if possible

(b) For an older child:

1 Bend the child forwards and give five sharp slaps between the shoulder-blades

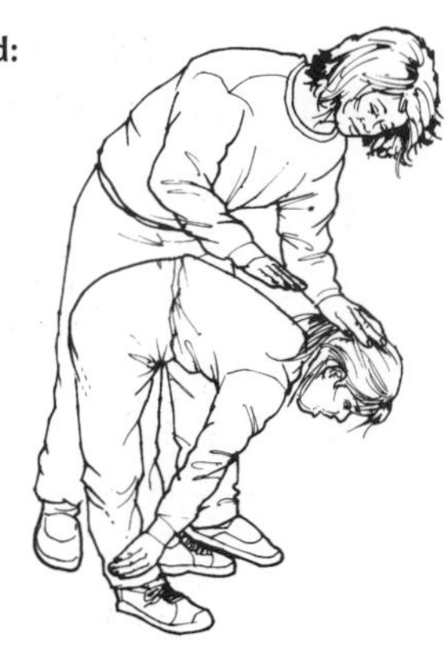

2 Lay the child on their back and give five downward thrusts (see page 327)

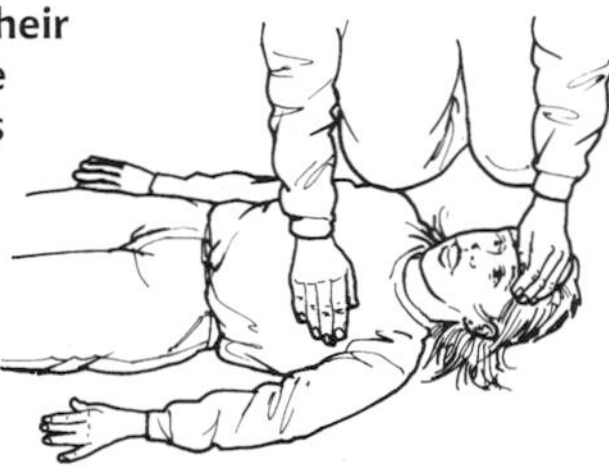

3 Check the mouth and remove object if possible. If not, continue by giving five upward thrusts (see page 327)

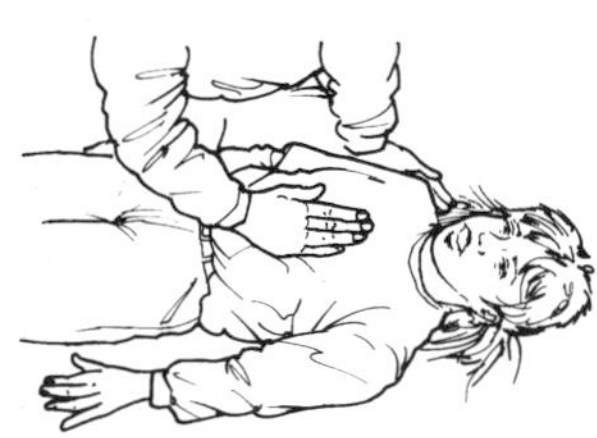

4 Check the mouth and remove object if possible

5 If object cannot be removed, call for medical aid
Continue the process, starting with 1 again, until the object can be removed or help arrives.
(With an older child, the back slaps can be given by turning them on to their side.)

Dealing with (a) a small child and (b) an older child who is choking

Progress check

What should the first aid box in a child-care establishment contain?

What is the emergency procedure for dealing with a child who is choking?

What is the first aid treatment for a nosebleed?

How long should burns be cooled with cold water?

What does RICE stand for in connection with the treatment of sprains?

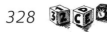

FIRST AID BOX

All establishments and homes should have a first aid box that is easily accessible and contains all the items shown below.

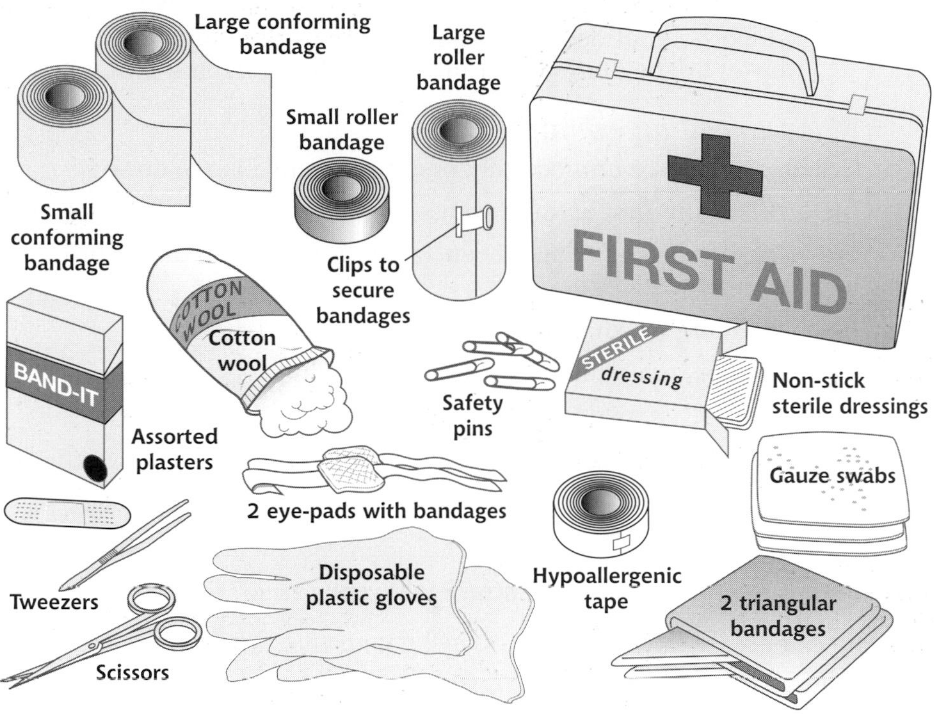

The contents of a first aid box

Asthma

Asthma attacks are very frightening for children – the airways go into spasm, making breathing difficult, especially breathing out. The typical picture is of a child leaning forwards with a hunched posture, gasping for breath – taking air in but unable to blow it out. Speech is impossible during an attack.

IMMEDIATE ACTION

If an undiagnosed child has an asthma attack, call an ambulance. In the meantime, follow the steps below.

Management of an asthma attack

- Reassure the child.
- Encourage relaxed breathing – slowly and deeply.
- Loosen tight clothing around the neck.
- Sit the child upright and leaning forward against a support, such as a table, supporting themselves with their hands in any comfortable position.
- Stay with the child.
- Give the child their bronchodilator to inhale – two doses – if they are known asthmatics.
- Offer a warm drink to relieve dryness of the mouth.

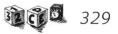

- Continue to comfort and reassure.
- When the child recovers from a minor attack they can resume quiet activities.
- If the condition persists, call for an ambulance and contact parents.
- Report the attack to the parents when the child is collected. If the child is upset by the episode, parents should be contacted immediately.

When to call an ambulance

Call an ambulance immediately, or get someone else to do so if:

- this is the first asthma attack
- the above steps have been taken and there is no improvement in 5 to 10 minutes
- the child is exhausted
- the lips, mouth and face are turning blue.

Progress check

What happens during an asthma attack?

How would you recognise an asthma attack in a young child?

How would you deal with a child who is having an asthma attack?

When would you consider it necessary to call an ambulance?

Diabetes

key term

Hypoglycaemia
low levels of glucose in the blood

Because this condition arises when there is a disturbance in the way the body regulates the sugar concentrations in the blood, **hypoglycaemia** (too little sugar in the blood) or hyperglycaemia (too much sugar in the blood) may occur. Both conditions will eventually lead to unconsciousness, but hyperglycaemia usually develops slowly, so it is most likely that a diabetic child will experience episodes of hypoglycaemia.

HYPOGLYCAEMIA

This may result from too much insulin, not enough food, illness or unusually vigorous exercise. Signs include:

- irritability and confusion
- loss of co-ordination and concentration
- rapid breathing
- sweating
- dizziness.

Management of a hypoglycaemic attack

If the child is conscious:

- sit the child down and stay with them

- give sugar, for example glucose tablets, chocolate or a sugary drink, such as Lucozade.

The condition should improve within a few minutes:

- If so, offer more sweetened food or drink.
- Inform parents who should seek necessary advice to stabilise the condition. Parents must be informed of any hypoglycaemic attack because it could indicate the need for adjustment to the diet and/or insulin.

If the child is unconscious:

- put them in the recovery position (see page 324).
- call an ambulance, ensuring that somebody stays with the child at all times.

It is good practice to carry glucose tablets or a sweetened drink when accompanying a child with diabetes on a school trip or a swimming lesson.

Case study . . .

. . . a hypoglycaemic attack

Sally is 6 years old and she is diabetic. Her condition is controlled by insulin injections in the morning before school and in the afternoon after school. She is aware of controlling her diet and knows which foods she can eat.

Sally's class have just started to go swimming on Tuesday afternoons and she is very excited. She is so busy chatting about swimming at lunchtime that she only eats a small amount of her school dinner. Sally trips up the top step when getting out of the pool, and is very slow to get her clothes on, buttoning her blouse the wrong way. The teacher, Miss Brown, notices that her face looks damp when she gets on the bus and that she is breathing quickly. She looks pale and starts to cry quietly. Miss Brown always carries a packet of dextrose tablets in her bag and she offers them to Sally. After sucking two tablets, Sally seems more in control. She stops sweating and by the time the bus arrives back at school, she feels much better. Sally climbs down the bus steps and into the classroom to eat some digestive biscuits and drink a carton of milk.

1. *What signs of hypoglycaemia was Sally displaying?*
2. *What did the teacher do to remedy the situation?*
3. *What caused this attack?*

Progress check

What is the role of the child-care worker during a hypoglycaemic attack?

What action should be taken if you are not sure whether the child is hyperglycaemic or hypoglycaemic?

Why is it so important to report any hypoglycaemic episodes to parents?

Febrile convulsions

A febrile convulsion is a type of fit or seizure, which occurs as a direct result of a raised body temperature. They usually occur in children between the ages of 6 months to 5 years at the beginning of an illness – children are vulnerable because the developing brain cannot cope with the sudden increase in temperature. A child who has had one febrile convulsion is more likely to have another one.

SIGNS

- loss of consciousness
- rigidity (stiffness) of the body
- twitching movements of the body and/or face – eyes may roll back
- possible incontinence of urine or faeces.

The child may regain consciousness briefly and then sleep or lapse straight into a deep sleep. They will probably be confused and irritable when they wake up.

MANAGEMENT OF A FEBRILE CONVULSION

- Stay with the child throughout the convulsion and prevent them damaging themselves, by falling out of bed for example. *Do not interfere* with the process of the convulsion – allow it to take its course.
- Ask a colleague to send for the doctor if possible.
- Put the child into recovery position when movements have stopped – loosen tight garments.
- Gently reassure the child if they regain consciousness before sleeping.
- Call the doctor when the convulsion is over, if this has not been done already.
- Continue efforts to reduce the temperature, i.e. tepid sponging and removing clothing.

The doctor may prescribe antibiotics to fight bacterial infections and may prescribe sedatives to be given if the temperature increases again to prevent future attacks.

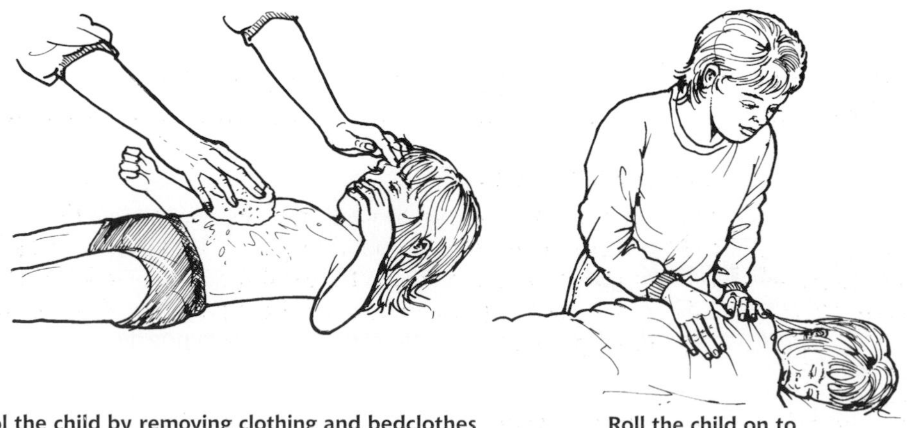

Cool the child by removing clothing and bedclothes
Sponge with tepid water until temperature falls
Roll the child on to
their side and cover with a sheet

Dealing with a febrile convulsion

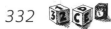

Case study . . .

. . . febrile convulsion

Geraldine had completed a first aid course for children at her local college before taking up her new post as playworker at the local out-of-school club. She thought she should be prepared for any accidents the children may have in the playground or elsewhere. She thoroughly enjoyed the new job. At the end of the first month she joked with her colleagues that she was pleased not to have found any need for her first aid skills.

One evening, a few of the children were watching a video, sitting on beanbags on the school hall floor. Frazer, who had seemed a little under the weather, suddenly rolled off his cushion on to the floor and began to convulse. Geraldine immediately went to his side and stayed with him. She checked his airway was clear, but did not interfere with the progress of the convulsion. One of her colleagues reassured the other children and took them into another play area. Another child-care worker telephoned Frazer's parents to tell them what was happening and request that they come to collect him as soon as possible. The parents agreed that the doctor should be contacted. Frazer had never had a convulsion before and although Geraldine had not taken his temperature, she could feel that Frazer was hot. He settled off to sleep on the beanbags when the convulsion was over.

1. *What had happened to Frazer?*
2. *What did Geraldine do immediately to help Frazer?*
3. *How did her colleagues support her?*
4. *What else could be done to reduce Frazer's temperature?*

Progress check

What is a febrile convulsion?

What are the possible signs of a febrile convulsion?

What action should the child-care worker take when a child suffers a febrile convulsion?

How can a child's temperature be reduced?

Workplace policies and procedures

INFORMING PARENTS

Parents must be informed of all injuries, however minor, which occur to their child, with as much detail as possible about how the injury happened. This ensures continuity of care between the establishment and home – the child may need to talk about their experiences with their parents who are then prepared to deal with any consequences.

key term

Accident book
legal documentation of all accidents and injuries occurring in any establishment

ACCIDENT BOOK

Every accident should be recorded in an **accident book** to comply with health and safety regulations.

The information recorded in the accident book should include:

- time and date of the accident
- name and address of the injured child or adult
- the location of the accident
- who was involved and what happened (details of witnesses)
- details of the injury
- any treatment that was given
- who was informed of the accident.

Accident books should be kept safely for at least 3 years.

Progress check

Why is it important to inform parents about any accidents their child is involved in?

What information should be recorded in an accident book?

How long should accident books be kept for?

Now try these questions

What action should a child-care worker take if they find an unconscious child in the playground?

Explain why a comprehensive knowledge of first aid is important for child-care workers.

Describe the workplace health and safety policies and procedures in your establishment.

key terms

You need to know what the key terms and phrases in this chapter mean. Go back through the chapter and find out.

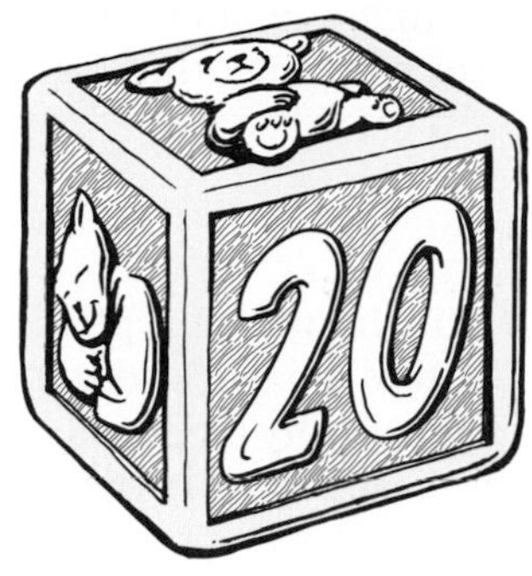

CHILDREN IN HOSPITAL

Sick children are often cared for at home, as it is better for the child to be in familiar surroundings and with their main carers. Children usually go into hospital for short stays for specific treatment and return home as soon as possible.

This chapter will cover the following topics:

- *preparation for admission*
- *play*
- *children with life-threatening or terminal illness.*

Preparation for admission

A large number of children have to go into hospital at some stage in their lives; many go into hospital as emergency admissions so it is important that all children get to know about hospitals. Children often see ambulances and play with toy ones and this will give an opportunity to talk about hospitals. You may pass a hospital in the car or on the bus and can point out the building. There are lots of books about hospitals that you can look at and read with children. In child-care settings the imaginative play area can be used to give opportunities for hospital play or play about doctors and clinics, children can handle 'medical equipment' and try on uniforms. Role play will enable them to try out the situation in a protected environment. Do not wait until the child is going to be admitted before making them familiar with hospitals. This familiarity will help if a child does have to go in to hospital with little or no warning.

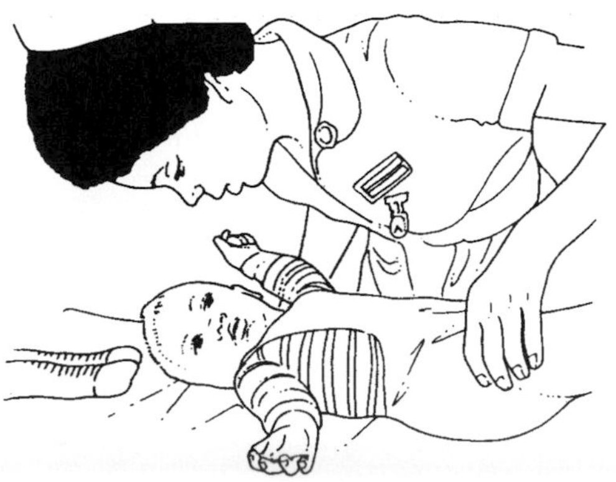

A large number of children have to go into hospital at some stage in their lives

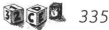

PLANNED ADMISSIONS

Despite general preparation, the prospect of hospital admission can be frightening for the child and the parents or carers. Planned admissions have the advantage of contact with doctors and nurses in the outpatients department. Visits to the ward may be arranged before admission. A hospital booklet especially for children is an important source of information. It may contain pictures of children or a familiar toy such as a teddy participating in hospital activities. It will also have pictures of things that a child is likely to see, like a thermometer or stethoscope.

PREPARING AT HOME

At home the child can be helped to understand what will happen by playing at hospitals. A few days before admission the child should be told clearly and honestly what may happen. Any questions should be answered as truthfully as possible in a way that the child can understand. The child should be assured that parents or carers will be able to arrange to stay overnight and visit whenever possible. How much a child can be told or will understand will depend on their age. Older children may enjoy packing and unpacking their case, choosing favourite toys to bring into hospital, especially if they have a cuddly toy they like to hold. Any special name for these things should be mentioned to the ward staff.

Case study . . .

. . . emergency admission

Jamie is 5 and has been admitted to hospital as an emergency with bad stomach pains and being very sick. Jamie's GP thinks that he might have appendicitis. The doctor at the hospital thinks that this is likely, but as Jamie's condition has improved since his arrival, she is going to observe him for a while and do some more tests. Jamie's Mum was able to come to the hospital with him and they are waiting for his Dad to come. Jamie is feeling a bit better and tells his Mum about how he had played at hospitals at his nursery and how one of his friends had told all the children about how he had been into the hospital when he broke his arm. He remembered how they had all done drawings on his plaster. After a while Jamie got anxious and told his Mum that he didn't want to stay in hospital and wanted to go home. He said the hospital pyjamas were uncomfortable and that his pet rabbit would be missing him. Jamie's Mum comforted him and said that the nurses had told her that she could stay all the while and that she would be sleeping at the hospital with Jamie. She said that when his Dad came he would be bringing Jamie's own pyjamas and his favourite teddy, and that Roy from next door was going to take special care of his rabbit. After this Jamie settled down and even had a little sleep until his Dad came.

1. *What had happened at nursery that helped Jamie to feel more familiar with hospital?*
2. *What did his Mum do to help him settle down more easily?*
3. *If Jamie has to have an operation for his appendicitis, how will the staff help him to understand what is going to happen?*

IN HOSPITAL

Positive reminders

Continuing links with home are important even when a child has parents or carers who are resident or visit frequently. There are ways to provide children with reminders of home:

- familiar possessions, such as clothes, toys, cuddlies
- a photograph for the child's locker

- something familiar belonging to the mother, father and other carers
- letters and cards, to be put up where the child can see them.

Emotional reactions

Children's reactions to being in hospital will be affected by the severity of their illness. The acutely ill child may have little awareness of their surroundings; the less ill child will react sensitively to the environment. The two factors that most affect the child's feelings are age and degree of dependence on parents or carers. Babies and pre-school children are most secure if the parent or carer is with them for all or most of the time; 4 to 8 year olds are beginning to be independent but need a lot of reassurance. They need to have a parent or carer with them, particularly during the more stressful parts of their hospital stay.

Children who are separated from their parent or carer during a stay in hospital may show all the signs of acute distress.

These are:

- *distress* or protest shown by crying, and expressions of anger about being left
- *despair*, where the child fears that their carer might not return and becomes listless, disinterested and refuses to play
- *detachment,* where the child becomes convinced that their carer will never return and their behaviour becomes erratic.

Play

Any severe anxiety may have short-term or longer lasting effects on a child's emotional development. Anxiety associated with being in hospital must be anticipated, recognised and reduced to a minimum. Play can be a valuable way of doing this and there are a variety of opportunities, some of which are outlined below:

- *In the community* – parent and toddler groups, playgroups, nurseries and primary schools can provide play things with a hospital box, toys and books. Children can be encouraged to act out their experiences, in imaginative play and role play. Topics such as 'People who help us'; visits from the school nurse, health visitor or other health personnel will be helpful familiarisation for children. NAWCH (National Association for the Welfare of Children in Hospital) provides information for parents and children about local facilities.
- *Outpatients* – play should be available in outpatients, and children attending can be encouraged to participate by attractive and interesting provision; this helps to reduce children's own anxiety level and that of their parents.
- *In the ward* – when settling in, familiar favourite toys and treasured objects should always be brought into the ward and kept with the child. Most children's wards in hospitals have a play room where a qualified play leader will provide suitable activities, stories and videos for use in the play room and at the bedside.

key term

Regression
responding in a way that is appropriate to an earlier stage of development

PLANNING PLAY

Sick children need to play. but they may not make the effort or have the ability to create suitable play activities for themselves. As mentioned in Chapter 18, in the section on caring for sick children at home, concentration may be lacking, they may tire easily and they may **regress** and revert to a former level of behaviour.

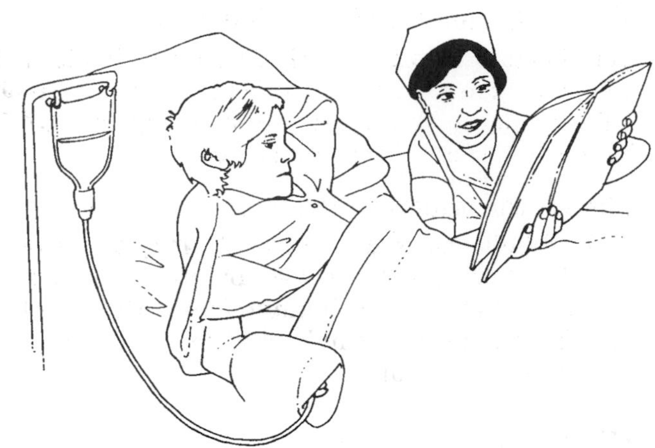

Sick children may lack concentration and tire easily

A variety of play needs to be offered; some children because of their previous experience may need support to play and be messy. Those who are immobile will need individual play. The child should be able to take part fully in the activity. The best play builds on the familiar, fits the child's abilities and stimulates with something new.

THE CHILD CONFINED TO BED

Children who have to stay in bed, because they are very ill, or because their treatment means that they cannot get up, will need appropriate activities that will interest them. These could include, talking, reading, being read to, board games, tapes of stories, videos and hand-held computer games. Variety is the essential ingredient, as children who are ill frequently have short attention spans.

key term
Supine
lying on the back

Supine

Lying **supine** means that vision is restricted. Mirrors can help here, and pictures, posters and mobiles will make the area above the child's head more interesting. Books, listening to stories, tapes and talking, and some board games will be possible, but using the arms for all activities in this position is very tiring.

On the side

If the child has to lie on her side, then activities with play people, animals, board games and trains are possible.

key term
Prone
lying face down

Prone

Lying **prone** more activities are possible, especially if the child is supported on a special frame. The child can then paint, read and play board games.

Sitting up

Children may be confined to bed but able to sit up, for example if they are on traction. They may have lots of energy, which can be released through clay and dough play or a hammering activity.

The child with an intravenous infusion (IV)

An IV may limit mobility but not confine the child to bed. When the IV is set up care is taken not to use the dominant arm. This leaves the more skilful hand free for play. Wherever possible, move the child to where the activities are going on. Suitable activities will include painting, board games, small toys, anything that does not require two hands. If in doubt, try it out one-handed yourself first.

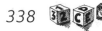

The child needing intensive care

Very ill children may show little interest in play but it is still important to continue visual and aural stimulation. Singing, reading, mobiles, pictures and talking to the child about everyday things are very important. A favourite comfort object needs to be in sight, even if it cannot be held.

The child requiring isolation

A child being nursed in a cubicle may see little of other children. Any visitors, usually adults, may have to wear gowns and masks. As a result, the child will need the carers to spend much more time in the cubicle initiating and joining in with the play. Toys and games will have to stay in the cubicle. Washable toys and water play are especially useful.

THE WARD PLAY ROOM

Many children's wards and departments have their own play rooms with a qualified child-care worker, who will provide play to meet the needs of the children who use it. A full range of play and learning opportunities will be available, with skilled staff to support the children and their parents and carers. In many hospitals there will be a qualified teacher to support the continued learning of school-aged children.

Children with life-threatening or terminal illness

The death of a child seems to be more difficult to accept than the death of an adult. Many people feel that children, with all their future before them, are a far greater loss than an adult who has already lived a full and useful life. The death of a child today, when there are so many ways of preventing death, is far more of a tragedy than in the days when many children died in infancy.

A CHILD'S PERCEPTION OF DEATH

Children have many experiences of death in a broad sense. Loss and separation are also a part of many of their experiences. How they think about these things depends on how the adults close to them react and on the explanations they give. Death is often a subject that is not spoken about and the thought is pushed away, when the need is to think through ideas in order to be able to answer children's questions. The idea of death is complex and is built up over many years. The child's understanding will be limited by:

- previous experience
- language development
- grasp of the concept of time
- intellectual development.

Children who are dying often have very clear images, fears and concerns about death. Adults may say that a child does not know, but many children do realise they are dying and the crucial difference is whether they have the chance to express their feelings or not. To say that a child does not talk about death could mean that the child has had no *chance* to talk, usually because the adults are finding this too difficult.

The young child, under 7, thinks that death is reversible, a state of sleep or separation, from which the person could return. Perhaps the main fear for the young child who is dying is thinking about separation and going into a darkness where there is no one familiar to give love and comfort. Children will express their fears in different ways; they may want close physical comfort and someone to listen and talk to them. At other times, they may express their fears in anger. Their anger can often be directed at the person they love and trust the most. This can often be very hard for loving parents and carers to understand, but it is an indication of the child's feelings of trust in them.

ADULT REACTIONS TO THE DEATH OF A CHILD

Parents' emotions affect the care they give to their dying child and to the rest of the family. Frequently parents experience a range of emotions:

- *Initial shock* – parents and carers may suspect that their child has a life-threatening illness, but the confirmation of this will produce reactions of shock, disbelief, numbness and panic; they may not take in any of the explanations and afterwards may say that no one explained.
- *Confusion* – this is a common reaction, often caused by parents or carers suddenly losing the role they thought they had, that of bringing up a child.
- *Fear* – part of the confusion is because of a gripping physical, emotional fear; there is a feeling of being trapped and being unable to cope with the unknown.
- *Anger* – this arises from the feelings of unfairness that the child is dying; the feelings of anger are often very powerful and it can take very little to trigger them off.
- *Guilt* – parents and carers often take the death of a child as a punishment for something they have done, but this is often unrelated to the child's illness.

STAYING IN THE FAMILY

Children with terminal illness very rarely die in hospital. Families are supported so that they can care for their child at home. Each family can decide upon their own plan of care in consultation with the care team. The family can be in frequent contact with the home-care nurse who acts as the consultant to the family in providing care for their child. During the home visits, home-care nurses also provide emotional support to the child's family. Although families are apprehensive about their child dying at home, good support and a feeling of being in control in familiar surroundings will often create the best and most comfortable circumstances for all the family.

Now try these questions

In what ways can you raise children's awareness of hospitals?

What are the advantages of a planned admission to hospital?

List some of the ways in which children might express their fear of hospital.

What is the role of the home-care nurse?

Describe suitable play for a child who has to stay in bed.

Why is it important for a child's parent or carer to remain with them while they are in hospital?

How can parents and carers be supported while their children are in hospital?

key terms

You need to know what the key terms and phrases in this chapter mean.
Go back through the chapter and find out.

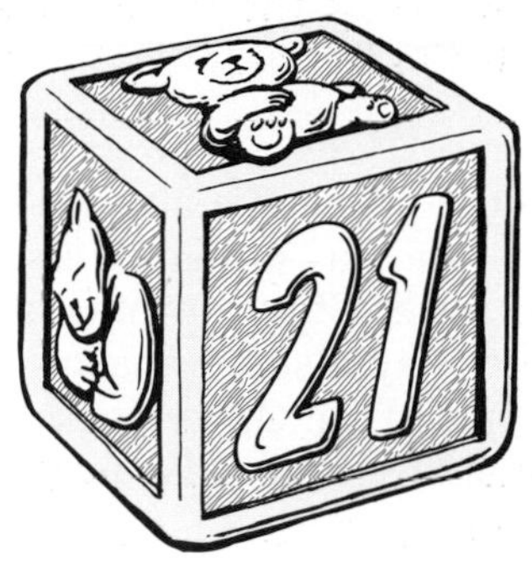

COMMON ILLNESSES AND CONDITIONS

Some childhood illnesses and conditions are long term (chronic), and require child-care workers to have a special degree of knowledge and understanding to support the child and the family through some very difficult times. In order to do this effectively child-care workers must be able to offer, not only appropriate care for a particular illness or condition, but also an understanding of the emotional effects on the child, parents and family.

This chapter will cover the following topics:

- asthma
- autism
- cerebral palsy
- cleft lip/and or palate
- coeliac condition
- cystic fibrosis
- diabetes
- Down syndrome
- epilepsy
- haemophilia
- hearing impairment
- hydrocephalus
- muscular dystrophy (Duchenne)
- phenylketonuria
- sickle cell anaemia
- spina bifida
- visual impairment.

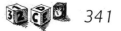

Asthma

key term

Asthma
difficulty in breathing, when the airways in the lungs become narrowed; triggered by allergies, infections, exercise and emotional upset

CAUSES

Asthma (reversible airways obstruction) is a condition in which the airways in the lungs become narrowed. Allergy to certain substances, such as pollen, house dust mite or pet hair, causes the lining of the airways to swell. Children may also be allergic to certain foods, for example, peanuts. There may also be spasm of the airways causing further narrowing, restricting the supply of air. Other factors such as infection, exercise, the weather, cold air or emotional upset may also precipitate attacks.

CHARACTERISTICS

Breathing becomes difficult as the airways go into spasm and the child wheezes and is breathless. The airways may also become narrowed when the linings swell and by increased secretions of mucus. Attacks vary in severity. In a severe attack, breathing becomes very difficult and the child is anxious and afraid. Between attacks breathing is normal. Severe asthma attacks are serious and can be fatal.

DIAGNOSIS

Diagnosis is made by observing the attacks. Skin tests may help identify the allergen.

key terms

Bronchodilator (reliever)
a drug that helps the airways to expand, used to treat asthma

Preventer
drug given on a regular basis to prevent asthma attacks, often given by inhaler

TREATMENT AND PROGRESS

The usual form of treatment is to give drugs called **bronchodilators,** which help the airways to relax and dilate (widen or expand). These are commonly called **relievers** and are given by inhaler so that the drug is breathed in and goes straight to the affected air passages. Drugs can also be given in tablet or linctus form. It is important to try to prevent attacks by avoiding allergens and situations that are known to be problematic. Drugs called **preventers** can also be given by inhaler on a regular basis to help to prevent attacks occurring.

Relievers are given in blue inhalers; preventers are given in brown/orange inhalers.

MANAGEMENT OF AN ASTHMA ATTACK

- Reassure the child.
- Stay with the child.
- Encourage relaxed breathing.
- Give the child their reliever inhaler.
- Sit the child upright in a comfortable position.
- Keep calm and continue to comfort and reassure until the attack subsides.
- You may need to call and ambulance (see page 330).

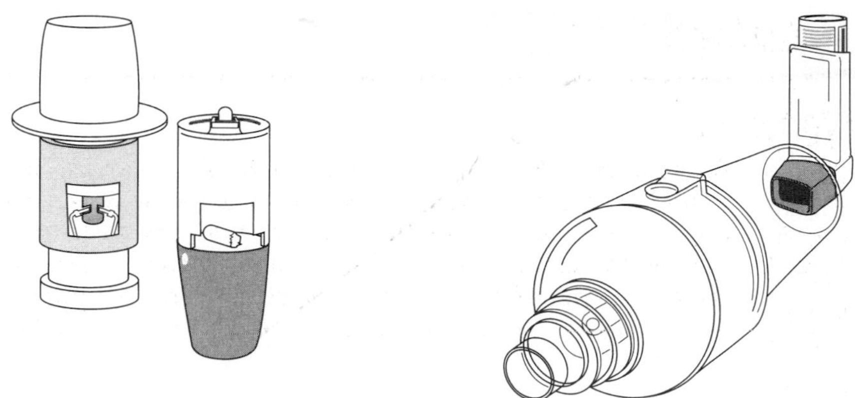

Different types of inhaler used by asthma sufferers

Case study . . .

. . . asthma and allergy

Amy is a lively little 4 year old who enjoys coming to the nursery three times each week. She celebrated her birthday just recently with a lovely party, inviting all her new friends from the nursery. She was especially happy because she had been given lots of presents, including a kitten from her granny. Amy loved the kitten and played with it all day and it came into her bedroom to sleep at night.

Several weeks after her birthday, the staff at the nursery noticed that Amy seemed to get out of breath very quickly. Her mother had also noticed that she had noisy breathing and had developed a cough at night.

What is Amy showing symptoms of?

What new circumstances in Amy's life could have caused her symptoms?

What treatment may help her?

For further information about how to manage an asthma attack, see Chapter 19 Responding to Emergencies.

Autism

CAUSES

A child with **autism** has difficulty in relating to other people and making sense of the social world. The primary cause is unknown. Autism occurs in all parts of the world and usually begins from birth.

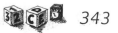

CHARACTERISTICS

key term
Autism
difficulty in relating to other people and making sense of the social world

An autistic child may:

- lack awareness of other people
- pay more attention to objects than people
- have a problem in using non-verbal and/or verbal communication
- may not develop language
- lack imagination and the ability to play
- repeat activities and have uncoordinated body movements
- have learning difficulties.

Some autistic children may have an ability in which they excel, such as drawing.

DIAGNOSIS

Diagnosis is made by observation of the child's progress. Parents or carers often recognise that their child is behaving differently from an early age. They are frequently frustrated that no diagnosis is made. The things they notice may include lack of eye contact, difficulty with feeding, screaming, lack of motor co-ordination, resistance to change.

TREATMENT AND PROGRESS

Treatment is centred on modifying the child's behaviour. Consistent one-to-one care requires patience and skill on the part of all the family members. Pre-school activities are important. Respite care and long-term provision are helpful in enabling young people to gain some independence.

Cerebral palsy

key term
Cerebral palsy
a disorder of movement and posture; part of the brain that controls movement and posture is damaged or fails to develop

CAUSES

Cerebral palsy is a disorder of movement and posture; the part of the brain that controls movement and posture is damaged or fails to develop. There are many causes that may occur before, during or after birth. These include:

- the mother catching rubella during pregnancy
- lack of oxygen to the brain of the baby before or during birth
- Rhesus incompatibility (for more on this, see the section on Practice of antenatal care on page 434)
- pre-eclampsia (you will also find more on this in the section on Practice of antenatal care on page 433)
- birth injury
- accidents or infections after birth.

CHARACTERISTICS

The term cerebral palsy covers a wide range of impairment. There are three main types of impairment of movement:

- *spasticity*, where the movements are stiff, the muscles are tight and the limbs are held rigidly and turned in towards the body
- *athetosis*, when the limbs are floppy, movements are frequent and involuntary, especially when attempts are made to make the movements purposeful
- *ataxia*, where there is a lack of balance and poor co-ordination.

Cerebral palsy may affect and involve one or more limbs.

DIAGNOSIS

Diagnosis is made by observing the child's progress associated with a history of possible brain damage.

key term

Conductive education
a teaching method aimed at enabling motor-impaired children to function in society

TREATMENT AND PROGRESS

No way has been found to repair the damage to the brain. Early assessment is very important. Therapy needs to be individual and works at maximising the child's potential; it may involve physiotherapy, speech therapy, occupational therapy or **conductive education**. Equipment can aid communication, mobility and independent living.

Progress check

What substances might affect the airways of a child who has asthma?

What other factors might bring on an asthma attack?

What is a bronchodilator?

What are the characteristics of a child with autism?

What are the three main types of impairment of movement that might occur in a child with cerebral palsy?

Which part of the body is damaged or impaired if a child has cerebral palsy?

Cleft lip and/or palate

key term

Cleft lip or palate
a structural impairment of the top lip, palate or both

CAUSES

A **cleft lip or palate** is a structural impairment of the top lip, palate or both. The development of the lip and/or the palate fails to take place in the early weeks of fetal life.

CHARACTERISTICS

The failure of the development of the top lip and palate may occur in different ways:

- the lip only may be affected and will be divided into two or three sections by one or two clefts
- the palate only may be divided into two or three sections by one or two clefts

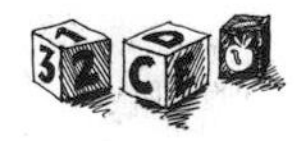

- the lip and the palate may both be divided into two or three sections by one or two clefts.

DIAGNOSIS

Diagnosis is made by the examination of all babies at or soon after birth.

TREATMENT AND PROGRESS

Treatment varies depending on the extent of the impairment; it can be lengthy and involve a series of operations to repair the gaps in the lip and palate. In general, the lip is repaired first, the palate later. Feeding will need careful management, and speech therapy may be required. The medical team treating the child will work closely together to produce the best results. Progress is individual and positive, with good results in many instances.

Coeliac condition

key terms

Coeliac condition
a metabolic disorder involving sensitivity to gluten; there is difficulty in digesting food

Metabolic
related to the process of digesting, absorbing and using food

Gluten
a protein found in wheat, rye, barley and oats

CAUSES

Coeliac condition is a **metabolic** disorder involving sensitivity to **gluten** (a protein found in wheat, rye, barley and oats); there is difficulty in digesting food. There is thought to be a familial tendency to the disease. The lining of the small intestine is sensitive to gluten and the resulting damage reduces the ability to absorb nutrients from the food broken down by the digestive process.

CHARACTERISTICS

The child exhibits signs of malnutrition and does not gain weight and grow normally. The child may also be irritable, have pale, bulky, foul-smelling stools, and may vomit.

DIAGNOSIS

Diagnosis in children is made by observation of the failure to grow and gain weight satisfactorily, particularly after weaning on to foods containing gluten. Diagnosis is also by biopsy and examination of tissue taken from the intestine.

TREATMENT AND PROGRESS

A diet free of gluten must be followed. Gluten is found in many foods but the Coeliac Society produces food lists to help parents and carers. Foods like meat, fish, fresh fruit and vegetables are gluten-free, while anything containing flour contains gluten. The intestine usually recovers and the child will begin to grow normally.

Progress check

Describe three ways in which the development of the lip and/or palate can be affected.

What substance in the diet is a child with coeliac disease sensitive to?

Which part of the digestive tract is affected by the coeliac condition?

Cystic fibrosis (CF)

key term

Cystic fibrosis
an hereditary, life-threatening condition affecting the lungs and digestive tract

CAUSES

Cystic fibrosis is an hereditary and life-threatening condition that affects the lungs and the digestive system. It is a recessively inherited condition. For the child to be affected both parents must carry the CF gene. (For more on this, see the section on Recessive inheritance on pages 294–6.)

key terms

Pancreas
a gland that secretes insulin and enzymes that aid digestion

Enzyme
a substance that helps to digest food

CHARACTERISTICS

Mucus throughout the body is thick and sticky and the airways in the lungs become clogged. There are breathing difficulties, coughing and repeated chest infections. The **pancreas** fails to develop properly and mucus clogs the ducts, affecting the flow of **enzymes** into the digestive tract. Food is not digested and absorbed properly. The child fails to gain weight and grow satisfactorily.

DIAGNOSIS

Family history and genetic counselling may mean that prenatal diagnosis is possible. A blood test is carried out on the 6th day after the birth as part of routine screening. Later, diagnosis is by observation of the baby's symptoms, followed by a sweat test and/or a blood test.

TREATMENT AND PROGRESS

The treatment is aimed at:

- keeping the lungs free from infection, with antibiotic therapy
- respiratory education and therapy to expel mucus and keep the lungs clear
- pancreatic enzymes taken with every meal; a high-protein diet with vitamin and mineral supplements is prescribed.

Treatment is time-consuming, but children gradually become more independent and are able to manage and understand their condition.

Diabetes

key term

Diabetes
a condition in which the body cannot metabolise carbohydrates, resulting in high levels of sugar in the blood and urine

CAUSE

Diabetes occurs when the pancreas gland produces insufficient amounts of **insulin** or none at all, resulting in high levels of sugar (glucose) in the blood. Insulin controls the amount of glucose in the body; its absence results in abnormally high levels of glucose in the blood and urine.

There are two types of diabetes:

- Type 1, usually starting before 30 years of age and requiring insulin injections
- Type 2, common in older people and controlled with diet and medication.

CHARACTERISTICS

Early symptoms of diabetes are excessive thirst, frequent passing of urine; children may lose weight. Complications include visual impairment, kidney damage and

key term

Insulin
a hormone produced in the pancreas to metabolise carbohydrate in the bloodstream and regulate glucose

problems with circulation. Untreated diabetes will lead to the insulin levels dropping; unconsciousness and coma quickly follow.

DIAGNOSIS

Diagnosis is by observation of the child's symptoms, and by testing the blood and/or urine for sugar.

TREATMENT AND PROGRESS

For children, treatment is by injections of insulin together with a carefully controlled diet that restricts the amount of carbohydrate that can be eaten. Children quickly learn how to test their own blood and/or urine and keep a record of the results. They also learn how to give their own insulin. To keep healthy requires regular meals, regular insulin, regular exercise and regular medical supervision. Once the child and family have adjusted to the need for regular treatment and diet, a full and active life is possible.

key term

Hypoglycaemia
low levels of glucose in the blood

One of the possible complications that may occur when a child is in your care is **hypoglycaemia** – low levels of glucose in the blood.

Signs of hypoglycaemia:

- irritability
- confusion, loss of co-ordination and concentration
- rapid breathing
- sweating
- dizziness.

Management of a hypoglycaemic attack:

- Stay with the child.
- Give glucose to drink if the child is conscious and able to swallow.
- If the child is unconscious, put them in the recovery position (see Chapter 19, Responding to Emergencies) and get someone to call an ambulance. Stay with the child.

Case study . . .

. . . recognising signs and symptoms of diabetes

Ben is 5 years old and has just started at his local infants school. He had not been coming to school long before his mother became worried about him. She came into school to discuss the situation with the class teacher and the nursery nurse. Ben's mum had noticed that he was always tired these days, having previously been a really lively boy. He had lost his appetite, but seemed to need a lot more to drink. His mum wondered if this was why he had wet the bed a few times. Ben's class teacher and nursery nurse had noticed that Ben seemed to be unable to concentrate, he also seemed to be drowsy and sweaty at times. Ben's mum was taking him to the family doctor that evening.

1. *List Ben's symptoms.*
2. *What do you think might be wrong with Ben?*
3. *How will a diagnosis of Ben's condition be made?*
4. *What is the likely treatment for Ben's condition?*

Down syndrome

key term

Down syndrome
a condition caused by an abnormal chromosome, which affects a person's appearance and development

CAUSE

Down syndrome (previously Down's syndrome) is caused by an abnormal chromosome; usually chromosome 21.

CHARACTERISTICS

Down syndrome may affect the child's appearance and development. The condition may be identified soon after birth by the presence of typical characteristics. Not all the children will show all the characteristics to the same degree, but they may include some of the following:

- almond-shaped eyes
- short hands and feet – the hands may have a single palmar crease
- small jaw, so that the tongue appears large
- poor muscle tone
- poorly developed nose, sinuses and lungs, with increased susceptibility to infections.

There may be other impairments, such as heart disease.

key terms

Amniocentesis
a sample of amniotic fluid is taken via a needle inserted into the uterus through the abdominal wall; used to detect chromosomal abnormalities

Chorionic villus sampling (CVS)
A small sample of placental tissue is removed via the vagina; used to detect chromosomal and other abnormalities

DIAGNOSIS

Pre-natal tests are available for high-risk groups. The most common is **amniocentesis**, which is carried out after the 16th week of pregnancy. **Chorionic villus sampling (CVS),** carried out at 8 to 11 weeks of pregnancy, can also be used to detect Down syndrome. Diagnosis can also be made by observation of the characteristics after birth.

TREATMENT AND PROGRESS

Treatment is given to respiratory tract infections and any other impairment that may affect the child. There is assessment and help with areas of development that may be affected. A stimulating environment and positive attitude help the children reach their full potential.

Progress check

What is the cause of cystic fibrosis?

How is a child with cystic fibrosis affected?

What causes diabetes?

What is the treatment for Type 1 diabetes?

What is the cause of Down syndrome?

Describe one test carried out in pregnancy to detect Down syndrome.

Epilepsy

key term

Epilepsy
recurrent attacks of temporary disturbance of the brain function

CAUSE

Epilepsy is a condition in which there are recurrent attacks of temporary disturbance of brain function. It may be caused by severe injury, stroke or brain tumour. It may occur spontaneously or be triggered by stimuli such as flickering lights, fever or drugs. There may be a familial tendency towards the condition.

CHARACTERISTICS

Epilepsy can take many different forms. The condition is different for each child and ranges from disturbances in consciousness that are scarcely noticeable, such as mild sensations and lapses of concentration, to severe seizures with convulsions.

DIAGNOSIS

Diagnosis is by observation and history of seizures (fits), by EEG (electroencephalogram), which measures the electrical activity of the brain. Tests are also undertaken to exclude other causes.

key term

Anti-convulsant
a drug that is given to prevent fits

TREATMENT AND PROGRESS

Anti-convulsant drugs are used to control the seizures. Care is important so that obvious dangers are avoided and to ensure that medication is taken regularly. Fear and misconception have always reinforced the stigma of epilepsy, so the child will need plenty of understanding and support. Most children with epilepsy go to mainstream schools.

Recognising major epilepsy

A fit progresses through the following stages:

- sudden falling into unconsciousness
- rigidity and arching of the back
- jerking movements
- breathing may cease
- froth or bubbles round the mouth
- bladder or bowel control lost
- regains consciousness within a few minutes
- feels dazed or confused
- may need to sleep.

Managing an epileptic attack

- Clear a space around the child.
- Protect the head with padding.
- Do not restrain or put anything in the mouth.
- When the convulsions have stopped, check airway and breathing.
- Put in the recovery position (see Chapter 19, Responding to Emergencies).

- Stay with the child at all times and reassure.
- If the child has never had a fit before, if they fit again, or remain unconscious for more than 10 minutes, call an ambulance.

Haemophilia

key term

Haemophilia an inherited blood disorder, where there is a defect in one of the clotting factors

Haemophilia is an inherited blood disorder where there is a defect in one of the clotting factors. It is inherited through the female line, but causes bleeding only in the male.

CHARACTERISTICS

Bleeding will occur for much longer than normal after an injury; it may occur spontaneously into joints and elsewhere in the body; bruising is common. The child may experience severe pain when bleeding occurs into a joint.

DIAGNOSIS

Diagnosis is made by knowing the family history, followed by prenatal tests such as chorionic villus sampling; and by observation of the symptoms after birth.

TREATMENT AND PROGRESS

Haemophilia centres provide treatment and support. Treatment is given with injections of the appropriate clotting factor. Progress will depend on a balance being achieved between adequate protection and allowing the child to grow up into a well-adjusted healthy adult. Although the chance of bleeding is always present, it is important that child-care workers enable children with haemophilia to take part in normal activities as far as possible.

Hearing impairment

key term

Hearing impairment either conductive deafness or nerve deafness; ranges from slight hearing difficulty to profound deafness

CAUSES

Causes of **hearing impairment** include:

- heredity
- impairment of the cochlea nerve
- maternal rubella in pregnancy
- congenital defects
- head injury
- otitis media (infection of the middle ear)
- infections such as meningitis
- toxic action of drugs, such as streptomycin
- blockage of the ear canal by wax or other foreign bodies.

CHARACTERISTICS

There is a wide range of impairment affecting a substantial proportion of people in the UK. Hearing impairment falls into two main categories:

- **conductive deafness**, an interruption to the mechanical process of conducting sound through the ear drum and across the middle ear
- **nerve deafness**, which is damage to the cochlea (part of the inner ear), the auditory nerve or the hearing centres in the brain; the range of impairment is very wide, from slight loss to profound deafness.

key terms

Conductive deafness
deafness caused by an interruption to the process of sounds passing through the eardrum and the middle ear

Nerve deafness
deafness caused by damage to the inner ear, or to the nerves, or hearing centres in the brain

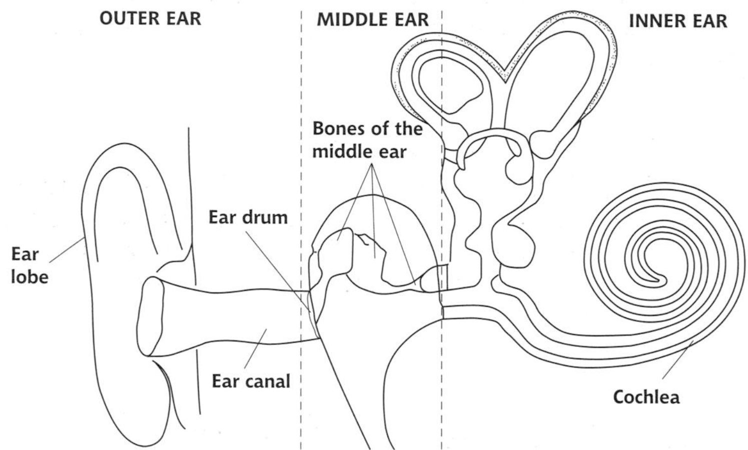

The structure of the ear

DIAGNOSIS

Initially parents or carers often suspect a hearing difficulty. Diagnosis is by hearing tests; the first hearing test is usually at 7 months, but testing is possible at any age. (See Chapter 15, The Promotion and Maintenance of Health.)

TREATMENT AND PROGRESS

Conductive deafness can often be treated by removing blockages, treating infections and some surgical treatments. Nerve deafness is much more difficult to treat but a cochlea implant has recently become available.

Early diagnosis is very important. Child-care workers need to be aware that most children will experience hearing loss at some time, usually caused by middle ear infections related to colds. Carers need to be aware and supportive.

Progress check

What should you do if a child in your care has a major epileptic convulsion?

What is the cause of haemophilia?

What are the two main types of deafness?

When is a child's hearing first normally tested?

What is the most common cause of a middle ear infection?

Hydrocephalus

key term

Hydrocephalus
a condition involving an increase in the fluid surrounding the brain, often associated with spina bifida

key term

Cerebro-spinal fluid
the fluid surrounding the brain and spinal cord

CAUSE

Hydrocephalus is an increase in the fluid surrounding the brain. The cause is not known but it is often associated with spina bifida.

CHARACTERISTICS

Cerebro-spinal fluid (surrounding the brain and spinal cord) increases because it is unable to drain in the usual way. The head becomes larger and in a small baby the fontanelles and sutures may widen. Increasing pressure on the brain causes pain and brain damage.

TREATMENT AND PROGRESS

Early diagnosis is by measuring the head circumference. The introduction of a valve (shunt) allows the cerebro-spinal fluid to drain satisfactorily. Early detection stops damage to the brain. The child should then be able to make progress, although frequent hospital visits and susceptibility to repeated infection may be a problem.

Muscular dystrophy (Duchenne)

key term

Duchenne muscular dystrophy
a condition involving progressive destruction of muscle tissue, only affecting boys

CAUSE

Duchenne muscular dystrophy is a life-threatening condition involving progressive destruction of muscle tissue. The condition only affects boys and is an abnormality of the X chromosome inherited through the female line (see Chapter 16).

CHARACTERISTICS

Duchenne is the most common and most severe type of muscular dystrophy. At birth there is usually no sign of disability. Later clumsiness in walking, frequent falls and difficulty in running become evident. Muscle weakness is slowly progressive so that everyday activities become more difficult. As walking becomes impossible, a wheelchair will be needed. Eventually the muscles of the hands, face and respiration are affected, and respiratory tract infections usually prove fatal.

DIAGNOSIS

Diagnosis is made by knowing the family history. Prenatal tests, such as amniocentesis, can be used to detect Duchenne muscular dystrophy. There will also be observation of the above characteristics after birth.

TREATMENT AND PROGRESS

Parents or carers may often know that there is a problem early on. Treatment is aimed at maintaining mobility and independence for as long as possible. Parents or carers and families will need information and support. The child will need to be able to discuss his feelings and have long-term support to understand the progressive nature of his condition. Child-care workers will need to support and maintain mobility and independence for as long as possible.

Phenylketonuria (PKU)

key term

Phenylketonuria (PKU)
a metabolic impairment that prevents the normal digestion of protein; recessively inherited

CAUSE

Phenylketonuria (PKU) is a metabolic impairment that prevents the normal digestion of protein. It is recessively inherited (see Chapter 16 for more on this). A child will develop PKU if both parents carry and pass on one altered PKU gene. There is an inherited defect in an enzyme, called phenylalanine hydroxylase. This means that the child cannot use the amino acid phenylalanine, which is part of protein, in the usual way. This substance builds up in the body and causes progressive brain damage.

CHARACTERISTICS

If left untreated, the high levels of phenylalanine that build up in the body will damage the developing brain. All areas of development may be affected.

DIAGNOSIS

key term

Guthrie test
on the sixth day after birth, a sample of the baby's blood is taken, usually by pricking the heel, to test for phenylketonuria, cystic fibrosis and cretinism

All babies born in the UK are screened for PKU by a blood test. This test is called the **Guthrie test** and is taken on the 6th day after birth and after the baby has had some milk feeds (breast or formula). The midwife takes a sample of the baby's blood, usually by pricking the heel. This blood test is also used to detect other possible problems such as hypothyroidism, which is an endocrine disorder where the thyroid gland is not working properly.

TREATMENT AND PROGRESS

Early diagnosis means that babies with PKU can be given a diet in which the amount of phenylalanine is carefully controlled. The treatment is complex but with support the children can learn to manage their diet and be independent.

Progress check

Describe hydrocephalus.

What is the cause of Duchenne muscular dystrophy?

Who may be affected by Duchenne muscular dystrophy and why?

Describe the test for PKU.

If a child has PKU, which of the main food groups needs to be modified?

Sickle cell anaemia

CAUSE

Sickle cell anaemia (or sickle cell condition) is an inherited condition of **haemoglobin** formation. If a child inherits sickle haemoglobin from one parent, they will have *sickle cell trait*, which is symptom-free. If, however, a child inherits sickle haemoglobin from both parents, they will have sickle cell anaemia.

key terms

Sickle cell anaemia
an inherited condition of haemoglobin formation

Haemoglobin
a red oxygen-carrying protein containing iron, present in the red blood cells

CHARACTERISTICS

Sickle cell anaemia causes bouts of anaemia, pain, jaundice and infection, called *crises*. Painful crises are caused by the red cells in the blood changing their shape from the normal round shape to a crescent or sickle shape. The sickle cells clump together and block the smaller blood vessels causing pain and swelling. Pain is common in the arms, legs, back and stomach. There may be swelling of the hands and feet. The sickle cells are also removed more quickly from the bloodstream, causing anaemia.

DIAGNOSIS

Diagnosis is made by knowing the family history, prenatal tests and a specific blood test after birth, and by observation of any symptoms.

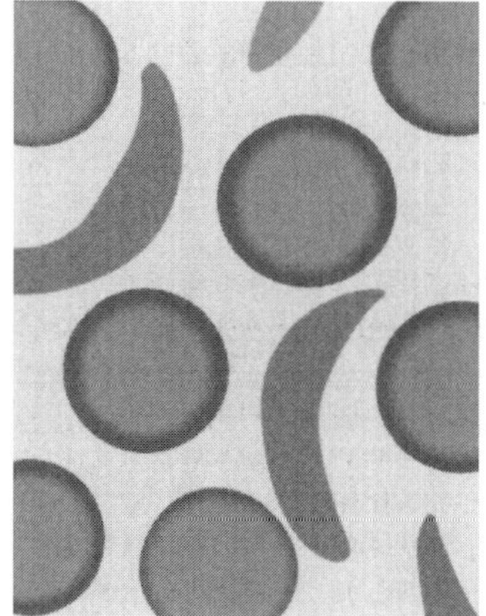

Normal and sickle red blood cells

TREATMENT AND PROGRESS

Prompt recognition and treatment are important. Carers will aim to maintain good general health and diet and arrange for early treatment of infections, keeping the child warm and dry with plenty of rest. Blood transfusions may be needed. Support and understanding are needed particularly during crises. Co-operation between home, school and hospital will give the child the best opportunity to manage the condition and become independent.

Spina bifida

key term

Spina bifida
a condition in which the spine fails to develop properly before birth

CAUSE

Spina bifida occurs when an area of the spine fails to develop properly before birth. There is a gap in the bones of the spine leaving the contents of the spinal cord exposed. The fault can occur anywhere on the spine. The precise cause is not known, but there are thought to be environmental and genetic factors that prevent the normal development of the bones of the spine.

CHARACTERISTICS

There are two main forms of spina bifida:

- *spina bifida occulta*, in which the skin is intact – this rarely causes disability
- *spina bifida cystica*, which has two types:
  - *meningocele*, in which there is a fluid-filled sac on the back, where the fluid and membranes of the spinal cord protrude through the gap in the bones of the spine
  - *mylomeningocele*, in which the sac contains spinal fluid and the nerves of the spinal cord.

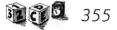

Mylomeningocele is the most severe form. As a result there is some degree of paralysis below the lesion.

DIAGNOSIS

Diagnosis is by prenatal blood tests, ultrasound scan and/or amniocentesis.

TREATMENT AND PROGRESS

Treatment is by closure of the lesion and prevention of infection. There will also be treatment of associated hydrocephalus (see above). Ongoing support is needed to enable the child to take part in all the usual activities for their age, such as playgroup, nursery or mainstream school.

Visual impairment

key term

Visual impairment impairment of sight, ranging from blindness to partial sight

CAUSES

Visual impairment may be present at birth (congenital) or may occur later. The causes of congenital blindness include infections in pregnancy, such as rubella and syphilis, optic nerve atrophy or tumour. Causes after birth include cataract, glaucoma and infections such as measles and the herpes virus. There are some hereditary conditions such as retinitis pigmentosa.

CHARACTERISTICS

There are three main categories of visual impairment:

- blind
- partially sighted and entitled to use the services appropriate to blind people
- partially sighted.

The experience of visual loss is very different for those who become blind and can use their experience of sight, from those who are born blind.

DIAGNOSIS

The condition is usually detected early as parents or carers recognise the lack of response to visual stimuli and eye contact. Later, vision tests may confirm earlier problems.

TREATMENT AND PROGRESS

Early diagnosis is followed with support, practical information and time for families to adjust. Spectacles and contact lenses are valuable aids for some partially sighted children. Carers will need to encourage exploration and independence. The Royal National Institute for the Blind has a full range of support services, including education advice services, specialist schools and a wide range of supporting aids, books in Braille, Moon and talking books. Progress towards independence will vary with individual children.

Progress check

What happens to the red blood cells if a child has sickle cell condition?

What causes a painful crisis in sickle cell anaemia?

Briefly describe spina bifida.

What are the three main types of spina bifida?

What are the early signs of visual impairment?

Now try these questions

A child in your care has asthma. How could you ensure that the risk of an asthma attack is reduced? Describe how you would manage an asthma attack.

What is the Guthrie test? When is this test done and what conditions does it detect?

What important points would you need to consider if you were caring for a child with sickle cell anaemia.

Describe the causes of hearing impairment.

Describe the stages of a major epileptic attack.

key terms

You need to know what the key terms and phrases in this chapter mean. Go back through the chapter and find out.

Unit 6: Play, Curriculum and Early Learning

This unit will enable you to recognise the different types of children's play and the links between play and learning. You will learn about your own role and that of other adults in promoting children's learning and how to provide a positive environment that allows this to take place. You will also learn about statutory requirements regarding the structure and content of the curriculum and the context in which current approaches to the curriculum have developed.

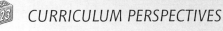

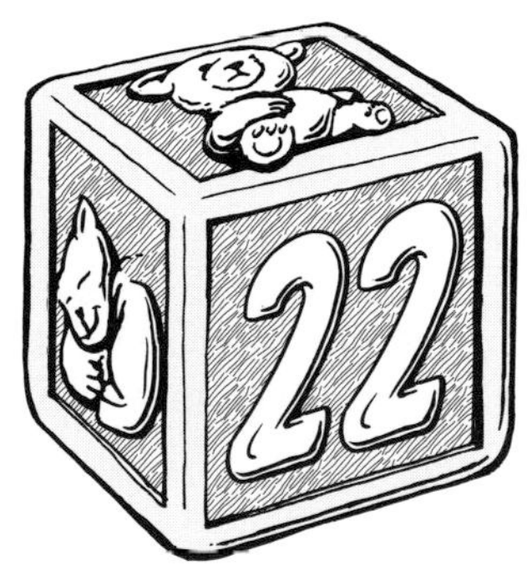

PLAY

Young children and babies need to acquire many skills and to find out about the world they live in. They do this through relentless exploration of their environment and constant practising of their developing skills. Adults call this play. To enable children to get the most out of their play, it is important that people who are involved with children understand the value of play and how to organise play opportunities.

This chapter will cover the following topics:

- *why is play a good way of meeting young children's needs?*
- *types of play*
- *the role of adults in play.*

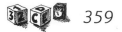

Why is play a good way of meeting young children's needs?

key term

Self-esteem
liking and valuing oneself

- Play occurs naturally in young children. It is therefore familiar to the child, a link between home and the establishment they are in. It is a way to harness what the child is already able to do to help their learning.
- Play cannot be wrong. It therefore provides a safe situation for the child to try out new things without the fear of failure. This is important for the child's development of a positive **self-esteem**.
- Play provides the opportunity for repetition. One of the important ways that learning takes place is through repetition. Play provides the opportunity for the child to practise and consolidate new skills in an enjoyable, familiar and interesting way.
- Play provides the opportunity for extending learning. A carefully structured play environment will provide opportunities for learning across a wide ability range. For example, sand can be a soothing, sensory experience and also provide the opportunity for a child to begin to learn about capacity and volume. A child's skills can therefore develop in a familiar situation, one where there is no competition between the physical skills and the intellectual and language skills.
- Play provides the opportunity for a child to practise and perfect their skills in a safe environment. Through play situations, children can also try out new skills. This can be done within a safe environment as the child can opt out of the play situation when they want.
- Play is always at the child's own level, so the needs of all children within the group can be met. It is important therefore to make sure that there is a range of play materials and equipment to enable all children to participate at their own level. Adult intervention in a child's play is necessary to move them on to the next developmental level.

Progress check

How do children and babies find out about the world?

Why is play familiar to children?

Why is play safe for children?

Why is repetition in play important for children?

How can play meet the needs of all the children in the group?

key term

Physical development
the development of bodily movement and control

WHAT CHILDREN LEARN THROUGH PLAYING

Young children need to develop a whole range of skills. These need to be practised and developed through the opportunity to repeat them in concrete situations. The skills that a child needs to develop can be categorised into a number of areas to make them easy to understand and learn (see the figure below), but it is important to remember that children's development cannot be divided up in the same way. All the areas of development are dependent upon one another.

SOCIAL DEVELOPMENT
The development of skills needed to interact with other people in both individual and group settings.

EMOTIONAL DEVELOPMENT
Concerned with the development of healthy expression and control of feelings and emotions. This includes feelings about self. This is called self-esteem.

THE DEVELOPING CHILD

PHYSICAL DEVELOPMENT
The development of bodily movement and control. It can be divided into two main areas: gross motor and fine motor skills.

LANGUAGE (LINGUISTIC) DEVELOPMENT
The development of communication through speaking or British Sign Language; this includes non-verbal communication. It is also the development of early reading and writing skills.

COGNITIVE (INTELLECTUAL) DEVELOPMENT
The development of thinking and learning skills; it includes the development of concepts, problem-solving skills, the imagination, creativity, memory and concentration.

The developing child

key terms

Gross motor skills
whole body and limb movements, co-ordination and balance

Fine motor skills
small finger movements and manipulative skills, hand–eye co-ordination

Play provides the opportunity for all these skills to be developed. It also has the advantages of being familiar to the child, secure in that mistakes are not permanent and always at an appropriate level. It is also enjoyable and provides the opportunity for the repetition of skills necessary to learning.

Physical development

Physical development is the growth, development and control of bodily movements. Children need to practise these skills by repeating them over and over again. Physical development includes:

- **gross motor skills** – whole body and limb movements, co-ordination and balance
- **fine motor skills** – small finger movements, manipulative skills and hand–eye co-ordination.

Case study . . .

. . . developing fine motor skills

As part of their ongoing assessment of the children, staff in the nursery noted that, overall, the children in the group needed to work at their fine motor skills. The staff decided to work towards doing some sewing with each child. They planned a series of activities, linked to the sewing, to develop the children's manipulative skills and their hand–eye co-ordination. Over a term, alongside all the other activities, the children were encouraged to:

- play with lacing boards and tiles
- thread beads, cotton reels and buttons
- play with peg boards
- do some weaving
- complete simple sewing boards, with laces and bodkin needles.

Finally, when staff felt that they were likely to succeed, each child was introduced to sewing.

1. *Why is sewing a good way to develop fine motor skills?*
2. *Why did the staff plan activities linked to sewing for the children to attempt first?*

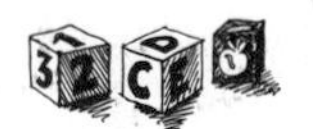

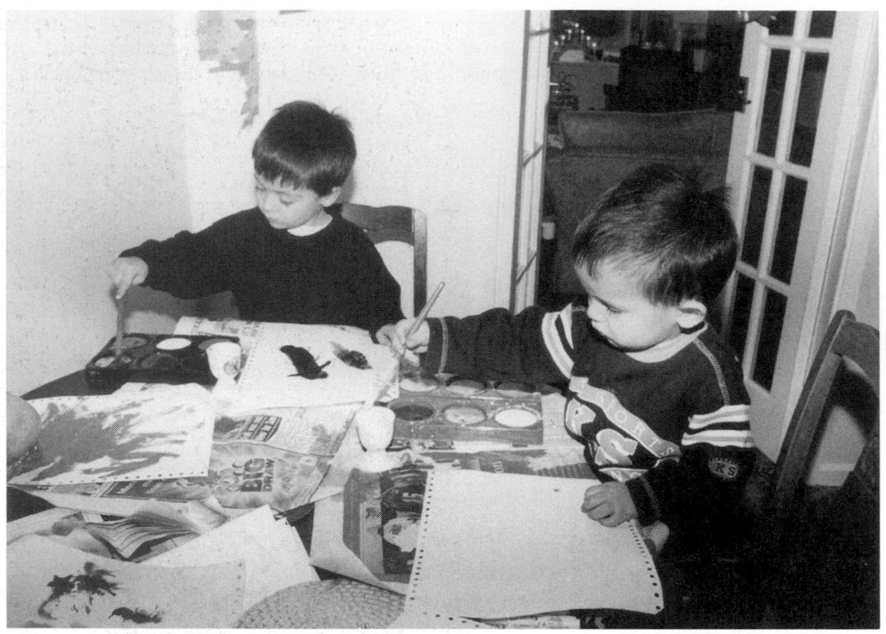

Painting activities contribute to the development of fine motor skills

Outdoor play

Outdoor play is an important aspect of physical development. It provides the opportunity for a range of physical skills to be practised and developed, but there are many other benefits:

- fresh air and exercise that aid growth and development
- space, which allows children to release energy; this provides a contrast to indoor areas within an establishment where physical movement needs to be restricted
- the opportunity to make a noise; indoors low levels of noise need to be maintained. Outdoors children can make far more noise, which may help them to adapt to the usual necessary restrictions
- a different time scale – more space may result in longer play sequences. The space is usually not required for other activities and fewer restrictions are necessary
- adjustment to the school environment; play outside is familiar to most children. It allows a feeling of freedom. Nursery children can get used to playtime
- discovery of the environment; children can experience different materials (leaves, twigs, pebbles, stones). Outdoor play provides a rich sensory experience where children can develop awareness of many concepts, for example wind, rain, temperature, light and shade, smell, water, heat and cold.

Outdoor play needs to be as carefully planned as all other play activities. Issues that need to be considered include safety, staffing, space, storage, opportunities for all skills to be developed and all children to be involved over a range of abilities and needs.

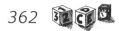

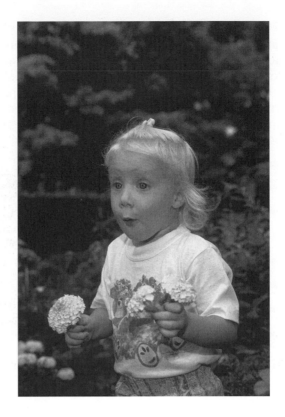

Children can experience different materials in an outdoor environment

> **key term**
>
> **Cognitive development** the development of thinking and understanding, which includes problem solving, reasoning, concentration, memory, imagination and creativity; also called intellectual development

Cognitive development

Cognitive development (or intellectual development) is the development of thinking and learning skills. It includes the development of concepts, problem-solving skills, creativity, imagination, memory and concentration. Play provides the opportunity for the early stages of all these skills to be developed.

A painting activity, for example, may develop the following skills:

- Concepts of colour, size, shape, properties of water, mixing, thick, thin, wet and dry.
- An opportunity to work through problems of how to stop the paint running, how to mix colours, how to stop the paintbrush dripping, what size to draw to fit everything on to the page. These may seem like simple problems, but the child is developing skills that can be applied elsewhere.
- An opportunity to use creative and imaginative skills. Children choose what to paint and develop their own ways of representing their ideas. Again, the skills necessary to enable them to do this can be transferred to other situations where the child needs to think through ideas or problems and develop personal responses to them.
- Children are encouraged, by being involved in an absorbing and enjoyable activity, to use their memory and develop their skills of concentration by finishing what they started.

Through play, therefore, children have the opportunity to acquire, practise and consolidate intellectual skills that form the basis of later learning. This can be done in a secure, familiar and enjoyable environment.

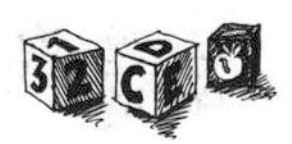

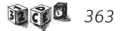

key terms

Language development
the development of communication skills, which includes non-verbal communication, reading and writing, as well as spoken language; also called linguistic development

Non-verbal communication
non-spoken communication, for example, bodily movements, eye contact, gestures and facial expression; sometimes used to enhance or replace speech

Language development

Language development (or linguistic development) is the development of communication skills. This includes verbal skills (talking) and **non-verbal communication** skills (gesture, eye contact, body movements), reading and writing. Early language development is mainly concerned with expressive language (spoken or signed). Written language and reading are later skills. Again, like all other skills, expressive language skills are acquired, practised and refined through use. As children play they use expressive language for many things:

- describing
- discussing
- reporting
- imagining
- predicting
- asking and answering questions
- practising new words
- forming and maintaining relationships.

To enable children to learn and practise their spoken language they need:

- good role models
- the opportunity to speak and to practise their speech
- adults who are sensitive to both their present level of development and the next stage.

Play provides the opportunity for children to interact with adults and other children to hear and see language, and to practise and develop their own skills. Interaction can occur during any activity or experience.

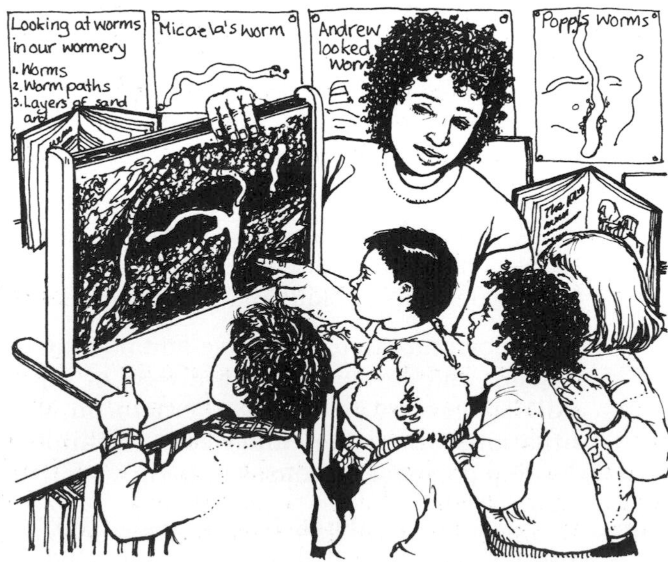

Talking with others is necessary for children to pick up language and to adjust and refine their language skills

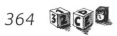

Non-verbal communication

As well as verbal or expressive language, children acquire non-verbal communication skills through play. These are bodily movements, gestures, eye contact, facial expression, and so on. Non-verbal communication sometimes replaces speech, for example a finger on the lips indicating a command to be quiet. It also forms part of what we are saying when speaking, for example pointing to emphasis a point, facial expression reflecting what is being said. The meanings of these non-verbal signs are understood in the same way as spoken language. They have a powerful impact, and when the non-verbal clues are misunderstood, the meaning of what is being said can be misinterpreted. (It is important to realise that there are cultural differences in the meanings of some non-verbal signs. This can also lead to misinterpretation of what is being said or meant.)

Children's interaction with others in their play provides the opportunity to observe, learn and practise these non-verbal communication signs. For example, a child can become other people in a role play and adopt their use of spoken language, tone of voice and non-verbal signs. They can observe the effect these have on others and adapt and change them as they wish. This is all done in the knowledge that the child can opt out of the play at any time if they begin to feel uncomfortable in the role.

Case study . . .

. . . using communication skills in imaginative play

Sarah and Christopher were playing in the imaginative play area, which was a shop. Sarah was the shopkeeper and Christopher the customer:

Sarah	Can I help you?
Christopher	Yes, some people are coming to my house for tea and I need to buy some food.
Sarah	We have got bread and beans. Do your friends like beans on toast?
Christopher	I think so. There are hundreds of my friends coming so I will need lots of food.
Sarah	OK. We have got huge tins in our shop. How many will you need?
Christopher	Twenty hundred.
Sarah	There you are. Fifteen pence please.

1. *How did Sarah and Christopher use language in this interchange? (Refer to the list above.)*
2. *Which non-verbal signs may they have used?*
3. *How may this activity have helped their development?*

Developing an understanding of reading and writing

Children also need opportunities to develop an understanding of reading and writing. Play provides this opportunity. For example, if notepads, pencils, menus, pricelists and notices are provided in an imaginative play area that is a cafe or restaurant, children have the opportunity to develop early reading and writing skills. By imitating what they have seen in cafes or restaurants, they may pretend to read the menus, make marks on the paper to represent writing when taking orders and refer to pricelists. This puts reading and writing into a realistic context where children can begin to understand the importance of these skills. Older children who have acquired some reading and writing skills can further develop them in similar play situations.

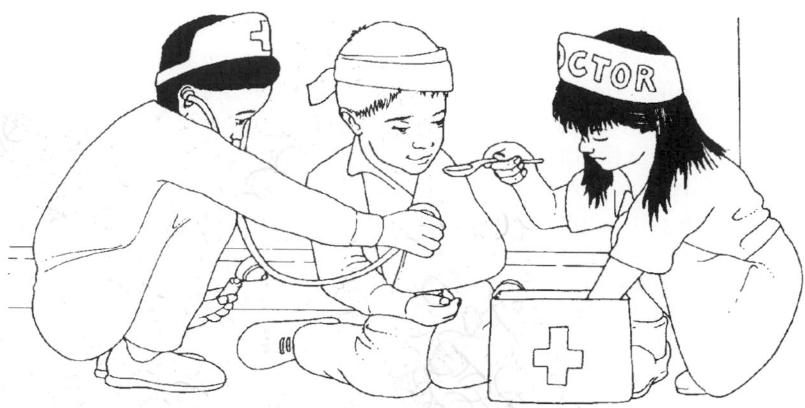

A child can become other people in a role play, but opt out of the play at any time if they begin to feel uncomfortable

key term

Emotional development the development of the healthy expression and control of feelings and emotions. This includes feelings about oneself

Emotional development

Emotional development includes the development of the healthy control and expression of feelings and emotions. These are learned skills and are often culturally defined. Emotional development is also concerned with the development of feelings about self (self-esteem).

Feelings exist and cannot be changed. It is the behaviour that results from the feelings that can be modified. Through play, children have the opportunity to explore feelings that they have. They have the opportunity to experiment with responses to their feelings. Play enables children to express positive feelings openly and begin to develop ways of expressing difficult feelings in acceptable ways.

Case study . . .

. . . expressing and exploring emotions in imaginary play

Amelia's mummy had just had a new baby. Initially she was excited and spoke a lot about the baby and what she did to help look after her. Once this initial excitement had died down, the staff noticed how she would role play being her mummy over and over again.

In the home corner, with a friend, Amelia would be the mummy and her friend became Amelia. They looked after the baby together. However, in role, Amelia would tell her friend that she was too tired to play and that they couldn't go to the park now because the baby needed to be fed. During this play, Amelia instructed her friend to cry when she was told that she couldn't do something that she wanted to do. Amelia responded by sighing a lot, putting her arm around her friend and kissing her, and sitting her on her knee to comfort her.

1. *Why do you think Amelia wanted to play like this?*
2. *What are the benefits of this role play?*

Play can also be a positive **self-concept** builder. The way that we feel about ourselves has a large impact on all aspects of our lives. It is therefore important that children develop a positive self-esteem. Play is familiar and natural to them and so is not a threatening experience – as we have already said, play cannot be wrong. Children play at their own level and so the risk of constant failure is minimised. This

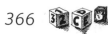

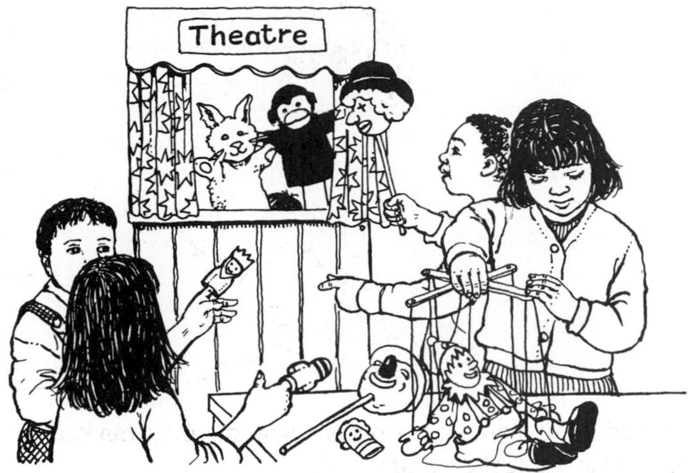

Imaginative play enables children to feel what it is like to be somebody or something else

key term

Self-concept (or self-image) the image that we have of ourselves and the way we think that other people see us

familiar positive environment gives them the opportunity to develop a positive sense of their achievements and to begin to feel good about themselves. This in turn affects their later development.

key term

Social development the growth of the ability to relate to others appropriately and become independent, within a social framework

Social development

Social development is concerned with the development of skills that enable children to get on successfully with other people. Social skills enable a child to become a reasonable, acceptable and effective member of a community. These skills are learned through interaction with other people. It is a life-long process. Young children need to begin to acquire skills such as:

- sharing
- taking turns
- co-operating
- making and maintaining friendships
- responding to people in an appropriate way.

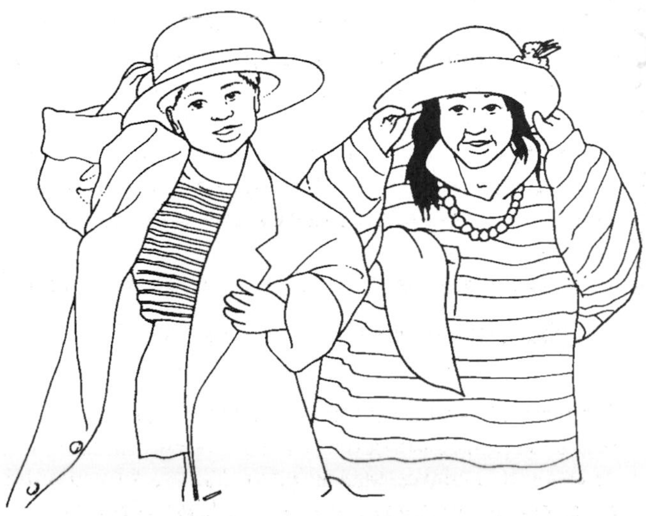

Play is also a positive self-concept builder

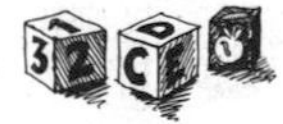

Play acts as a bridge to social skills and relationships. It provides children with the opportunity to interact with others, both adults and children, at an appropriate level. This in itself helps children acquire the necessary skills for getting on with others and becoming part of a group. Through play, children are also given the opportunity to practise and perfect social skills in situations that are not permanent. The activity, game or experience will finish, but the social skills used will eventually be remembered. In this way the child is not made to feel inadequate as new skills are acquired.

The development of social play

How children play within the group follows a developmental pattern. Progress through the stages of development depends upon having the opportunity to play with other children. As children learn and develop social skills these are taken into account in their play. The pattern is summarised in the figure below.

key terms

Solitary play
a child plays alone

Parallel play
a child plays side-by-side with another child but without interacting; their play activities remain personal

Associative play
play begins with other children; children make intermittent interactions and/or are involved in the same activity although their play remains personal

Co-operative play
children are able to play together co-operatively; they are able to adopt a role within the group and to take account of others' needs and actions

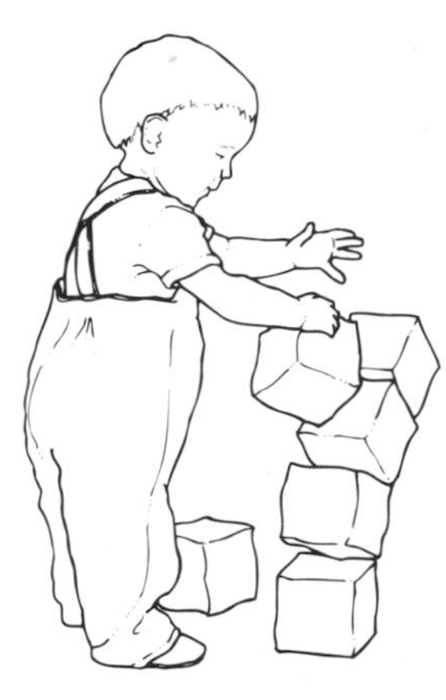

1 Solitary play

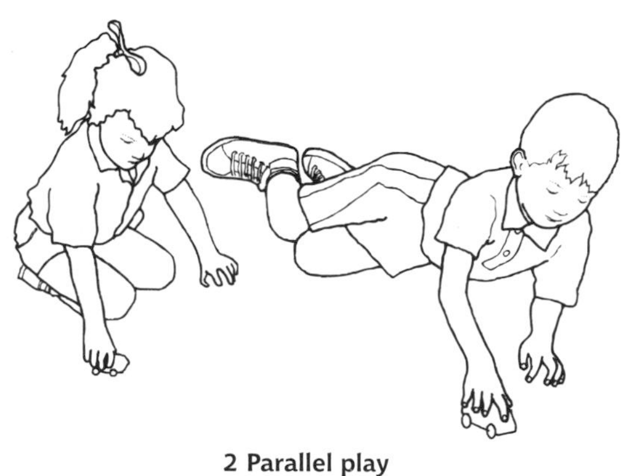

2 Parallel play

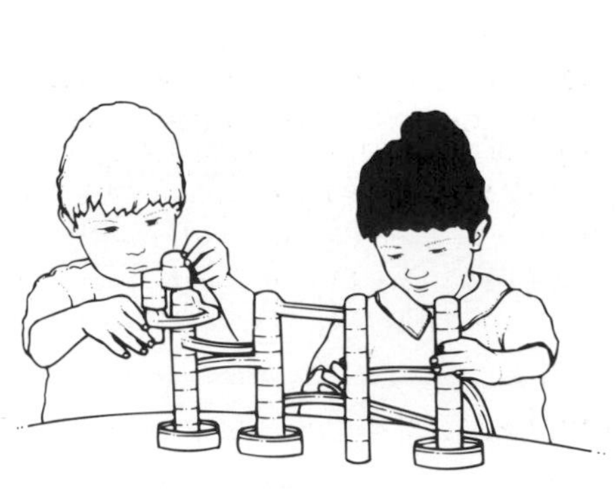

3 Associative play

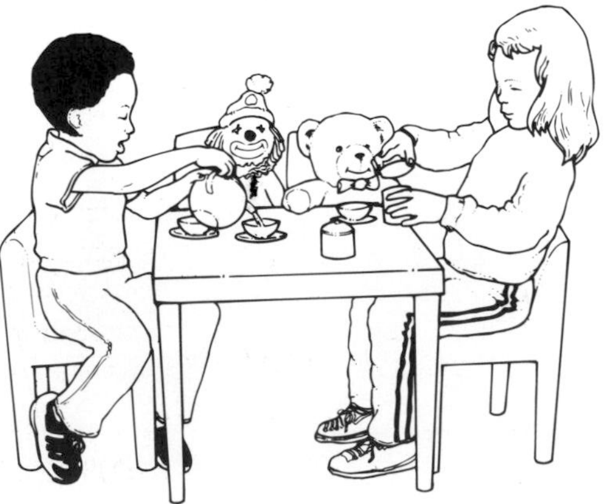

4 Co-operative play

The development of social play

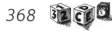

Progress check

How does play contribute to the development of fine and gross motor skills?

Why is outdoor play beneficial to children?

What needs to be considered when planning outdoor play?

What is intellectual development?

How can play contribute to the development of intellectual skills?

What is language development?

How can play help language development?

What are:
(a) verbal skills? (b) non-verbal skills?

List the ways in which children may use language when playing.

What is emotional development?

List some ways in which play can contribute positively to a child's emotional development.

What is self-image (or self-concept) and why is it important?

What are social skills and why are they important?

How are social skills acquired?

Why is play a good way for children to develop these skills?

Types of play

Children's play can be divided up into a number of types of play. It is important to realise that these are adult divisions of play. Children's relentless exploration of their world flows through one activity or experience to another. These divisions are sometimes necessary for effective planning, resourcing and monitoring of children's play and development.

Different settings will use different ways of identifying and categorising play activities and experiences. Outlined below are some of the types of play that may be used in different settings.

It is important that a range of play activities are provided for children to ensure that there are opportunities for all the necessary skills and concepts to be developed, and that their experiences are broad and balanced. Each area of play should be provided regularly with sufficient repetition of activities to enable children to practise and consolidate skills and concepts.

CREATIVE PLAY

Creative play includes:

- play with natural materials such as sand, water, wood, clay and dough
- painting
- collage
- exploration of sound with percussion instruments.

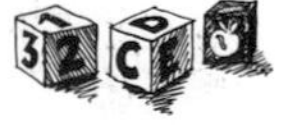

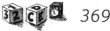

A creative activitiy involves expression of imaginative ideas. These ideas should be the child's ideas. Teaching children skills, for example how to weave, is an important part of their learning, but it is not creative as children are not expressing their own ideas.

For an activity or experience to be creative it should have a number of the following features:

- use of the imagination
- begin with an open-ended outcome
- be a personal expression of ideas
- be unique in its process and product
- have the process as equally important as the product.

Very young children will need to explore materials to become familiar with them, and to develop and use their emerging skills. They need the time, space, materials and encouragement to develop their ideas, skills and knowledge. Older children, who are familiar with the materials, will need the challenge of finding creative ways of producing an item, for example, box modelling to create a moon buggy.

PHYSICAL PLAY WITH LARGE EQUIPMENT

Young children need opportunities to develop, practise and refine bodily movement and control. These include:

- whole body and limb movements
- co-ordination
- balance.

This control of bodily movement enables children to develop skills such as running, climbing, kicking, skipping, hopping, throwing, catching, swimming and riding a bike.

Play with large equipment, both indoors and outdoors, provides opportunities for practice and consolidation of skills. As with creative development young children need lots of time and space to explore and experiment with the equipment. Older children will need and enjoy a physical challenge, for example building a den big enough for three children, weaving through posts on a bike or skipping ten times without stopping.

All children need a variety of opportunities to ensure a range of skills are developed. For example:

- large bricks and other large construction equipment
- den making and building equipment
- hoops and ropes
- large and small balls
- bats and rackets
- scrambling tubes
- balancing beam
- tricycles and bikes
- climbing frame.

IMAGINATIVE PLAY

Imaginative play is activities and experiences that enable children to use their imagination. These may be art and craft activities or pretend play activities. What is important is that children can develop their own imaginative ideas. Young children need the time, space, resources and, when appropriate, sensitive adult intervention, to express their thoughts and ideas. There are opportunities for this in many activities:

- domestic play, for example in a home corner
- role play, for example, Goldilocks in the three bears' house
- play with dolls
- dressing up
- small world play, for example, a model farm or hospital
- outdoor pretend play, for example, a climbing frame is a boat and the playground sea with sharks in it
- play with large and small construction equipment
- art and craft activities where the children are free to think of and develop their own ideas.

MANIPULATIVE PLAY

Manipulative play is play that enables children to practise and refine their motor skills. Children need a lot of practice at these skills. The range of activities and experiences offered should enable children to work at different levels and provide opportunity for increasingly effective use of tools and equipment.

Many activities provide the opportunity for practice and refining these skills at all levels. Their effectiveness can be assessed by whether children are able to practise and refine their skills at their own level, for example within a group of children there may be some who cannot yet build a tower of bricks while others may be building complex buildings. This group will need activities that provide opportunities for practice for some children and challenging opportunities for others.

Activities for developing manipulative skills include:

- threading
- jigsaws and puzzles
- large and small construction
- free drawing with a variety of crayons and pencils
- free painting
- dough and clay work
- dressing and undressing dolls and themselves.

The role of adults in play

Adults have an important role in children's play to ensure that the maximum benefit is gained from it. The adult needs to plan and prepare the activities carefully. They also need to interact with the children during the activity and monitor what is happening through observation. The adult's role in play is summarised in the figure below.

What are the children's developmental levels?
What are the special needs of children within the group?
Which skills do the children need to develop?
How much space is available?
How much time is available?
What are the staffing levels and expertise?
Is there a current theme or topic?
Does the planning reflect cultural diversity?
What activities do the children enjoy?
Are there any safety issues to be considered?

The children:

- Does the play provided meet their needs?
- Who is playing with which activity? Is this significant?
- What interaction with the child/children is appropriate?
- How can the children's play be extended?

The activity:

- Is the activity appropriate for the group of children?
- Is it attractively presented?
- Is all the necessary equipment available so that the children can be as independent as possible?
- Was there enough time and space for the children to play with the activity successfully?
- Was the adult's time and expertise made full use of?

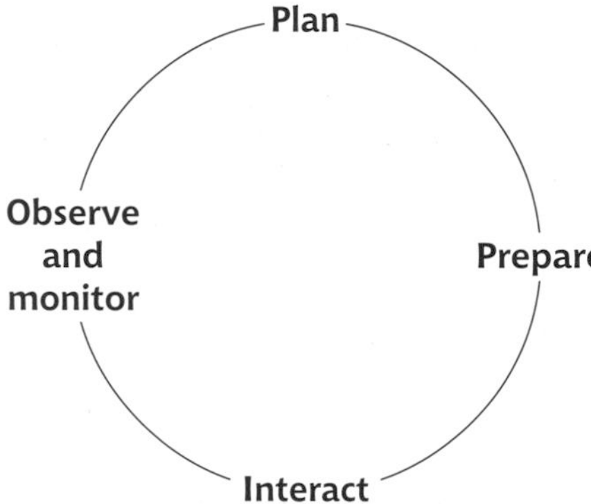

The activity needs to be attractive and easily accessible to the children.
Is all the necessary equipment available?
Is the activity presented in an inviting way? This may include beginning the activity to suggest ways of doing it to the children.
Is there enough space, time and adult help available to enable the child to be successful at the activity?
Is the area safe?

Ways of interacting with the children include:

- joining in the children's play
- playing alongside the children
- providing a commentary on the play
- suggesting new or different ideas for the play
- introducing different equipment to extend the play
- discussing the activity prior to or after the play
- observe the play without direct intervention, allowing the child/children to develop their own ideas.

The role of the adult in children's play

THE PLAY ENVIRONMENT

- The entrance to the centre gives the first impression that parents, children and visitors gain of your work. A welcoming entrance with displays of children's work and interesting and current information about the centre will all contribute to a positive impression. The notices should reflect the linguistic diversity within a setting to enable all visitors to have access to the information. If the entrance is also used as a waiting area and there is space, try to provide some chairs.
- The outdoor area provides for an important aspect of children's learning and should be planned with care. A tarmac or paved space that is large enough for the navigation of wheeled toys should be available and, where possible, a grassy area with space for growing things. Safety will be an important consideration and fences and gates must be secure.
- Cloakrooms, washbasins and lavatories should be easily accessible and child-sized to promote increasing independence.
- Displays can be an important educational tool in the pre-school setting and their use will also add to the attractiveness of the environment. Children's

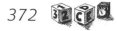

work, well mounted and displayed with care, shows them that you value the children's achievements and enables them to feel positively about these achievements themselves. Displays can be a stimulus to further learning and will also, at a glance, demonstrate to parents and visitors what the children have been working on. Use walls, windows, ceilings – whatever is appropriate in your setting. If you have to pack everything away at the end of every session it might be possible to use fold-up screens for display.

A welcoming entrance creates a positive impression:

- Furniture, carpets and curtains will all add to the attractiveness of the environment and make it a pleasant place to work in. In a child-centred environment, these items should be chosen with children in mind, particularly with regard to size and durability.
- Children need plenty of space in which to play but often a large open space is not conducive to the most purposeful types of play. Providing a number of separate areas for different types of activity through strategic positioning of pieces of furniture will enable children to concentrate more readily. This approach allows for flexibility too as the overall make-up of space can be altered easily as required.
- An attractive environment invites children to participate.

Case study . . .

. . . organising space for play

A pre-school group was set up in a spare classroom of a local primary school. The room was large and airy, and had its own access to an outside play area. The pre-school workers provided a wide range of activities and encouraged children to move freely between them. They noticed that very few of the children settled into the activities for any length of time, with some spending less than a minute at activities. The room seemed very noisy and children were having to be frequently reminded to stop racing around the room.

The pre-school workers decided to borrow some surplus furniture from the school stores and experimented with setting up the room in a different way. Quiet areas such as the book corner and the puzzle table were situated away from the door to the outside play area and the rest of the room was divided into discrete but accessible areas using the furniture as dividers, supplemented by drapes and curtains in some areas. This arrangement gave the impression of separate spaces but allowed the staff to oversee what was going on in each area.

Individual members of staff were allocated to particular activities within the room and were responsible for children working within those areas. The children stayed longer at the activities and had the opportunity to develop their play there, often supported by an adult. The noise level was affected too, as the positioning of the furniture had cut down on the run-through routes and the fabrics absorbed some of the sounds.

1. *Look at your own setting. Could you organise the space differently?*
2. *If you organised your setting differently, what effect would this have?*

Space should be organised so that all children can participate fully:

- You may need to make adjustments for, say, a child who is blind or one who uses a wheelchair.

- Paint, clay, sand and water need to be near sinks where possible, and on safe and durable floor covering.
- Keeping doors and windows accessible should be a consideration, as should the need for children to circulate freely within the area.
- In centres where meals are served, thought should be given to provision of a dining area. Children staying for day-long sessions may also require an appropriate space for rest and sleep.

The physical environment must be a safe place for children and adults. Health and Safety Regulations must be adhered to, with staff taking responsibility, checking the premises for hazards regularly and ensuring prompt action is taken where necessary.

Providing and organising resources

Most pre-school centres would include provision for activities in the following educational areas:

- a creative or craft area, to include a range of activities
- a construction area for both large and small equipment
- provision for role play, including other kinds of socio-dramatic play as well as home-corner play
- an area for malleable materials, such as dough, clay, Plasticine, etc.
- miniature world play, such as play people, farms, cars, dolls' houses, etc.
- outdoor play, to include imaginative play as well as climbing, running, pedalling, etc.
- puzzles and games
- natural materials such as sand, water, clay, earth and wood
- a writing area where children experiment with different writing media and use writing meaningfully
- a book area
- an area for technology including, in some centres, provision for information technology
- an area for larger group interaction, often the home carpet or corner.

It is through these areas of activity that all aspects of the curriculum can be presented to children in a way that takes into account their individual capabilities and preferences:

- The resources provided for use in the above areas should support the full range of learning needs. Variety in provision will maintain interest in the area. However, this should be balanced by children's need to become familiar and confident in using certain types of resources. For example, if Lego is offered only occasionally in the interests of variety, then children will not have sufficient opportunity to explore all its possibilities.
- Staff should decide on spending priorities when it comes to resource allowances, as some areas may require more substantial and expensive attention than others.
- Criteria need to be set when selecting resources. Safety will obviously be a primary concern, as will quality and durability. Equipment that can be used in a variety of ways will provide for versatility and is good value for money when

budgets are limited. Consideration should be given to the promotion of equal opportunities through the selection of resources. (You will find more on Anti-bias in activities in Unit Ten.)

- Organisation of resources is an important consideration. A High Scope delivery of the curriculum (see Chapter 23) will require resources to be organised in a way that allows children to select the items they need and then return them to their place after use. Whatever the method of curriculum delivery, children will become more independent if they are able to locate the equipment they need and if they are involved in putting it away afterwards. To this end, it will be helpful if resources are stored where they are accessible to children and labelled appropriately.
- Resources need to be regularly maintained, cleaned and checked for damage. Anything that is incomplete, unhygienic or beyond repair should be discarded.

THE ROLE OF THE ADULT IN MANAGING THE LEARNING ENVIRONMENT

The role of the adult in managing the learning environment could be summarised as follows:

- to plan and prepare the environment so that it meets the individual learning needs of each child in the group
- to be aware of the learning opportunities that each activity provides
- to welcome and encourage children to the session and into specific activities
- to interact with children in ways that focus on the learning potential of the materials and activity
- to provide for balance in the range of activities experienced by individual children – this will involve monitoring children's choices and encouraging them into activities that are generally avoided
- to observe and evaluate the response to activities and use this in future planning
- to supervise the area and maintain safety during the session
- to ensure that all children can join in and that none are intimidated or bullied
- to monitor noise levels so that the atmosphere is conducive to purposeful play
- to care for the learning environment so that it continues to offer a welcoming and stimulating experience.

Children gain a great deal from the involvement of adults in their play. Child-care workers should watch children closely and take every opportunity to involve themselves as appropriate.

Progress check

What considerations should be borne in mind when planning the learning environment?

How can the organisation of the learning environment promote children's independence?

How does the organisation of the learning environment influence the curriculum and the curriculum influence the learning environment?

Outline the role of the adult in managing the learning environment.

Now try these questions

Why is play a good way of meeting young children's needs?

Describe the range of skills and concepts that a child can develop through play.

What is the role of the adult in children's play?

What should be considered when planning a play environment?

key terms

You need to know what the key terms and phrases in this chapter mean.
Go back through the chapter and find out.

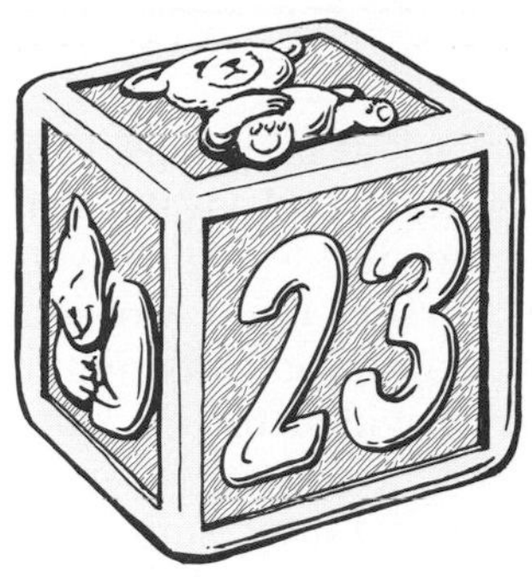

CURRICULUM PERSPECTIVES

This chapter looks at various approaches to the early years curriculum and considers how these approaches are informed by what is known about the ways in which children learn. It then looks at statutory requirements concerning the content of the curriculum and makes links to the role of the curriculum in promoting equality of opportunity. (You may find it helpful to read this chapter in conjunction with Chapters 9 Cognitive development, 10 Language development, 22 Play and 24 Curriculum areas.)

This chapter will cover the following topics:

- *current context*
- *influences and curriculum models*
- *statutory requirements for the curriculum*
- *equal opportunities and the curriculum.*

Current context

key terms

Curriculum
the content and methods that comprise a course of study

Child-centred
with the child at the centre, taking into account the perspective of the child

Experiential
achieving through experience

A 'course of study' is the simple dictionary definition of **curriculum**. But in the early years, the term curriculum carries more than this simple academic definition implies. The curriculum also transmits the values of the setting and those who work within it. Through it, children learn about themselves and their place in the world.

Studies of the way that children learn, and Piaget's work in particular, indicate that concepts are best understood through actual experiences, in effect, that children *learn by doing*. These theories have had a significant influence on the way that we organise early years provision and have led to an approach to learning that takes into account the child's individual capabilities and interests (**child-centred**) and which is achieved through experience (**experiential**). Piaget's work provides a rationale for play as an appropriate medium for young children's learning, because it provides opportunities for children to develop understanding through first-hand experiences. Thus, the role of play in providing a developmentally appropriate curriculum for young children is emphasised in current statutory guidance.

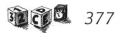

Case study . . .

. . . making a rainhat for teddy

An activity was set up for the 5 year olds in the class to work at in groups. Children were provided with a range of different fabrics, a bowl of water and a water squirter. They were asked to examine all the fabrics carefully and decide which would be most suitable to use to make a rainhat for teddy. The nursery nurse worked with the children at the table getting them to talk about what a rainhat was required to do and also encouraging them to use the equipment provided to test out their choices.

After some time spent squirting water on each of the fabric samples, they were able to eliminate most of the samples as no good for keeping teddy dry and then were able to decide on a 'best choice' from those that were left. Later on that day they were able to test out the rainhat that they had made by taking teddy out during a heavy shower. By the end of the session they had gained a considerable understanding of the concept of absorbency and were beginning to develop their own methods of scientific enquiry. They also experienced a sense of achievement and satisfaction at being able to follow the task all the way through to completion.

1. *Why was this a successful activity for the children?*
2. *What do you think the children learned from this?*
3. *How did the adult support children's learning here?*
4. *An adult could tell children about absorbency and the properties of fabrics. Would this enable them to understand this concept?*

In most settings the environment is carefully organised so that children have the maximum opportunity for hands-on experience. Equipment will be accessible so that they can make choices and follow up interests, fostering a responsibility for their own learning. A number of activities will be available at any one time and the atmosphere buzzes with busy noise. Children will be involved in planning and working collaboratively, both with adults and with each other, and will be encouraged to contribute their own ideas. Staff monitor progress, interact with children and plan and provide for the next learning activity.

This current approach to the curriculum assumes that if children engage with and enjoy what they are doing, then their learning will be both effective and meaningful.

Progress check

What do you understand by the term 'curriculum'?

How does our current approach to the early years curriculum differ from that of the past?

What is experiential learning?

How has Piaget's work influenced the way that we provide for young children's learning?

Influences and curriculum models

In order to understand current approaches to children's learning, it is helpful to look at some of the influential figures in early education and also to look at a range of ways in which the curriculum is approached.

FRIEDRICH FROBEL (1782–1852)

Froebel pioneered an approach to early childhood learning that emphasised the importance of providing children with a wide range of experiences to enable them to develop an understanding of themselves and the world around them. He believed that play was a highly significant activity for young children and advocated a structured play approach to young children's learning.

MARGARET MACMILLAN (1860–1931)

Macmillan is acknowledged as one of the pioneers of nursery education. She recognised the importance of early education to all children but was aware that many children living in poor communities did not have access to nursery education. She recognised that unhealthy and malnourished children found it difficult to learn and therefore focused her attention on improving their health. Nursery education, she believed, could compensate for the deficits in some children's lives. Her open-air schools emphasised the importance of play, both outdoors and indoors. Macmillan also encouraged parental involvement, recognising the important role that parents play in supporting their children's learning and development. This is considered to be an important element of current early education practice.

SUSAN ISAACS (1885–1948)

Isaacs's work was based on her own observations of children at nursery school. Through these, she analysed and identified the role of play in promoting intellectual growth, in particular identifying the breadth of individual differences in children's development and the need for the curriculum to cater for these.

The work of these pioneers and the curriculum models of Montessori, Steiner and High Scope, examined below, have much in common. All are based on an understanding that children learn through active involvement with their environment and that this is often best achieved through the medium of play. They all acknowledge that childhood is a sensitive learning time and that children are highly receptive to all experiences. Where they differ is in the emphasis placed on the various elements of the curriculum and on the methods used.

The influence of these approaches is not limited to the relatively small number of centres that have adopted them in their entirety: some elements of all of these approaches can be recognised in much of what is considered 'mainstream' provision.

MONTESSORI EDUCATION

Montessori education is named after its founder, Maria Montessori, who devised an approach to learning based on her observations of the children she worked with. The child is at the centre of the Montessori method. She believed that children learn best through their own spontaneous activity and that they have a natural inquisitiveness and eagerness to learn. The role of the adult is to provide a planned environment that will allow the child the opportunity to develop skills and concepts.

Montessori classrooms follow a similar pattern. Furniture is child-sized, including long, low cupboards from which children select their own materials. There are rugs so that children can sit on the floor, and the classroom is bright and light with pictures on the wall, and plants and flowers around the room.

Central to the Montessori method are the didactic (teaching) materials. These consist of blocks, beads, cylinders and rods provided for the children to play with. Experimentation with these materials allows the children to discover and understand basic concepts for themselves. There is no time limit to this exploration; the children continue until satisfied. To achieve this, the materials are:

- simple – though not easy – so that the child can understand them and the observant adult can decide when to become involved
- inherently interesting
- self-checking, so that the child knows whether they have succeeded without the need for adult intervention.

Children's exploration of the didactic materials remains an important part of the Montessori curriculum, although this is usually presented alongside a broader range of experiences.

In a Montessori classroom, the adult's role is considered to be that of 'director', that is to keep children's interest through guiding, but also to withdraw so that the children do things for themselves and develop a sense of independence and self-confidence. The director observes the individual children and notes the stage achieved on records that relate to the didactic materials. The director will then determine what activities are suitable for the next steps in each child's learning and guide the child towards them.

STEINER EDUCATION (THE WALDORF SCHOOLS)

Steiner education is based on the educational philosophy of Rudolf Steiner. He did not believe that the purpose and focus of education should be a narrow teaching of skills that are required for society's economic growth, but rather that the true purpose of education was to allow the individual's impulses and talents to unfold. Steiner felt that as children learn from what happens all around them, the environment had the most significant influence on the child, and that this included experiences and interactions with other people, as well as the physical environment. Steiner believed strongly in the need for children to develop their own inner world, valuing creativity and self-expression most highly. The Steiner method encourages these qualities through activities such as drawing, dancing, music, movement and all kinds of fantasy and pretend play. Eurhythmy – whole body rhythmical movement – is also valued as an important means of creative self-expression.

A Steiner kindergarten will have many or all of the following features:

- items made from natural materials, wherever possible
- toys and articles that can be used in an open-ended, imaginative way
- a room that is pleasing to the child, with factors such as light and use of colour considered
- plenty of paper, pens and modelling clay provided
- large boxes, pieces of carpet and lengths of fabric for children to develop their own role- play themes
- a garden where children can come into contact with the natural cycle of planting, tending and harvesting.

The adult's role in the Steiner system is that of provider and guide. The adult should not initiate play but become involved where appropriate. Steiner believed that children learn through imitation and interaction. Therefore, the good behaviour of adults towards one another and towards children serves as a powerful role model to influence children's own standards of behaviour.

Although Steiner's approach may appear unconventional in the current educational climate, it should be noted that education in the Steiner system does not preclude children from achieving conventional educational targets, such as success in public examinations, alongside the Steiner aims of developing individual talents.

HIGH SCOPE

> **key term**
>
> **Compensatory education**
> a programme or initiative that is offered to those who might be likely to experience disadvantage in the education system

High Scope is an approach to the early years curriculum that was developed in the US in the 1960s as part of the Headstart **compensatory education** programme. It has been shown to have good results, particularly in terms of developing in children a sense of responsibility for their own learning and actions. Follow-up research, which has tracked those children involved in the original High Scope project for 30 years, has shown that this type of pre-school experience has had a positive effect on the participants well into their adult lives, which is indicated by their social and economic well-being. The High Scope approach has been adopted by a number of centres in the UK, not necessarily as part of a compensatory programme, but because its principles are recognised as developmentally appropriate for young children.

High Scope is characterised by the following themes:

- *The daily routine* – this comprises the Plan–Do–Review approach, where children are required to indicate to an adult what they are going to do during a session (plan), to carry out this plan during the 'worktime' part of the session (do) and then to recall what they have done (review). This recall time will often include some kind of representation such as a drawing, or showing the work, or describing what's been done. Recall may be incorporated into 'small group time' when children are involved in structured, adult-led activities. Also incorporated into the daily schedule will be sessions of outside time – usually focused on vigorous activity – and circle time, when the whole group get together to sing, discuss or play games.
- *Room and equipment organisation* – the room is arranged for particular activities in distinct work areas, usually with a book area, a construction area, a home area and an art area. All equipment and materials are stored and clearly labelled so that children have independent access to them.
- *Key terms, concepts and experiences* – the curriculum is designed to develop a range of key experiences and cognitive skills, and the child's progress is reviewed with reference to these. Key experiences provide the focus for adult–child interaction. These may be specifically planned for small group time or arise incidentally during a worktime. It is the adult's responsibility to guide play and talk in such a way as to draw these key experiences into focus.
- *The role of the adult* – the role of the adult in the High Scope curriculum is to encourage, demonstrate and to assist but not to dominate. The adult creates a framework for learning that values and acts upon the children's initiatives and interests.

This approach actively involves children in decisions about their learning and fosters responsibility and independence.

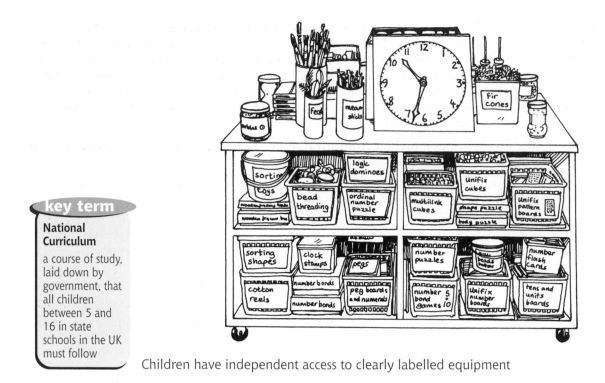

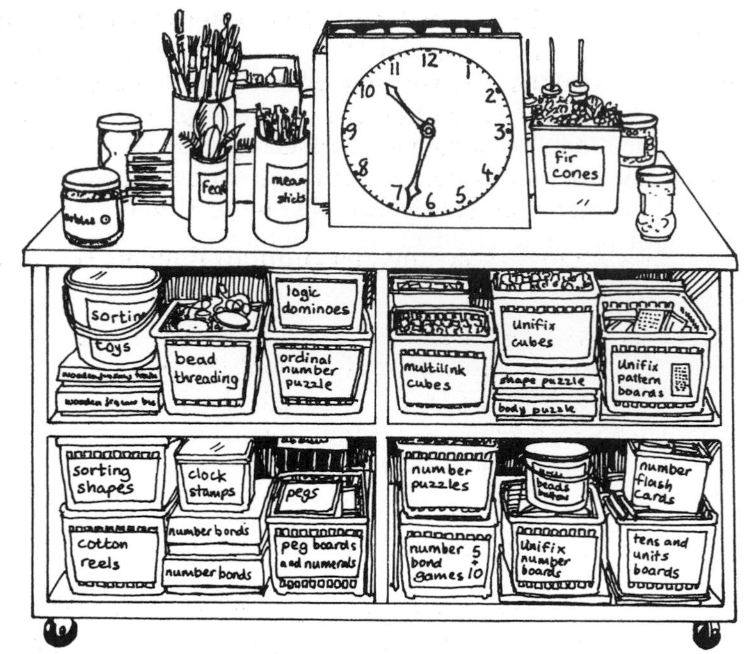

Children have independent access to clearly labelled equipment

key term

National Curriculum
a course of study, laid down by government, that all children between 5 and 16 in state schools in the UK must follow

Progress check

Outline the curriculum models described above.

What similarities are there in the various approaches?

What are the features of the High Scope approach? How does this approach develop responsibility?

Statutory requirements for the curriculum

This section summarises the statutory (laid down by law) curriculum requirements in the UK for state schools and for nurseries and other settings who are in receipt of government grant for the provision of education.

THE NATIONAL CURRICULUM

key term

Foundation Stage
the introductory stage of the National Curriculum, for children from 3 until year 1 of Key Stage One

The **National Curriculum** was introduced in England and Wales as part of the 1988 Education Reform Act (a similar Act relates to Scotland). The main points of relevance to the early years can be summarised as follows:

- The National Curriculum is compulsory for all children between the ages of 5 and 16 in all state schools (this includes special schools).
- There is a **Foundation Stage** of the National Curriculum, introduced in September 2000, with separate curriculum guidance (the **Early Learning Goals**) compulsory for all settings receiving public funding (**nursery grant**) for the education of 3 and 4 year olds.

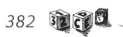

key terms

Early Learning Goals
what most children will achieve in the six areas of learning, by the beginning of Key Stage One

Nursery grant
public funds paid to settings in the private and voluntary sector for the education of 3 and 4 year olds

- At Key Stages One to Four, the curriculum comprises the following subjects: English, mathematics and science (plus Welsh in Welsh-language schools), design and technology, information and communication technology (ICT), history, geography, art and design, music, physical education, with a modern foreign language introduced at Key Stage Three. Priority is given to the three core subjects of English, mathematics and science. In addition, teaching in religious education must be provided.
- Subjects are divided into **attainment targets**, each with a programme of study.
- The curriculum is divided into four key stages, with the Foundation Stage for children between 3 and 6 years. The programme for Key Stage One is followed for six terms, in years 1 and 2 of compulsory schooling, with children transferring to Key Stage Two at the beginning of the school year after their 7th birthday.
- At the end of each key stage, children's progress in the core subjects is assessed by Standard Assessment Tasks (SATs) and, at Key Stage One, also by teacher assessment. The child's progress is then reported and discussed with parents. School results are aggregated and published. Information about the performance of individual children is not made public.

key term

Attainment targets
the different elements of a curriculum area; for example, the attainment targets for English are speaking, reading and writing

Some effects of the National Curriculum and its implications for child-care workers

The importance of science and technology in the early years was emphasised by the National Curriculum. In-service training and investment in equipment have given staff the opportunity to plan and deliver these subjects with increased confidence.

Planning a programme to meet the requirements of the National Curriculum has encouraged staff to work collaboratively. Nursery nurses and classroom assistants have much to contribute here.

Evidence needs to be gathered to support teacher assessment. This may mean observations of the children as well as items of work. Everyone who works with the children will have a part to play in collecting this.

Children (and parents) may become anxious at the prospect of formal assessment at the age of 7. Child-care workers must take time to reassure both and avoid putting pressure on children.

Young children learn most effectively through child-centred and experiential methods. These have been shown to be the most appropriate methods for delivering the National Curriculum too, particularly at the Foundation Stage, although research has also demonstrated the effectiveness of some whole-group teaching.

The content and structure of the National Curriculum has been changed a great deal in a relatively short space of time. Concerns have been raised that the curriculum for Key Stages One and Two is overloaded and that inadequate time is available for developing the key skills of literacy and numeracy. With the introduction of the **National Literacy Strategy** (1998) and the **National Numeracy Strategy** (1999) to dovetail with the requirements of the revised National Curriculum (2000), these important areas have been emphasised.

key terms

National Literacy Strategy
government guidance (1998) for the structure and content of a daily hour-long literacy lesson for children from Reception to Key Stage Two

National Numeracy Strategy
government guidance (1999) for the structure and content of a daily 45-minute numeracy lesson for children from Reception to Key Stage Two

THE NATIONAL LITERACY STRATEGY

The literacy strategy or literacy hour, as it is often known, was introduced in September 1998 and is a key feature of a government drive to meet improvement targets in children's literacy. It is not additional to the National Curriculum but should be seen as a recommended approach to teaching some of the reading and writing requirements for English at Key Stages One and Two. The daily literacy hour should be made up of the following elements:

- around 15 minutes spent with the whole class on text work, often on a big book, fiction or information
- a further 15 minutes spent on word level work, which, at Key Stage One, comprises phonics, spelling and awareness of rhyme and sounds
- for around 20 minutes on small group work, where teachers lead guided reading or writing. Generally the teacher focuses on a group of between four and six children daily, while the others work independently on specific tasks to promote literacy
- the final 10 minutes spent as the plenary session, which brings the group together to reflect on and consolidate what they have learned.

At reception age, the guidance recommends that children are introduced to all the elements of the strategy, though not necessarily one after the other in a single hour.

(Adapted from: the *National Literacy Strategy: Framework for Teaching Literacy from Reception to Year 6*, DfEE,1998.)

THE NATIONAL NUMERACY STRATEGY

The numeracy strategy was introduced in September 1999 as part of a government initiative to raise national standards in numeracy. It provides a structured daily mathematics lesson of between 45 minutes and one hour for all pupils of primary school age. The framework stands alongside the National Curriculum requirements for mathematics at Key Stages One and Two. As with the literacy strategy, schools are not compelled to follow the numeracy strategy but, in practice, most schools in the state sector do so. The guidance recommends that children at Reception age have some daily focused time on mathematics in order to prepare them for the 45-minute daily lesson introduced in year 1. It identifies a particular approach to the teaching of mathematics and suggests that the time is organised as follows:

- an introduction with the whole class, usually with counting, finger games, number rhymes and songs
- some teaching of the whole class on the main mathematics topic of the day
- group activities, which may mean everyone at the same activity simultaneously in small groups or may be achieved through a focus on the chosen aspect of mathematics developed through a range of play activities and supported by adults working alongside the children
- a session with the whole class to extend and consolidate through discussion and questioning, what they have been learning and to recognise and praise progress.

(Adapted from: the *National Numeracy Strategy: Framework for Teaching Mathematics from Reception to Year 6*, DfEE, 1999.)

Within both the literacy and numeracy strategies, there is a clear role for classroom assistants working alongside teachers in supporting both groups and individual children through the various elements of the sessions.

THE CURRICULUM FOR THE FOUNDATION STAGE – THE EARLY LEARNING GOALS

The curriculum for the Foundation Stage of the National Curriculum, the Early Learning Goals, was introduced in September 2000 (see pages 386–8 for a listing of the Early Learning Goals). It is so called as it is designed to lay the foundations for children's later learning with the goals for the end of the Foundation Stage, providing a clear bridge to the programme for Key Stage One. All settings receiving public funding for the education of children pre-Key Stage One, either by claiming nursery grant or through direct funding in maintained schools, must follow the curriculum for the Foundation Stage. No distinction is made between the types of setting: private day nurseries, playgroups, family centres, nursery schools and nursery classes and Reception classes in primary schools, all are required to provide the full curriculum. Settings are required to base their 3 to 5+ curriculum on a programme that works towards developing children's skills and concepts, so that they can achieve the goals by the beginning of year 1 at Key Stage One. The curriculum is divided into the following six areas of learning:

- personal, social and emotional development
- communication, language and literacy
- mathematics
- knowledge and understanding of the world
- physical development
- creative development.

key terms

'Stepping stones'
indication of the steps children need to take from 3 years towards the early learning goals at 5+

Baseline assessment
an assessment of a child's capabilities currently undertaken on entry to school at 5 years

As with the National Curriculum, these requirements were derived from what was considered to be good early years practice for this age group. For each area of learning, there is a statement that defines the skills and concepts, the goals, which young children need to develop by the *end* of the Foundation Stage (see the chart on pages 386–8). Comprehensive guidance (QCA 2000) identifies the '**stepping stones**' to provide that will enable children from 3 onwards to make progress towards the goals. There is no formal assessment for the Foundation Stage, although establishments are expected to make regular assessments of the progress of individual children as part of their provision. However, it is likely that **baseline assessment**, currently applied on children's entry to school at 5, will be revised and rescheduled for the end of the Foundation Stage.

Progress check

What does the term 'statutory' mean with regard to the curriculum ?

Which settings must follow the Foundation Stage of the National Curriculum?

What are the six areas of learning defined in the Early Learning Goals?

Which subjects are studied by children at Key Stage One?

When are children assessed by SATs? What happens to their scores?

Equal opportunities and the curriculum

The curriculum can be a powerful tool in promoting **equal opportunities**. Child-care workers have a responsibility to present the curriculum in a way that includes and enables all children and that reflects the experiences of all sections of society. The planning and delivery of the curriculum must provide for equality of opportunity, irrespective of race and culture, gender, socio-economic background or

EARLY LEARNING GOALS

PERSONAL, EMOTIONAL AND SOCIAL DEVELOPMENT

- Continue to be interested, excited and motivated to learn
- Be confident to try new activities, initiate ideas and speak in a familiar group
- Maintain attention, concentrate, and sit quietly when appropriate
- Respond to significant experiences, showing a range of feelings when appropriate

- Have a developing awareness of their own needs, views, feelings and be sensitive to the needs, views and feelings of others
- Have a developing respect for their own cultures and beliefs and those of other people
- Form good relationships with adults and peers
- Work as part of a group or class, taking turns and sharing fairly, understanding that there needs to be agreed values and codes of behaviour for groups of people, including adults and children, to work together harmoniously
- Understand what is right, what is wrong and why
- Consider the consequences of their words and actions for themselves and others
- Dress and undress independently and manage their own personal hygiene
- Select and use activities and resources independently
- Understand that people have different needs, views, cultures and beliefs, which need to be treated with respect
- Understand that they can expect others to treat their needs, views, cultures and beliefs with respect

COMMUNICATION, LANGUAGE AND LITERACY

- Interact with others, negotiating plans and activities and taking turns in conversation
- Enjoy listening to and using spoken and written language and readily turn to it in their play and learning
- Sustain attentive listening, responding to what they have heard by relevant comments, questions or actions
- Listen with enjoyment and respond to stories, songs and other music, rhymes and poems and make up their own stories, songs, rhymes and poems
- Extend their vocabulary, exploring the meanings and sounds of new words
- Speak clearly and audibly with confidence and control and show awareness of the listener, for example by their use of conventions such as greetings, 'please' and 'thank you'
- Use language to imagine and recreate roles and experiences
- Use talk to organise, sequence and clarify thinking, ideas, feelings and events
- Hear and say initial and final sounds in words and short vowel sounds within words
- Link sounds to letters, naming and sounding the letters of the alphabet
- Use their phonic knowledge to write simple regular words and make phonetically plausible attempts at more complex words
- Explore and experiment with sounds, words and texts
- Retell narratives in the correct sequence, drawing on language patterns of stories
- Read a range of familiar and common words and simple sentences independently
- Know that print carries meaning and, in English, is read from left to right and top to bottom

EARLY LEARNING GOALS CONTINUED

- Show an understanding of the elements of stories, such as main character, sequence of events, and openings, and how information can be found in non-fiction texts to answer questions about where, who, why and how
- Attempt writing for different purposes, using features of different forms, such as lists, stories and instructions
- Write their own names and other things such as labels and captions and begin to form simple sentences, sometimes using punctuation
- Use a pencil and hold it effectively to form recognisable letters, most of which are correctly formed.

MATHEMATICS

- Say and use number names in order in familiar contexts
- Count reliably up to 10 everyday objects
- Recognise numerals 1 to 9
- Use developing mathematical ideas and problems to solve practical problems
- In practical activities and discussion, begin to use the vocabulary involved in adding and subtracting
- Use language such as 'more' or 'less' to compare two numbers
- Find one more or one less than a number from one to 10
- Begin to relate addition to combining two groups of objects and subtraction to 'taking away'
- Use language such as 'greater', 'smaller', 'heavier' or 'lighter' to compare quantities
- Talk about, recognise and recreate simple patterns
- Use language such as 'circle' or 'bigger' to describe the shape and size of solids and flat shapes
- Use everyday words to describe position
- Use developing mathematical ideas and methods to solve practical problems.

KNOWLEDGE AND UNDERSTANDING OF THE WORLD

- Investigate objects and materials by using all of their senses as appropriate
- Find out about, and identify, some features of living things, objects and events they observe
- Look closely at similarities, differences, patterns and change
- Ask questions about why things happen and how things work
- Build and construct with a wide range of objects, selecting appropriate resources, and adapting their work where necessary
- Select the tools and techniques they need to shape, assemble and join materials they are using
- Find out about and identify the uses of everyday technology and use information and communication technology and programmable toys to support their learning
- Find out about past and present events in their own lives, and in those of their families and other people they know
- Observe, find out about and identify features in the place they live and in the natural world
- Find out about their environment and talk about those features they like and dislike
- Begin to know about their own cultures and beliefs and those of other people

EARLY LEARNING GOALS CONTINUED

PHYSICAL DEVELOPMENT

- Move with confidence, imagination and in safety
- Move with control and co-ordination
- Travel around, under, over and through balancing and climbing equipment
- Show an awareness of space, of themselves and others
- Recognise the importance of keeping healthy and those things which contribute to this
- Recognise the changes that happen to their bodies when they are active
- Use a range of small and large equipment
- Handle books, objects, construction and malleable materials safely and with increasing control.

CREATIVE DEVELOPMENT

- Explore colour, texture, shape, form and space in two or three dimensions
- Recognise and explore how sounds can be changed, sing simple songs from memory, recognise repeated sounds and sound patterns and match movements to music
- Use their imagination in art and design, music, dance, imaginative and role play and stories
- Respond in a variety of ways to what they see, hear, smell, touch and feel
- Express and communicate their ideas, thoughts and feelings by using a widening range of materials, suitable tools, imaginative and role play, movement, designing and making, and a variety of songs and musical instruments.

(From *Qualifications and Curriculum Authority, Curriculum Guidance for the Foundation Stage*, DfEE, 2000)

key term

Equal opportunities all people participating in society to the best of their abilities, regardless of race, religion, disability, gender or social background

disability. It must also consider how best to develop the potential of children who are more timid or aggressive or more confident than others in their group. Treating all children the same will not provide for equality of opportunity. We must recognise that some children in our society are more likely to experience disadvantage than others and that some **positive action** might be necessary to enable them to succeed. This is an important consideration when planning the curriculum. (Further explanation, with practical examples of this important aspect of the child-care worker's role is discussed in Unit Two, Work with Young Children.)

Now try these questions

key term

Positive action taking steps to ensure that a particular individual or group has an equal chance to succeed

Explain why a child-centred approach to children's learning is appropriate for the early years.

How does the High Scope approach to curriculum delivery promote children's independence?

Describe how the Foundation Stage of the National Curriculum prepares children for the next stages of learning.

key terms

You need to know what the key terms and phrases in this chapter mean. Go back through the chapter and find out.

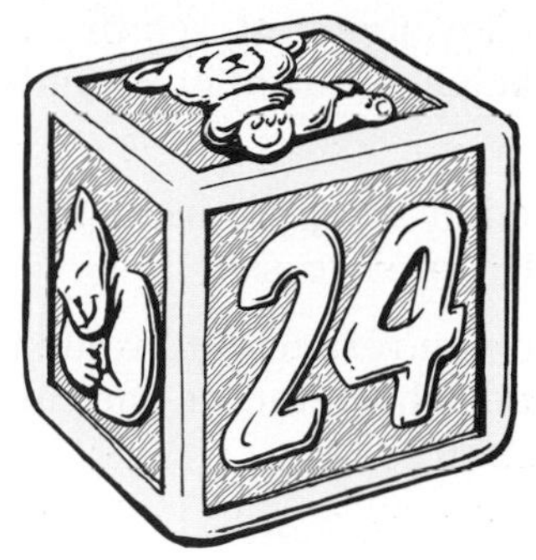

CURRICULUM AREAS

This chapter looks at the elements that go together to make up the curriculum for the early years and suggests some of ways in which the child-care worker can support children's learning in these areas. Although examined separately in this chapter, these subjects will not be taught in isolation, but will be presented as part of an integrated and balanced programme of learning. (You may find it helpful to read this chapter in conjunction with Chapters 12 Emotional and Social Development and 23 Curriculum Perspectives.)

This chapter will cover the following topics:

- *personal, social and emotional development*
- *early literacy*
- *children's books*
- *developing maths*
- *science and technology*
- *history and geography*
- *creativity*
- *physical activities.*

Personal, emotional and social development

Personal, emotional and social development permeates the whole early years curriculum. It is not a discrete subject area in itself, but is concerned with the skills and attitudes that enable children to develop a strong sense of their own worth and become successful members of society. As these are crucial aspects of children's development and have an impact on their ability to learn, it is important that issues of personal and social development are understood and considered seriously by child-care workers in the programme they provide and in their interactions with children. This area of children's development is discussed in detail in Chapter 12, but there are some points that are appropriate to consider here to ensure that the curriculum effectively promotes children's personal, emotional and social development.

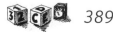

SELF-ESTEEM

This is an important element in emotional and social development, relating to the individual's assessment of their own worth. This can be encouraged in a number of ways:

- by providing tasks and activities that are pitched at an appropriate level for the child, challenging but offering an opportunity for success
- in your interactions with children, showing that you respect and value them for themselves, through praising their efforts and achievements and through sensitive intervention that allows a child to succeed
- by encouraging children to be independent and use initiative, for example being able to select and extend an activity and then be responsible for clearing it away
- by providing positive images for all children with regard to gender, ethnicity and disability, thus encouraging children to value their own cultural background and identity
- in the daily routine and the way that the setting is organised. A regular routine enables children to predict what is likely to happen and this consistency will foster feelings of security and confidence. An environment where resources are stored at child level and accessible to children will allow children to be independent in their choice and use of equipment.

INTERPERSONAL SKILLS

Interpersonal skills enable us to get along with other people. Young children find it difficult to see the world from another's point of view and need to be given opportunities to develop social empathy, that is to be able to tune into other people's viewpoints and act accordingly. They need to develop skills in:

- forming and maintaining friendships
- sharing and taking turns
- responding appropriately to others
- being sensitive to other people's feelings
- expressing their own feelings appropriately
- understanding appropriate behaviour.

Child-care workers can help children to develop these skills through the range of experiences and activities they provide, but also through the ways that they interact with children and positively encourage their social behaviour. Examples include the following:

- being a good role model. Children model their behaviour on what they experience and should see their child-care workers demonstrating respect for and sensitivity to others
- planning activities that require children to co-operate and share, such as mural painting, large jigsaws and games, and by interacting with the children to support this
- encouraging children to share and take turns and monitoring that this happens, for example with popular items of equipment
- providing activities, such as role play and small-world play, that give children an opportunity to begin to experience the world from another perspective

- allowing children opportunities to express their feelings in appropriate ways. A child may wish to stretch and punch at clay to get rid of angry feelings, or curl up in a corner with a blanket if sad or overwhelmed. The death of a nursery pet will provoke sadness and an opportunity to grieve
- supporting children's developing social skills by praising those who co-operate and show consideration for others, providing a model for other children.

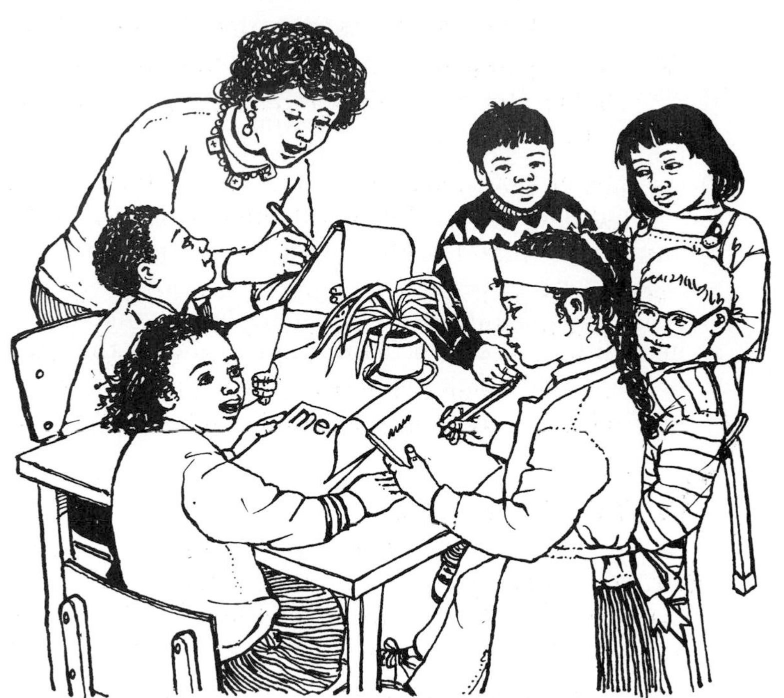

Plan activities that require children to co-operate and take turns, and interact to encourage this

MORAL DEVELOPMENT

This is concerned with developing an understanding of right and wrong. Young children cannot be expected to consider their actions and attitudes and their impact on others in the same way that older children do, but by the pre-school years, children are beginning to become aware that their actions and attitudes affect other people and that the rules governing and shaping behaviour have to be kept. Initially children will accept rules; for example, you cannot snatch the doll from another child, because someone powerful and significant is enforcing the rule. However, eventually the child will understand the reasons why the rule exists and begin to internalise them as moral values.

Even quite small children can begin to understand about rules if they:

- are few in number and are easily recalled
- express the values, ethos and expectations of the setting
- are understood by everyone in the establishment, including parents
- are consistently applied
- are modelled by staff members.

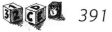

Case study . . .

. . . establishing the rules

As part of a topic on 'Ourselves', the role play area was presented as a doctor's surgery. The children had helped to collect the resources for the area and were looking forward to playing in it. On the first morning that it was available, many children wanted to play in it and this resulted in it being too full. At circle time, the child-care worker discussed this with the children and they all agreed that it was unsatisfactory. The problem was that there were too many children playing at the same time. After some discussion, they decided that the problem would be solved if they limited the number of children who could play in the area at one time. They also decided that they needed a sign to show that only four children could be in the area at any one time. The following day some of the children made a sign showing four people. They showed it to the other children and then hung it up at the entrance to the surgery.

A few days later, at circle time, they talked about how well the rule was working and decided that it was now easier for to play in the doctor's surgery and so the rule was better for everyone.

This collaborative way of establishing a rule demonstrated to the children the necessity of rules. Their involvement meant that they could see the problem and helped to identify a solution. In this way, they could start to understand the reason for rules.

1. *Identify the ways in which the nursery nurse helped the children to establish this rule.*
2. *Why is it important that the children were involved?*
3. *How could the staff involve children in establishing other necessary rules?*

Progress check

Explain why personal, social and emotional development is such an important part of the curriculum.

How can the child-care worker help children to develop a positive view of themselves?

Explain how children's interpersonal skills can be encouraged.

What activities can help children become aware of another person's perspective?

How can children be helped to understand the need to have and keep to rules?

Early literacy

key term

Literacy
the aspects of language concerned with reading and writing

We live in a literate world, in a society that values reading and writing (**literacy**). Consequently, a great deal of emphasis is placed on becoming competent in these areas. Children begin to notice and respond to this literate world long before they begin the formal process of learning to read and write. Their environment contains many examples of writing, from the signs in the supermarket and on the bus ticket, to the postcard from Granny and the bedtime story book. Through their everyday experiences, children become familiar with the product of writing. When they see someone take a telephone message or write a cheque, they become aware of the process of writing too. These experiences have an impact; once children realise that writing carries meaning, they have taken their first step towards becoming literate.

LEARNING TO READ AND WRITE

Learning to read and write is a long and complex process for most children. They will need to learn skills and rules and have plenty of practice to consolidate them. If children have already begun to enjoy books, then it is likely that this will spur them on and give them a reason to persevere.

By the age of 5, many children will have a sight vocabulary of a number of words. Most will recognise their own name; many will be able to write it. Formal instruction in reading and writing will often begin in a pre-school environment alongside other, less formal, experiences and activities that contribute to the development of reading and writing skills. These include activities that involve any or all of the following:

- *hand–eye co-ordination and fine motor skills* – you need to control a pencil to write
- *visual discrimination* – it is important to be able to distinguish one word or letter from another
- *sequencing* – the order of the letters or words affects the meaning
- *auditory discrimination* – hearing the difference between sounds and combinations of sounds helps reading
- *use of symbols* – reading and writing are representational forms in which one thing, a combination of letters, stands for something else.

Also very important at this stage is using reading and writing as a meaningful part of play, for example, 'reading' the menu in the café or 'writing' a telephone message in the home corner.

Remember that reading and writing are essential tools for later learning. They are used and practised in every area of the curriculum.

Reading

key terms

Look and say
an approach to reading that relies on recognition of the shape or pattern of a word

Phonics
an approach to reading that is based on recognition of sounds

There are basically two approaches used in the teaching of reading:

- **look and say**
- **phonics**.

Look and say involves the recognition of whole words by their shape. Words are often written on flashcards and children will attempt to memorise them, often practising at home. Children can then read simple stories comprised of the words that they have learned. They recognise words from their shapes, from the look of them. The shortcoming of this approach is that early readers will have no way of recognising words that they have not yet learned.

Phonics breaks down words into sounds and encourages the sounding out of words. Children are encouraged to pick out patterns in the sounds of words, noticing rhymes and rhythms. This disadvantage with this method is that English is not phonically regular – a letter may make one sound in one word and a completely different sound in another. It is not very rewarding for the early reader to be limited to phonically regular words that can be sounded out. On the other hand, a knowledge of phonics will give children a good strategy for attempting unfamiliar words.

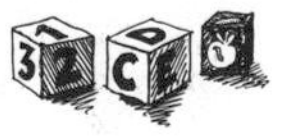

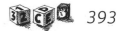

There is some debate over which is the most effective method and a combination of both is usually applied. However, the National Literacy Strategy emphasises a phonic approach to reading and through the Foundation Stage and into Key Stage One, children will be encouraged to learn letter sounds and then the sounds that letters make when combined with others.

Reading schemes or 'real books'?

Reading schemes are carefully structured and graded. A limited number of words is introduced in each book and there is much repetition of these words. The same characters usually appear in a number of books so children have the opportunity to become familiar with them.

Critics of reading schemes say that the stories are contrived and that the language of the books is stilted. They advocate the use of 'real books' for readers, that is picture books and story books that represent good children's literature. They maintain that interesting books make children want to read and that this motivation brings success. Critics of the 'real books' approach say that children miss the step-by-step structure and may choose books that are beyond their capabilities.

Most settings use a mixture of both reading schemes and 'real books', adjusting their approach to what best suits the individual child alongside the preference of the teacher.

How can you help?

Early readers need lots of practice. When you listen to children read you can help them by:

- giving them your attention
- finding a place with minimal distractions
- giving the child thinking time
- helping when necessary – sometimes a bit of encouragement or a clue, for example 'What's that sound?', 'What's happening in that picture?' can help the child move on
- talking about the book and getting them to talk to you – the child may lose the sense of a story when reading it word by word
- monitoring and recording their progress – you may notice that a child is not doing very well on a particular book, so suggest something else, as different approaches suit different children
- alerting them to patterns in words and sounds
- being positive about their achievements.

You might also be involved in making special individual books for children. These usually consist of photographs of the child with simple text about themselves, their family and so on, mounted on card and bound in some way. These are very popular and are often the first books that children get to read.

Remember that reading is a complex skill that may take years to achieve. As with all skills, some children will grasp it easily and progress quickly, while others find it more difficult.

Case study . . .

. . . a book for Nathan

Nathan, at 5+, was showing himself to be a very reluctant reader. While most of the other children in his class were making progress with the early levels of the reading scheme, he seemed uninterested. When Maria, the nursery nurse, tried to interest him in the books, he replied that they were boring and just for babies. She decided to involve him in making a special book, just for him. They spent some time together talking about him and what he liked to do and his favourite things. Maria took some photographs of Nathan and found other illustrations from magazines, and she made a book using these pictures and simple text that was all about Nathan and presented it to him. Nathan was very pleased with his book and worked hard with Maria to read the text. Maria followed this up with another book, this time about Nathan's pets. After a few weeks, he began to express an interest in the other reading books around the classroom.

1. *Why do you think Nathan rejected the reading books?*
2. *Why was Maria's approach successful?*
3. *Why is it important to encourage reluctant readers early on?*
4. *What could you learn from this case study?*

Writing

Children begin writing by making marks. To adults this may appear to be meaningless scribble, but to the child it is a telephone message, a letter to Santa, their name. During their early years in school, children need to learn the rules and conventions of writing. It becomes an important tool that they use to communicate with themselves and with the outside world.

The conventions of writing that children need to learn are as follows:

- *Letter formation* – children need to know how to form letters correctly and consistently. This means where you start and where you finish and requires a great deal of practice. Children also learn to recognise the feel of a letter when they write it. Tracing in the air and in sand helps to reinforce this.
- *Orientation* – in English (and many other languages) this means writing (and reading) from left to right and from top to bottom. Bilingual children may have experienced a written language, Urdu or Hebrew for example, that is oriented differently.
- *Spacing* – groups of letters go together to form words and spaces separate these words. Spacing words correctly needs practice.
- *Spelling* – children need to learn that there is a standard way of spelling words. However, excessive concentration on this at the very early stages will limit and inhibit children's writing.
- *Punctuation* – this is a skill acquired later, but children notice punctuation early on in their reading and begin to introduce it into their writing. It also includes the appropriate use of upper and lower case letters.

Children's writing is not just about the technical skills listed above, it is about content too. Sometimes children become overwhelmed by these technical skills and this affects the content of their writing. A child who is limited to the words that they can spell correctly or who is afraid to make a mistake will not become involved in or enjoy writing. It will become a task to be completed because an adult demands it. A sensitive adult will watch the child's progress and introduce the need for correct spelling at the right stage, ensuring that child retains confidence in their writing abilities.

Teaching writing

Writing is taught in a variety of different ways. All approaches will ensure that children learn to form letters correctly and develop fluency in their handwriting style. Some schools favour an approach where the child writes completely on their own and then reads the writing back to an adult who may then identify something with the child that can be discussed. This approach is known as **emergent writing** (or developmental writing). It enables children to get on with what they want to write without waiting for an adult to show them the correct way to write a word. Critics say that technical accuracy takes longer to establish with this method. Other schools place an earlier emphasis on accuracy, with children relying on adults for correct spelling at an early stage, with independent writing coming later. Critics of this approach say that children become over-dependent on adults and may not have the confidence to make their own attempts. Of course, there are merits in both approaches and most schools will strike a balance with the aim of producing children's writing that shows both independence and accuracy.

key term

Emergent writing
an approach to writing that encourages children to write independently; also known as developmental writing

Case study . . .

. . . emergent writing

The Reception class had been working on a topic about minibeasts, which had involved searching for wildlife in the school garden and examining the animals closely. The school encouraged independent writing by valuing children's emergent writing. After the session in the garden with the microscopes and bug-boxes, the children were encouraged to write about their investigations. Katy was engrossed and spent a long time over her writing. When she had finished, she took it to her teacher and read out her writing to her.

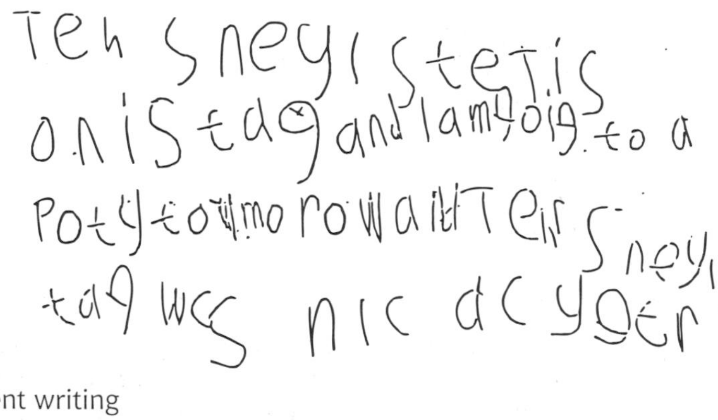

Katy's emergent writing

This is what she read: 'The snail's teeth is on its tongue and I am going to a party tomorrow and the snail's tongue works like a cheese grater.'

1. *What purpose was Katy using her writing for?*
2. *What did she gain from this exercise?*
3. *What was the teacher's role here?*
4. *Refer back to the section on the conventions of writing above. Which of the conventions of writing has Katy grasped?*

How can you help?

- Sit with children and help them form letters correctly. Left-handed children may need particular help.
- Be a good role model. Let children watch you making notes for your file, filling in a register and so on, so they see that writing is a part of everyday life.
- When you write for children, make sure that your writing is clear, legible and accurate. If children are going to copy your writing, make sure that it is large enough.
- Talk to children about their writing; use it in displays. Let them know that you value it.
- Present children with a variety of writing tasks, not just stories. Get them to make shopping lists, record experiments, write letters and invitations.
- Show children that writing can be found in many different places. Collect examples – involve children in this – and make a display of comics, cereal boxes, bus tickets, labels, and so on.
- Help children to present their writing in different ways, such as making books, using a word processor.

Progress check

What does the term literacy mean? Why is it important that children become literate?

Why is it important that children have an understanding of the purposes of reading and writing?

What are the differences between the phonic method and the look and say approach to teaching reading?

Why is it important that children learn the conventions of writing?

What is emergent writing?

Children's books

Books are an important and integral part of the early years curriculum. They are provided in all nurseries and classrooms. Reading and story time are part of each day. Some children also have books at home and read with parents and carers. This early experience of books is very important in establishing positive attitudes to books and to reading.

WHY ARE BOOKS IMPORTANT?

Books and stories are an important part of children's development. Outlined below are some of the main skills that can be developed and nurtured. Books and stories can be introduced to very young children. Although the child may not fully understand the story, a quiet, intimate time reading with a parent or carer forms a positive association for the child. This in turn helps to establish a habit of reading and listening to stories that has many benefits for the child.

Language development

Language is learned: the more exposure a child has to different patterns in language, the richer their own language is likely to be. Initially this will be expressive (spoken) language, later read and written language. Listening to stories and talking about books enables young children to listen and respond to the sound and rhythm of spoken language. This is important to speech development at all levels. Initially children need to recognise the sounds and rhythms that occur in their language; once this has been established they need to practise and refine their use of spoken language.

Listening to stories can also extend a child's vocabulary. As long as most of the language in the text is familiar to the child, new, imaginative language can be introduced. The child will begin to understand these new words by their context, that is, how they are used and linked with the story line and the pictures.

Experience with books and story telling is also an important part of a child's early understanding of symbols. A child who has contact with books begins to understand that the squiggles on the page represent speech. This is a vital skill in the development of reading and writing.

Emotional development

Books and stories are enjoyable. They give children the opportunity to express a whole range of positive emotions. They provide a rich imaginative world that can be a source of great pleasure to the child, and through identification with the characters and the story line children can develop and practise their own responses to events and experience situations and feelings that are beyond their own life experiences. This can be done in a safe environment where the child has an element of control over events.

Cognitive development

Books, if carefully chosen, can provide a powerful stimulus to the imagination of a child. They can encourage interesting and exciting thoughts and ideas. The development of imagination is an important part of being creative. Creative thoughts and ideas are an important part of the quality of life and necessary to the development of society.

Books can also introduce children to a wide range of concepts. Repetition and varied contexts enable children to develop their understanding of the world that they live in. Listening to stories, recalling and sequencing the events are also positive ways of extending young children's concentration span and memory.

Social development

Books and stories are more than just the presentation of a sequence of events; they carry in them a whole range of messages about how a society functions. This includes acceptable patterns of behaviour, expectations of groups within the society and moral codes of right and wrong. Children pick up these messages. It is therefore vital that books for young children portray a positive view of society and the people within that society. This positive view of the world contributes towards young children developing a balanced and constructive outlook on life.

Group story time and sharing books contribute to the development of social skills of sharing, turn taking and co-operating with others. Children begin to learn that they have to take other people's needs and wishes into account. Story time can also provide children and adults with the opportunity to build and maintain relationships. If a cosy and comfortable environment is provided it offers a sense of closeness and intimacy for the children and adults involved.

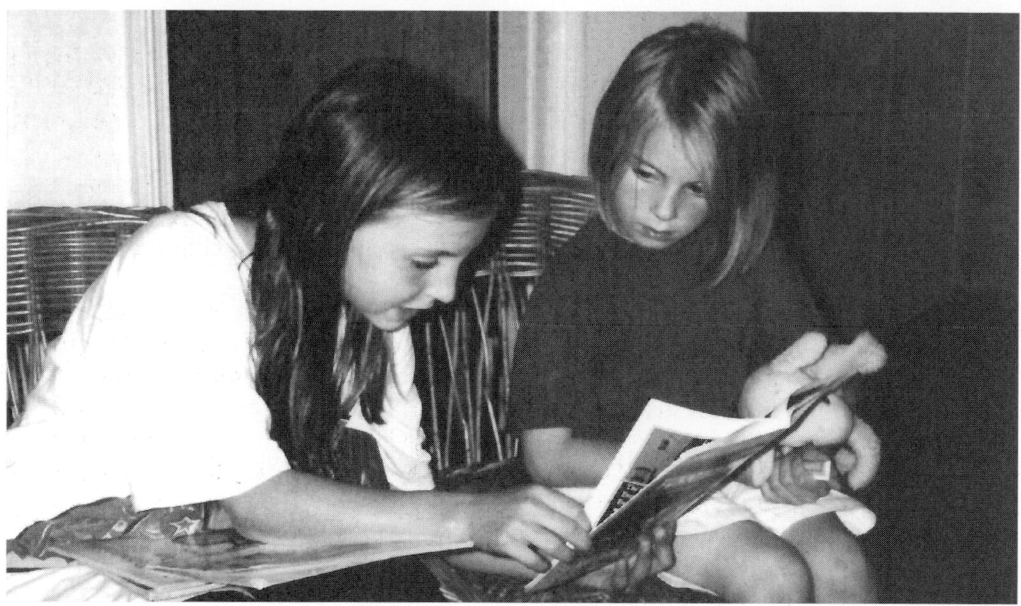

Sharing books contributes to the development of social skills

CHOOSING CHILDREN'S BOOKS

It is important that children's books are chosen carefully. Children have different needs and interests at different stages of their development. The maximum benefit can be gained if the book chosen meets the child's needs. All children are individual and will have different needs, likes and dislikes. This needs to be taken into account. There are, however, some general points to consider when choosing a book for a young child and these are listed in the table below.

PLANNING STORY TIME

Story time needs to be planned as carefully as any other activity for children. The following points should be considered for all story telling, whether on a one-to-one basis, or in a small or large group:

- Choose a book that is appropriate to the child/children involved, considering their interest and their concentration span.
- Allow the child to see the pages as the story is being told.
- Point to the words as you read them, demonstrating left-to-right tracking and identifying individual words as you say them. This will help children to develop aural reading and writing skills.
- Tell the story enthusiastically; showing that you are enjoying it.
- Talk about the book after you have read it through, and follow on with songs and rhymes that link to the subject.

When telling a story to a group of children you also need to think about:

- *the area* – it should be cosy, quiet, warm, comfortable
- *the structure of the session* – introduction, story, discussion topics and questions, rhymes or songs appropriate, where possible, to the story

Books are a powerful way of influencing children's views about the society they live in. Books for children must, therefore, reflect positive images of all sections of society, in both the text and the illustrations.

0–3 YEARS

- Picture books are appropriate for this age range, especially for children under 1 year.
- Where there is text, it needs to be limited, especially for children aged 0–1.
- The pictures need to have bright colours and bold shapes.
- The pictures need little detail. They need to be simplified so that they are easily identified – the most obvious features stressed.
- Children enjoy familiar themes, for example families, animals.
- The complexity of pictures and text can be increased for children aged 2+.
- The context of the story time is as important as the book itself; the cosy, close and intimate time gives children a positive association with books and reading.

3–5 YEARS

- Repetition is important – for language development and for the enjoyment of the sound and rhythm of language.
- Books need to be reasonably short, to match children's concentration span.
- Books need minimum language with plenty of pictures that relate to the text.
- Popular themes are still everyday objects and occurrences.

5–7 YEARS

- A clearly identifiable story and setting are important.
- Children's wider interests, experiences and imagination should be reflected in themes.
- The characters can be developed through the story.
- Language can be richer – playing with rhyme and rhythm, the introduction of new vocabulary and the use of repetition for dramatic effect.

3–7 YEARS

- Illustrations still need to be bold, bright and eye-catching, but can be more detailed and have more meaning than pure recognition.
- Sequenced stories become popular – with a beginning, middle and end.
- The story line needs to be easy to follow, with a limited number of characters.
- Repetition is important so that the reader or listener can become involved in the text.
- Animated objects are popular – children can enter into the fantasy.
- Children enjoy humour in stories, but it needs to be obvious humour, not puns or sarcasm.

Guidelines for choosing books for young children

key term

Story sack
an aid to story telling that contains puppets, games or other activities linked to the story

- *visual aids* – a storyboard, puppets and other props will encourage participation and understanding, with **story sacks,** which contain puppets, games or other activities linked to a particular story, being particularly effective
- *behaviour management* – how will you manage the behaviour to minimise interruptions and to make sure that all children can be involved in the session?

Progress check

Why is it important to introduce books and stories to young children?

How can books and story telling contribute to children's all-round development?

How can books and stories influence children's view of the society that they are growing up in?

What criteria should be used when selecting books to use with children?

Why should an area for telling a story be cosy, quiet, warm and comfortable?

What are the benefits of using visual aids in story telling?

Developing maths

Maths in the early years should be approached primarily through practical activities that children will be able to relate to and understand. Children who 'do' maths through first-hand experiences are most likely to develop confidence and understanding in the subject. Much of what children experience in activities will involve an element of maths. This may be something that is planned, for example measuring sunflowers to find out which is tallest, or it may arise incidentally, perhaps when a child is sharing out birthday sweets. The child-care worker needs to be aware of the mathematical potential of any situation and be prepared to extend and develop this through interactions with the children.

Remember that many adults feel nervous about maths, perhaps recalling negative experiences from their own schooldays. It is important that this negative attitude is not passed on to children.

In Reception classes, children will be introduced to the National Numeracy strategy, building up to the full daily lesson in year 1. It is important that a firm foundation is laid in children's early mathematics where understanding is developed from practical experiences before more abstract calculation is required.

WHAT IS MATHS?

Maths is all around us and children have many mathematical experiences in their everyday lives before they begin the formal study of maths.

Maths is much more than figures and formulae.

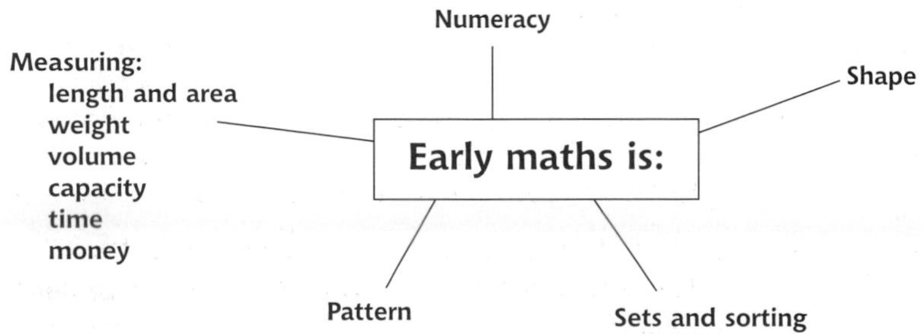

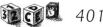

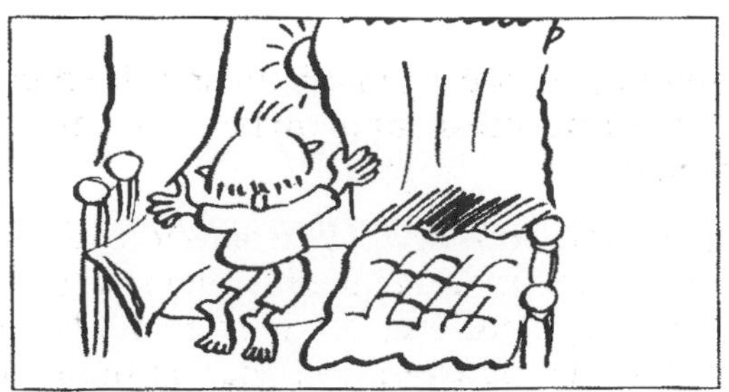

1. Getting up. Is it still dark? (Time; making logical deductions)

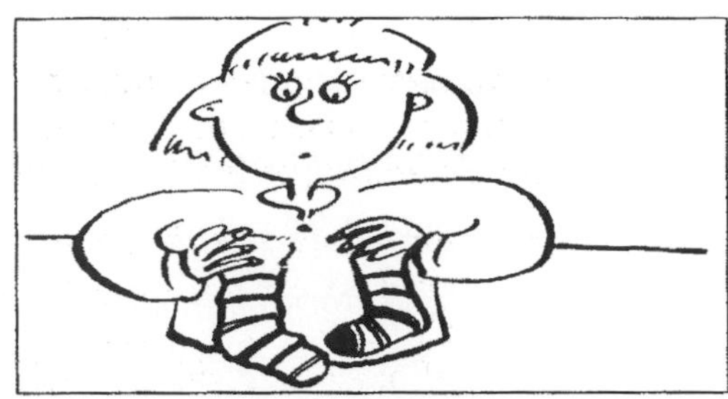

2. Getting dressed; putting clothes on in the right order. Are these socks a pair? (Sorting, sequencing, matching)

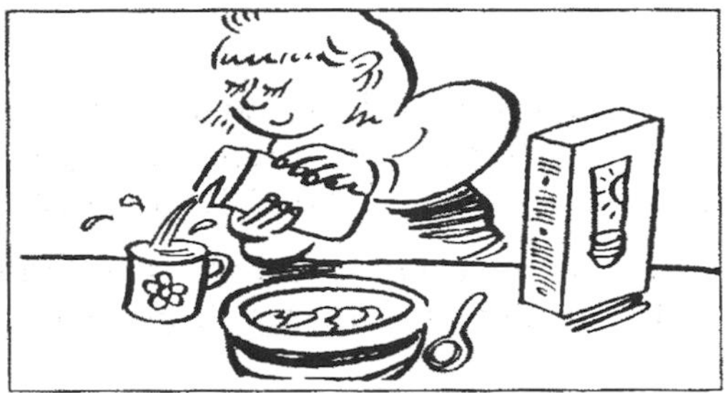

3. Having breakfast; pour cornflakes into a bowl and juice into a cup. Ooops! Don't spill it! (Estimating quantity, volume)

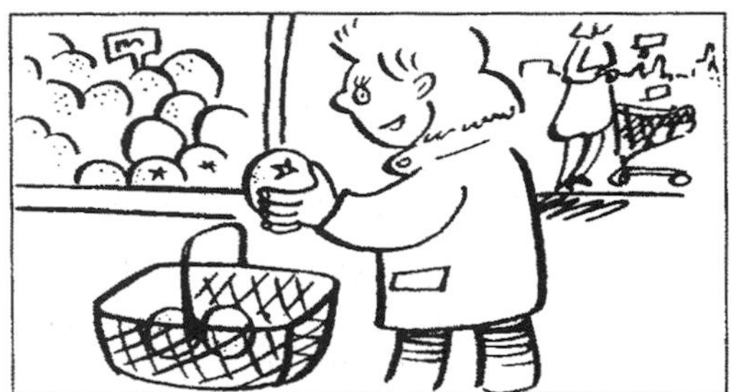

4. Going shopping. How many oranges? A large packet or a small packet? How much does it cost? (Counting, size, money)

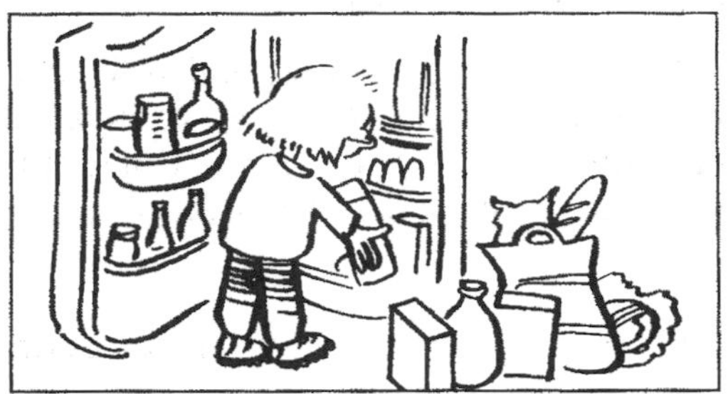

5. Unpacking the bags. Where will these boxes fit? What goes in the fridge? (Sorting, shape, size)

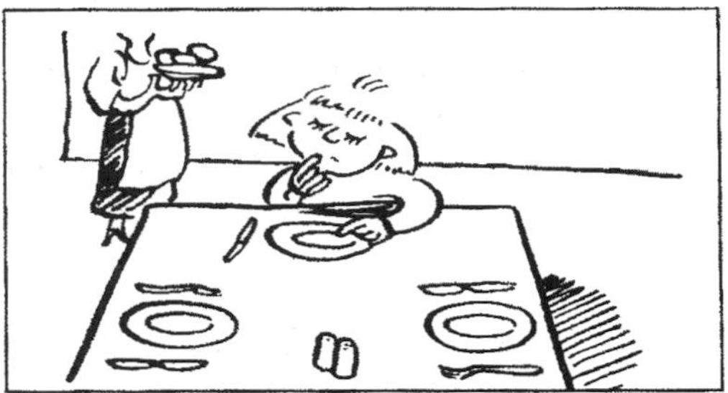

6. Laying the table. How many places? Are there enough plates? How long before we eat? (Matching, counting, time)

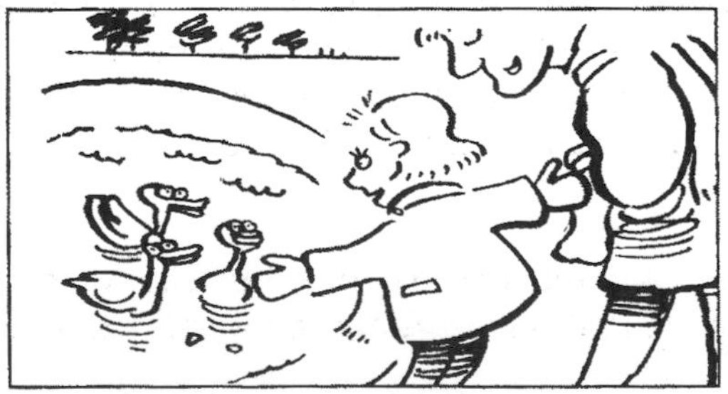

7. Out for a walk. How far is it? Have I seen more buses or more lorries? How many ducks on the pond? (Estimating, comparing, counting)

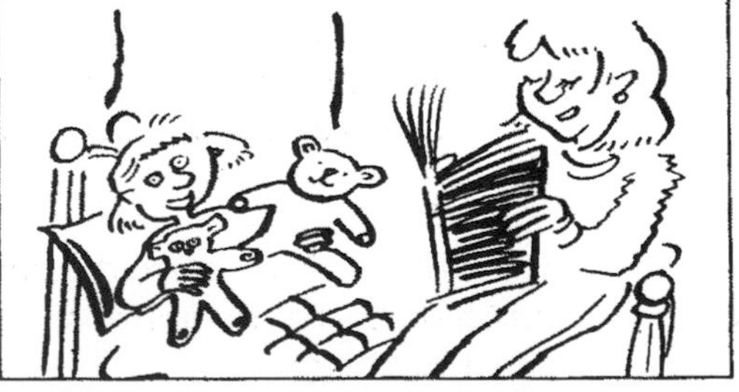

8. Bedtime. Can I have one more story? I'll have the big teddy and the little teddy. How long is it till morning? (Number, size, time)

Mary's mathematical day shows how maths is contained in children's everyday experience

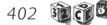

Numeracy

Numeracy includes counting, estimating, recording numbers and the four rules of number – addition, subtraction, multiplication and division – and, later, an understanding of fractions and decimals.

- *Activities* – taking every opportunity to count, for example children in the class, coats on the pegs, bottles in the crate; matching one thing to another, children to chairs, saucers to cups; linking number symbols to groups of objects; dividing apples into halves, quarters and sharing them out; using real objects to add to, take away, share. As they develop an understanding of number, children will begin to recognise numerals and use symbols to record their work.

Shape

Children need to be able to recognise shapes in both two and three dimensions. They need to learn about the properties of shapes, for example that cylinders roll, cubes have right angles, how they fit together and the space that they occupy.

- *Activities* – identifying shapes in the environment; drawing around shapes; sorting junk and modelling with it; making shapes with playdough or clay; building with bricks.

Sets and sorting

Children need to be able to sort objects into sets and explain why they belong there. This contributes to the development of their logical abilities.

- *Activities* – sorting with structured sorting apparatus and with collections of shells, beads, etc.; sorting for colour, for shape, for more complex attributes, for example, making a set of animals that live on farms. Older children will begin to record their findings on diagrams and in other ways.

Pattern

Pattern occurs both in number and in shape. It is an important mathematical concept that lays the foundation for algebra. The essential features of a pattern are that it is regular and predictable.

- *Activities* – looking for pattern in the environment, for example in brick walls, on floor tiles, on fabrics and also in nature, in animal markings and in plant life; making patterns with beads, bricks and other materials including painting, printing and collage; copying and continuing patterns with bricks, beads and peg boards and also using computer software.

Money

As for numeracy, but additionally children will become familiar with coins and understand about equivalence, that is that one coin may be worth the same as, say, ten other coins.

- *Activities* – making shops in the classroom and buying and selling; counting real money, for example milk or trip money; handling play money and sorting coins; making a collection of price tags, receipts, etc.

Time

Children need to understand that time can be measured and to be familiar with how we measure time. At about 7 years, we expect children to be able to read the time from both analogue and digital clock faces. They also need to be able to sort events into past, present and future.

- *Activities* – talking about daily routines; filling in daily calendars; using all kinds of timers to measure, for example, how many jumps in a minute, etc.; using movable clock faces. Stories such as *Sleeping Beauty* deal with the passing of time and can be helpful to children's understanding of this concept.

Weight

Children need to be able to use non-standard (a book weighs as much as three apples) and standard (grams and kilograms, pounds and ounces) measures. They need to be able to apply the concept of equivalence (equal weight) and be able to make comparisons based on weight.

- *Activities* – practical experience of holding things and talking about *heavy* and *light*, then *heavier than*, *lighter than*; cooking activities using non-standard (cups, spoons) or standard measures; using balance scales to weigh first with non-standard, then with standard measures (balance scales provide clear evidence of equivalence that the children can see); investigation of other types of scales.

Length and area

Children need to be able to estimate and measure length and area using non-standard as well as standard measures. They need to be able to select the most appropriate unit of measurement for the task.

- *Activities* – measuring with hand spans, strides, pencils, etc.; measuring using standard measures, rulers, tapes, trundle wheels; measuring and making charts of height – who is tallest?, who is smallest? – ordering: smallest to tallest, tallest to smallest; drawing around hands, feet, children on squared paper and counting the squares; covering box models with paper and estimating how much is needed.

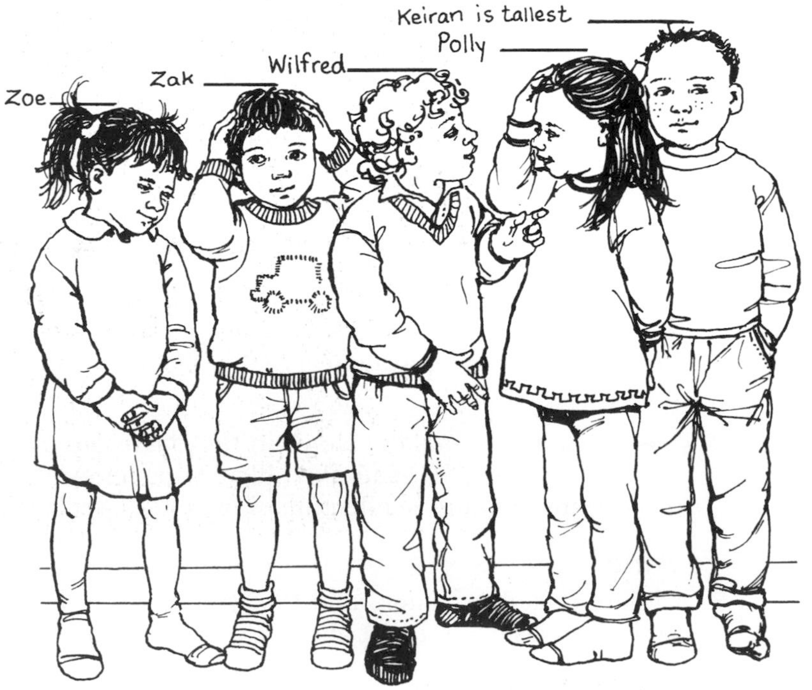

Get children to measure and compare heights

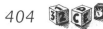

Case study . . .

. . . measuring the playground

The children in the nursery had been talking about measuring. They had taken part in a number of different measuring activities, using hand spans, strides, pencils, bricks and conkers. A group of the older children wanted to measure the playground. After some discussion, they settled on using pencils as their unit of measurement, placing a number of pencils end to end. The task proved too much for them and they soon gave up. At group time later that morning they talked about their difficulties and, together with the nursery nurse, decided on other ways of going about the task in the afternoon.

1. *Why did this prove such a difficult task for the children?*
2. *What would you have suggested to help them?*
3. *What did the children learn from this unsuccessful attempt?*

Capacity and volume

This is a difficult concept for young children to grasp. They need to understand that capacity and volume can be measured using non-standard as well as standard measures. They need to be able to compare containers of different sizes and shapes and to make comparisons about their capacity.

- *Activities* – filling buckets, beakers, containers with sand or water. Posing problems – how many cups to fill a bucket? Using standard measures to compare the capacity of other containers; 'real life' questions – how many beakers can you fill from a squash bottle?

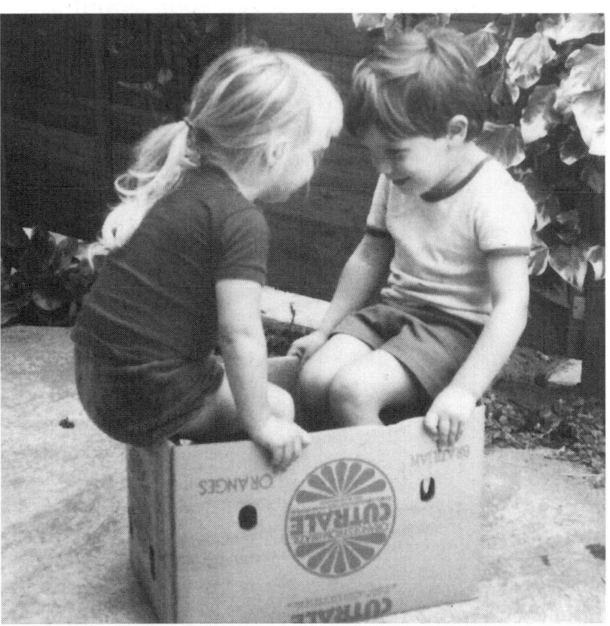

How can we fit into this box?

How can you help?

- Encourage and explain. Many children take a while to grasp new ideas.

- Talk to the children about their work. Introduce mathematical language, *more than*, *less than*, etc. Name shapes accurately.
- Use everyday experiences to reinforce mathematical learning, for example counting stairs, sharing biscuits, laying the table.
- Be aware of the mathematical potential of activities and experiences and develop children's understanding.
- Observe progress on an individual level and use this to plan the next step.

Progress check

How should early maths be approached?

What are the elements of early maths?

Why is it vital to promote positive attitudes to maths in the early years?

Why is it important to give children practical experiences to develop their mathematical understanding?

How can the adult promote children's mathematical development?

Science and technology

Children are naturally curious about themselves and about the world they inhabit. Good early years provision will harness this curiosity, providing the foundation for children's scientific understanding. Science and technology are aspects of the 'Knowledge and understanding of the world' programme of learning in the Early Learning Goals and have separate programmes of study at Key Stage One of the National Curriculum.

WHAT IS SCIENCE?

There are many situations in which the young child can be a scientist. Here are some examples:

- *the natural world* – caring for plants and animals, looking at the seasons, caring for the environment, life cycles, work on growth, ourselves
- *natural materials* – discovering the properties of water, wood, clay, sand, air, and so on
- *creative materials* – identifying the science in painting, collage, junk modelling, music
- *the physical world* – using magnets and batteries, investigating light and colour with lenses and mirrors, looking at movement and forces
- *chemistry* – combining substances, watching changes, e.g. in cooking.

Science is not approached in isolation. In the pre-school years, it is an integral part of many of the activities provided routinely, such as outdoor play, construction, sand, water, paint. In school, scientific themes will be developed through topic work.

How can you help?

The adult's role in promoting the growth of children's scientific understanding is crucial. Their role is to:

- provide a rich and stimulating environment for the children
- interact and question the children, encouraging them to think, to pose questions and to solve problems for themselves
- help children decide on ways to try out their ideas, including ways of designing a fair test
- help children to organise their understanding of what has happened, that is, to draw conclusions and to form concepts
- encourage children to record their findings using a variety of methods including talking, drawing, making tables, writing
- monitor children's progress and provide opportunities to extend learning.

Case study . . .

. . . planting seeds

The year 1 class were to plant some bean seeds as part of their work around the theme of growing. Sally, the nursery nurse, gathered a small group of children together to talk about what they were going to do. She wanted the children to understand that living things would only grow if they received the care that they needed.

They looked at the seeds carefully, examining them with magnifying glasses. The children were encouraged to describe them, commenting that they were hard and shiny. They talked about what they would do to make them grow. Some of the children had experience of growing things at home and were keen to make suggestions. They all agreed that the beans needed soil and water to grow, but they couldn't decide on whether they needed a warm place or a cool place and whether it should be light or dark. Eventually they decided that they would try out a number of places. They would plant all the seeds in soil and keep them moist, but would put one pot in the fridge (cool and dark), one in the cupboard (warm and dark), another on the window-sill (warm and light) and the last outside (cool and light). They marked on the calendar when they'd planted them and examined them every week on the same day, recording their seed's progress by drawing it on the right pot on the weekly progress sheet.

After three weeks, Sally got the group together and asked them to look at the seeds in the pots and decide which had grown most successfully. They were then able to decide, from their experience, what conditions were best for growing seeds. They recorded their decision on the final progress sheet and used the school camera to record the 'evidence'.

1. *What did the children learn about the principles of scientific investigation from this activity?*
2. *Why was it important that the children were able to follow through their own ideas about growing?*
3. *How were children's observational skills developed here?*
4. *How did the adult support the children's learning through this activity?*
5. *Think of some other activities that would encourage children to develop early science skills.*

TECHNOLOGY AND ICT

Technology for the early years is closely linked to science. It involves the use of tools and materials in practical projects. Children need opportunities to plan and design, as well as to make. As their experience increases, their designs will become more complex. In this area of learning, the adult's role is to give the children access to a range of materials and to encourage them to complete and evaluate their projects. This will include the teaching and practising of techniques such as cutting, joining things and sewing, as well as encouraging the children in their projects.

Technology should be available for use by children to support their learning across the curriculum. They will have access to a range of equipment, for example, cassette recorders, cameras, electronic keyboards, televisions and video recorders.

Information and communication technology (ICT), involving the use of computers, is now very much a part of the early years curriculum. Children will become familiar with the operation of the equipment and work with software programs specially designed to meet their learning needs. In our electronic age, it is expected that children become familiar with information and communication technology, and use it to support their learning across all areas of the curriculum.

Progress check

What kinds of activities will allow children to develop scientific understanding?

What is the role of the adult in promoting children's scientific understanding?

Why is it important that children be encouraged to ask questions?

What is the adult's role in asking and answering questions?

In what ways can children record their investigations and findings?

What does early years technology consist of?

How can children use information and communication technology to support their learning across the curriculum? Give examples.

History and geography

History and geography will be included in any thematic approach to the early years curriculum. There are National Curriculum programmes of study for history and geography at Key Stage One. In the Early Learning Goals, these subjects are part of the programme for 'Knowledge and understanding of the world'.

HISTORY

The concept of time is not an easy one for young children to grasp. 'A long time ago' to a small child could be last week or years ago. However, there are some ways of making the notion of the past meaningful to children:

- Order and sequence events in their own lives, for example looking at photographs of themselves as babies and toddlers and comparing with the present day.

- Comparisons with 'then' and 'now' can be very successful, particularly if children have a chance to handle objects from the past and make a direct comparison with now, for example, comparing the dolly tub with an automatic washing machine.
- Many museums run excellent programmes that get children to experience, say, a Victorian schoolroom, complete with costumes and tasks.
- Getting older people to talk to children about the past can be helpful. Children can question their own parents and grandparents for insights about the recent past.
- Old newspapers and photographs can provide useful starting points. Children might search for clues and put the pictures in chronological order.

Case study . . .

. . . toys then and now

The nursery's topic for the term was 'Toys'. The children had been looking at their own toys and investigating what they were made of and what they could do with them. To develop the topic further, the nursery teacher brought in a selection of her own toys from 20 years ago, and asked the children's parents and grandparents if they had any toys that could be borrowed. They were all examined very thoroughly and the children commented on how different these toys were from their own. To further the investigation, the teacher was able to borrow a small collection of Victorian toys from a local museum. The children were fascinated when their teacher described how children would play in the street with whips and tops and would roll hoops along the gutter. When one child asked why the children hadn't been knocked over by cars while playing with their toys, the nursery teacher showed the children a photograph of the period so that they could judge the danger from traffic for themselves.

1. *Why was this an appropriate starting point for historical investigation?*
2. *Why do you think it was important that the children had a chance to handle the toys?*
3. *What do you think the children understand about the Victorian period as a result of this activity?*

GEOGRAPHY

The geography curriculum encourages children to investigate the physical and human features of their immediate surroundings and, from this basis, to learn about the wider world. The following activities would contribute to this understanding:

- making simple maps, perhaps of home-to-school routes
- reading simple maps by following directions and identifying features
- looking at similarities and differences in locations, for example between a city school and a village school – many schools 'twin' to achieve this
- providing opportunities to look carefully at the local environment, giving children a chance to recognise different uses of land and to notice changes. Children could also be asked to suggest how their environment could be improved

- noticing and recording the weather and acknowledging its importance and that of the seasonal cycle.

As children learn through direct experience with the world, much of this learning should be achieved by going out into the local environment. This may be to observe certain features, such as buildings or ponds, or to experience certain conditions, such as wind or snow. The adult's role here is to focus children's observation and to draw their attention to relevant features in the environment.

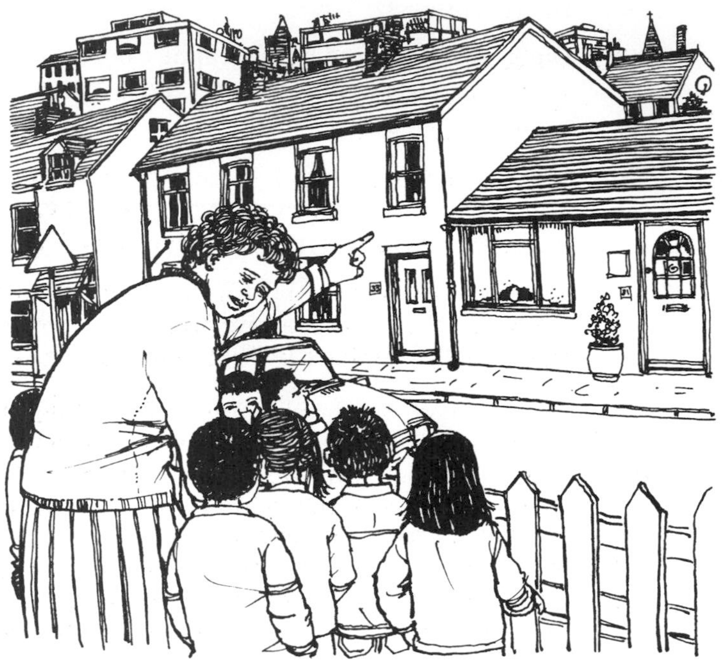

The adult can draw children's attention to relevant features in the environment

Progress check

Why is the concept of history difficult for young children to grasp?

List some of the ways in which history can be made relevant to young children.

What does the early years geography curriculum consist of?

Why is it important that children should go out and observe their environment?

Suggest some experiences that would contribute to children's geographical understanding.

Creativity

Creativity involves the expression of ideas. Creative activities provide children with a means of communication with themselves and with the outside world. Creative activities are those that value the process as well as the product of any endeavour. Opportunities for children to be creative, to develop their own ideas through a variety of media, should be provided throughout the early years.

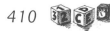

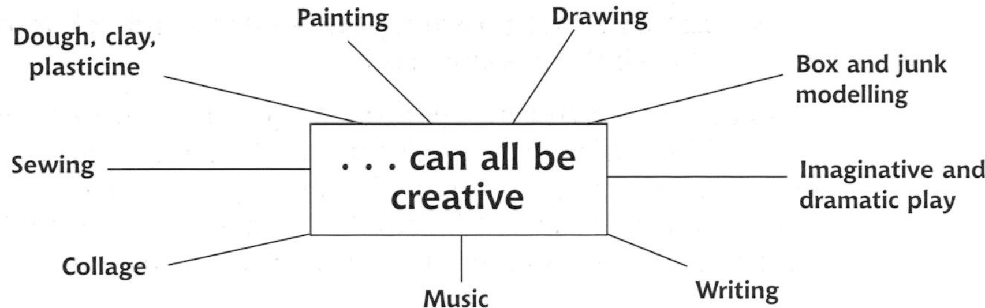

PROVIDING FOR CREATIVITY

> **key term**
> **Creativity**
> the expression of ideas in a personal and unique way, using the imagination

The way an activity is presented affects how much scope it offers for **creativity**. Consider the following activities:

1. Children have been asked to make a collage using natural materials they collected on an autumn walk. Paper and glue are available and the children are interpreting this brief in a number of ways.
2. Children are busy cutting around circles of paper. They are then sticking them on to an outline drawing of a clown on a piece of paper. They are matching the circles for size to spaces on the paper.

The first activity gives the children an opportunity to develop their own ideas, to be creative. The second activity, which is also a collage activity, is getting the children to practise the skill of cutting, and is developing their concepts of size and shape. This activity provides an opportunity for children to develop valuable skills, but it does not allow them to be creative.

What we expect from children and what we provide for them in creative activities needs to be linked to their developmental stage. At the early stages they will explore and experiment with the materials, using them in a random manner. They finish quickly and then move on to something else. As they become more experienced, they build up a repertoire of skills and techniques that they can then apply creatively. They will work for a longer period at an activity and show more concern for the end product.

Good early years provision will ensure that all aspects of children's creative development are catered for. A stimulating environment will encourage children to take part in a wide range of experiences, giving them opportunities to explore and experiment.

PROVIDING FOR DRAWING AND PAINTING

By the time they come to the child-care setting, children are likely to have widely varying experiences of drawing and painting. Most children will have had opportunities to use different types of drawing media and some will be familiar with paint. However, it is not helpful to assume that all children have had common experiences.

Drawing

A variety of drawing media will allow children to discover different properties and applications. The following would provide a range of effects:

- *Pencil* – offer thick and thin, carbon and coloured.
- *Charcoal* – demonstrate the techniques associated with the medium.
- *Chalk* – white and coloured chalks offer different effects and textures.
- *Wax crayons* – provide different thicknesses and textures.

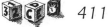

- *Felt and fibre-tip pens* – provide a wide range, including those where the colours blend together.
- *Pastels* – oil and water pastels produce a wide range of effects, although they are expensive and fragile.

Painting

The way that painting is provided for will depend on the space available and, to some extent, on the budget. With this in mind, here are some general points:

- *Provide a variety of paints* – include powder paint, redimix paint in squeezy bottles and finger paints. Mix paint with glue or paste for different effects.
- *Provide a variety of brushes and tools* – include thick and thin brushes, decorators' brushes for large areas. Introduce tools that can be used with paint such as sponges, corks, old toothbrushes and straws and demonstrate these techniques.
- *Provide a variety of paper* – give children the chance to paint on different surfaces, rough, smooth, shiny, corrugated. Cut paper to different sizes and shapes and offer a range of colours.
- *Consider the space* – large-scale works will need some floor space. Try to offer easels as well as tables so that children can discover how paint behaves in a vertical plane.

Providing for collage

Collage involves sticking two-dimensional or three-dimensional materials, such as fabrics, paper, twigs and feathers, and introduces children to a variety of textures.

- *Supply the correct adhesive* – children will soon become frustrated trying to stick carpet with wallpaper paste!
- *Collect and store a stimulating range of materials* – get children and parents to help.
- *Organise storage so that materials are accessible to children* – vet all materials for safety.
- *Present materials that are themed*, for example natural materials or shiny things. Choosing from within a theme can provide a framework for children to work within.
- *Provide a variety of surfaces for children to stick on to* – card, board, fabric, etc.
- *Teach children different tearing and cutting techniques*, and provide effective scissors.

Providing for box and junk modelling

Working in three dimensions presents another challenge to children's creativity as it provides them with more problems to solve.

- Collect sufficient materials to allow the children maximum flexibility.
- Store materials in an organised and accessible way.
- Demonstrate and resource a variety of joining techniques. As well as glue, include Sellotape, treasury tags, split pins, staples, cutting flaps and hinges.
- Provide enough space and time for the activity.
- Protect the models when they are at the fragile, wet stage.

Clay, dough and other malleable materials

Using these media provides another means of creative expression. Children will need time to familiarise themselves with the materials before they become aware of their potential. They will practise techniques of cutting and rolling and experiment with tools. These materials can be combined with others with contrasting textures, such as pebbles, fir cones and shells. For some malleable materials, baking and firing will extend the activity further.

MUSIC

The early years environment should provide children with opportunities to listen and respond to music and to make their own music. As well as fostering an appreciation of music, this will provide children with another channel for communication and self-expression.

- *Provide opportunities for children to listen to music* – introduce a wide range of musical styles, classical, contemporary, electronic. Choose music that is culturally diverse. Alert the children to the characteristics of music – pitch, tone, pace – and listen for phrases that recur.
- *Teach children songs and rhymes* – include all sorts of rhymes, traditional, funny, number, and from all over the world. Encourage children to recognise the rhythm in songs and rhymes. Introduce clapping and simple instrumental accompaniment.
- *Get children to move to music* – create a mood with music or use music to tell a story and get children to respond. Introduce children to different styles of dance and encourage children to respond to music with their bodies through dance.
- *Encourage children to make their own music* – for maximum variety, provide commercially produced instruments alongside the children's home-made ones. Let children tape their own music to use in their play or to share with their parents.

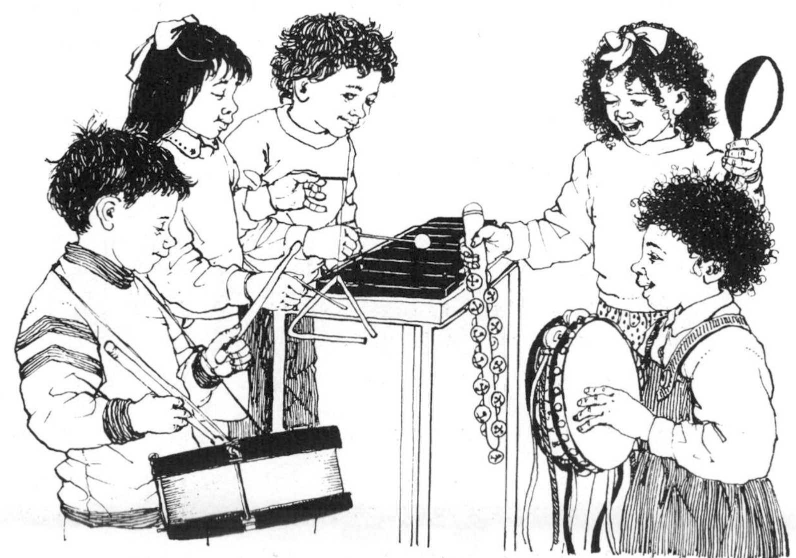

Give children an opportunity to make their own music

IMAGINATIVE AND DRAMATIC PLAY

Most settings will provide for a range of imaginative play opportunities. There is usually an area for domestic play and other provision for imaginative role play such as a café or hospital. Children will be able to create their own scenarios in construction areas and with small world play. Dressing-up clothes are often available, either linked to a theme or as a separate activity. Sand and water and other messy activities may also provide a focus for children's imaginative play.

Imaginative play provides children with a means of communication with others and themselves. It can also give them another perspective on the world and the role they play in it.

To encourage imaginative play:

- Vary home corner provision, maintaining a balance between new and familiar equipment.
- Plan imaginative play areas to link with any theme that might be developed.
- Ensure dressing-up clothes are easy to put on. Provide hats, bags and other accessories and a mirror for children to admire themselves in.
- Provide for large brick play. This often involves collaboration and complex story lines.
- Show children that you value their imaginative play by talking to them about it and join in, if appropriate, and extend and challenge sensitively.
- Present small world play in varied ways, sometimes on playmats, sometimes in the sand, sometimes in with the bricks.
- Plan for imaginative play outside too. Tents can be made from blankets and drapes. Chalk markings on the playground can trigger all kinds of games.
- Give children the time and space to develop their own imaginative play. Encourage them to use resources in their own unique ways.

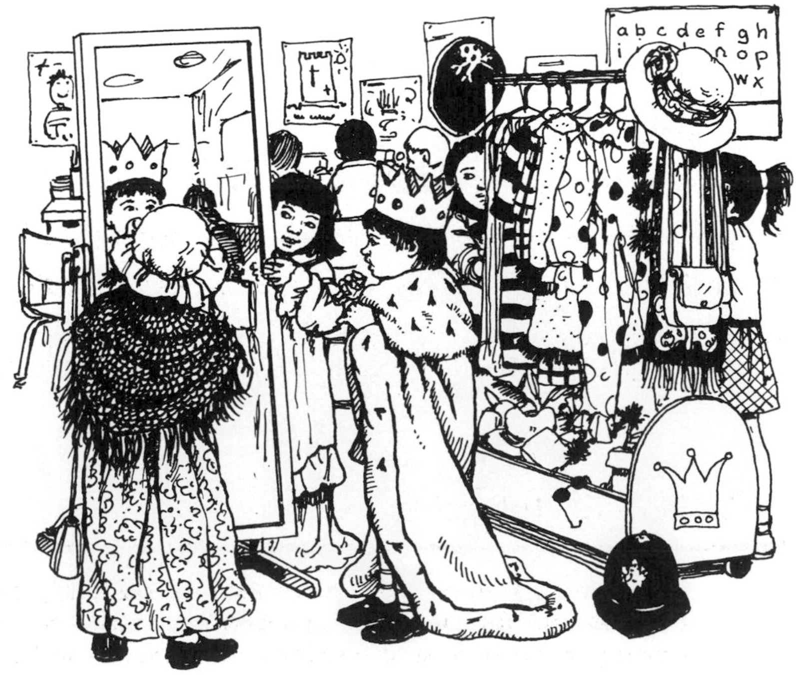

Children enjoy admiring themselves in a mirror

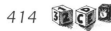

THE ROLE OF THE ADULT IN DEVELOPING CHILDREN'S CREATIVITY

Provision

- Select and present materials and equipment appropriate to the stage of development of the child, for example thick brushes for 3 year olds, finer ones for 7 year olds.
- Organise storage of materials so that they are accessible and easily maintained.
- Introduce new materials. They can act as a stimulus to children's ideas.
- Display children's work with care, showing that you value their own efforts.

Planning

- Give time and space to creative activities.
- Organise experiences that will act as a stimulus to creative activities.

Working alongside

- Encourage the child.
- Do not judge by adult standards. Value the child's work for its own sake.
- Do not do it for the child. You will make him dissatisfied with his own efforts and dependent on you.
- Children may be affronted if you ask 'What is it?'. 'Could you tell me about it?' might be better!
- Teach children techniques. Children's creativity may be hindered if they lack the skills associated with the activity.

Progress check

What is creativity?

What kinds of activities allow children to explore their creativity?

Why are creative activities important to children's development?

Make a list of the points that you should consider when providing for children's creativity?

How can adults support the development of children's creativity?

Physical activities

Physical activities are a vital part of the early years curriculum. They are important for the health and development of children and may also provide a starting point for leisure activities. All nurseries will provide regular opportunities for vigorous outside play. This kind of play is important for all areas of development, not just the physical (see Chapter 22, Play).

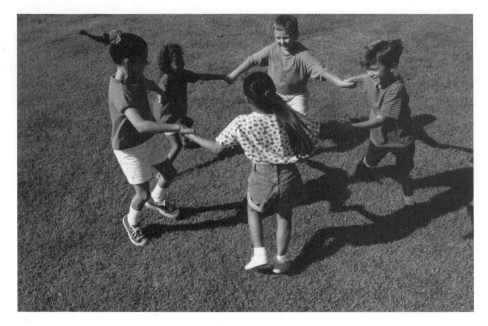

Vigorous outdoor play contributes to all areas of development

Many centres will provide some or all of the following as part of the PE curriculum:

- Gymnastics sessions that include floorwork as well as the use of large and small apparatus. Children often work with a theme in mind, for example moving on different parts of the body. They are encouraged to set targets for themselves. Some younger children might find the large apparatus daunting and adults should be sensitive to this and allow the child to stand by and watch until ready to join in. Children also have a part to play in the setting up and putting away of equipment; adequate supervision is vital here.
- Opportunities for dance to live or recorded music. Dance styles from a variety of cultures may be introduced, sometimes by demonstration.
- Games and games skills will be introduced during the early school years. These could be indoor or outdoor sessions. Younger children may have difficulty remembering rules but can usually manage simple games. Large team games are not suitable at this stage as the children spend too much time waiting. Remember that there can be quite significant differences in children's physical co-ordination, balance and manual dexterity at this age and this range needs to be catered for in any skills sessions.
- Equipment is important too: a beanbag is easier to catch than a tennis ball; a full-size football is too big for a small child. Make sure that all children take part. They will not enjoy playing the game if they have not had a chance to learn the skills.
- Swimming may be offered in areas where facilities are available. Children who have not experienced swimming before may be frightened at the prospect and need reassurance. If staffing is adequate, an adult in the water will help too. Sessions need to be short but frequent and children should never be forced into situations if they feel unsure.

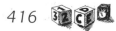

- In school, playtime will provide another opportunity for physical activities, often without the direction of an adult. Some children organise themselves in complicated games; others will enjoy just running around. Children new to the situation and used to the organisation and adult interaction of the nursery playground, may find the frenetic activity of the school playground frightening and will want to find a quiet place to observe until they feel more secure.

Remember to allow plenty of time for changing both before and after PE sessions, as many children will need help.

Case study . . .

. . . learning to swim

Dominic's class were to have a regular trip to the swimming baths once a week for the summer term. Many of the 6 and 7 year olds were regulars at the baths, but Dominic had never been before. The class teacher talked to the whole class about what they would be doing and reminded children to bring their swimsuits and towels for the session.

Although Dominic felt quite excited on the bus, when he got to the side of the pool he was too frightened to get in. Seeing the other children jumping in and splashing, obviously enjoying themselves, made him feel worse. His teacher told him to wrap himself up in his towel and find a place where he could watch. He didn't need to worry about going into the pool today.

Before the next session, the teacher had a word with Gina, one of the nursery nurse students on placement at the school, and arranged for her to go swimming with the group and join them in the water. Dominic started off on the side of the pool as before, but 5 minutes from the end of the session Gina managed to persuade him to sit with his legs dangling in the water, splashing and kicking.

Week by week, Dominic became more adventurous and, with Gina's help, by the end of the term he was spending the full time in the pool and asking his mum to take him swimming at the weekend.

1. *Why was the class teacher right to respond to Dominic's fears in the way that she did?*
2. *What would have happened if Dominic had been forced into the water?*
3. *Why do you think Gina's approach was successful in calming Dominic's fears?*

Progress check

Why is vigorous play important for children's development?

What kinds of physical activities are provided in school?

Why is it important to teach games skills to children?

How should you deal with children who are reluctant to join in with some physical activities?

Now try these questions

How can the child-care worker promote the development of children's writing?

What mathematical concepts could be introduced to children as part of a biscuit-making activity?

What points would you bear in mind when selecting books for 3 to 5 year olds?

Describe how you would promote children's creativity in painting?

How can you present the concept of history to children in an accessible way?

key terms

You need to know what the key terms and phrases in this chapter mean. Go back through the chapter and find out.

Unit 7: Work with Babies in the First Year of Life

In this unit you will learn about conception, antenatal care, birth and the care of young babies. This unit also covers the principles of promoting development and learning. On successful completion of this unit you should be able to identify how to practise safely and provide a positive, caring environment for babies. You should also understand how to promote a positive relationship with primary carers and be able to recognise and meet the needs of babies being cared for during the day in a group or domestic setting.

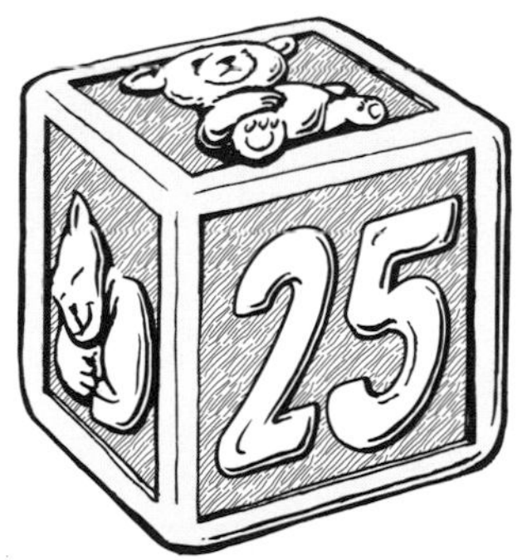

CONCEPTION, FETAL DEVELOPMENT AND ANTENATAL CARE

Growth and development of the baby begins well before the actual birth. Preparation by the prospective parents and good preconceptual care has a strong influence on future growth and development. Growth and development begins in the uterus at conception and continues throughout the 40 weeks of pregnancy and proceeds according to a set timetable. During this time there are many good and harmful influences that can affect growth and development. Good antenatal care helps to ensure the health of the mother and the unborn baby.

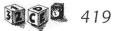

This chapter will cover the following topics:

- *the male and female reproductive organs*
- *the menstrual cycle*
- *the development of the ovum*
- *fetal growth and development*
- *preconceptual and antenatal care*
- *pregnancy.*

The male and female reproductive organs

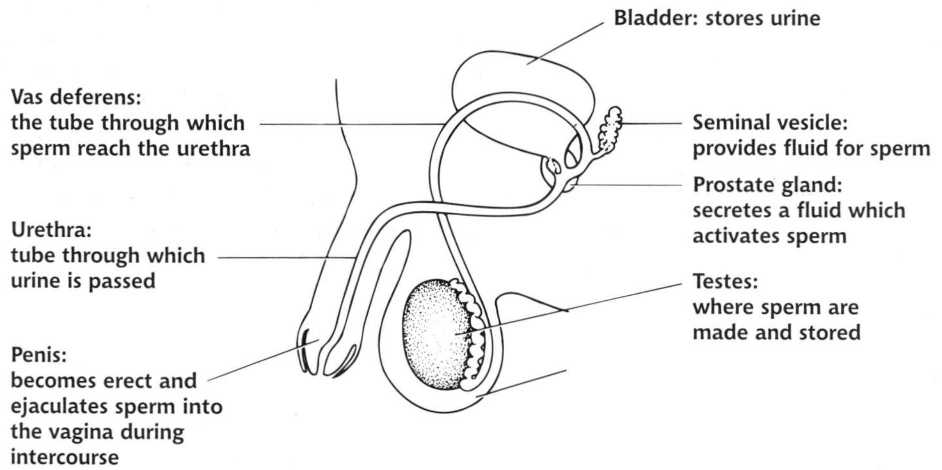

The male reproductive organs

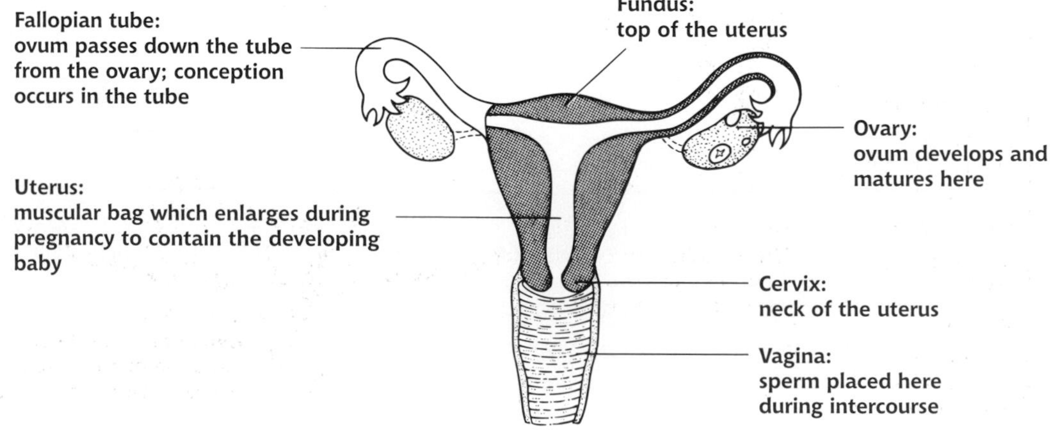

The female reproductive organs

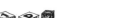

Progress check

What is the name of the narrow opening between the uterus and vagina?

What is the function of the prostate gland?

Where does the ovum develop?

What is contained in the scrotum?

Where does conception take place?

The menstrual cycle

key terms

Menstrual cycle
the process of ovulation and menstruation in sexually mature, non-pregnant women

Ovum
egg produced by the ovary

Uterus
part of the female reproductive tract; the womb

Sperm
the mature male sex cell

Conception
occurs when sperm fertilises a ripe ovum

Oestrogen
a hormone produced by the ovaries

Progesterone
a hormone produced by the ovaries

Endometrium
the lining of the uterus

Vascular
well supplied with blood vessels

The **menstrual cycle** concerns the production of a ripe **ovum** by the ovary and the preparation of the **uterus** to receive it. If the ovum is fertilised, by a **sperm**, after it has been released from the ovary then **conception** takes place. The menstrual cycle usually takes about 28 days to complete, but this will vary from woman to woman. The menstrual cycle is controlled by two hormones (chemical messengers) called **oestrogen** and **progesterone,** which are produced by the ovary. The first part of the cycle (called proliferation) is stimulated by oestrogen: the **endometrium** (the lining of the uterus) is reconstructed. The second part of the cycle (known as secretion) is stimulated by progesterone and the endometrium becomes thickened and **vascular** (well supplied with blood vessels) in order to nourish the fertilised ovum. In the pre-menstrual phase (called regression) the endometrium stops growing 5 to 6 days before menstruation.

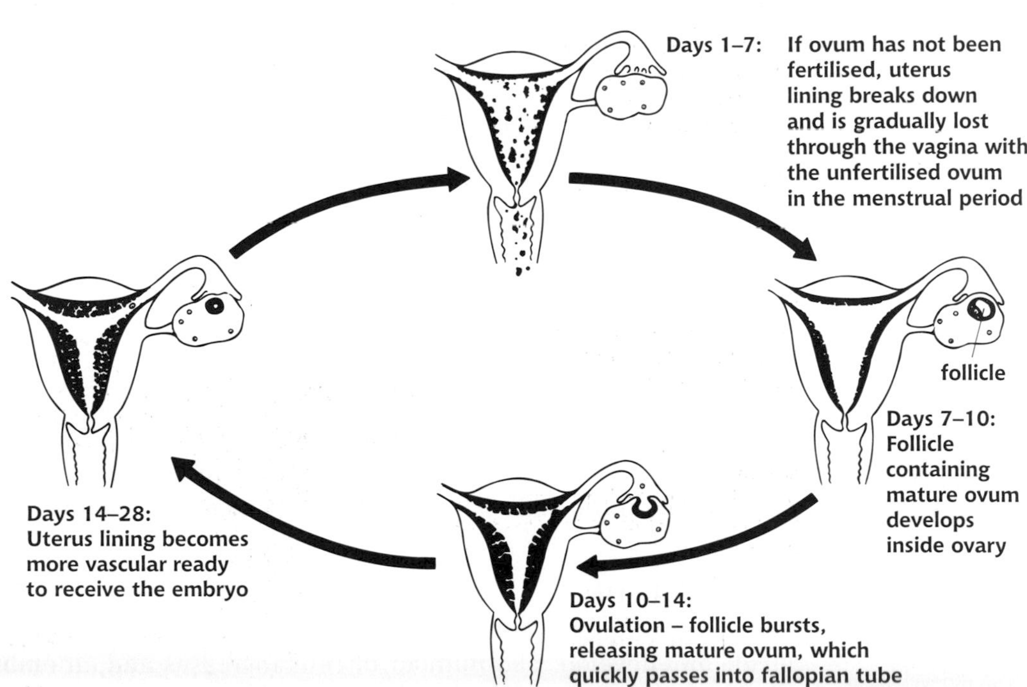
Days 1–7: If ovum has not been fertilised, uterus lining breaks down and is gradually lost through the vagina with the unfertilised ovum in the menstrual period
follicle
Days 7–10: Follicle containing mature ovum develops inside ovary
Days 10–14: Ovulation – follicle bursts, releasing mature ovum, which quickly passes into fallopian tube
Days 14–28: Uterus lining becomes more vascular ready to receive the embryo

The menstrual cycle

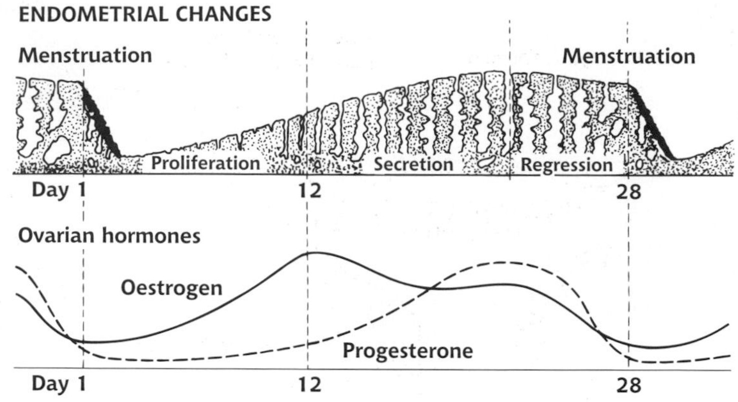

The influence of the ovarian hormones

Progress check

What is a hormone?

Which two hormones does the ovary produce?

When, in the menstrual cycle, does ovulation take place?

What happens to the endometrium if the ovum is not fertilised?

Where does the ovum develop?

The development of the ovum

key term

Implantation
occurs when the fertilised ovum settles into the lining of the uterus

key terms

Embryo
term used to describe the developing baby from conception until 8 weeks after conception

Placenta
structure that supports the baby as it develops in the uterus

At around day 12 of the menstrual cycle, a woman's ovaries release one ripe ovum. The ovum quickly passes into the Fallopian tube. During intercourse mature sperm from the male are deposited at the cervix in the female. The sperm are contained in a fluid called semen. If intercourse takes place around the time the ovum is released, the first active sperm to reach the ovum in the Fallopian tube will penetrate the outer shell and fertilise the ovum. Conception will have taken place. As soon as this happens the outer shell of the ovum becomes resistant to any other sperm so that only one sperm is allowed to fertilise the ovum.

When the ovum and sperm unite at fertilisation, genetic information from both partners combines to create a new individual. The fertilised ovum immediately begins to divide, first into two cells, then into four. It continues to divide in this way as it passes down the Fallopian tube to arrive in the uterus. The uterus lining has been preparing to receive it. The ball of cells settles into the uterine lining. This is called **implantation** and happens at around day 21 of the menstrual cycle.

IMPLANTATION

Once it has implanted into the lining of the uterus, the fertilised ovum continues to divide and develop. The number of cells increases and an **embryo** forms. Besides producing the embryo, the fertilised ovum also gives rise to the **placenta**, **umbilical cord** and **amnion**. These structures are developed for the support of the baby and they leave the uterus with the baby at birth.

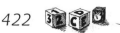

key terms

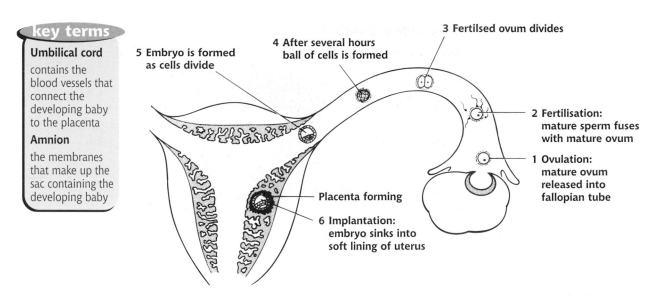

Umbilical cord contains the blood vessels that connect the developing baby to the placenta

Amnion the membranes that make up the sac containing the developing baby

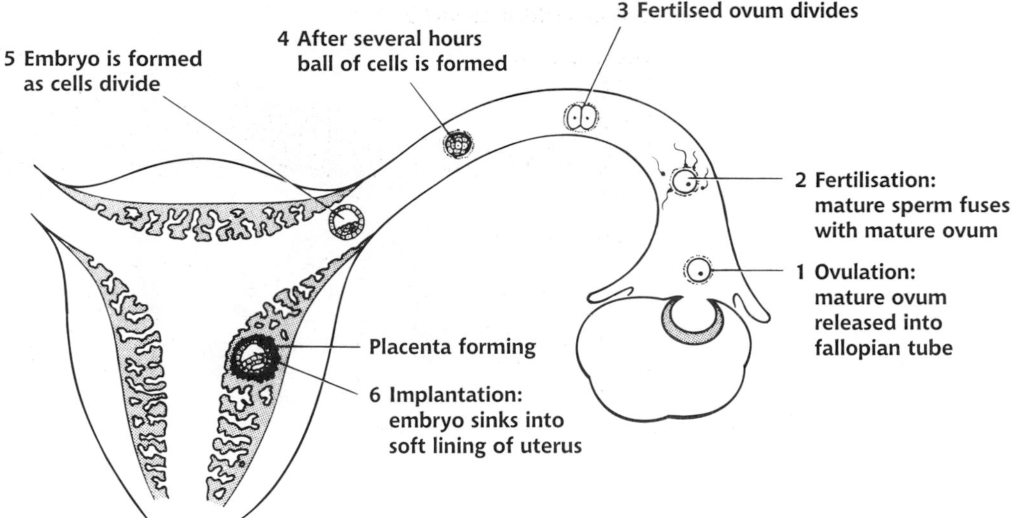
3 Fertilsed ovum divides
4 After several hours ball of cells is formed
5 Embryo is formed as cells divide
2 Fertilisation: mature sperm fuses with mature ovum
1 Ovulation: mature ovum released into fallopian tube
Placenta forming
6 Implantation: embryo sinks into soft lining of uterus

The stages leading to implantation

key term

Fetus the term used to describe the baby from the eighth week after conception until birth

- The developing baby until 8 weeks after conception is called the embryo.
- The developing baby from 8 weeks after conception until the birth is called the **fetus**.

Case study . . .

. . . becoming pregnant

Rosa and Damon have a stable relationship and would like to have a baby. Rosa has a normal menstrual cycle lasting about 28 days. Rosa has not, so far, become pregnant but this month she has missed her normal menstrual period and is now 2 weeks past the date that this should have happened.

1. *Is it likely that Rosa is pregnant?*
2. *Describe what has been happening to the ovum since it was released from the ovary.*

THE PLACENTA

The life-support system of the embryo and the fetus is the placenta. The placenta has finger-like projections called villi. The villi fit closely into the wall of the uterus. The placenta is joined to the fetus by the umbilical cord. Inside the cord are an artery and a vein. The artery takes the blood supply from the fetus into the placenta, and the vein returns the blood to the fetus.

key term

Capillaries very small blood vessels

In the placenta are **capillaries** filled with the blood of the fetus. In the wall of the uterus are large spaces filled with the mother's blood. The blood of the fetus and the mother's blood do not mix; the wall of the placenta separates them, but they are brought very close together. The wall of the placenta is very thin. This allows oxygen and nutrients to pass from the mother to the fetus and waste products to be passed back to the mother for disposal.

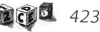

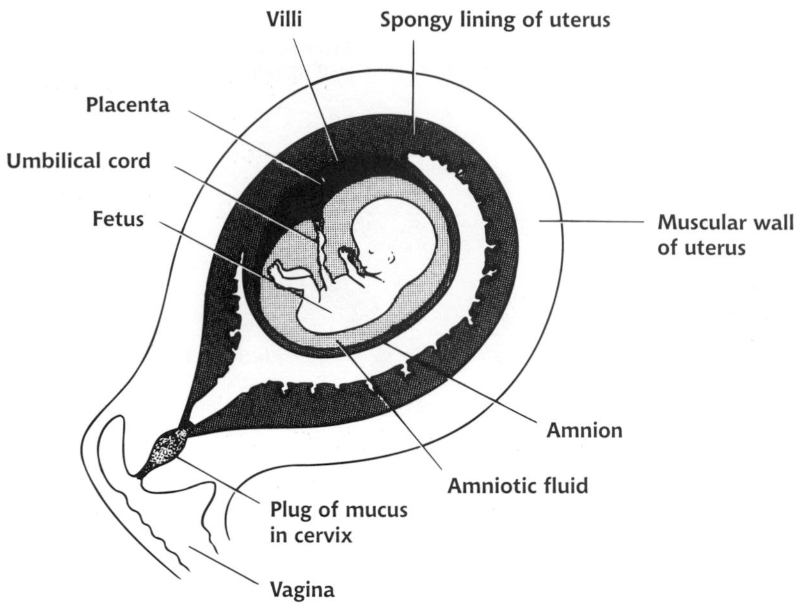

The developing fetus

Progress check

What does the ovum do immediately after fertilisation?

What is the term used to describe the developing baby until 8 weeks after conception?

What is the term used to describe the developing baby from 8 weeks after conception until birth?

How does the fetus exchange oxygen and nutrients with the mother?

What is the function of the umbilical cord?

Fetal growth and development

The growth and development of the embryo and fetus take place over the 40 weeks of pregnancy. The timetable of growth and development for all babies follows the same pattern. Any harmful influences during this time can result in abnormalities in growth or development.

4–5 WEEKS AFTER CONCEPTION

key term

Neural tube
cells in the embryo that will develop into the baby's spinal cord

Five weeks after conception is the time when most pregnant women are beginning to think that they are pregnant. Yet already the nervous system in the embryo is beginning to develop. Cells fold up to make a hollow tube, called the **neural tube**. This will become the baby's brain and spinal cord, so the tube has a head end and a tail end. At the same time the heart is forming and the embryo already has some of its own blood vessels. A string of these blood vessels connect the mother and the embryo and will become the umbilical cord.

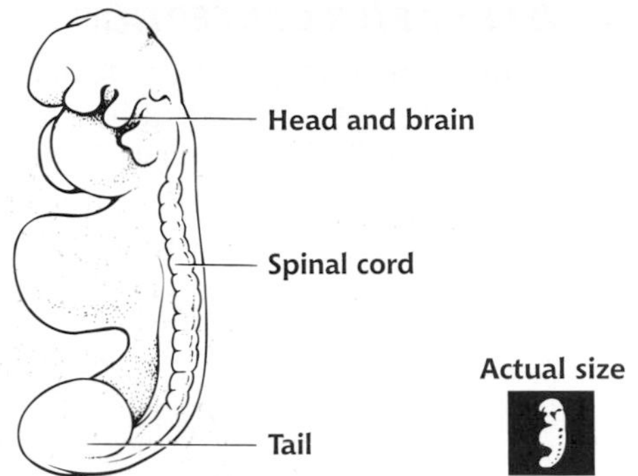

The embryo 5 weeks after conception

6–7 WEEKS AFTER CONCEPTION

The heart is beginning to beat and this can be seen on an ultrasound scan. Small swellings called limb buds show where the arms and legs are growing. At 7 weeks the embryo is about 8 mm long.

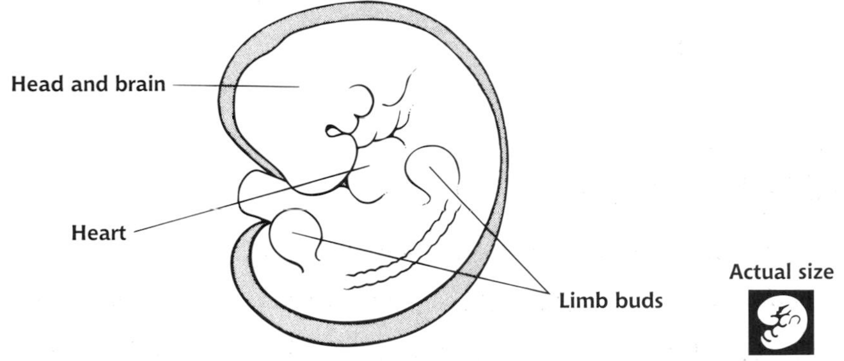

The embryo 6–7 weeks after conception

8–9 WEEKS AFTER CONCEPTION

The developing baby is now called the fetus. The face is slowly forming. The eyes are more obvious and there is a mouth with a tongue. The major internal organs (the heart, brain, lungs, kidneys, liver and intestines) are all developing. At 9 weeks the fetus is about 17 mm long from head to bottom.

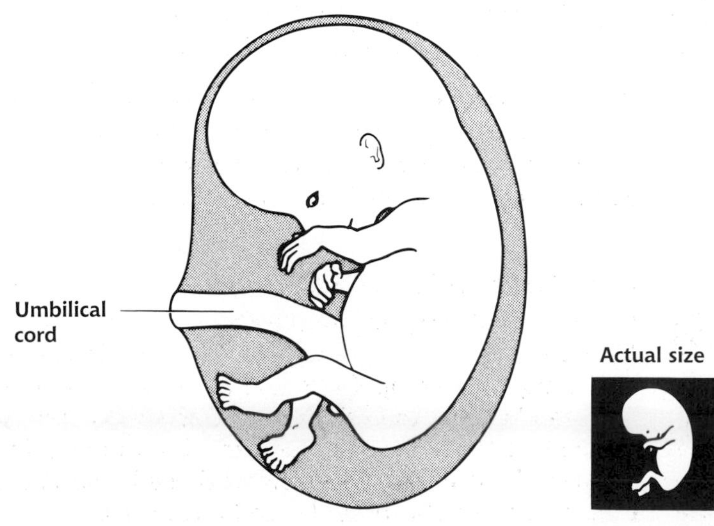

The fetus 8–9 weeks after conception

10–14 WEEKS AFTER CONCEPTION

Twelve weeks after conception the fetus is fully formed. From now on it has to grow and mature. The fetus is already moving, but the mother cannot feel these movements. By about 14 weeks the heartbeat is very strong and can be heard using an ultrasound detector. The heart rate is very fast – about 140 beats per minute. At 14 weeks the fetus is about 56 mm long from head to bottom.

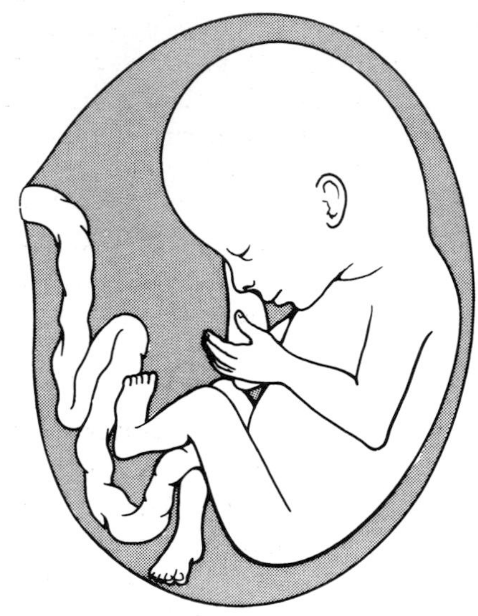

The fetus 10–14 weeks after conception

15–22 WEEKS AFTER CONCEPTION

The fetus is now growing quickly. The body has grown bigger so that the head and body are more in proportion. The face looks much more human and the hair is beginning to grow as well as the eyebrows and eyelashes. Finger and toe-nails are now growing. The lines on the skin are now formed and the fetus has its own fingerprints. At about 22 weeks the fetus becomes covered in fine downy hair called **lanugo**. At about 18–22 weeks movements are first felt by the mother. If this is

> **key term**
> **Lanugo**
> fine hair found on the body of the fetus before birth and on the newly born infant

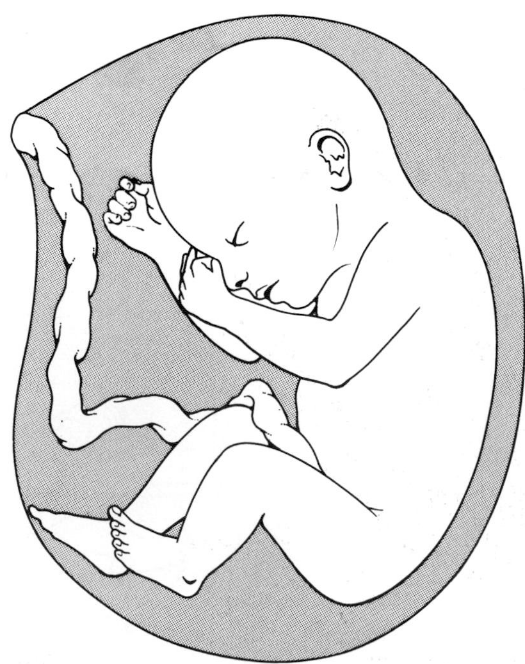

The fetus 15–22 weeks after conception

 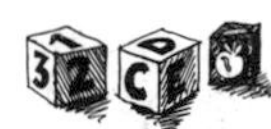

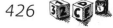

key terms

Vernix
white creamy substance found on the skin of the fetus, in the skin creases of mature babies and on the trunk of pre-term infants

Viable
capable of surviving outside the uterus

a second baby, movements are often felt earlier, at about 14–16 weeks after conception. At 22 weeks the fetus is about 160 mm long from head to bottom.

23–30 WEEKS AFTER CONCEPTION

The fetus is now able to move around and responds to touch and sound. The mother may be aware that the fetus has its own times for being quiet and being active.

The fetus is covered in a white creamy substance called **vernix**, which is thought to protect the skin as the fetus floats in the amniotic fluid. At about 26 weeks the eyes open. At 28 weeks the fetus is **viable**, which means that it is now thought to have a good chance of surviving if born. Many babies born before 28 weeks do survive, but often have problems with their breathing. Specialised care in Special Care Baby Units helps more babies born early to survive. At 30 weeks the fetus is about 240mm long from head to bottom.

31–40 WEEKS AFTER CONCEPTION

During the last few weeks the fetus grows and puts on weight. The skin, which was quite wrinkled, is now smoother and the vernix and lanugo begin to disappear. Ideally, the fetus moves into the head-down position, which is the safest position for the birth.

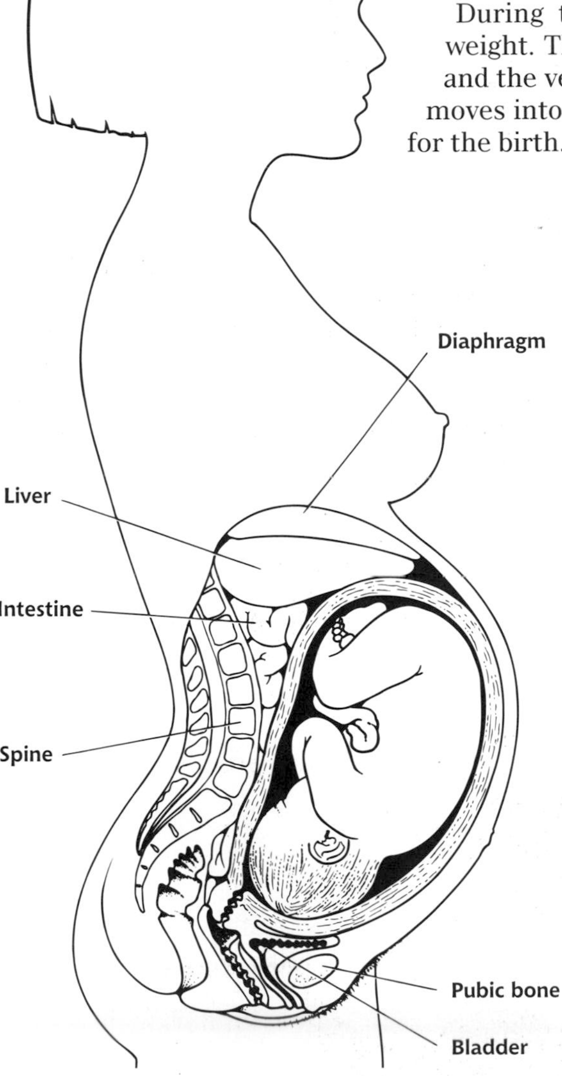

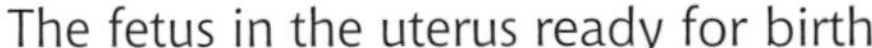

The fetus in the uterus ready for birth

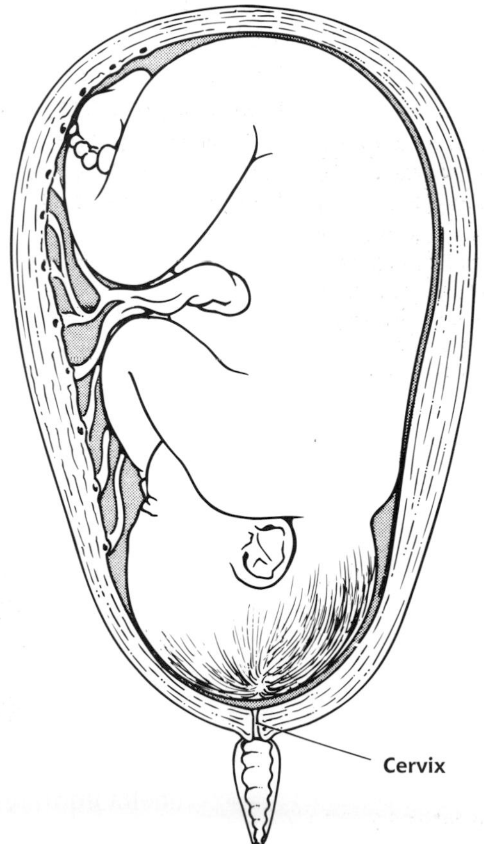

The fetus 31–40 weeks after conception

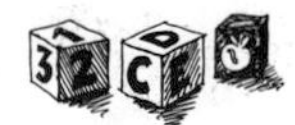

Progress check

What will the neural tube eventually become?

Name the fluid in which the fetus floats.

How long is the fetus at 9 weeks?

When is the fetus fully formed?

What is:

(a) lanugo? (b) vernix?

When does the mother first feel the fetus move?

When does the fetus respond to sound?

When do the eyes of the fetus open?

What is the best position for the fetus to be in ready for the birth?

Preconceptual and antenatal care

The health of the mother and that of the developing fetus are very closely linked. To give the fetus the best chance of developing and growing normally, a good system of antenatal care is needed. Preconceptual advice and care may also be available.

key term

Preconception the time between a couple deciding they want a baby and when the baby is conceived

PRECONCEPTUAL CARE

Preconception is the term used to describe the time between a couple deciding they would like to have a baby and when the baby is conceived. For the first few weeks of pregnancy, a woman may not realise that conception and implantation have occurred, because by the time menstruation stops the embryo is already growing rapidly inside the uterus. This is the time when future parents can make sure they are in the best of health so that their child has the greatest chance of growing and developing normally. In some places it may be possible to attend preconceptual care clinics for help and advice to prepare both partners for a healthy pregnancy. These clinics may be part of the local maternity services or part of the general practitioner service.

General health factors during preconceptual care

Basic screening checks are made at the preconceptual care clinic. The following areas of health may also be checked:

- weight
- blood pressure (BP)
- dental care
- cervical smear
- rubella immunity
- anaemia
- genetic counselling if there is a family history of an inherited condition.

Advice is given about the following:

- *Drugs* – any substance taken for its effect on the workings of the body is a drug. Alcohol is a drug; so is nicotine, which is present in tobacco; medicines prescribed by a doctor or purchased over the counter without a prescription; or drugs acquired illegally may all cross the placenta and affect the developing fetus.
- *Smoking* – it is much better for both parents to stop smoking before conception takes place. Smoking can lead to a higher risk of miscarriage, premature birth, low birthweight, stillbirth, sudden infant death syndrome (SIDS). It can also adversely affect male sperm.
- *Alcohol* – evidence suggests that moderate and high levels of alcohol consumption during pregnancy affect fetal growth and development. Excessive alcohol consumption in men can cause infertility and abnormalities in the sperm.
- *Medicines* – only those medicines prescribed by a doctor should be taken and only when the doctor has confirmed that they do not damage the fetus.
- *Illegal drugs* – all drugs are potentially dangerous substances. They are not only dangerous for a woman to take but could risk the life of a baby.

ANTENATAL CARE

Throughout pregnancy regular check-ups by a community midwife, a general practitioner, obstetric staff, or a combination of these carers, will make sure that the mother and the developing fetus are both fit and well. The health of the mother can be maintained or improved. Checks can be made on the growth and development of the fetus, and any problems, large or small, can be identified early. Pregnancy and delivery can be planned by the parents to suit their needs. The prime aim of antenatal care is to help the mother to a successful delivery of a live, healthy infant.

General health factors during antenatal care

Diet

A well-balanced diet is important at all times and especially in pregnancy. Women who are significantly overweight or underweight may have difficulty in conceiving, and should be given dietary advice about how to achieve a suitable weight before pregnancy begins. Eating disorders such as anorexia nervosa and bulimia must be treated.

A diet rich in vitamins, minerals and protein is preferable before conception takes place. Folic acid supplements should be taken for 3 months before a pregnancy begins and for at least 3 months after it has started. This mineral may help to prevent a neural tube defect, such as **spina bifida**. It is essential that the mother has good dietary advice and acts upon it before becoming pregnant and during the antenatal period. This advice should also include a warning to avoid soft cheeses and pate, which may contain the listeria virus (infection can result in damage to the fetus), and to cook food thoroughly to prevent toxoplasmosis (a parasite, which can attack the fetus, that can be found in undercooked meat).

key term

Spina bifida
a condition in which the spine fails to develop properly before birth

Communicable diseases

Sexually transmitted diseases (STDs), such as gonorrhoea and syphilis, can be detected and treated before pregnancy begins to avoid the possibility of the baby being affected. If they are not treated, babies can be born with congenital syphilis, which is eventually fatal. Gonorrhoea can cause blindness as the baby's eyes can be infected during delivery.

Human immunodeficiency virus (HIV – the virus that can cause AIDS) is not yet curable. Women who think that they may be infected with this virus need professional counselling to help them to decide whether to have a test or not. Women who are HIV positive can pass on the virus to their babies during pregnancy.

Lifestyle

The way women live their lives affects their general health; this includes the amount of exercise taken and the type of work done. Regular exercise and a stress-free environment will help to improve the general health and well-being of both partners.

Case study . . .

. . . preconceptual and antenatal care

Rosa and her husband Damon planned to start a family and they have worked together preconceptually to make sure their baby will have the best possible start in life. Rosa is now 13 weeks pregnant. She has had an uneventful pregnancy so far, and plans to carry on working for as long as she can. She has been attending the antenatal clinic at her GP's surgery regularly and last week she went to the maternity hospital for a regular antenatal appointment. Rosa is trying to do everything she can to make sure her baby will be born fit and healthy, and her husband Damon has supported Rosa all through her pregnancy.

1. *What steps could Rosa and Damon have taken before Rosa became pregnant to try to give their baby a good chance of growing and developing normally?*
2. *What important point in its development would Rosa's baby have reached at her last antenatal visit?*
3. *Describe the growth and development of Rosa's baby from now until the baby is born.*

Progress check

What is preconceptual care?

What health checks may be made at the preconceptual care clinic?

Why is it important to take folic acid supplements before pregnancy begins?

Why is smoking in pregnancy discouraged?

Why are soft cheeses and pate best avoided in pregnancy?

What problem could maternal gonorrhoea cause to the fetus?

Pregnancy

Pregnancy begins when fertilisation of the ovum and sperm takes place, usually in the Fallopian tubes. It is impossible for a woman to be aware of this happening inside her body. It is only after the embryo (fertilised ovum) has implanted in the wall of the uterus that the signs and symptoms of pregnancy appear.

These early changes noticed by the mother are caused by the action of the two female hormones, oestrogen and progesterone, produced by the ovary for the first 12 weeks of pregnancy and then by the mature placenta. Pregnancy is usually confirmed by using a simple urine test to detect **human chorionic gonadotrophin (HCG).** This a hormone produced by the implanted embryo, which is excreted in the mother's urine.

key term

Human chorionic gonadotrophin (HCG)
a hormone produced by the implanted embryo, which is excreted in the mother's urine; its presence confirms pregnancy

SIGNS AND SYMPTOMS OF PREGNANCY

Amenorrhoea

Amenorrhoea (stopping of menstruation) is a very reliable symptom of pregnancy in an otherwise healthy woman, who has had a regular menstrual cycle and is sexually active.

Breast changes

Breast changes that take place during pregnancy may include prickling, enlargement, darkening of the primary areola around the nipple and sometimes fluid may be expressed.

Frequent passing of urine

Due to hormonal action and the enlarging uterus, women need to empty their bladders more often in early pregnancy.

Fundal heights at various weeks during pregnancy

The growth of the uterus during the weeks of pregnancy

Nausea and sickness

Often referred to as 'morning sickness', nausea can occur at any time of the day or night, or be present all the time. This usually passes by the end of the third month.

Tiredness

Lethargy (lack of energy) is common in early pregnancy but usually improves as the pregnancy progresses.

Vaginal discharge

A white vaginal discharge, which is not offensive, is normal and is caused by increased hormonal activity.

Later signs of pregnancy

At 12 weeks, the uterus is above the pelvic bone and can be felt by a midwife or doctor.

At 16–20 weeks, the mother may begin to feel the baby move (fetal movements or quickening), and it is possible to feel parts of the baby when she is examined at antenatal clinic. The fetal heart can be heard using a stethoscope.

Progress check

What are the early signs of pregnancy?

What are the later signs of pregnancy?

THE KEY PRINCIPLES AND PRACTICE OF ANTENATAL CARE

The concept of antenatal care was introduced as recently as 1915, but was not available to all women free of charge until the National Health Service was created in 1948. Antenatal care has been largely responsible for the significant reduction in the maternal mortality rate and the reduction in the infant mortality rate.

Antenatal care alone cannot take all the credit for these large reductions. Improvements in living conditions since 1915 are also responsible for the improved health of the population; but people who live in poverty and are disadvantaged today still suffer from higher than average maternal and infant mortality rates.

PRINCIPLES OF ANTENATAL CARE

Antenatal care is care offered free of charge by professionals to a woman and her partner during pregnancy. The professionals might be the community midwife, general practitioner, health visitor or obstetrician, who specialises in care of the mother and unborn child. The care includes all aspects of health and social conditions to promote well-being. Its aims are:

- to maintain and improve health in pregnancy
- to find any abnormality as early as possible and treat it
- to prepare both parents for labour and a safe, normal delivery, which is a pleasurable experience
- to encourage breastfeeding
- a live, healthy mature baby who is happily accepted into the family
- health education of the parents.

PRACTICE OF ANTENATAL CARE

Early pregnancy

Women are encouraged to see their own doctor (GP) as soon as they think that they may be pregnant. The doctor may confirm their condition by doing a simple urine test for HCG (above). It is important to see a doctor as early as possible in pregnancy so that:

- a baseline of recordings and observations can be made – it is much easier then to see if any abnormalities occur later
- advice can be given about health and lifestyle to promote a healthy pregnancy.

The doctor should explain to the mother about the choices available to her regarding antenatal care and where she wants her baby to be born. If the woman chooses to have a hospital delivery, the doctor will refer her to the local maternity unit, and she will be sent an appointment to attend the booking clinic.

Booking clinic

The booking clinic is the first visit to the hospital antenatal clinic (ANC). A bed is booked for the time the baby is due. Several observations, tests and recordings are made at this clinic and the information is put into the woman's hospital notes.

History taking

At the booking clinic the following information will be gathered:

- *General particulars* – accurate records of the woman's name, age, address, GP and midwife are taken.

- *Present pregnancy* – calculation of the expected date of delivery (EDD). The woman is asked the date of the first day of her last menstrual period (LMP). Nine calendar months are counted forwards and 7 days added, for example: LMP: 1.1.99, add 9 months and 7 days, EDD: 8.10.99. Health during this pregnancy is assessed, for example the mother may report excessive sickness, vaginal bleeding or any other abnormality.
- *Previous pregnancies* – details of previous pregnancies are recorded, because this may affect the care given during this pregnancy.
- *Medical history* – any illnesses affecting the mother are recorded, especially if they may affect the baby, for example diabetes or heart disease.
- *Family history* – twins, multiple births, genetic conditions or medical problems are recorded.

The midwife's examination

At the booking clinic the midwife will make the following examinations:

- *Weight* – weight is recorded as a base measure for future weight gain. The average gain in pregnancy is 12–15 kg.
- *Height* – height may indicate the size of the pelvis.
- *Urine test* – the urine is tested for protein, ketones and sugar. These substances are not usually found in the urine; if they are present further investigation will be required.
- *Blood pressure (BP)* – this again provides a baseline for future recordings. High BP in pregnancy may be the first sign of pre-eclampsia.

Pre-eclampsia is a condition that only occurs in pregnancy. The signs of pre-eclampsia are:

- high blood pressure
- protein in the urine
- oedema (swelling of tissues), especially in the hands and feet
- rapid weight gain.

Mild pre-eclampsia is common and is treated with rest and careful monitoring by the midwife and doctor. Severe eclampsia can seriously harm the mother and baby – the only recourse may be to deliver the baby. This may be a very early delivery, and the baby will have the associated problems of prematurity and will probably be **light-for-dates** as well.

> **key term**
> **Light-for-dates**
> a baby who is smaller than expected for the length of the pregnancy (gestation)

Medical examination

A full medical examination will be performed by an obstetrician. This will include examination of:

- teeth
- breasts
- heart and lungs
- abdominal examination
- lower limbs, for varicose veins or swelling (**oedema**)
- internal vaginal examination to check the size of the uterus; an ultrasound scan will give an even more accurate assessment. A cervical smear will be done if necessary.

> **key term**
> **Oedema**
> swelling of the tissues with fluid

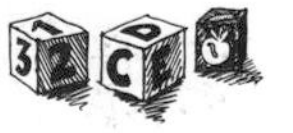

Blood tests

At this first visit to the ANC, a sample of blood is taken for a variety of tests:

- *ABO group and Rhesus factor* – with information from this test, blood can be cross-matched without delay in the case of anaemia or bleeding during pregnancy, when a transfusion may be needed. The four main groups are A, B, O and AB. In addition, there is a substance found in the blood of some humans called the Rhesus factor. About 85 per cent of the population are Rhesus positive and about 15 per cent are Rhesus negative. The baby inherits two Rhesus genes, one from each parent. The Rhesus positive gene D is dominant. The Rhesus negative gene d is recessive.

  During pregnancy fetal and maternal blood should not mix, but at delivery, or if a miscarriage has occurred, the baby's blood can enter the mother's system. If the mother is Rhesus negative and the baby Rhesus positive, the mother may react to the Rhesus factor in her baby's blood and make antibodies to attack the foreign cells (the Rhesus factor in the baby's blood).

  The amount of damage can vary, from mild **anaemia** and **jaundice**, to haemolytic disease of the newborn, which is very serious and may require an exchange blood transfusion. Fortunately, this situation is now very rare, because regular blood tests during pregnancy can detect antibodies in the mother's blood. An injection of Anti-D (anti-Rhesus factor) can prevent the further formation of antibodies and protect the baby.
- *Serology* – to detect syphilis (a venereal disease), which can be treated to prevent damage to the baby.
- *Haemoglobin* – the iron content of the blood is recorded and is taken at monthly intervals thereafter to detect early signs of anaemia.
- All mothers of African, Asian or Mediterranean descent have their blood tested for sickle cell disease and thalassaemia.
- *Rubella* – blood is tested for rubella antibodies.
- **Serum alpha-fetoprotein** *(SAFP)* – this test is taken at 16 weeks of pregnancy when a raised level of SAFP indicates that the baby may have spina bifida; this high level could mean, however, that it is a multiple pregnancy or that the date of the LMP is incorrect. An amniocentesis is offered to mothers with a raised SAFP, and a detailed ultrasound scan will usually be performed to check for twins, or more, and to examine the spine of the fetus.
- **Triple test** – this test may be offered to women over 35 years of age, or it may be requested. It measures levels of serum alpha-fetoprotein (SAFP), human chorionic gonadotrophin (HCG) and oestriol (placental hormones). In conjunction with maternal age, the test calculates the risk of the baby having Down syndrome and spina bifida. An amniocentesis may be offered to mothers if necessary.

key terms

Anaemia
a condition in which the blood lacks adequate amounts of haemoglobin

Jaundice
yellowing of the skin and whites of the eyes as a result of too much bilirubin in the blood

key term

Serum alpha-fetoprotein (SAFP)
a protein found in the maternal blood during pregnancy; a high level requires further investigation

key term

Triple test
an antenatal blood test to measure levels of serum alpha-fetoprotein (SAFP), human chorionic gonadotrophin (HCG) and oestriol

The co-operation (co-op) card

Every pregnant woman is given a co-operation card to record every antenatal assessment made by the community midwife, GP or obstetric staff. As its name implies, the card is to enable co-operation between all the providers of antenatal care, as well as the mother. She should carry it with her at all times because pregnancy is not predictable – a problem could occur at any time, even when out for the day or on holiday. Whoever cares for her will need to know the progress of the pregnancy so far, so that the best treatment can be offered. In some parts of the country a more detailed version of the co-operation card is used. This is a more detailed record held by the mother and reflects the style of hospital notes.

ANTE - NATAL RECORD

INVESTIGATIONS	DATE	RESULTS
A.B.O.Blood Group Rhesus Blood Group Antibodies WR/KAHN X-Ray Chest Other	24/8/98	A Rh + 3/1210668

IMPORTANT NOTE - in the event of a transfusion this record of the blood grouping should always be checked and cross-matching should always be carried out

HISTORY: Oedema, Headache, Bowels, Micturition, Discharge, Date of quickening

FIRST EXAMINATION — Date — Sig.
Height 5. 6".
Teeth, Breasts, Heart, Lungs, Varicose veins, Pelvis — NAD
Cervical smear Aug. 96

Special observations: Wishes to breasr feed
URINE CULTURE
CERVICAL CYTOLOGY
K.P. INDEX
SERUM ALPHA FOETO-PROTEINS 28/9/98 by GP
~~RUBELLA~~ A/B

EXAMINATION 33/37 week: Date; Head/Brim relationship; Pelvic capacity; Sig.

This patient is fit for inhalation analgesia. Date. Signature of Doctor

DATE	WEEKS	WEIGHT	URINE ALB SUGAR	B.P.	HEIGHT FUNDUS	PRESENTATION AND POSITION	RELATION OF P.P. TO BRIM	F.H.	OEDEMA	Hb	NEXT VISIT	SIG	NOTES e.g. antibodies, other tests, infections, drugs
26.7.98	7	57 kg	n ad.	95/60		—	—		nil			SB	Well
24.8.98	11	598	Nad	100/65	Just palp	—	—		Nil	12.6	2wk	Jo Haris	SAFP here
20.9.98	15	59kg	NAD.	94/60	16				nil		4 wk	SB	BKD MISS BAKER CHN
18.10.98	19	59kg	N AD.	100/60	19	—	—	FHH	nil		4 Wk.	SB	Well
5.11.98	Home visit Community midwife.				Home conditions suitable for 24hr discharge							Cateby	Breasts examined: satisf. Br care advice
15.11.98	22+	62½kg	NAD	95/60	23	—	—	FHH	nil		4 wk.	SB	
13-12-98	27	65kg	N.A.D.	100/60	27	Ceph.	Free	"	nil		4 wk.	SB	Well
10.1.99	31	69kg	NAD	90/50	31	Ceph.	Free	H	nil		31st Jan	SB	well - Asilone tabs.
19/1/99	32	67 kg	NAD	100/60	32	Vx mobile	LOT	FHH	nil	11.4	4wk.	RS	
31.1.99	34	67kg	NAD	90/50	34	Vx mobile		H	nil		2 wk.	SB	Well
6/2/99	36	69.35	NAD	100/60	36	Vx at brim	LOT	FHH	nil		2 wk.	RS	
21.2.99	37	69 kg	NAD.	90/54	37	"	LOT,	FHH	nil	11.7	1 wk.	SB	Well
28.2.99	38	69.5kg	NAD.	88/54	38	Vx.	LOT,	FHH	nil.		1 wk,	SB	Well
5-3-99	39	70.0 kg	NAD	95/55	39	Vx.			nil.		1 wk.		
13-3-99	39+	70.0	NAD	95/55	40	Vx.		✓	nil.		1 wk.	SB	Well

A co-operation (co-op) card

As the pregnancy progresses, it will be possible to record the fetal heart and feel the fetal parts when the mother is examined. The mother will begin to feel the baby move, at about 20 weeks for a first baby, and earlier for subsequent pregnancies because an experienced mother will recognise the sensation of fetal movement. These observations will be recorded at each antenatal visit on the co-operation card.

Visits for antenatal check ups are made regularly and progress will be monitored by the GP, community midwife and obstetric staff.

Common tests and investigations during pregnancy

Ultrasound scan

An ultrasound scan can be used to check the size and position of the fetus in the uterus, diagnose some fetal abnormalities and detect and confirm multiple pregnancies.

At 18 weeks of pregnancy women are offered a detailed scan for doctors to look at the structure of fetal organs.

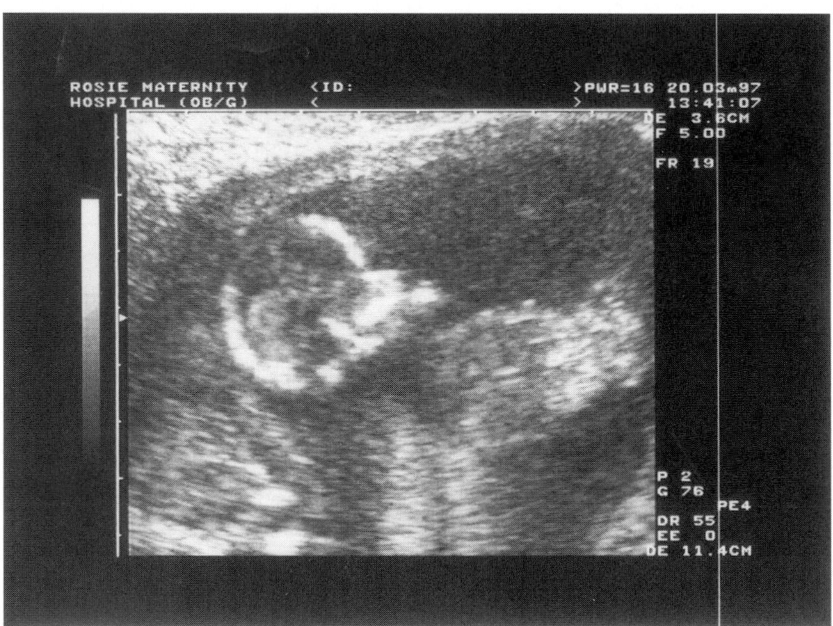

An ultrasound scan

Placental function tests

A healthy placenta is essential for a fetus to grow and develop normally. It is possible to test the health and strength of the placenta by checking the amount of pregnancy hormones it produces.

Amniocentesis

Amniocentesis involves the removal of a small sample of amniotic fluid from the uterus, via the abdominal wall. It may be performed after the 16th week of pregnancy, when it is possible to check that the chromosomes, including the sex chromosomes, are normal.

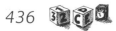

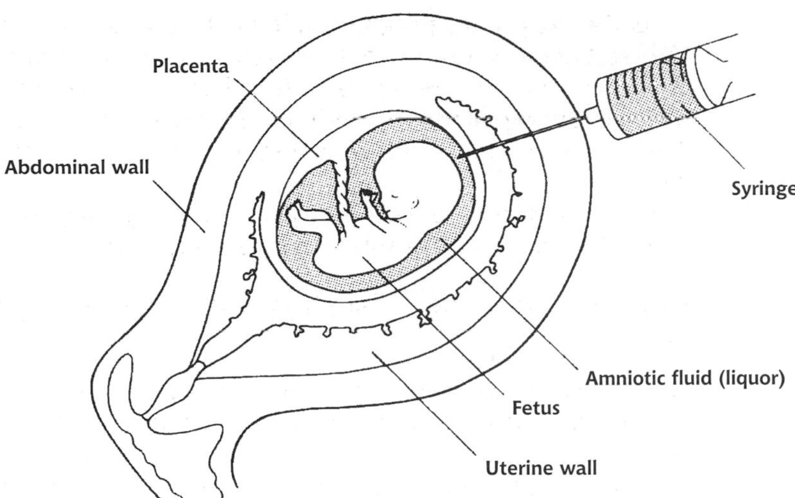

Amniocentesis

Amniocentesis may be offered to women who have:

- a history of chromosomal abnormalities, such as Down syndrome
- raised SAFP
- a history of sex-linked disorders, such as Duchenne muscular dystrophy
- passed the age of 35 years (the risk of chromosomal abnormalities, especially Down syndrome, increases with age).

Chorionic villus sampling

Chorionic villus sampling (CVS) is carried out between 8 and 11 weeks of pregnancy. With the help of an ultrasound scan to find the position of the placenta and the fetus, a small sample of placental tissue is removed via the cervix. CVS is used to detect inherited disorders such as Down syndrome, haemophilia, thalassaemia, sickle cell disease, cystic fibrosis.

It can also be used to detect the sex of the fetus if there is a family history of sex-linked conditions.

A couple may decide to terminate a pregnancy because of the results of amniocentesis or CVS. Whatever their decision, they will need a great deal of support and empathy from all the professionals involved in their care.

Professional guidance

The midwife, doctor and health visitor will provide a great deal of emotional support, as well as physical care. As the pregnancy progresses, they will be available to discuss, advise and give reassurance on any issues that may be causing the parents concern.

Parents will be invited to preparation for parentcraft classes towards the end of the pregnancy, when a mother who has been in employment will by that time be on maternity leave. These classes are organised by the local health authority and are run by the local midwife and/or health visitor in the health centre or hospital. They usually last for 2 hours and take place once a week for 6–8 weeks, and include evening sessions that the mother's partner can attend. A wide range of relevant topics will be covered.

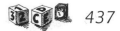

Progress check

What are the principles of antenatal care?

List some of the observations that are recorded on the co-operation card.

Assuming that the following dates are the first day of the last menstrual period (LMP), work out the expected date of delivery (EDD): 25.12.2001; 6.5.2001; 29.1.2002.

What tests are made on the urine sample?

Describe oedema.

Explain the purpose of:

(a) ultrasound scan (b) blood test for serum alpha-fetoprotein (SAFP)

(c) amniocentesis (d) chorionic villus sampling (CVS).

Who can give professional guidance during pregnancy?

Now try these questions

Copy these diagrams of the male and female reproductive organs. On the male diagram label the following parts: vas deferens; scrotum; penis; prostate gland; testes; urethra. On the female diagram label the following parts: vagina; fundus; uterus; Fallopian tube; cervix; ovary.

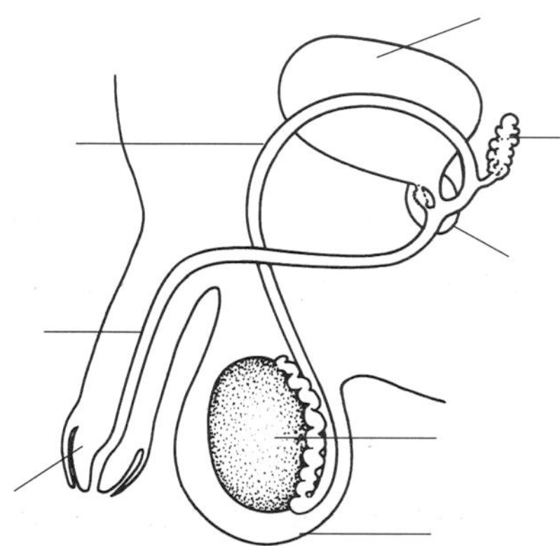

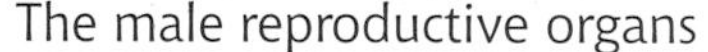

The male reproductive organs

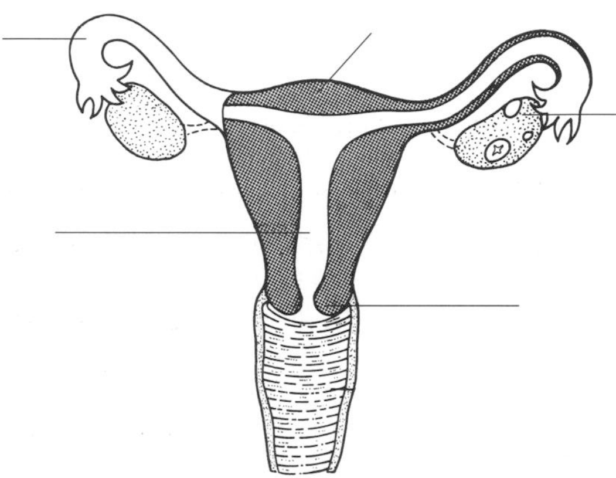

The female reproductive organs

Describe the development of the fertilised ovum, from conception until implantation in the wall of the uterus.

Why are good pre-conceptual care and good antenatal care important?

Describe the blood tests taken in pregnancy and when they are taken.

What is the value of the co-operation card?

key terms

You need to know what the key terms and phrases in this chapter mean. Go back through the chapter and find out.

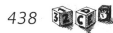

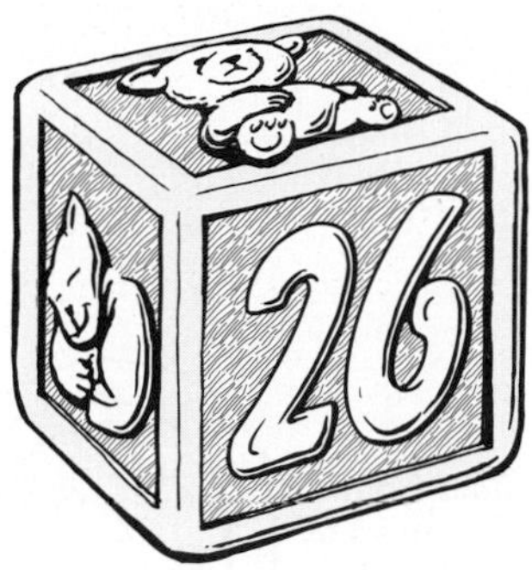

BIRTH, POSTNATAL CARE AND LOW BIRTHWEIGHT BABIES

Labour and delivery follow the weeks of growth and development in the uterus. The immediate care given at birth and the subsequent postnatal care given to the baby are crucial to future development.

This chapter will cover the following topics:

- *the birth process*
- *immediate care at birth*
- *postnatal care*
- *low birthweight babies.*

The birth process

key term

Labour

the process by which the fetus, placenta and membranes are expelled from the birth canal

Labour is the process by which the fetus, placenta and membranes are expelled through the birth canal.

Signs that labour has started:

- the onset of strong and regular contractions
- a 'show' – the discharge of blood-stained mucus from the vagina
- 'waters breaking' – rupture of the membranes, resulting in some amniotic fluid escaping via the vagina.

One, or any combination of these, may indicate that labour has begun. A woman should contact her midwife for advice as soon as she thinks that she may be in labour. The rupture of the membranes may allow infection to enter the uterus, so she should contact the hospital immediately if the baby is to be born there.

key term

Term

between the 38th and 42nd week of pregnancy

NORMAL LABOUR

A normal labour will have the following characteristics:

- It starts spontaneously (naturally) without any help from the doctor or the use of drugs.
- It starts at **term**, that is between 38 and 42 weeks of pregnancy.

- There is a cephalic (head-first) presentation.
- It is completed in 24 hours.
- The baby is born alive and healthy.
- There are no complications.

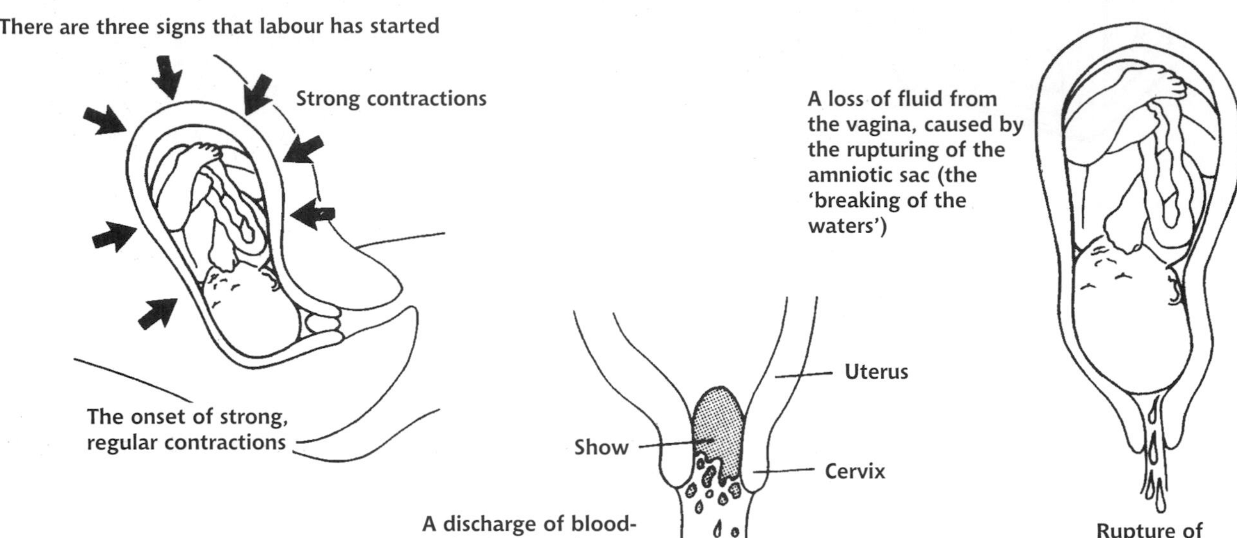

The onset of labour. There are three signs that labour has started

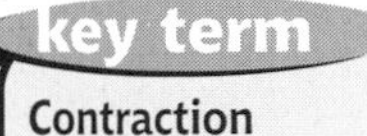

A loss of fluid from the vagina, caused by the rupturing of the amniotic sac (the 'breaking of the waters')

Contraction
involuntary, intermittent muscular tightenings of the uterus

STAGES OF LABOUR

Labour is divided into three stages.

Stage 1

The first stage of labour begins with the onset of regular uterine **contractions**, during which the cervix dilates (widens or gets larger) to allow the baby to be delivered. It ends with full dilatation of the cervix, when it is about 10 cm dilated and cannot get any bigger.

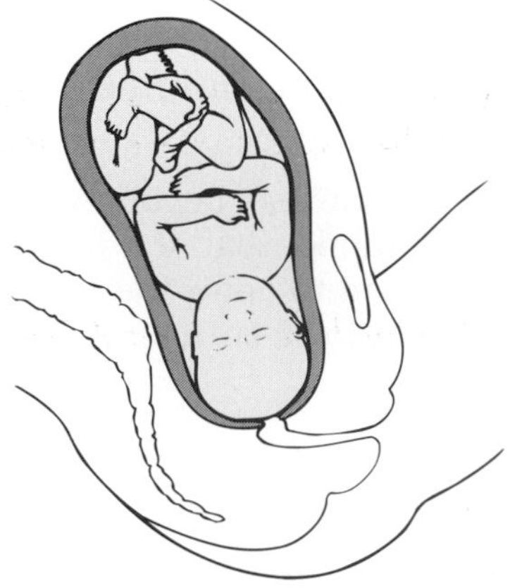

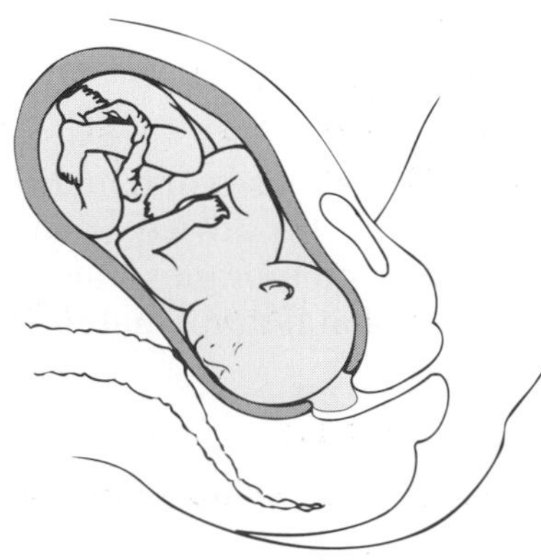

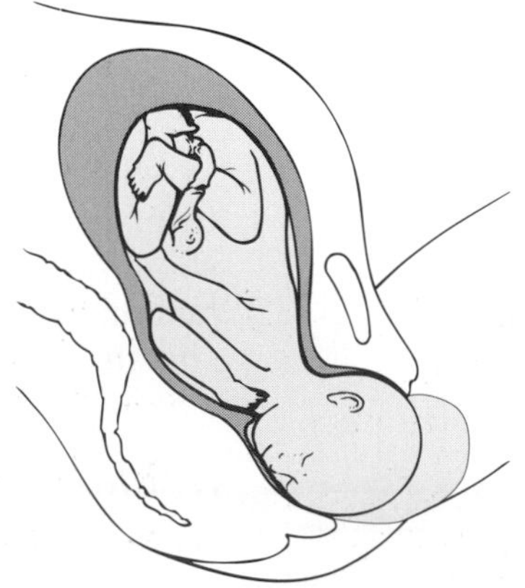

When the cervix is fully dilated, the head is about to be delivered

The first stage of labour

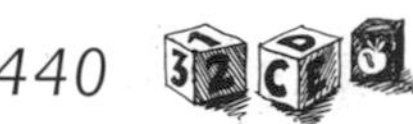

Stage 2

The second stage of labour begins with full dilatation of the cervix and ends with the birth of the baby.

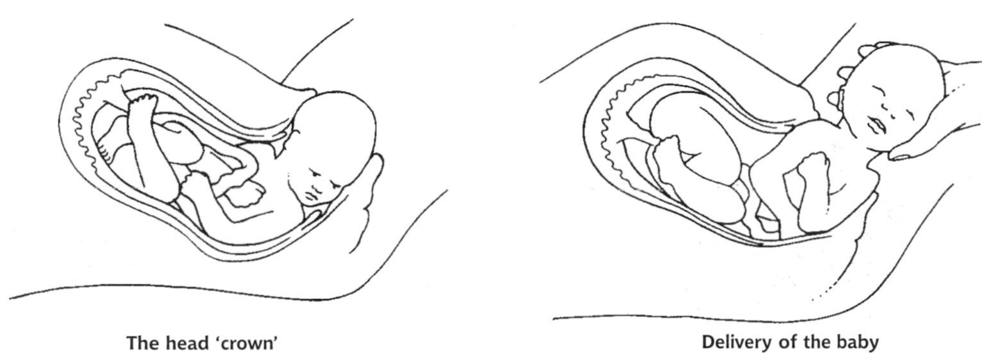

The second stage of labour

Stage 3

The third stage begins with the birth of the baby and ends with the complete delivery of the placenta and membranes.

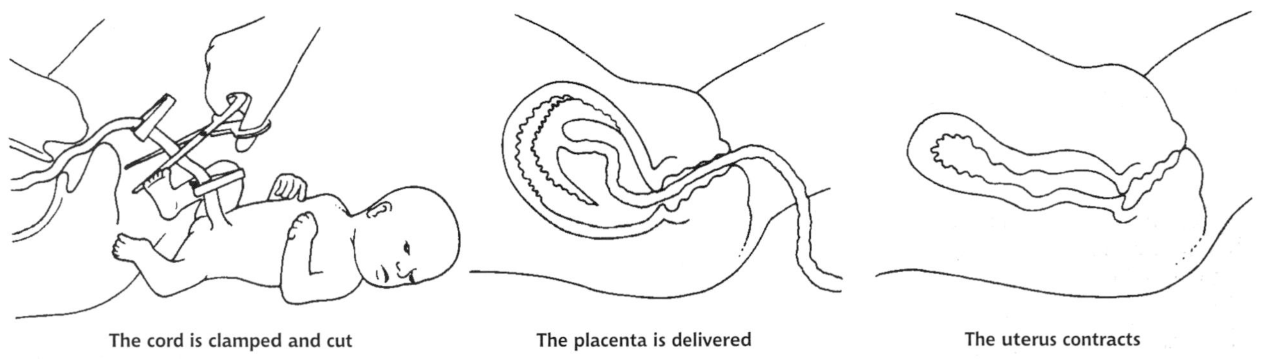

The cord is clamped and cut
The placenta is delivered
The uterus contracts

The third stage of labour

TYPES OF DELIVERY

Some babies and mothers need help with the birth process, and some type of medical intervention may be necessary to make sure that both mother and baby are healthy at the end of labour.

> **key term**
>
> **Induction**
>
> starting labour by artificial means, for example by breaking the waters or giving hormones to stimulate contractions

Induction

Induction means starting labour by artificial means. Labour may need to be induced if:

- the baby is very overdue
- the mother is ill, for example with pre-eclampsia
- the placenta is failing.

Labour may be induced by rupturing the membranes and/or giving artificial hormones to stimulate contractions.

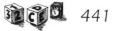

key term

Episiotomy
a cut to the perineum to assist the delivery of the fetus

Episiotomy

An **episiotomy** is a cut made in the perineum (the area between the vagina and the rectum) during the second stage of labour. It is done for two main reasons:

- to allow the baby to be delivered more quickly if there is any indication of fetal compromise
- to prevent a large tear.

key term

Forceps
spoon-shaped implements to protect the baby's head and assist in the delivery of the fetus

Forceps delivery

Delivery may be with **forceps** if the baby is becoming distressed. Forceps are spoon-shaped and fit around the baby's head so that the doctor can help with the delivery of the head.

Ventouse extraction

A **ventouse** extraction involves the use of a cup-shaped instrument that fits on to the baby's head and is attached to suction equipment. The baby is gently helped down the birth canal with the help of suction.

key term

Ventouse
a suction cup applied to the fetal head to assist delivery

Caesarean section

A **Caesarean** section is a surgical operation to remove the baby, placenta and membranes via the abdominal wall. It may be performed when the mother is awake, but under an epidural anaesthetic or spinal block, which prevents any feelings of pain. Some women may prefer to have a general anaesthetic. Caesareans are performed for many reasons. Some are 'elective', which means that they are done before labour starts, and some are done as an emergency procedure because of an abnormality occurring during labour.

key term

Caesarean
delivery of the fetus via an abdominal incision

Pain relief in labour

The best form of pain relief in labour is having a positive attitude and knowing what is happening. Women who have been to parentcraft/relaxation classes usually cope well, and their partners are aware of how best to help. Having a familiar hand to hold, a sympathetic midwife and remembering breathing techniques may help to prevent the use of analgesics (painkillers) and anaesthetics. The following forms of pain relief are, however, used by many women:

- *pethidine* – a strong drug that can be injected every four hours, to take the edge off contractions
- *nitrous oxide and oxygen (NO_2 and O_2)* – a gas the mother can breathe in to help with contractions; she controls the amount she takes, so that she cannot be given too much
- **epidural** – the injection of a painkilling drug into the space around the spinal cord; it numbs the pain of contractions by anaesthetising the nerves that carry sensations to the brain. This type of anaesthetic does not harm the baby and leaves the mother fully conscious
- **transcutaneous nerve stimulation (TENS)** – consists of equipment that produces electrical impulses that block any sensations of pain before they reach the brain; the equipment is loaned to the mother before labour begins so that she can start to use it as soon as she thinks that labour has begun. It is most effective if it is started very early in labour
- *water birth* – enabling the mother to use a bath of warm water can provide pain relief during the early stages of labour.

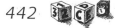

key terms

Epidural
anaesthetic injected into the epidural space in the spine to numb the area from the waist down

Transcutaneous nerve stimulation (TENS)
an electronic device to help control pain in labour

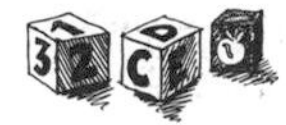

Progress check

What are the three signs that labour has begun?

What do you understand by 'normal labour'?

What are the three stages of labour?

Why may labour be induced?

What is an episiotomy?

What types of pain relief may be offered in labour?

Immediate care at birth

ESTABLISHING RESPIRATION

As soon as the head is delivered, the midwife will wipe the baby's nose and mouth so that when the first breath is taken it is not contaminated with mucus or blood. Most babies breathe spontaneously, but specialised equipment is available in the delivery room for resuscitation if necessary.

MAINTAINING BODY TEMPERATURE

Babies are wet at birth and lose heat very quickly. That is why hospital delivery suites are so hot. It is important to dry the baby as quickly as possible, usually by wrapping her in warm towels to be cuddled by her mother. Radiant heaters over the cot will warm it in preparation for the baby.

The temperature of the baby is taken within an hour of birth using a rectal or digital thermometer.

BONDING

It is extremely important that the parents have close contact with their new baby, so that their relationship can begin positively. Bonding can be encouraged by:

- the mother helping with the delivery, by holding the baby's shoulders and lifting him out
- the baby being delivered into the mother's arms, or on to her tummy if possible
- the mother or her partner cutting the umbilical cord if they wish – this is a symbolic gesture of the start of a new life
- the mother being encouraged to breastfeed as soon as possible after delivery, if that is her chosen method of feeding.

IDENTIFICATION

The baby will be labelled immediately after she is born by attaching small bracelets to one wrist and one ankle. These labels contain the name and hospital number of the mother and the date and time of birth. The baby's cot will also be labelled.

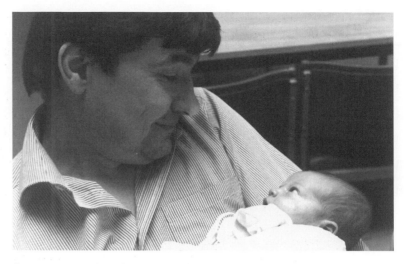

It is extremely important that the parents have close contact with their new baby

OBSERVATIONS

The Apgar score

While all this is happening, the midwife will be closely observing the baby. She will be looking at the vital signs:

- heart rate
- respiration
- muscle tone
- response to stimulus
- colour.

key term

Apgar score a method of assessing the newborn baby's condition by observing the vital signs

From observing these specific areas she will be able to assess the **Apgar score**. This is an internationally used system for assessing the condition of babies at birth. Each of the five areas above is observed and the baby is given a score of 0, 1 or 2 points according to their condition. These points are added to give a maximum score of 10. (See the table below.)

The Apgar score

Sign	0	1	2
Heart rate	Absent	Slow (below 100)	Fast (above 100)
Respiration	Absent	Slow, irregular	Good, crying
Muscle tone	Limp	Some flexion of extremities	Active
Response to stimulus (stimulation of foot or nose/mouth)	No response	Grimace	Cry, cough
Colour	Blue, pale	Body pink/dusky, well oxygenated; extremities blue	Completely pink/healthy colour, well oxygenated

The heart and respiratory rate are the most important factors.

Babies of black, Asian or mixed parentage are a dusky pink colour at birth, because the melanin under the skin, which is responsible for their eventual colour, has not yet reached its full concentration. All babies are assessed by monitoring the oxygenation of the blood to the skin.

The test is first performed when the baby is 1 minute old, then 5 minutes later, and every 5 minutes afterwards until the maximum of 10 is achieved. A score of 8 to 10 indicates that the baby is in good condition at birth. The Apgar score may be referred to later in childhood if the child shows any signs of developmental delay that may have been caused by their poor condition at birth. A record of the score is kept in the child's health records held by the parents, the health visitor and later by the school nurse.

Measurements

The baby will be weighed soon after birth and the weight recorded in kilograms.

The circumference of the head is also recorded to give a baseline reading against which to measure future growth.

Temperature

The temperature is taken to ensure that the baby is warm enough.

Stools and urinary output

It is very important that the midwife observes and records whether the baby has passed urine, and passed meconium (a greenish-black soft stool). Failure to do one or either of these things indicates an abnormality, which will need investigation.

EXAMINATION

A detailed examination of the baby in the presence of the parents will be made.

General observations

The midwife will check for regular, effortless breathing and skin colour – a healthy bloom will indicate that blood is circulating oxygen around the body.

All babies are varying shades of pink at birth, regardless of their racial origin. There may be **lanugo** (soft, downy hair mainly found in pre-term babies, but some may still be present in babies born at term). Vernix caseosa is a white, greasy substance that protects the skin in its watery environment in the uterus. In mature babies, it may be found in the skin creases, but may also be present on the trunk if the baby is premature.

The midwife will note the baby's activity, whether the limbs are moving.

> **key term**
>
> **Lanugo**
> the fine hair found on the body of the fetus before birth and on the newborn infant; mainly associated with pre-term babies

Detailed observations

The head

Fontanelles and suture lines are felt; the eyes are examined to confirm their presence and that formation is normal. The ears are checked for skin tags and the mouth for cleft lip and palate.

The arms and hands

The arms and hands are checked for full movement; fingers are counted and webbing (rare) noted.

The body

An umbilical cord clamp is applied; external genitalia are noted and checked.

The anus is checked by taking the temperature. With the baby in prone (face down), the back is examined to look for any evidence of spina bifida. There may be an open lesion (wound) or a small dimple to signify the presence of a hidden lesion.

> **key term**
>
> **Mongolian blue spots**
> smooth, bluish-grey to purple skin patches consisting of an excess of pigmented skin cells

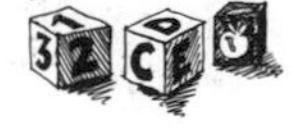

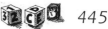

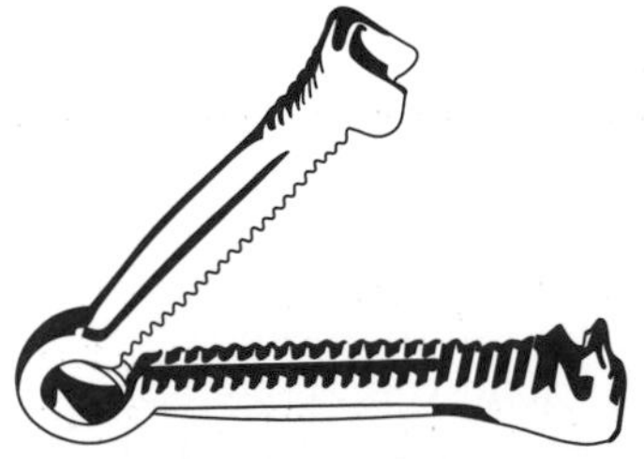
An umbilical cord clamp

key term

Talipes
an abnormal position of the foot, caused by the contraction of certain muscles or tendons

The baby may have **mongolian blue spots**, areas of blue tingeing to the skin which look like bruising. They are commonly found at the base of the spine (the sacrum), although they can be anywhere on the body. They are usually found in babies of Asian, African-Caribbean or Mediterranean descent, or in babies of mixed race. They disappear before the age of 5 years, but should be recorded to prevent any later allegations of child abuse.

The legs

The baby's hips are tested for congenital dislocation. Leg movements are noted, to exclude paralysis, and **talipes** (an abnormality of the foot) is noted. The toes are counted.

Within 24 hours of birth the baby should be examined by a paediatrician (a doctor who specialises in the care of children). This check will include listening to the heart and lungs and palpating (feeling) the abdominal organs.

Progress check

What immediate care is given to the baby at birth?

Why are delivery rooms kept very warm?

Why is the Apgar score such an important observation?

What measurements of the baby are recorded after birth?

What is a baby's first stool called?

What is lanugo?

What is vernix caseosa?

What is a mongolian blue spot?

Case study . . .

. . . a normal delivery

Jocelyn has just delivered her second baby. It was a much easier birth this time – her partner, Barry, was with her and she appreciated his presence and concern throughout. The first stage only lasted 4 hours and, after 20 minutes of pushing, their son, Jake, was born. When the head was delivered, the midwife encouraged Jocelyn to feel his head and to help to lift his shoulders out with the next contraction. The baby was placed on Jocelyn's abdomen and Barry cut the cord, supervised by the midwife. Jocelyn was cuddling the baby when the midwife told her that his Apgar score was 9 at 10 minutes, but she was too busy counting his fingers and stroking his hands to ask for an explanation.

1. *What did the midwife and parents do to encourage bonding during the delivery?*
2. *How else can bonding be encouraged?*
3. *How would you explain the Apgar score to Jocelyn?*

Postnatal care

SECURITY IN OBSTETRIC UNITS

Most hospitals now employ strict security measures to keep babies safe during their hospital stay. These measures include the use of locks on ward doors, video cameras to record what happens in hospital corridors and wards, extra security personnel, and electronic tagging of babies to monitor their whereabouts and to prevent abductions.

DAILY OBSERVATION AND CARE

Registered midwives have a legal right and responsibility to examine all mothers and babies for a minimum of 10 days after birth. They may continue to visit for 28 days, if necessary.

During the first 24 hours, most abnormalities and illnesses will be identified. It may be considerably longer before some disabilities, such as deafness or developmental delay, are confirmed. Daily observations, as well as noting temperature, respiration and feeding patterns, should include the following areas.

> **key term**
> **Milia**
> 'milk spots' – small white spots on the noses of newborn babies caused by blocked sebaceous glands

The skin

Many babies have **milia** (tiny, white, milk spots) over the nose. These disappear in time, but occasionally they become infected and need treatment.

Birthmarks may appear in the first few days after birth; not all are present at birth.

> **key term**
> **Meconium**
> the first stool passed by the newborn – a soft, black/green motion present in the fetal bowel from about the 16th week of pregnancy

Stools

Meconium is the first stool passed by the baby. It is dark green and sticky, composed of the contents of the digestive tract accumulated during fetal life. After milk feeds, it becomes greenish-brown, then yellowish-brown. These are called *changing stools*, as the last of the meconium is excreted together with the waste products of the milk feeds. This normally takes place around the 4th day.

The stools of a breastfed baby are typically watery, bright yellow and passed three or four times a day (although the frequency will vary). There is little or no odour. Those of a bottle-fed baby are firm, paler, putty-like, with odour. Green stools occur naturally in some babies, depending on the mother's diet if she is breastfeeding, or the type of artificial milk. Yellow or green, watery, frequent stools may indicate gastro-enteritis. Small, dark green stools are usually due to underfeeding.

> **key term**
> **Sticky eyes**
> a discharge from the eyes in the first 3 weeks of life

The eyes

Sticky eyes (ophthalmia neonatorum) are common, because a new baby cannot yet produce tears. They are easily treated with antibiotic drops if discovered early. The eyes are examined daily and cleaned, using separate swabs for each eye.

> **key term**
> **Thrush**
> a fungal infection of the mouth and/or nappy area

The mouth

The mouth is checked for oral **thrush**, a common fungal infection. It looks like milk residue on the tongue and cheeks.

The umbilical cord

The cord should be checked daily and kept clean and dry to avoid infection. The cord stump usually drops off by the 6th day.

Feeding

Whether breastfed or bottlefed, babies will establish their own routine. Demand feeding when the baby is hungry rather than on a strict 4-hourly schedule (see Chapter 29) is recommended.

Bathing

Babies can be bathed daily and the midwife will teach the new mother the correct procedure. However, topping and tailing (washing the face, hands and bottom) is quite adequate with a full bath every 2 or 3 days, if this fits in more easily with the home routine.

Crying

All babies cry in the early weeks, as it is their way of communicating their needs. Crying is usually caused by hunger, thirst, soiled or wet nappy, discomfort from wind pains, being too hot or too cold. Further advice should be sought if crying is felt to be excessive or unusual.

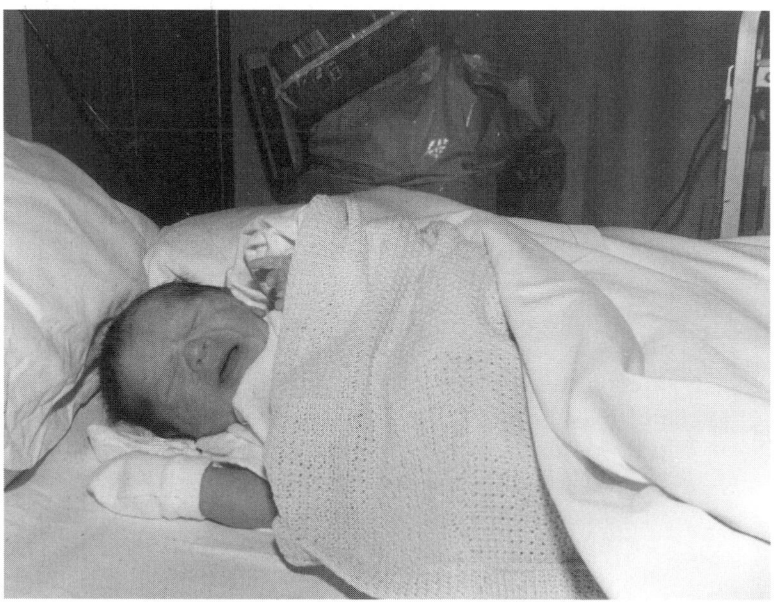

All babies cry to communicate their needs

> **key term**
>
> **Screening**
> checking the whole population of children at specific ages for particular abnormalities

> **key term**
>
> **Guthrie test**
> on the 6th day after birth, a sample of the baby's blood is taken, usually by pricking the heel, to test for phenylketonuria, cystic fibrosis and cretinism

SCREENING TESTS

Various **screening** tests are performed in the early neonatal period to check for specific abnormalities that can be successfully treated if detected early enough.

The Guthrie test

The **Guthrie test** is performed on the 6th day of milk feeding, to detect phenylketonuria (PKU) and cystic fibrosis. A sample of blood is obtained by pricking the baby's heel. This sample is also checked for levels of thyroxine so that hypothyroidism (cretinism) can be treated.

Barlow's test

This hip test is performed by the midwife and later by the doctor, to check for congenital dislocation of the hip. The health visitor will repeat the test, and so will the GP when the baby has a 6-week medical and development check.

 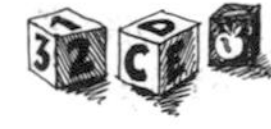

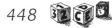

Low birthweight babies

key terms

Low birthweight
babies born prematurely (pre-term) or below the 10th centile for their gestation, usually weighing less than 2.5 kg at birth

Pre-term
a baby born before 36 completed weeks of pregnancy; also referred to as premature

Light-for-dates
a baby who is smaller than expected for the length of pregnancy (gestation)

Not all babies are born at term; some are born early and an increasing number of these are surviving because of improved neonatal care. **Low birthweight** babies can be divided into two main categories:

- **pre-term** *(premature)* – these babies are born before 37 completed weeks of pregnancy, i.e. at 36 weeks' gestation or less
- **light-for-dates** *(small-for-dates)* – these babies are below the expected weight for their gestational age – the length of the pregnancy, according to percentile charts.

Some babies are both premature *and* light-for-dates. There is a greater chance of a baby surviving if he weighs more than 2.5 kg.

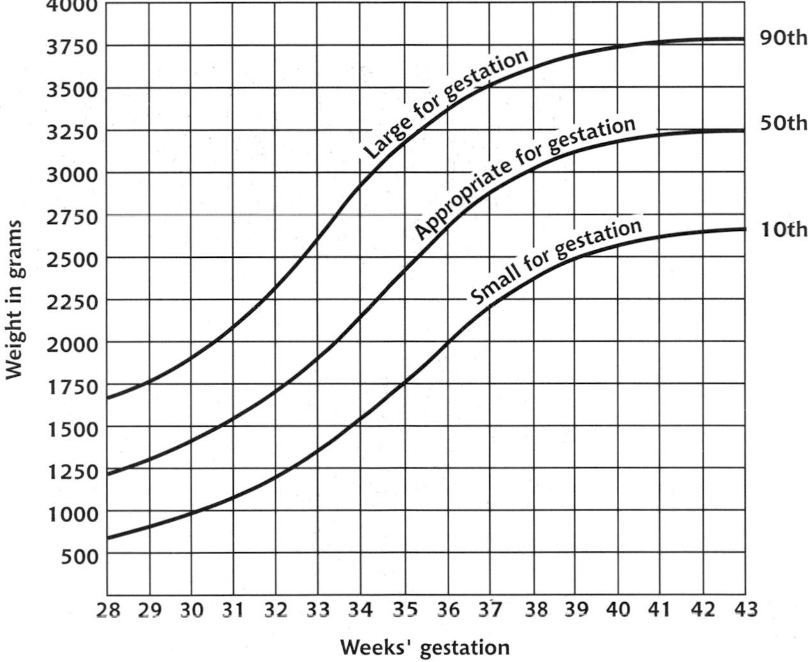

A percentile chart showing weight and gestation

PRE-TERM BABIES

Pre-term (or premature) babies are immature and are not yet ready to survive alone outside the womb. They have a better chance of survival if their weight falls between the 90th and 10th percentile.

Characteristics of pre-term babies

There are several characteristics common to pre-term babies:

- The head is even larger in proportion to the body than usual.
- The face is small and triangular with a pointed chin.
- The baby looks 'worried'.
- They may be reluctant to open their eyes.
- The sutures and fontanelles are large.

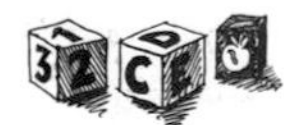

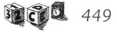

- The skin may be red.
- The veins are prominent.
- The baby may be covered in lanugo.
- The limbs are thin.
- Nails are soft.
- The chest is narrow.
- The abdomen is large.
- The umbilicus is low-set.
- There are small genitalia, poorly developed.
- Muscle tone is floppy.
- Arms and legs are extended.
- They are feeble and drowsy.
- Reflexes are poor, the baby may be unable to suck.

Causes of prematurity

Causes of premature delivery are often unknown, but are more common in mothers who smoke and in those with pre-eclampsia or with a multiple pregnancy. Prematurity is also associated with poverty and deprivation, which may indicate the importance of a good diet and healthy lifestyle in pregnancy.

Complications of prematurity

key term

Birth asphyxia failure of the baby to establish spontaneous respiration at birth

Complications which might arise for a pre-term baby are:

- **birth asphyxia** – pre-term babies may be slow to breathe at birth due to an immature respiratory centre in the brain
- *respiratory problems* – immaturity of the lungs may make breathing difficult
- *intracranial haemorrhage (bleeding in the brain)* – fragile blood vessels in the brain may bleed easily. This may cause long-term damage.

The care of premature babies is a highly specialised field; they are prone to many difficulties. For example, like all babies they cannot control their temperature, but the smaller the baby the greater the risk of hypothermia. They are more likely to become jaundiced or anaemic and are vulnerable to infections. Some pre-term babies do survive and develop well, but some suffer long-term damage as a direct result of their prematurity.

Possible effects on development are:

- *generalised developmental delay* – this 'global' delay may affect all areas of development, with milestones being achieved at a much later age, if at all
- *specific developmental difficulties* – there may be a particular problem with one area of development, such as motor or communication skills
- *sensory loss* – blindness and deafness are much more common in children who have been born very early.

SPECIAL CARE BABY UNIT (SCBU)

Some pre-term infants will require the specialised care of the SCBU to provide the highly skilled and technological support that they need. These units are usually divided into high-dependency and low-dependency areas.

key term

Incubator
an enclosed cot that regulates temperature and humidity

High dependency

In the high-dependency area, babies are cared for in **incubators**. Incubators are enclosed, transparent cots. They automatically adjust the temperature to maintain the baby's body temperature at 36.5 to 37.2°C. Babies may be covered with a heat shield and dressed in hat, mittens and bootees to retain their warmth, providing that this does not prevent observation of their condition. An apnoea mattress will monitor their breathing and an alarm will sound if respiration stops or becomes irregular.

Small, pre-term babies are handled as little as possible but very gently. They are fed and cared for through perspex doors in the side of the incubator. Strict attention to hygiene in the SCBU helps to prevent infection.

Low dependency

As the baby's condition improves, they are transferred into the low-dependency area where they are nursed in a cot. Progress is monitored before discharge to the postnatal ward or home.

SUPPORT FOR PARENTS

At the time of birth the mother may be able to hold the baby for a short time before transfer to the SCBU. She and her partner can visit the baby at any time, and will be encouraged to touch and stroke the baby and hold its hand. Parents are always supported and encouraged to provide as much care as possible – early contact and touching is essential to promote bonding.

Progress check

For how long after a birth does a midwife have the responsibility to visit a mother and baby?

What are milia?

Describe the typical stool of:

(a) a breastfed baby (b) a bottlefed baby.

Why are a baby's eyes vulnerable to infection?

What is demand feeding?

When is the Guthrie test performed? Why is it done?

What are the two categories of low birthweight babies?

Why is the birthweight of a baby important?

What may be the cause(s) of prematurity?

What are the characteristics of pre-term babies?

What effects may prematurity have on future development?

What specialised care is provided in a SCBU ?

Why is parental involvement so important if a baby is in SCBU ?

Now try these questions

What are the common signs that indicate that labour has started?

Briefly describe the three stages of labour.

Describe the role of the Special Care Baby Unit.

What are the particular needs of pre-term and low birthweight babies?

Describe the available forms of pain relief during labour.

key terms

You need to know what the key terms and phrases in this chapter mean. Go back through the chapter and find out.

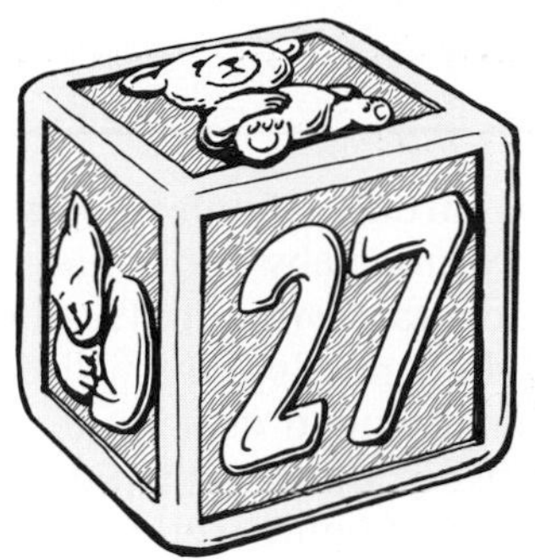

PROMOTING DEVELOPMENT AND LEARNING

The early development of the baby will be strongly influenced by the care, stimulation and the close, secure physical contact given by the significant adults in their lives. This chapter will cover the following topics:

- *early development*
- *the role of play and playful experiences in encouraging development.*

Early development

There are wide variations in the ages at which babies will develop particular skills. It is important to remember that all children develop in a very individual way and that their progress should be measured against:

- what is typical for their age range
- cultural/biological origin
- parental/genetic background
- social group
- gestational age
- level of stimulation
- medical background
- their own achievements, that is whether or not any new skills have been learnt by them within a period of time.

It is important to remember that all areas of development are linked and dependent on each other, and should not be viewed in isolation.

There is detailed information about the development of the baby from birth to one year in Unit Four, The Developing Child.

The role of play and playful experiences in encouraging development

All babies need to be stimulated in order to progress through the developmental stages. Stimulation can be as simple as talking to a young baby and achieving or maintaining eye-contact. Babies need a lot of physical contact with adults, who will spend time with them, caring for them and meeting their needs. This will enable babies to communicate and feel secure. Above all, babies need close and secure contact with adults. It is through this trusted relationship that development will proceed and skills will be learnt. A feeling of security and of being well cared for is essential for a child to reach its full potential.

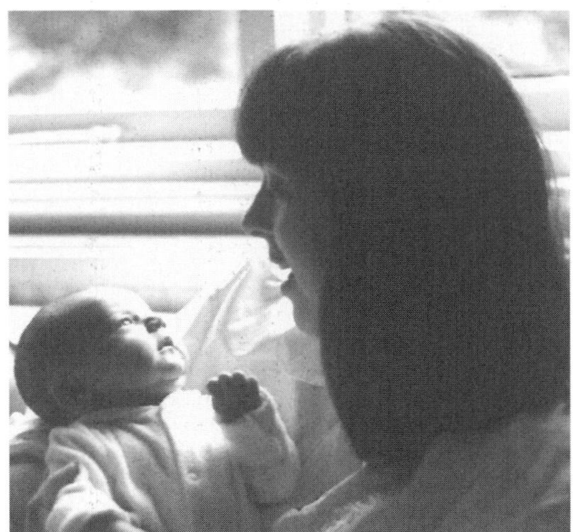

Babies are fascinated by human faces

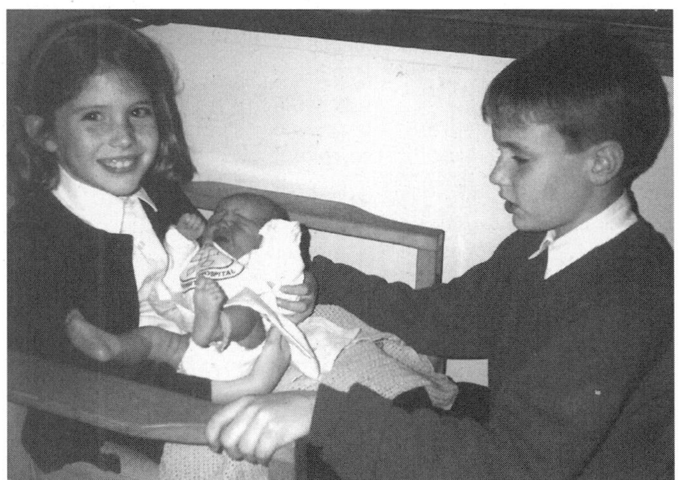

Babies need physical contact with their close family

PROMOTING DEVELOPMENT AND LEARNING

The table set out opposite summarises activities and the role of play, playful experiences in overall development and toys that are appropriate for the different ages and stages of development.

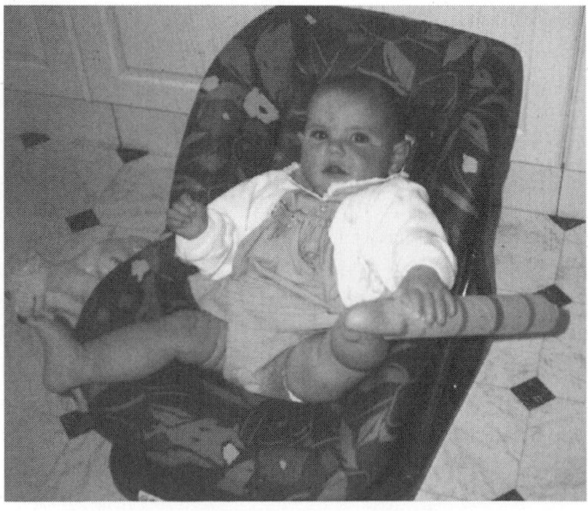

At 6–9 months babies will sit unsupported for longer periods

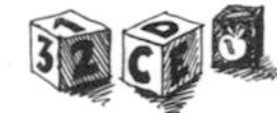

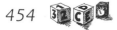

Methods of stimulating development

Age	Area of development	Stage of development	Stimulating activities/toys
0–3 months	Gross motor	Head control developing; kicking legs with movements becoming smoother and more symmetrical in supine; enjoys being held sitting; begins to support head and chest on forearms in prone	Time for lying on the floor to kick and experiment with movement; opportunity to be without nappy or clothing to encourage co-ordination; change positions from prone to supine so that the baby feels comfortable in either; sitting supported on carer's knee and in bouncing cradle
	Fine motor	Fascinated by human faces; grasp reflex diminishing; outwards direction of development progressing; trying to co-ordinate hands and eyes to control environment; finger play: beginning to discover the hands; may begin to hold objects for a few moments when placed in the hand	Bright, colourful objects to encourage focusing within the visual field of 20–25 cm, e.g. mobiles, watching the washing line, pictures of faces around the cot, toys with facial characteristics; opportunity to watch what is happening around her; use of noise to attract attention, e.g. rattle placed in her hand or objects strung over the cot, which make a noise when touched; baby-gym, or other objects within reach of waving arms
	Hearing and speech	Recognises main carer's voice; vocalising in conversational pattern; beginning to look for the origin of the sound; cries to indicate need	Opportunity to bond with main carer and recognise their voice; lots of physical contact and cuddles with loving conversations which maintain eye contact and give the baby the opportunity to respond; carers need to show lots of pleasure when they do; enjoys being sung to
	Social and play	Smiles from about 5 to 6 weeks; enjoys all caring routines and responds to loving handling; imitates some facial expressions; beginning to recognise situations, e.g. smiles, vocalises and uses total body movement to express pleasure at bathtime or feeding time	Lots of contact with adults and children to widen the social network, but mainly with primary carer, to strengthen the bond; routines for meeting needs to ensure security and comfort; stimulating areas of development, as above; opportunity for eye contact and to watch faces and mimic them, e.g. sticking tongue out

Methods of stimulating development continued

Age	Area of development	Stage of development	Stimulating activities/toys
3–6 months	Gross motor	Head control established; beginning to sit with support; rolling over; playing with feet in supine, and raising head to look around; supporting head and chest on extended forearms in prone; weight bearing and bouncing when held standing	Opportunity to practise sitting, on carer's knee, then protected by cushions for a soft landing when she topples! Physical play: bouncing on the knee with suitable songs, rough and tumble on the bed, rolling and bouncing (NB Never leave a baby alone on the bed or other high surface); carer's knee is ideal gymnasium at this age: some babies love to stand and bounce up and down for long periods of time; baby bouncer may be useful purchase; time to practise and experiment skills on the floor
	Fine motor	Beginning to use palmar grasp and transfer objects from hand to hand; watches all activity with interest; moves head around to follow people and objects	As baby is finding her hands, toys which rattle are essential; as she holds an object, the noise it makes will attract her attention and she will see the clever thing she is doing; colourful, small, safe toys which can be grasped by tiny fingers are invaluable, e.g. soft animals, box of bricks, chiming ball, home-made toys, e.g. transparent plastic bottles with coloured water inside or half-filled with sugar or dried beans which rattle (lid must be tightly on and baby supervised); old plastic cotton reels strung together provide useful tactile experience; baby needs things to reach out for and things to hit
	Hearing and speech	Turns immediately to familiar sounds; screening hearing test may be performed from 6 months onwards; tuneful vocalisations, sing-song sounds, laughs and squeals with pleasure; responds to different emotional voices in carer	Lots of physical contact and play using songs and voice; conversations with carers and others, who give baby time to respond, reinforce responses by showing pleasure and repeating sounds; enjoys listening to nursery rhymes and finger games with tune and rhythm; 'This little piggy' and 'This is the way the farmer rides' encourage listening and fun
	Social and play	Beginning to put all toys in mouth to explore them and investigate the world object by object; recognising objects which make a noise, trying to utilise them; finding the feet as a source of investigation and pleasure; enjoys strangers if they are friendly and gentle	Safe, non-toxic toys to put in the mouth; some babies may enjoy finger feeding too; make bean bags with various fillings, e.g. dried peas, crunchy cereals, to give oral experience; make books suitable for chewing, using photographs and/or pictures in plastic covers; waterproof bath books useful purchase; opportunity to play and investigate both alone and in the company of other children

Methods of stimulating development continued

Age	Area of development	Stage of development	Stimulating activities/toys
6–9 months	Gross motor	Can sit unsupported for lengthening periods of time; may begin to crawl; may stand and cruise holding on to furniture or other stable objects; some may begin to walk with hands held or even alone	Needs to be given time to play on the floor, placed in sitting position, with support until stability is established; fun toys big enough to see and attract attention, just out of reach to stimulate mobility, but not enough to increase frustration; surround baby with toys in sitting position to encourage balance skills as he reaches to grasp to sides and the front; time spent bouncing on feet and encouraging strength in legs; stable furniture for baby to pull to stand
	Fine motor	Visually very alert to people and objects; developing pincer grasp with thumb and index finger; uses index finger to poke and point; looks for fallen objects	Needs lots of exciting visual activity, e.g. going to the park, shopping; toddler group good opportunity for observing other children play; smaller objects can be introduced with supervision, (remember that everything will go into the mouth), e.g. small pieces of biscuit or bread, hundreds and thousands to encourage a pincer grasp and yet be safe to eat; build towers of bricks to be knocked down with glee; look at picture books, encouraging baby to point at familiar objects with you; encourage baby to look for and find items 'lost' over side of high-chair, to help make sense of the world and cause and effect, e.g. something dropped does not disappear for ever
	Hearing and speech	Babbles loudly and tunefully, repeating sounds again and again, e.g. da da da; beginning to understand commonly used words and phrases, e.g. No, Bye bye; varies volume and pitch depending on mood, whether happy or cross; still cries for needs	Talk to baby about what is happening all the time; repeat their interpretations of words; sing repetitive songs, encouraging them to vocalise with you; finger rhymes encourage language; read books together, naming objects; encourage imitations of verbal and non-verbal language; name objects and people baby points at
	Social and play	Now wary of strangers; plays games like Pat-a-cake, Peep-bo; claps and waves; offers toys to others; finger-feeds; attempts to use cup and/or bottle; looks for partly hidden toys	Games and activities to encourage language development also stimulate play and social skills; as baby now discovers values of objects, she will need things that respond differently when same thing is done to them, e.g. ball will roll when pushed, brick will not; biscuit will crumble when squeezed, bread will not, toys that squeak, bricks that do not; safety mirror in plastic frame to allow the baby to recognise herself; post table-tennis balls down kitchen-roll tube; toys or safe household items that can be banged to make a noise, wooden spoon, saucepan or xylophone; babies are beginning to make music and be delighted by achievements

Methods of stimulating development continued

Age	Area of development	Stage of development	Stimulating activities/toys
9–12 months	Gross motor	Will now be mobile, crawling, bottom-shuffling, bear-walking or walking; may be able to crawl upstairs; mobility has frustrations as well as pleasures: baby can reach areas previously out-of-bounds, so needs attention in providing suitable playthings within reach	Large-wheeled toys fun to push around, brick-trolley or similar push-along toy to help develop skills of getting around corners, reversing, etc.; small climbing frames used with supervision to increase balance and co-ordination; swimming; walking outside with reins
	Fine motor	Mature pincer grasp; throws toys deliberately; points to desired objects; bangs toys together	Pull-string musical box or similar to encourage dexterity and also teach cause and effect; nesting toys, building bricks, etc. will encourage balance and concepts of shape, size and colour; roll balls for baby to fetch, she will soon roll them for you; tin or basket filled with interesting objects to take out and put back in; plastic jars and bottles with removable lids to encourage investigation of what is inside, or simple delight at removing lid
	Hearing and speech	Understands several words and phrases; obeys simple commands; lots of vocalisations with sounds for certain objects, e.g. dud may mean cup	Talk to baby constantly, repeat names of people and objects, sing songs, games and rhymes, read stories with familiar situations and few characters; baby must be surrounded by language to develop communication skills effectively
	Social and play	Usually loving and affectionate, likes to be near someone familiar; can drink from cup with a little help; tries to use spoon; likes to put objects in and out of containers; participates in routines	Make sure that care is consistent and familiar; give opportunity to learn to feed, e.g. allow practice with cup and spoon, regardless of inevitable mess; valuable for sensory experience; offer lots of opportunity for play with interaction from adults, e.g. taking turns, stop and go; baby sometimes acquires a new skill by making something happen by mistake – if it is fun he will want to do it again; adult must observe this and reinforce positive actions; opportunity to watch and imitate others, perhaps in routine domestic chores; small dustpan and brush or similar to encourage this and make help valued; needs own equipment, e.g. flannel, toothbrush, cup, spoon to foster feeling of personal identity, and encouragement to take part in caring routines

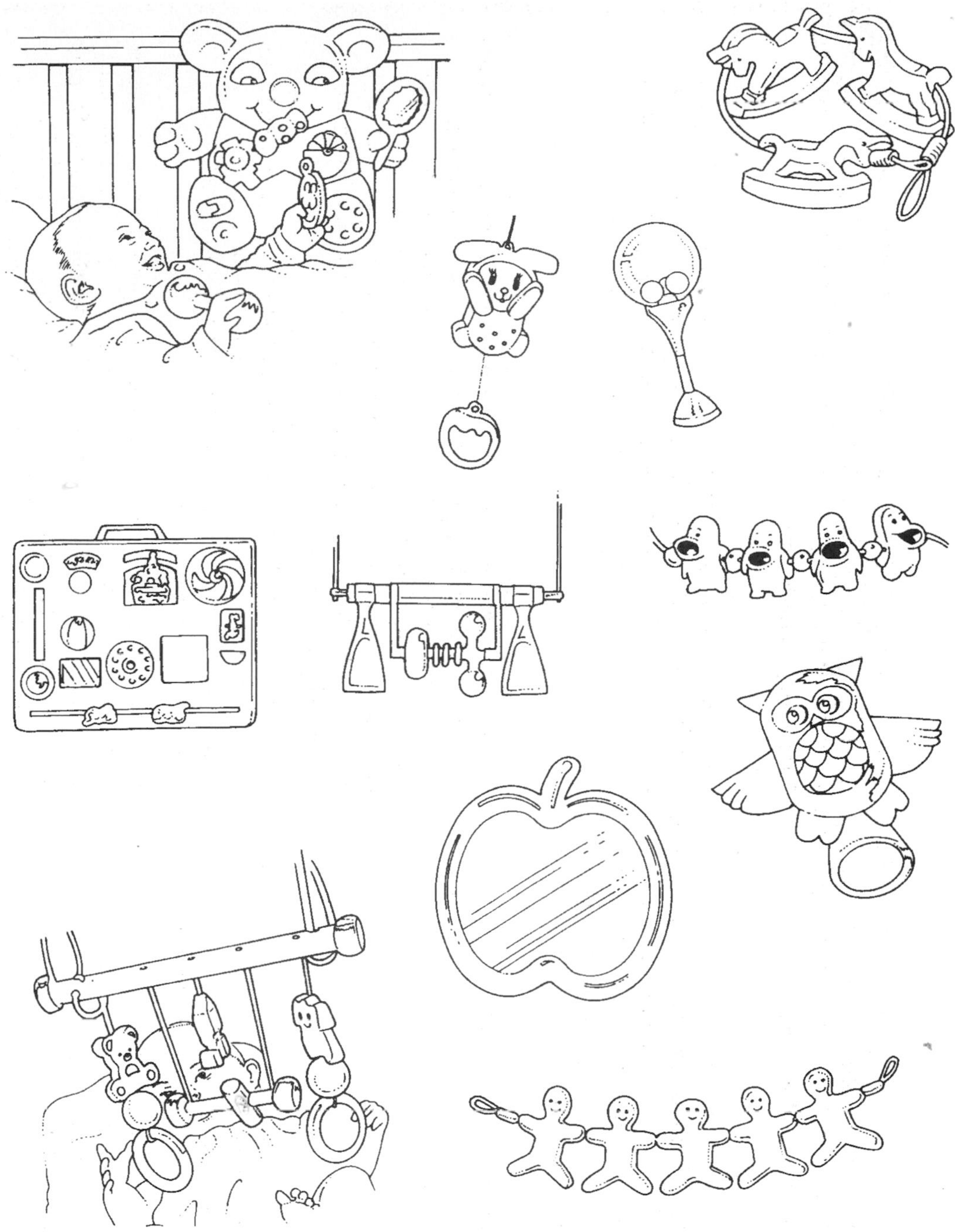

Some stimulating toys for a baby's pram or cot

All methods of stimulating development can be achieved without great financial cost. The most important factor is the quality of adult–baby interaction. Parents and carers should spend time talking and playing with a baby. It is important to remember that babies need to repeat activities and experiences in order to acquire skills before they move on to the next stage and child-care workers will need to be patient and allow babies to progress at their own pace. Not all families can afford frequent shopping trips to purchase the latest toy or aid to development. A little ingenuity and imagination, combined with an awareness of safety, can provide a multitude of learning experiences with everyday household articles.

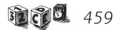

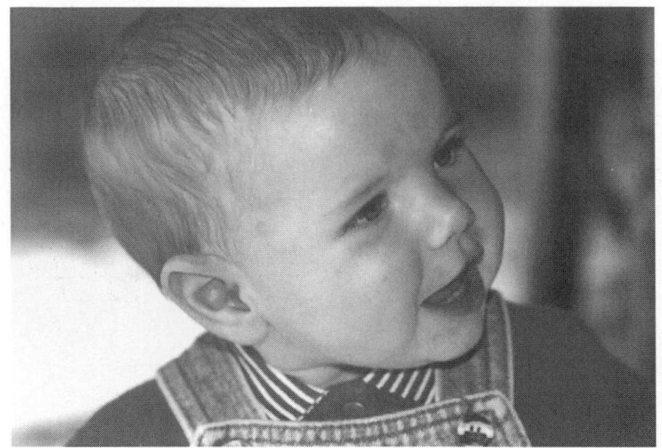

At 6–9 months babies show a real interest in their surroundings

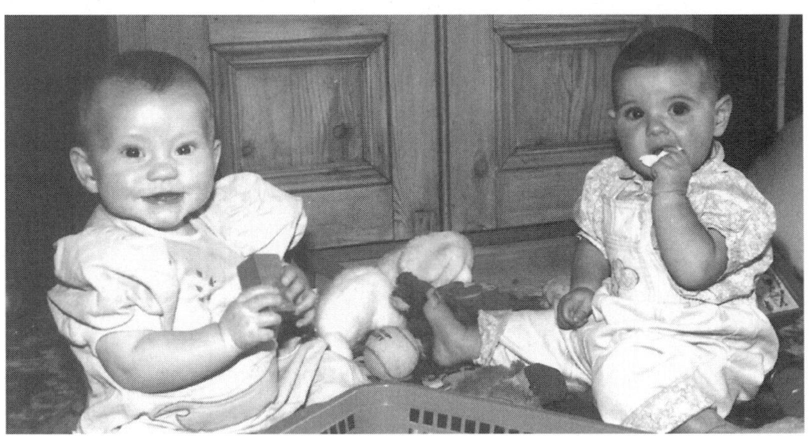

Everyday household articles can easily provide learning experiences

Now try these questions

What factors should be taken into account when assessing development?

Why is adult/baby interaction especially important to a young baby?

How could you stimulate:

(a) gross motor development from birth to 3 months?

(b) fine motor development from 3 to 6 months?

(c) social play from 6 to 9 months?

(d) hearing and speech from 9 to 12 months?

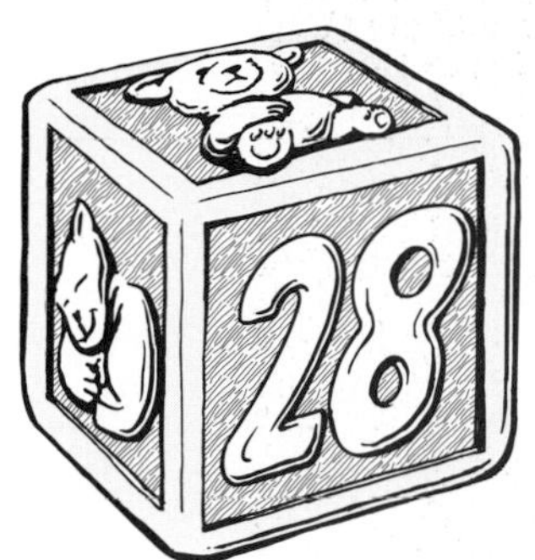

POSITIVE CARE AND SAFE PRACTICE

In the first year of life, babies require care that will meet their individual needs and the particular needs of all infants. All babies are unique and special and, because of their age and stage of development, they require highly skilled care from their parents or qualified child-care workers. This chapter explains the value of specialised types of care and equipment used in the first year of life.

This chapter will cover the following topics:

- *the importance of care routines*
- *care of the skin and hair*
- *commonly encountered signs and symptoms of illness*
- *sudden infant death syndrome (SIDS)*
- *positive health for babies*
- *equipment*
- *clothing for the first year.*

The importance of care routines

Babies are completely dependent on an adult to meet all their needs. Although babies' needs are generally the same, the manner in which they are met will differ in the first year. All babies are different – some will sleep well, others will not; some are happy and contented, others not. Caring adults need to be flexible and patient, to accept change and be aware of how and when these changes may occur. Child care and education workers need to be aware that child care practice varies and that it is important to know about and respond to the needs of the primary carers.

The emotional and physical needs of babies and young children can be summarised as follows.

- *Emotional needs* are:
  - continuity and consistency of care
  - physical contact

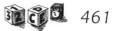

  - security
  - socialisation
  - stimulation.
- *Physical needs* are:
  - food
  - warmth, shelter, clothing
  - cleanliness
  - rest, sleep, exercise
  - fresh air, sunlight
  - safety and protection from injury and infection
  - medical intervention if necessary.

Babies will eventually settle into a routine that meets their need for food. The regularity of feeding and the urgency with which a baby signals its hunger is the basis of any routine in the early weeks. Feeding the baby on demand is often the most satisfactory method. As babies get older, they will sleep for longer at night, although some babies require a night feed or drink well into the second or third year. There are no rules controlling how babies behave: they are all individuals with very individual needs.

As the baby begins to sleep for longer at night, they will probably stay awake for longer periods in the day, until by the end of the first year they may only have one long, or two shorter, sleeps during the day. This increasing wakefulness provides the opportunity to develop in all areas, with good care and stimulation. It also gives the carer the opportunity to perform the caring routines that the baby will enjoy if they are treated with affection, patience and understanding.

Care of the skin and hair

See Chapter 5 for more general information on care of the skin and hair. It is important to give careful attention to caring for a baby's skin and hair, because:

- the baby is very vulnerable to infection
- the skin must be able to perform its functions.

As well as giving attention to keeping adequately clean, this routine care includes frequent observation of the condition of the skin for any rashes or areas of soreness.

DAILY CARE

Babies do not need to be bathed every day. They are not active enough in the early months to require their hair and whole body to be washed more than two or three times a week. Some carers prefer to bath the baby every day so that it becomes part of the routine, whether in the morning or evening. As babies get older a daily bath will become part of the daily routine.

Bath-time gives an ideal opportunity to talk and play with the baby. Topping and tailing can, however, be equally pleasurable, and is more reassuring for young babies who can feel insecure when their clothes are removed and they are submerged in water.

TOPPING AND TAILING

Topping and tailing involves cleaning the baby's face, hands and bottom.

Preparation

Collect all the necessary equipment:

- a bowl of warm water
- a separate bowl of cooled, boiled water for the eyes in the first month or so
- cotton wool balls
- baby sponge or flannel
- towel
- change of clothes
- nappies
- creams, if used
- blunt-ended nail scissors.

Method

- Lie the baby on a towel or changing mat.
- Remove outer clothing, if it is to be changed.
- Gently wipe each eye with a separate cotton wool ball, moistened with cooled boiled water, from the inner corner to the outer (nose to ear).
- Wipe the face, neck and ears with cotton wool balls.
- Make sure that the baby is dry, especially where the skin rubs together, such as in the neck creases.
- Clean the hands, using a sponge or flannel. Check that nails are short and that there are no jagged edges that the baby may scratch with. Cut them straight across.
- Remove the nappy and clean the bottom area, using cotton wool or a separate flannel. *Always* wipe from the vulva/scrotum to the anus – front to back direction. If the baby has soiled the nappy, soap is advisable to clean the area. Wet wipes may be used, but these may sometimes cause soreness.

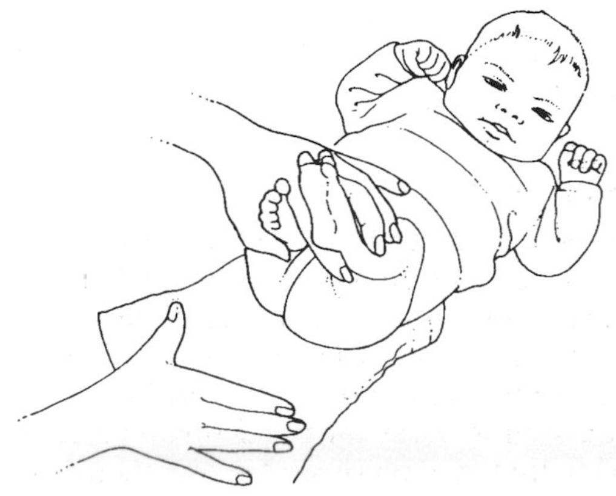

Topping and tailing

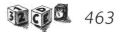

- Replace a clean nappy, after the bottom has been thoroughly dried.
- Replace clothing

BATHING

Bathing should eventually become a 'fun' time for the baby and carer, but there are nevertheless some conditions that are essential:

- The room should be warm – at least 20°C.
- The water should be warm – at body temperature, 37°C.
- Always put the cold water in the bath first.
- Collect all the equipment together before starting the bath.
- Never leave a young child alone in the bath – babies can drown in just 1cm of water.
- After the bath, ensure that the baby is completely dry, especially in the skin creases, to prevent soreness.

Safety in the bath

As the baby gets older, it may feel more comfortable in a sitting position in the bath. Constant physical support must be given to prevent the baby from sliding under the water, or feeling insecure. Such an experience could put a baby off bathing for a considerable time. A non-slip bath mat is a wise investment for safety. As the baby gets older, standing may seem fun. This should be discouraged, as serious injuries could result from a fall.

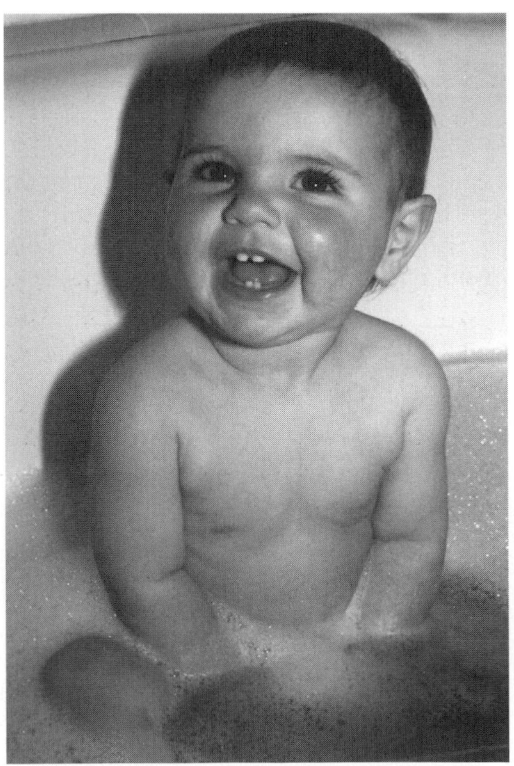

Bath time is fun

Bath-time is fun

If the baby is safe in the bath, she will feel secure and begin to enjoy the experience. There are many toys available for the bath, and many can be improvised from objects around the house. Empty washing-up liquid bottles will squirt water; squeezed sponges make a shower. But in the first year a baby is more interested in physical contact and play. Blowing bubbles, tickling, singing songs with actions will all amuse and give pleasure. Hair washing can be fun too. If the baby is accustomed to getting her face wet from an early age, hair washing should be easy. If it proves difficult, leave it for a couple of days. Wipe over the head with a damp flannel and gradually reintroduce the hair washing gently, using a face shield if necessary. Above all, never let this area become a battle. It is not that important and may create a real fear of water that could hinder future swimming ability.

Progress check

What are a baby's emotional needs?

Why do babies settle into different routines?

Why is it important to give careful attention to caring for a baby's skin and hair?

How often do babies need to be bathed?

What is topping and tailing?

What temperature should the bath water be?

What is the most reliable method of testing the temperature of the bath water?

Which important safety precautions should be taken when bathing a baby?

Why is it important to ensure that bath-time is an enjoyable experience?

NON-INFECTIOUS SKIN PROBLEMS

Cradle cap

Cradle cap is a fairly common condition affecting the scalp, especially the area around the anterior fontanelle (soft spot). It is a scaly, greasy or dry crust appearing by about 4 weeks and disappearing by 6 months. It is probably caused by unnecessary fear of rubbing that area of the scalp. Prevention is by washing the hair once or twice a week, and rinsing it very thoroughly. If it becomes unsightly or sore, the crust can be removed by special shampoo.

Heat rash

Heat rash is caused by over-heating and appears as a red, pin-point rash that may come and go. The treatment is to remove surplus clothing, bath the baby to remove sweat and to apply calamine lotion to reduce the itching and make the baby feel comfortable.

Eczema

Eczema is fairly common in babies, especially if there is a family history of allergies. It begins with areas of dry skin, which may itch and become red, and scaly patches. Scratching will cause the skin to weep and bleed. Cotton scratch mittens should prevent this. The treatment is to avoid perfumed toiletries; use oil such as Oilatum in the bath and an aqueous cream instead of soap. Biological washing powders and some fabric conditioners can irritate the condition, so use a gentle alternative. Cotton clothing is best, and try to prevent the baby scratching if possible. The GP should be consulted if the condition is severe or causing distress.

Nappy rash

Nappy rash usually begins gradually with a reddening of the skin in the nappy area; if this is not treated it will proceed to blistering, spots and raw areas, which may bleed. It is extremely uncomfortable for the baby, who will cry in pain when the nappy is changed. Causes of nappy rash are:

- a soiled or wet nappy left on too long – this allows ammonia present in urine to irritate the skin
- concentrated urine (a result of the baby not drinking well)

- an allergy to, for example, washing powder, wet-wipes, baby cream
- infection, for example thrush
- inadequate rinsing of terry nappies
- use of plastic pants, which do not allow the skin to breathe.

Treatment is as follows:

- Remove the nappy.
- Wash the bottom with unperfumed baby soap, rinse and allow to dry thoroughly.
- Let the baby lie on a nappy with the bottom exposed to the air.
- Leave the area free of nappies as often as possible, as contact with fresh air will help the healing process.
- Change the nappy as soon as the baby has wet or soiled it, at least every 2 hours.
- Do not apply any creams unless the bottom is completely dry; creams can cause nappy rash by sealing dampness in.
- Do not use plastic or rubber pants.

If there is no improvement, the carer should consult the health visitor or GP.

Progress check

What may cause cradle cap? How should this condition be treated?

How can heat rash be avoided?

If heat rash does occur, how should it be treated?

List three measures that can be taken to reduce the severity of eczema.

List five possible causes of nappy rash.

How may this condition be treated?

NAPPY CARE

There are two main types of nappy:

- terry nappies
- disposable nappies.

The choice of nappy is based on personal preference. The factors to consider are as follows:

- *Cost* – terry nappies involve a larger initial cost (24 will be needed), but are thought to be cheaper in the long term, especially if they are used for a subsequent baby as well. Research shows that this may be misleading, however, as the cost of electricity for washing (and sometimes drying), sterilising solution, washing powder, nappy liners, nappy pins, plastic pants and nappy buckets must also be considered. The cost of disposable nappies may prevent them from being changed as often as they should be.

- *Time* – disposable nappies certainly take less time generally.
- *Hygiene* – disposable nappies need to be disposed of in a hygienic way and many are simply put out with the household rubbish where they pose a hazard to the environment. Terry nappies need to be disinfected before washing, although some areas have a nappy laundering service.

Both types of nappy are quite adequate if they are used with care. Whichever type is used, babies should be changed 3 to 4 hourly, at each feeding time, and between if they are awake and uncomfortable. Avoid using nappy creams unless necessary. Clean the baby's bottom with water, baby soap, baby lotion, wet-wipes or baby oil. Make the experience fun; never show disapproval. Talk to the baby and let them enjoy some freedom without the restriction of a nappy.

Case study . . .

. . . nappy rash

Hamish is 6 months old. He is teething and has had a bout of diarrhoea. He has just completed a course of antibiotics for a chest infection. Hamish has now developed a nappy rash; his bottom and scrotum are red and sore and he cries every time his nappy is changed. His childminder is very gentle with him and washes his bottom carefully at every change and applies a thick layer of petroleum jelly to protect his delicate skin. This is not helping and Hamish's mother notices that his bottom is bleeding slightly.

1. *What might have caused Hamish's nappy rash?*
2. *Why do you think the petroleum jelly was not successful?*
3. *What treatment would you suggest to help to clear up the condition?*

Progress check

What different types of nappy are available to parents?

What are the advantages and disadvantages of using terry nappies?

List the advantages, and possible disadvantages, of using disposable nappies.

How should the baby's bottom be cleaned when the nappy is changed?

CARE OF BLACK SKIN

All babies may have dry skin, but it is especially common in black children and should be given special care. The following are general guidelines:

- Always add oil to the bath water and do not use detergent-based products, as these are drying.
- Massage the baby after the bath, using baby oil, massage gel or almond oil. This is a wonderful experience for both parties!
- Observe the baby frequently for signs of dryness and irritation – scaly patches need treating with a moisturising cream.
- Beware of sunshine – black skin is just as likely to burn as white skin. Always use a sun block on a baby's skin in the sun, and a sun hat.

- Wash the hair once a week, but massage oil into the scalp daily, as the hair is prone to being brittle and dry.
- Comb very curly hair with a large-toothed comb.
- Avoid doing tight plaits in the hair as this can pull the hair root out and cause bald patches.

Progress check

How can a child-care worker try to prevent dry skin in children?

How can the skin be protected from damage by the sun?

What special care does black hair need to keep it supple and healthy?

Commonly encountered signs and symptoms of illness

Because young babies cannot say when they feel unwell, or where there is pain, it is very important to be able to recognise the signs of illness. Babies can become seriously ill very quickly, and the advice of a doctor should be obtained whenever there is any concern about a baby's state of health.

Babies usually recover very quickly too, with the correct treatment.

The signs to look out for are as follows:

- *The baby looking pale and lacking energy* (babies with black skin look paler than usual) or *looking flushed and feeling hot*, due to a high temperature.
- *Loss of appetite* – a baby on milk alone may refuse feeds or take very little; an older baby may refuse solid foods and only want to suck from the breast or bottle.
- *Vomiting persistently after feeds and in between* – this should not be confused with normal regurgitation of milk after feeds. Projectile vomiting in a baby of 4 to 8 weeks may be a sign of **pyloric stenosis**. This is caused by a thickening of the muscle at the outlet of the stomach to the small intestine. The baby feeds and the stomach fills with milk, which cannot pass through the narrowed outlet to the small intestine. The baby then vomits to empty the full stomach. The doctor should be consulted urgently.
- *Diarrhoea* – persistent runny, offensive stools, which may be green, yellow or watery, should be treated immediately; babies can dehydrate very quickly.
- *Sunken* **anterior fontanelle** – this is a serious sign of dehydration, perhaps after a period of vomiting and/or diarrhoea or insufficient fluid intake due to loss of appetite.
- *Bulging anterior fontanelle* – the 'soft spot' is visible as a pulsating bump on the top of the baby's head, and is caused by increased pressure inside the skull; this requires urgent medical treatment.
- *Crying constantly and cannot be comforted* – this may occur with any other sign(s) of illness; the cry may be different from any of the usual cries.
- **Lethargy** – the baby lacks energy and may seem to regress (go backwards) in development.

key terms

Pyloric stenosis
a thickening of the muscle at the outlet of the stomach to the small intestine – milk cannot pass through the narrow outlet into the small intestine

Anterior fontanelle
a diamond-shaped area of membrane at the front of the baby's head. It closes between 12 and 18 months of age

Lethargy
lacking energy, tired and unresponsive

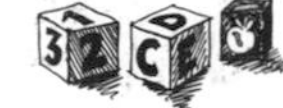

- *Rash* – if the baby develops a rash and has any other signs of illness, consult the doctor; a rash alone may be due to heat or allergy. It may be possible to treat this without medical intervention.
- *Persistent cough* – coughing is very distressing to a baby and carer; if it does not improve, or is associated with any other signs of illness, the doctor should be consulted.
- *Discharge from the ears, or if the baby pulls at the ears and cries* (especially if there are any other signs of illness) – a doctor should be consulted. Ear infections are common in young children and should be treated promptly to avoid damage to the hearing.
- *Changes in the stools or urine* – apart from changes due to diarrhoea (loose, frequent stools) and dehydration (scanty urine output), other changes may be observed. The stools or urine may contain blood or pus, the stools may become bulky and offensive. Stools should be observed for colour, consistency and frequency, and any abnormality recorded and investigated – it may be due to a change in diet. Any concerns should be reported to the doctor, preferably with a sample.

Progress check

Why is it important for child-care workers to be able to recognise the early signs of illness in a baby?

What is projectile vomiting a sign of?

What changes to the anterior fontanelle are serious signs of illness?

If a baby who is generally well develops a rash, what are the possible causes?

What changes in the stools and urine of a baby could indicate illness?

Sudden infant death syndrome

key term

Sudden infant death syndrome (SIDS) the unexpected and usually unexplained death of a young baby

Sudden infant death syndrome (SIDS) is the unexpected and usually unexplained death of an infant. It was previously called 'cot death syndrome' because the baby is usually found in the cot after failing to wake for a feed. This may occur between 1 week and 2 years of age, but around 3 months is the most common age.

CAUSES OF SUDDEN INFANT DEATH SYNDROME

Research has not isolated a particular cause, but has established that there are some risk factors linked to SIDS:

- overheating
- smoking
- being generally unwell in the few days prior to the death
- being put down to sleep on the stomach.

SIDS is commoner in:

- winter months
- boys
- premature babies
- low birthweight babies.

PREVENTION OF SUDDEN INFANT DEATH SYNDROME

There are four basic guidelines which, when adopted, reduce the risks of a cot death:

- Put the baby to sleep on their back in the cot, pram or buggy to prevent them from rolling over on to the tummy.
- Do not allow the baby to overheat.
- 'Feet to foot' in the cot – place the baby at the foot of the cot, with their feet touching the end. This prevents the baby from wriggling down under the covers and overheating, or suffocating.
- Do not use duvets – use a sheet and layers of blankets instead, because these can be adjusted to suit the temperature of the room. The ideal temperature for the baby to sleep in is 18°C.
- Keep the baby out of smoky atmospheres – it is preferable that people do not smoke in the rooms the baby uses. Parents should stop smoking during the pregnancy.
- The baby should be examined by a doctor if she is unwell in any way. If there is any concern it is better to be safe than sorry.

SUPPORT FOR PARENTS WHERE A BABY HAS DIED

Parents will go through the stages of grieving – initially feeling shocked and numb, unable to accept what has happened, confusion, anger, guilt and despair (see Chapter 20). They may want to talk and should be given every opportunity to do so.

A support network of families who have experienced the same trauma may be available via local voluntary groups. Professional counselling may be required.

There is a slightly increased risk that a second baby may also suffer SIDS and parents will be naturally anxious for the safety of their future children. Care of the Next Infant (CONI) is a programme set up to support parents who have lost an infant – to offer advice, practical help and reassurance.

The Foundation for the Study of Infant Deaths (FSIDS) recommend that parents keep their baby in their bedroom, in a separate cot, for at least the first 6 months.

Each cultural group has their method of child-rearing. In the UK, the rate of SIDS is lower among Asians. This may be because most Asian parents keep the baby in the parental bedroom through the night.

Progress check

Which babies are at most risk of SIDS?

What steps can be taken to reduce the risks of SIDS?

What support is available for parents who have experienced a 'cot death'?

Positive health for babies

Babies should be checked regularly by a professional carer to ensure that they are thriving and developing within the average range. This monitoring begins as soon as the baby is born, with the first examination by the midwife. A paediatrician will also examine the baby before they are discharged to go home. If the baby is born at home, the community midwife and GP will be responsible for these checks. The baby will be seen daily for the first 10 days by the midwife, who is responsible for her care. The GP should also visit the home to see the baby. When the midwife discharges the mother and baby (usually on the 10th day, if there are no problems), the health visitor will arrange to examine the baby. This 'birth visit' is usually at home. The health visitor will use her professional skills to decide how often the baby needs to be seen.

Regular surveillance of all babies is carried out by the primary health care team; there is more detailed information on this in Chapter 15.

CHILD HEALTH CLINICS

Throughout the first year of life, carers are encouraged to attend child health clinics with their baby. Here they can have the baby weighed, discuss progress with the health visitor and see the doctor if necessary. It is also an opportunity to meet other babies of a similar age and stage.

The immunisation programme is also commenced in the first year, at 2, 3 and 4 months. This is another opportunity for the baby to be observed, and for a carer to report progress and any difficulties.

SUPPORT GROUPS AND SERVICES

There are often local support groups for parents and carers with young babies. Groups of mothers who have met at relaxation classes may keep in touch and have regular meetings as a form of mutual support. The National Childbirth Trust, the La Leche League and hospital-based postnatal support groups are other alternatives. Gingerbread is a national organisation to help to support lone-parent families. There are probably others in your area.

There should be no need for anyone to sit at home worrying about a baby; there are lots of services and people who are very willing to help. However, there may be barriers, such as language, for example, which prevent people from using the services they are entitled to. In areas where there is a high proportion of people who do not speak English as their first language, specialist help is available, for example interpreters in clinics, leaflets printed in the relevant language and additional supportive home visiting by specially trained health visitors.

Progress check

Which professionals are responsible for the health care of babies?

What services are available at the child health clinic?

What are the benefits of social support groups for mothers?

How can mothers who speak English as an additional language be supported?

Equipment

Having a baby will necessarily incur some financial cost, unless the family has a baby already and has kept all the required items. Even so, they will need to ensure that the equipment is still suitable and safe to use. There are many factors to consider, the well-being of the infant being of prime importance. Some of these factors are outlined below.

SAFETY

All equipment bought, loaned or rented, new or second-hand, must comply with safety legislation and carry the BSI safety kitemark.

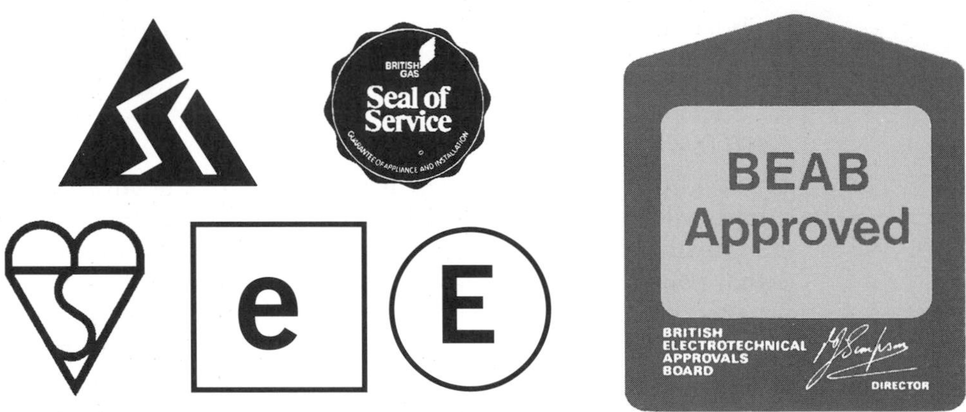

Marks of safety

ACCOMMODATION

The family may have plenty of space for large equipment, or may be living in a small flat, bedsit, or perhaps with extended family. Carers may need to consider, for example, how to cope with transporting the baby up several flights of narrow stairs.

ADAPTABILITY AND DURABILITY

Equipment that is to be purchased must be justified in terms of long-term usefulness and be strong enough to withstand normal wear and tear. A cot, for example, will be in use for 2 years and perhaps more. It should be strong enough to continue to be safe for this and subsequent babies.

Prams and pushchairs must be suitable for continued use as the baby becomes a toddler, to avoid having to replace it unnecessarily early.

ESSENTIAL ITEMS

All babies need:

- a place to sleep
- provision for feeding and hygiene routines, such as bathing and changing nappies
- to be safely transported.

The table below summarises the advantages and disadvantages of different types of essential items.

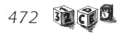

Essential items for sleeping and transport

Item	Features	Advantages	Disadvantages
To try to prevent avoidable cot deaths, current research recommends that all babies should sleep: • on their backs • without a pillow • without a duvet for the first year; sheets and blankets prevent overheating by removing a layer when necessary.			
Moses basket	Wicker basket with decorative lining and covers, with or without a canopy; usually with two handles for transport; may have a stand or be placed on the floor	Baby feels secure in small, enclosed space; easy to carry from room to room; looks pretty and appealing	Cannot be used to transport baby outside; unsafe for use in the car; unsuitable for older/heavier babies due to lack of internal space; may topple as baby moves around
Cradle	Wooden crib with rocking mechanism, either on rockers or suspended between two upright supports	As for Moses basket, except for ease of use between rooms; baby may respond well to being rocked to sleep	As for Moses basket
Carrycot	Rigid structure with mattress, waterproof cover and hood and carrying handles; covered in washable fabric or plastic	Enclosed space so baby feels comfortable and secure, used for night and daytime sleeping; easy to transport from room to room using handles; suitable for use outdoors, may be available with transporter (wheels) to convert to pram; restraining straps for transport by car	Babies will grow out of a carrycot sooner than a full-size pram; may be heavy and cumbersome to lift when the baby is older
Pram	Rigid, frame-built structure with hood and waterproof cover on wheels, with brakes, washable fabric, plastic or metal exterior and fabric interior with mattress; harness fixing points	Baby feels comfortable, safe and secure; can be used for sleeping downstairs at home; ideal for use outside, for journeys on foot or for letting the baby sleep in the fresh air; suitable for use in all weathers; large enough to carry the baby for the first year and longer; shopping tray makes transporting groceries easier; possible to transport a toddler as well on a specially designed pram seat	Unsuitable for getting up and down stairs, so alternative night-time sleeping arrangements required; may be a problem in a block of flats if lifts not working; unsuitable for transportation by car; may create storage problem in a small house/flat or bedsit

Essential items for sleeping and transport continued

Item	Features	Advantages	Disadvantages
Cot	A purpose-built sleeping area for a baby and toddler; should be strong and stable; bars should be no more than 7 cm apart to prevent hands, feet and head getting stuck; waterproof, safety mattress that fits tightly within the frame; dropside cots should have childproof safety catches; option of high or low mattress position, depending on age/stage of the baby	Safe, secure sleeping environment individual to each baby, whether room is shared or not	No disadvantages provided that all specifications under 'Features' are met
Rearward-facing baby car seat	Designed for safe car travel using standard inertia seat belts; contains harness to restrain the baby within it; carrying handle to move the seat to and from the car	Safe transportation in a car; easy to carry with a sleeping baby in it; back support for a very young baby; can be used from birth until about 9 months; useful for babies who need motion to get to sleep; can be used in the house as a first seat	Can be expensive; will need replacing with a fixed car seat at about 9 months; some models can be difficult to carry and attach car seat belts to
Bouncing cradle	Soft fabric seat for a baby from birth to about 6 months; may include a row of toys	Used from birth; baby can be transported from room to room and can see what is happening everywhere; babies can rock themselves to sleep; easy to wash fabric cover	Dangerous if left on a bed or worktop when the baby can bounce themselves off; not suitable when babies can sit unsupported
Carrying slings	Fabric baby slings, attached to the carer's body to enable the baby to be carried in an upright position on the chest	Baby feels comfortable and secure, can hear carer's heartbeat and feel body warmth; comfortable sleeping position; babies can be carried indoors and out, invaluable for fractious ones who find sleep difficult or crave constant contact; leaves two hands free to cope with a toddler or other children needing supervision and attention; allows carer to continue with routine tasks	May be difficult to put on and take off, depending on the mechanism; may strain the back as baby gets heavier; flat shoes and careful posture essential to prevent injury to the baby by falling

Essential items for bathing

Item	Features	Advantages	Disadvantages
Warmth is essential when bathing a new baby. A wall thermometer will ensure that the room is at least 70 °C before you start.			
Baby bath	Plastic, purpose-built baby bath, usually bought with a stand	Large enough to use until the baby is about 6 months; can be used in any room where there is sufficient heat; comfortable for baby and carer, who can sit in a chair to bath when the bathstand is in use	Limited life, and of little use when the baby is bathed in the big bath; difficult and heavy to carry when full of water; storage may be difficult in small accommodation
New washing-up bowl or storage box	Large plastic container	Can be used for its original purpose when no longer needed for bathing; easy to transport to a warm environment when full of water; large enough to bath a baby in the early weeks; avoids expense of purpose-built models	Baby will need to transfer to the big bath by 2–3 months

A large plastic bowl or box for bathing is efficient and cost-effective

Essential items for feeding

Advantages and disadvantages	Breast-feeding	Bottle-feeding	Other essential equipment
It is largely personal preference which will decide whether a mother will begin to breast- or bottlefeed her baby.			
The advantages and disadvantages of breast and bottlefeeding are discussed later in the chapter.	It is advisable to have some bottlefeeding equipment to provide extra water or fruit juices, even if the baby is being breastfed; two or three bottles and teats should be sufficient.	If the baby is being bottlefed, then eight to ten bottles and teats will be required to make up enough feeds for a 24-hour period.	Sterilising equipment will be essential, and a good supply of formula milk; there are many brands available

Progress check

Which factors need consideration when buying equipment for a new baby?

How should babies be put to sleep to try to prevent cot death?

What are the features of a Moses basket?

List the advantages of a carrycot.

Why should a bouncing cradle always be placed on the floor?

Clothing for the first year

key term

Layette
first clothes for a baby

LAYETTE

The **layette** is the first set of clothes provided for a baby. Some guidelines for purchasing baby clothes are given below:

- Avoid ribbons, ties and bows, which can trap tiny fingers and toes and be very difficult to take on and off. They may cause a strangulation hazard. Garments of a loose weave (for example, hand-knitted) can be similarly hazardous.
- Buttons are a dangerous choking hazard, as well as being fiddly for large fingers.
- Choose clothes that are easy to launder; babies need changing often.
- Natural fibres are the most comfortable; cotton, for example, is more absorbent than synthetic fabrics.
- Clothing should be comfortable, to allow for ease of movement, and not too tight, especially around the vulnerable feet. Clothes made of stretch fabric and with raglan sleeves make dressing and undressing much easier. Avoid suits with feet as it is tempting to continue using them after they have been outgrown. A footless suit with a pair of correctly sized socks is a better alternative.
- Garments should have a flame-retardant finish.

CLOTHING FOR A NEWBORN

- Six vests – bodysuits prevent cold spots and help to keep the nappy in place
- Six all-in-ones – babygros, preferably footless
- Three pairs of socks or bootees
- Three cardigans (matinée jackets)
- Hat – sun hat in the summer and bonnet for colder weather
- Outdoor clothing – type will depend on method of transporting the baby. A knitted pramsuit may suffice or a quilted all-in-one may be required
- Warm mittens and scratch mittens

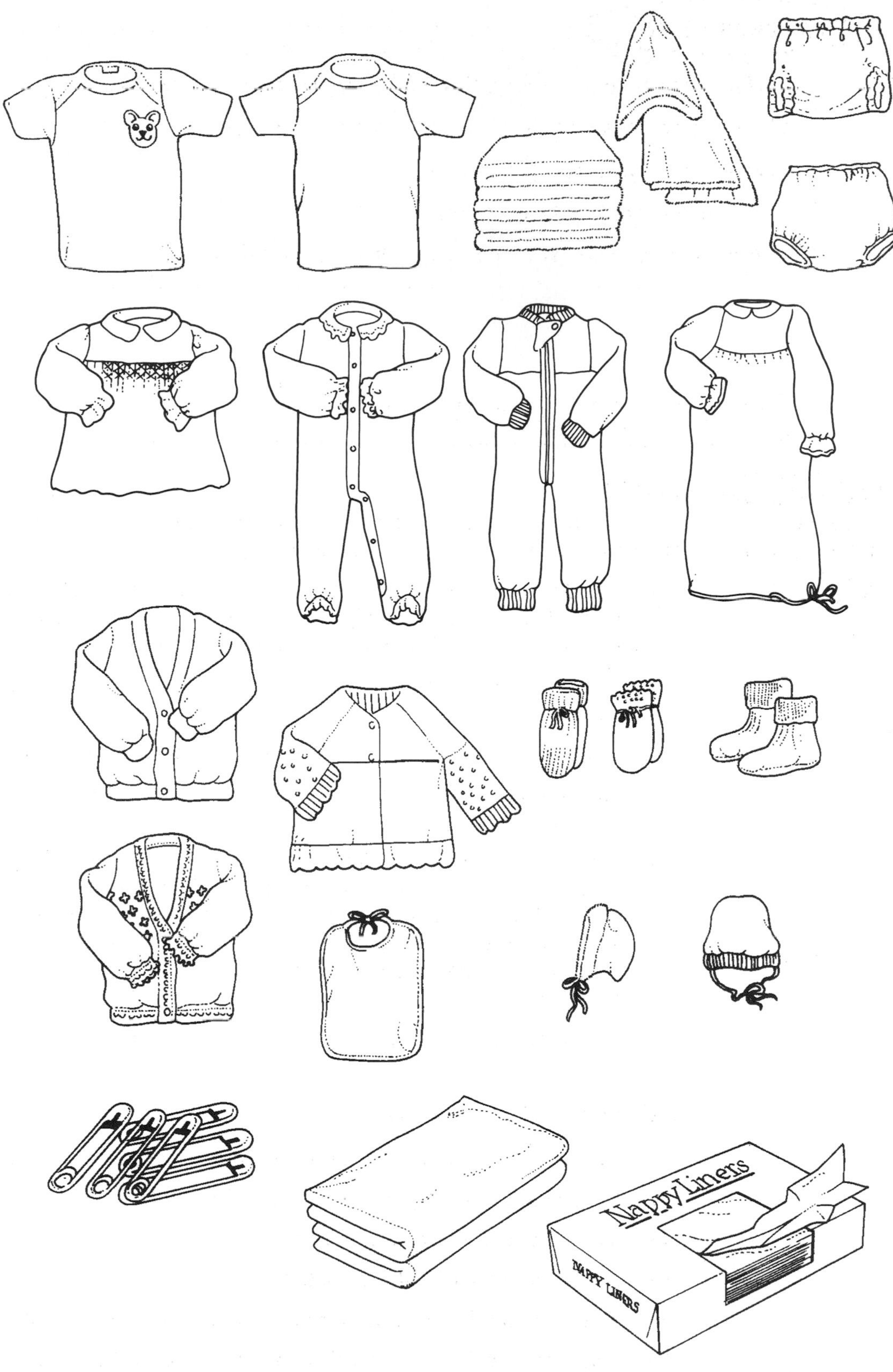

A baby's layette

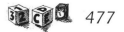

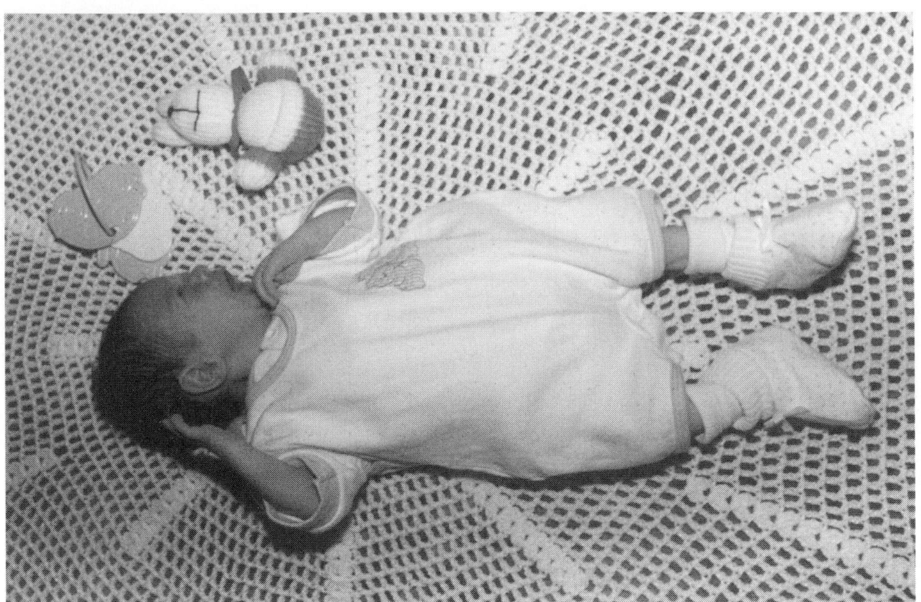

Clothing should be comfortable

Whether disposable nappies or terry nappies are to be used, a good supply is required. Do not buy more than one pack of first-size nappies until the baby is born and its size is known. Dial-a-nappy services are available in some areas.

Twenty-four terry nappies are sufficient, and will perhaps last for a subsequent baby. Nappy pins, nappy liners and plastic pants will also be required.

CLOTHING FOR THE FIRST YEAR

- Babies grow very quickly, so it is sensible not to buy too many clothes of the same size. There will be little chance to wear them all before they are outgrown.
- Shoes are unnecessary until a child needs to walk outside. Bare feet are preferable, even to socks, if it is warm enough and the flooring is safe.

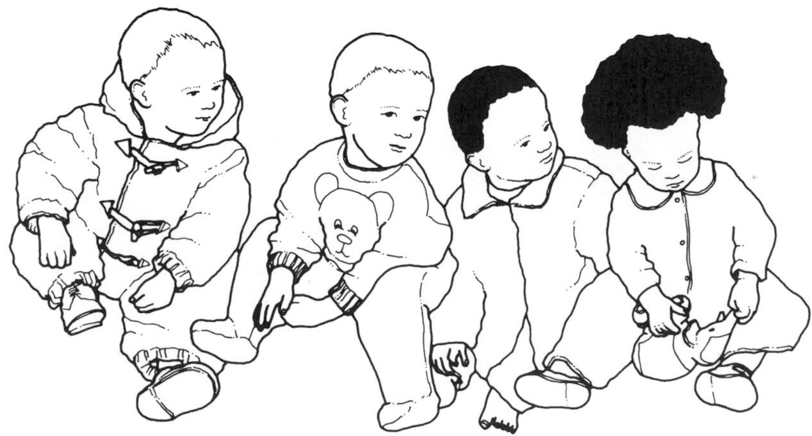

Clothing for the first year: garments should allow for ease of movement and be easily washable

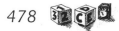

- Choose clothes that will help development and not hinder it; baby girls trying to crawl in a dress, for example, will become increasingly frustrated as they crawl into their skirts.
- Clothing needs will vary according to the season.
- Sort out clothes regularly and remove all that has been outgrown from the baby's drawers. This will prevent anyone who does not dress the baby often, trying to squeeze them into garments that are too small.

Now try these questions

Explain why it is important to observe babies, to monitor their health, in the first year.

Describe how a baby's physical needs may be met in the first year of life.

What are the signs and symptoms of eczema in young babies?

What support groups are available to families with young children in your area?

key terms

You need to know what the key terms and phrases in this chapter mean.
Go back through the chapter and find out.

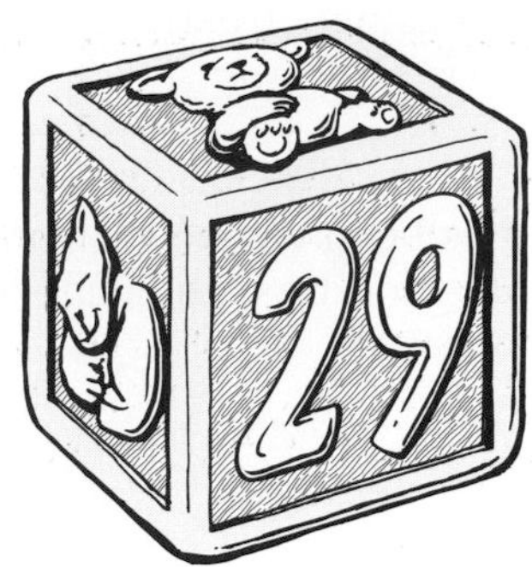

THE NUTRITIONAL NEEDS OF BABIES

Babies need to progress from being fed entirely on milk, either breast milk or formula milk, on to a mixed and varied diet that will provide all the required nutrients. This process usually takes place over the first year of life.

This chapter will cover the following topics:

- *feeding*
- *breastfeeding*
- *bottle (formula) feeding*
- *weaning.*

Feeding

All babies should be fed on milk only for at least the first 3 months of life, so parents must decide how the baby will be fed. The decision to breastfeed or bottlefeed is a very personal one. Most women have an idea of how they will feed their babies before they become pregnant. This may be influenced by how their mother fed them, how their friends feed their babies, health education at their school, the influence of the media and how they feel about their body.

There are advantages and disadvantages to both methods, but it is agreed that breast milk:

- is the natural milk for babies as it is the ideal source of nutrients for the first months of life
- should be encouraged as the first choice for infant feeding.

However, breastfeeding may not be possible for a number of reasons and women should not feel inadequate if they bottlefeed their babies.

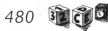

Breastfeeding

The primary function of the breasts is to supply food and nourishment to an infant. During pregnancy the breasts prepare for feeding. Successful breastfeeding does not depend on the size of the breasts; women with very small breasts can breastfeed just as successfully as those with large breasts.

Each breast is divided into 15–20 lobes containing alveoli, which produce milk. Each lobe drains milk into a lactiferous duct, which widens into an ampulla (small reservoir) just behind the nipple. It narrows before opening on the surface of the nipple.

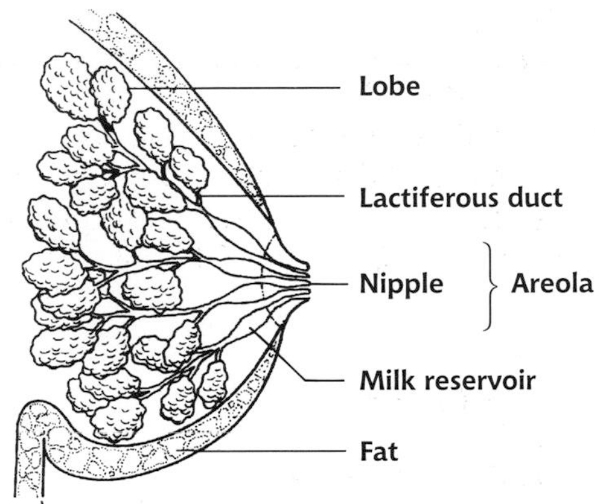

The structure of the breast

> **key term**
> **Colostrum**
> the first breast milk containing a high proportion of protein and antibodies

From the 16th week of pregnancy, the breasts produce **colostrum**. This will feed the baby for the first 2–3 days after birth. It is a thick, yellowish fluid that has a high protein content but is lower in sugar and fat than mature human milk. Only a few millilitres are produced at each feed but it satisfies the baby and is very easy for the new baby to digest.

On the 3rd or 4th day the milk comes in and a mother may notice that her breasts become fuller. Breast milk is not fully mature until about 3 weeks after birth.

ADVANTAGES OF BREASTFEEDING

- Breast milk from a well-nourished mother is the ideal food: it is made especially for babies. It contains all the right nutrients in exactly the right proportions to meet the changing needs of the baby. It is easily digested.
- Colostrum has a high concentration of maternal antibodies so it protects the baby from some infections.
- It is sterile (contains no germs) and reduces risk of infection.
- There are fewer incidences of allergies, for example asthma, in babies who are breastfed.
- It is always available at the correct temperature.
- It is more convenient: there are no bottles to prepare or heat.
- It is less expensive than purchasing modified milks.

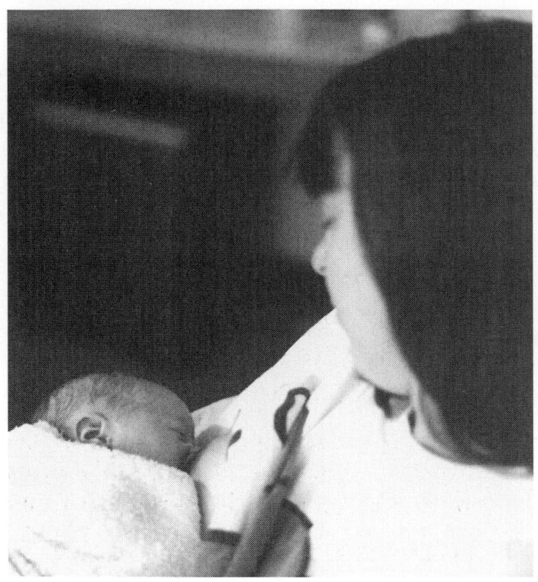

Breastfeeding

MANAGEMENT OF BREASTFEEDING

key term
Demand feeding
feeding babies when they are hungry in preference to feeding by the clock

key term
Complementary feeds
additional feeds as well as breast feeds

- **Demand feeding** (the baby is fed when hungry) is preferable to a strict regime of feeding by the clock. Babies have differing requirements and although they may feed often in the first few days, they will often have established their own 3 to 5 hourly feeding routine by 3–4 weeks. Some days they will require feeding more often – the only way they can stimulate the breast to produce more milk is by sucking for longer.
- Avoid giving **complementary feeds** in a bottle.
- The mother must be taking a well-balanced diet, especially high in fluids. Her diet will affect the composition of the breast milk and some foods may cause colic. The baby will not need extra vitamins if the mother is taking a healthy diet.
- Breastfeeding is tiring in the early weeks, so mothers should be encouraged to relax. Extra help at home until breastfeeding is established will benefit mother and baby.
- Allow the baby to finish sucking at one breast before offering the other. Avoid timing the feeds on each side because the more filling milk – the hind milk, with higher fat content – is the last to be expelled from each breast. This will help the baby to settle for longer between feeds.
- Breast milk can be expressed using the hands or a breast pump for use when the mother is unavailable. The expressed breast milk (EBM) can be stored for up to 3 months in a domestic freezer and offered in a bottle.
- Breastfeeding can continue for as long as the mother desires (feeding for even a few days is better than none at all). Weaning on to solid foods should begin between 4 and 6 months and milk consumption will gradually reduce.

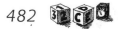

Bottle (formula) feeding

Most modern infant formulas (modified baby milks) are based on cows' milk, although some are derived from soya beans, for babies who cannot tolerate cows' milk. Manufacturers try to make the constituents as close to human breast milk as possible. All modified milks must meet the standards issued by the Department of Health. There are, however, basic differences between breast and modified milks. Cows' milk:

- is difficult to digest; it has more protein than breast milk, especially casein, which the baby may be unable to digest. The fat content is also more difficult to digest and this may cause wind or colic
- has a higher salt content; salt is dangerous for babies as their kidneys are not mature enough to excrete it. Making feeds that are too strong, or giving unmodified cows' milk can be very dangerous
- contains less sugar (lactose, needed by human infants) than breast milk.

ADVANTAGES OF BOTTLEFEEDING

The advantages of bottlefeeding are as follows:

- It is possible to see exactly how much milk the baby is taking.
- Fathers and other carers can help with the feeding regime, which may give the mother a chance for a good rest, especially at night; she may have more opportunity to go to work or pursue her own interests.
- The baby can be fed anywhere without embarrassment.
- It is less tiring for the mother in the early weeks.

PREPARATION AND STORAGE OF FEEDS

Equipment for bottlefeeding

All equipment for bottlefeeding must be thoroughly sterilised following the manufacturer's instructions on the sterilising solution bottle or packet. Equipment must be washed and rinsed before it is sterilised. Do not use salt to clean teats, as this will increase the salt intake of the baby if the salt is not rinsed off properly. Use a proper teat cleaner, which is like a small bottle brush. Feeds should then be made up according to the guidelines on the modified milk container. The following equipment will be needed:

- bottles (some have disposable plastic liners)
- teats
- bottle covers
- bottle brush
- teat cleaner
- plastic knife
- plastic jug
- sterilising tank, sterilising fluid or tablets, or steam steriliser.

There are some important points to remember when preparing bottlefeeds:

- Always wash your hands before and after making up feeds.
- Wipe down the work surface before preparing feeds.
- Rinse the feeding equipment with boiled water after it comes out of the sterilising fluid.
- Always put the water into the bottle or jug before the milk powder.
- Use cooled, boiled water to make up feeds.
- Demand feed, rather than time-feed, bottlefed babies. The primary carer should give the baby most of its feeds to encourage a close bond to develop.
- Wind the baby once or twice during a feed; check the size of the hole in the teat: if it is too small the baby will take in air as she sucks hard to get the milk, which will cause wind; if the teat is too large the feed will be taken too quickly and the baby may choke.
- Always use the same brand of baby milk; do not change without the advice or recommendation of the health visitor or doctor.

Never:

- add an extra scoop of powder for any reason
- pack the powder too tightly into the scoop
- give heaped scoops.

Doing any of these things will increase the strength of the feed and the salt intake. This will make the baby thirsty, so the baby will cry, more food will be given and increase the salt intake further. The baby can quickly become seriously ill.

Never:

- leave a baby propped with a bottle
- add baby cereals or other food to the bottle; when the baby is ready for solid feeding, it should be offered on a spoon.

How much milk?

Bottlefed babies should also be fed on demand and they usually settle into their own individual routine. New babies will require about eight feeds a day – approximately every 4 hours – but there will be some variations. A general guide to how much to offer babies is 150ml per kg of body weight per day (24 hours). For example:

- a 3 kg baby will require 450 ml over 24 hours
- a 4 kg baby will require 600 ml over 24 hours
- a 5 kg baby will require 750 ml over 24 hours.

The total is divided by the number of feeds a day to assess how much milk to offer the infant. When a baby drains each bottle, she should be offered more milk.

COLIC

Whether breastfed or bottlefed, some babies may experience colic, which is caused by air taken in during feeding or crying. This wind passes through the stomach and becomes trapped in the small intestines, resulting in contractions of the intestines that causes quite extreme pain.

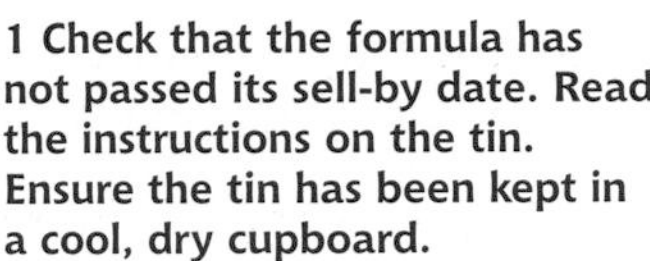

1 Check that the formula has not passed its sell-by date. Read the instructions on the tin. Ensure the tin has been kept in a cool, dry cupboard.

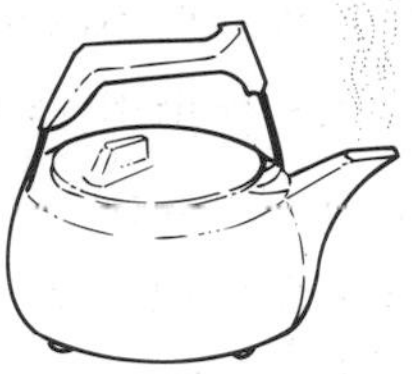

2 Boil some fresh water and allow to cool.

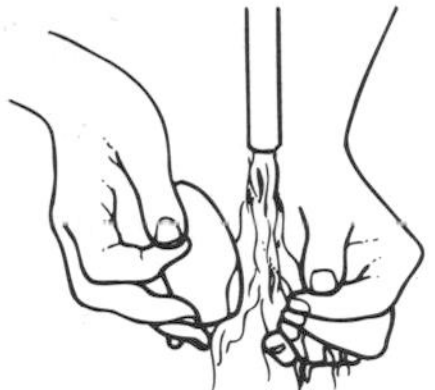

3 Wash hands and nails thoroughly.

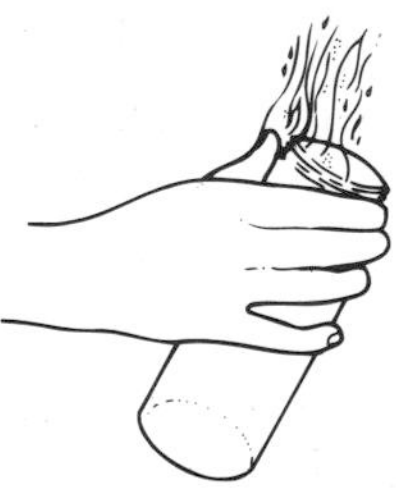

4 Take required equipment from sterilising tank and rinse with cool, boiled water.

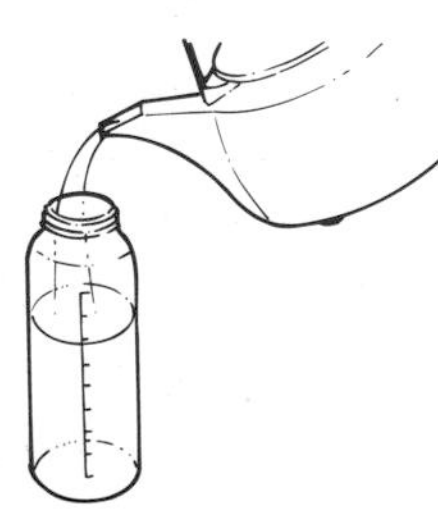

5 Fill bottle, or a jug if making a large quantity, to the required level with water.

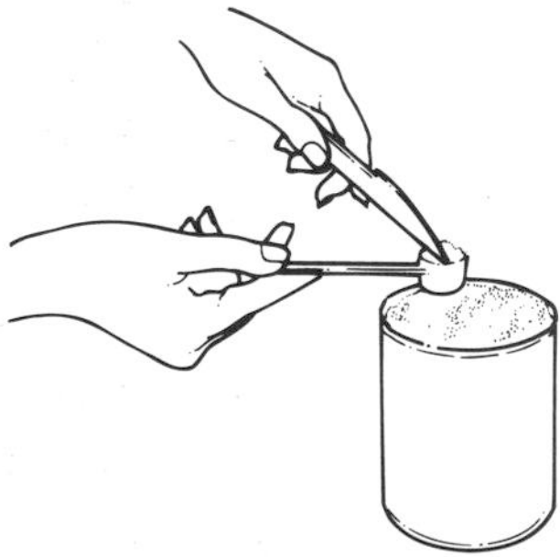

6 Measure the exact amount of powder using the scoop provided. Level with a knife. Do not pack down.

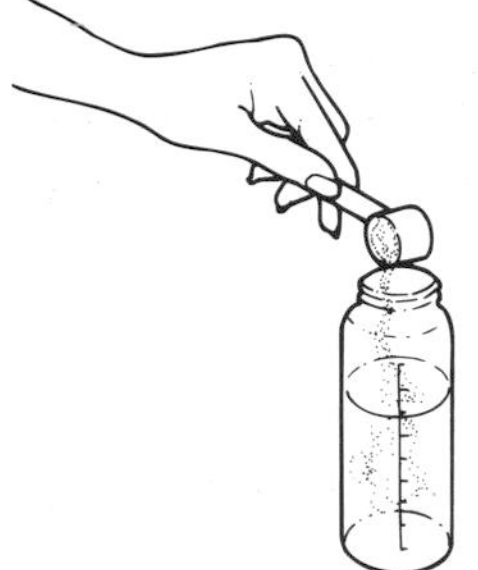

7 Add the powder to the measured water in the bottle or jug.

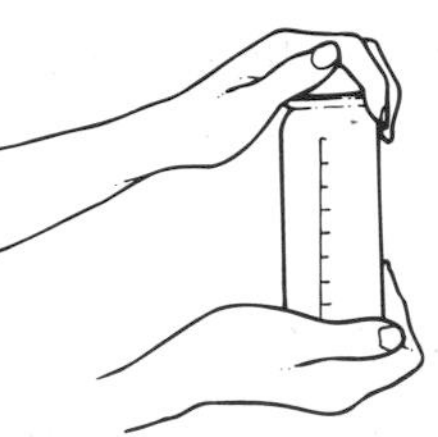

8 Screw cap on bottle and shake, or mix well in the jug and pour into sterilised bottles.

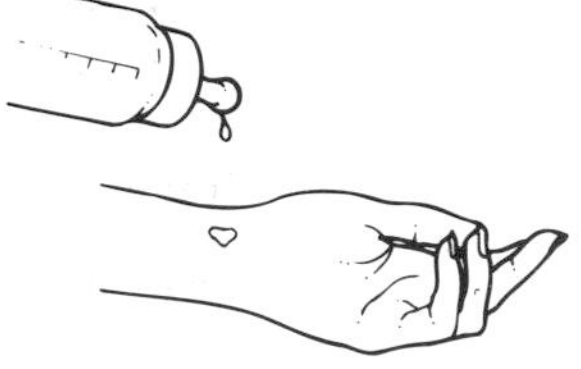

9 If not using immediately, cool quickly and store in the fridge. If using immediately, test temperature on the inside of your wrist.

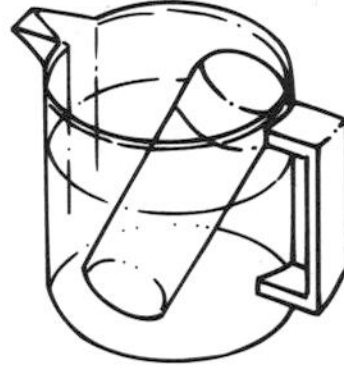

10 Babies will take cold milk but they prefer warm food (as from the breast). If you wish to warm the milk, place bottle in a jug of hot water. Never keep feeds warm for longer than 45 minutes, to reduce chance of bacteria breeding.

Note: whenever the bottle is left for short periods, or stored in the fridge, cover with the cap provided.

Making up bottlefeeds

Pain results in inconsolable crying, which is very distressing for parents and carers. Colic usually occurs between 2 weeks and 3 months of age. It is commonly known as '3-month colic' because that is the typical duration.

Milk should not be reintroduced into the baby's diet too quickly after a bout of gastro-enteritis. This could result in lactose intolerance and colic.

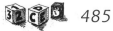

Signs of colic

The signs of colic are the baby crying, a reddened face, drawing knees up and appearing to be in pain. It is common in the evenings in breastfed babies. However, some babies are affected by colic both day and night.

It is unsafe, however, to assume that colic is to blame for all crying – exclude other possible causes. Any concerns should be discussed with the health visitor or doctor.

Care of a baby with colic

- Comfort the baby – pick them up and rub the back to dislodge any trapped wind.
- Lying the baby on the tummy on the carer's lap and rubbing the back usually helps.
- Rocking movements such as those created by car journeys, baby slings and walks in the pram may also help to relieve the pain.
- Some doctors advise breastfeeding mothers to monitor their diet to avoid foods that may exacerbate colic.
- Bottlefed babies should be winded regularly; check the teats for hole size and flow of milk – a small hole that does not allow much milk to flow will increase the amount of swallowed air.
- Homeopathic remedies are available from registered homeopaths. The GP may prescribe medicinal drops to be taken before a feed.

Progress check

How long should babies be fed on a milk-only diet?

What may influence a mother's decision to breastfeed or bottlefeed her baby?

Why is it generally agreed that 'breast is best'?

What is colostrum?

List the advantages of breastfeeding.

Describe what 'demand feeding' means.

What extra care must a breastfeeding mother take of her diet and her health?

List the advantages of bottlefeeding.

Describe the process of sterilising equipment and making up feeds.

How can you calculate how much milk to offer to a bottlefed baby?

What may cause colic in a young baby? How may this condition be treated?

Weaning

Weaning is a gradual process when the baby begins to take solid foods. This process should not be started before 3 months, and not later than 6 months.

WHY IS WEANING NECESSARY?

key term

Weaning the transition from milk feeds to solid foods

Milk alone is not nutritionally adequate for a baby over the age of 6 months. The baby has used the iron stored up during pregnancy and must begin to take iron in their diet. Starch and fibre are also necessary for healthy growth and development. Weaning also introduces the baby to new tastes and textures of food.

Babies at around 6 months are ready to learn how to chew food. The muscular movement helps the development of the mouth and jaw, and also the development of speech.

Mealtimes are sociable occasions and babies need to feel part of a wider social group. As weaning progresses, they learn how to use a spoon, fork, feeding beaker and cup. They also begin to learn the social rules in their cultural background associated with eating, if they have good role models; rules such as using a knife and fork, chopsticks, chewing with the mouth closed or sitting at the table until everyone has finished eating.

WHEN TO START WEANING

Between 3 and 6 months, babies will begin to show signs that milk feeds alone are not satisfying their hunger. There are no strict rules regarding the weight of the baby before weaning. The following are signs that the baby might be ready for weaning:

- still being hungry after a good milk feed
- waking early for feeds
- being miserable and sucking fists soon after feeding (this may also be a sign that the baby is teething)
- not settling to sleep after feeding, crying.

HOW TO WEAN

As young babies cannot chew, first weaning foods are runny so that the baby can easily suck it from a spoon. Start weaning at the feed at which the baby seems hungriest: this is often the lunchtime feed. Give the baby half their milk feed to take the edge off their immediate hunger, then offer a small amount of baby rice, puréed fruit or vegetables mixed with breast or formula milk to a semi-liquid consistency from a spoon.

The baby should be in a bouncing cradle or similar, but not in the usual feeding position in the carer's arms. There should be a relaxed atmosphere without any stress or distractions that might upset the baby. The carer should sit with the baby throughout the feed and offer their undivided attention. It may take a few days of trying for the baby to take food from the spoon successfully.

GUIDELINES FOR WEANING

- Never add salt to food, and never sweeten food by adding sugar.
- Do not give very spicy food; avoid chilli, ginger and cloves.
- First foods must be gluten-free, i.e. not containing wheat, rye or barley flour, because research shows that the early introduction of gluten could lead to the development of coeliac disease or other digestive problems in later life.
- Try different tastes and textures gradually – one at a time. This gives the baby the chance to become accustomed to one new food before another is offered. If a baby dislikes a food, do not force them to eat it. Simply try it again in a few days' time. Babies have a natural tendency to prefer sweet foods. This preference will be lessened if they are offered a full range of tastes.

- Gradually increase the amount of solids to a little at breakfast, lunch and tea. Try to use family foods so that the baby experiences their own culture and becomes familiar with the flavour of family dishes.
- As the amount of food increases, reduce the milk feeds. Baby juice or water may be offered in a feeding cup at some feeds. The baby still needs some milk for its nutritional value, and also for the comfort and security of feeding from the breast or bottle.

Cows' milk

After 6 months, babies may be given cows' milk in family dishes. They should not be offered it as a drink until they are over 1 year old. Milk drinks should continue to be modified milk or breast milk.

Iron

By 6 months, a baby's iron stores are low, so foods containing iron must be given. These include:

- liver
- lamb
- beans
- dahl (stewed lentils)
- green vegetables
- wholemeal bread
- cereals containing iron
- eggs, but these should not be offered until 12 months of age; because of the risk of salmonella, they must be hard-boiled and mashed.

Beef products should be avoided because of the risk of BSE.

WEANING STAGES

Stage 1

Early weaning foods are puréed fruit, puréed vegetables, plain rice cereal, dahl. Milk continues to be the most important food.

Stage 2

The baby will progress from puréed to minced to finely chopped food. Using a hand or electric blender or food processor is helpful to enable babies to enjoy family foods. Milk feeds decrease as more solids are taken. Well-diluted, unsweetened fresh fruit juice or herbal drinks may be offered.

Stage 3

Offer lumpy foods to encourage chewing. The baby may be offered food to hold and chew, such as a piece of toast or apple. A cup may be introduced. Three regular meals should be taken as well as drinks.

FEEDING DIFFICULTIES

Most feeding problems are caused by adults who are unfamiliar with the feeding or weaning process or who have unrealistic expectations of babies and children.

Problems may be avoided by following these guidelines:

- Be aware that weaning is a messy business; disapproval will prevent the baby from exploring and experimenting with food.
- Encourage independence by allowing the baby to use their fingers and offering a spoon as soon as the baby can hold one – it will eventually reach the mouth! Offer suitable finger foods too.
- Allow the baby to find eating a pleasurable experience.
- Babies have not learnt that courses conventionally follow a pattern and may prefer to eat them in a different order. Never start a battle by insisting that one course is finished before the next is offered. When the baby has had enough of one dish, calmly remove it and offer the next.
- Babies will normally want to eat, so refusing food could be a sign that a baby is ill. This may be a cause for concern or a minor illness, but if a baby normally eats well, refusing food should be taken as a serious sign and a medical opinion sought. Appetite will return once the baby is better.

key term

Food allergies reactions to certain foods in the diet

FOOD ALLERGIES

Food allergies can be detected most easily if a baby is offered new foods separately. Symptoms may include:

- vomiting
- diarrhoea
- skin rashes
- wheezing after eating the offending food.

The advice of a doctor should be obtained, and the particular food avoided.

Some babies may have cows' milk intolerance. If the baby is bottlefed, it may fail to thrive as expected, and should be referred to a paediatrician to confirm the condition. A dietitian will give feeding advice and should be consulted before weaning begins.

The allergy may be apparent in a breastfed baby and the mother may be advised to restrict the cow's milk in her diet. In all cases of cows' milk allergy, reintroduction should be carried out with medical supervision. There are substitute milks available, usually derived from soya beans.

More information about food allergy can be found in Chapter 7.

Progress check

What is weaning?

Why is weaning necessary?

How may a baby show that it is ready for weaning?

Describe the management of introducing the first solids.

Which foods are rich in iron?

Describe the weaning stages.

How can feeding problems be avoided?

What are the symptoms of food allergies?

Look at the picture overleaf and make a list of reasons for this baby's unhappiness about mealtimes:

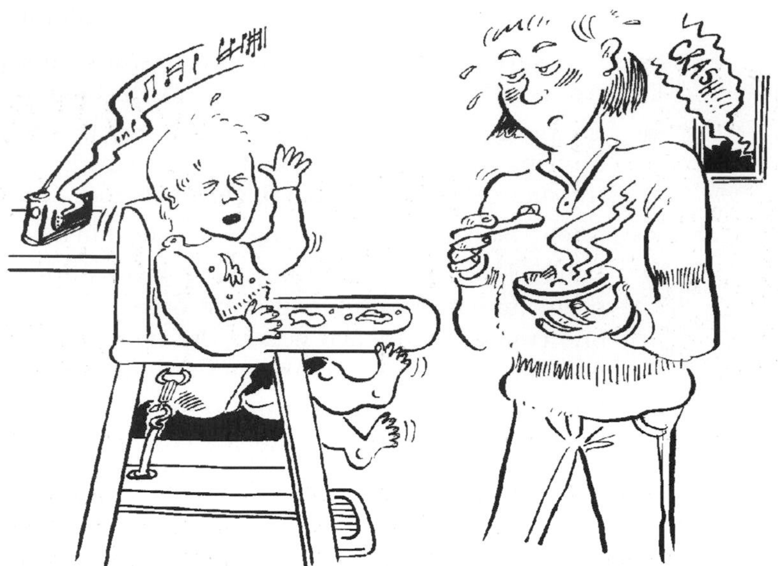

Distractions at feeding time

key terms

You need to know what the key terms and phrases in this chapter mean. Go back through the chapter and find out.

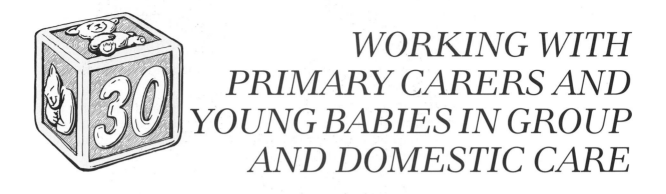

WORKING WITH PRIMARY CARERS AND YOUNG BABIES IN GROUP AND DOMESTIC CARE

During the first year of life primary carers are the most significant influence on babies' social, emotional, physical, linguistic and cognitive development. In addition, there is now substantial evidence highlighting the importance of the 'parenting' role to babies' subsequent health, well-being, educational attainment and social adjustment. However, the task of caring for a baby from 0 to 1 year is physically and emotionally demanding, often bringing significant changes to the economic and social lifestyle of the primary carers.

This chapter will cover the following topics:

- *the pressures on families and family life of caring for a baby*
- *building positive relationships with primary carers*
- *the particular requirements of young babies in group and domestic care*
- *the key worker system*
- *how babies learn through everyday interactions with their carers.*

The pressures on families and family life of caring for a baby

Despite 'parenting' being one of the most influential, demanding and challenging roles anyone can undertake, it is the one they are least likely to be formally prepared for or supported with.

SOCIAL PRESSURES

Many families experience pressures in their everyday lives. These are discussed in detail in Unit Nine and include the effects of disadvantage, the differences in the social, emotional and practical resources that enable some parents to cope more positively than others when under pressure, and the factors in some families that make babies and children more vulnerable to abuse.

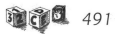

PERSONAL PRESSURES

The birth of a baby can bring particular pressures associated with:

- *loss of sleep by parents* – the tiredness experienced by some parents if their baby wakes frequently during the night can make ordinary, everyday tasks more difficult to achieve and exhaustion can lead to feelings of anxiety and stress
- *changes in the relationship between partners* – couples who have previously been accustomed to being the first person to receive each other's attention may at first find it difficult to adjust to the demands of a small baby who becomes the centre of their attention
- *being a lone parent* – an unsupported, lone mother (or father) may find the responsibility of caring alone for a baby initially overwhelming
- *the birth of a second or subsequent baby* – the demands of meeting the needs of the baby, together with those of older children who have different routines for eating and sleeping and other activities, can be difficult to adjust to
- *not having access to their extended family for support* – some people move around the country for their employment, leaving their family of origin and friends miles away and, as parents, lack their practical support when a baby is born.

Building positive relationships with primary carers

The role of the child-care worker may involve providing direct support and 'advice' to primary carers on an individual basis or through 'parenting groups', as well as indirect support through caring for their baby. It is also important that they know where they can advise primary carers to go to obtain more specialist advice and information outside their own knowledge and experience (see earlier references in this unit).

Childcare workers should:

- be aware of the statutory services
- become familiar with the range of formal and informal support groups and networks available to families with babies in the locality.

THE DIVERSITY OF CHILD-REARING PRACTICES

There is no blueprint for 'good parenting' and babies thrive in a wide range of family structures, with widely differing child-rearing practices. The child-care worker's role is to be non-judgemental about these differences and to avoid developing attitudes that cause them to stereotype parents whose lives and practices differ from their own. The worker's role includes providing continuity and consistency of care for babies, and this necessitates them working in partnership with parents. Such partnership involves recognising that primary carers usually know their own baby better than anyone else and learning from them about the particular personality and needs of their baby.

However, partnership with parents does not preclude the professional child-care worker discussing alternative care routines or child-rearing practices with parents, and using their own knowledge, training and experience to enrich the baby's experience, subject to the agreement of the primary carer. A child-care worker should only decide not follow the primary carer's wishes when it would place the welfare of the child at risk.

RELATIONSHIPS WITH PRIMARY CARERS

The term primary carer is used to describe the person or people who are the baby's 'first' carer. In most cases this is the child's mother and or father, but it may include other close relatives or substitute carers, such as foster parents.

An increasing number of parents resume employment outside their home soon after the birth of their babies. Deciding on the best care for their baby can be a difficult decision for parents and they will need to take time to research the alternatives. The demands of their employment and the cost of the different types of provision will be factors to be considered alongside personal preferences about how best to meet their baby's needs.

Such parents will expect 'value for money' but they may at times make unreasonable demands of carers, for example not turning up to collect their baby at the agreed time. A contract between them and the particular setting, making their mutual expectations of provision clear on both sides, will be helpful in maintaining positive relationships.

Some primary carers may demonstrate 'difficult' or challenging attitudes towards staff in child-care settings. This may be because they are unhappy about having been referred to a particular setting for help and support in caring for their baby.

It is important to try to build a positive relationship with all service users. The following are likely to promote positive relationships:

- assuming primary carers want the best for their baby
- listening with an open mind
- recognising and responding to the range of feelings primary carers may experience in entrusting their baby to the care of someone else
- adopting a non-judgemental approach
- empathising with primary carers' circumstances and way of life
- involving primary carers in the setting and in decision making about how the setting operates
- being willing to change the way things are done
- explaining and demonstrating an understanding of how to promote the development of babies and a genuine concern for the welfare and development of their baby.

Progress check

What social pressures may be experienced by the parents of young babies?

What particular personal pressures may the parents of young babies have to deal with?

What role in life are we least likely to receive preparation for?

In what circumstances might a child-care worker discuss alternative care routines or child-rearing practices with parents?

What approach should a child-care worker adopt towards the diversity of child-rearing practices that they might encounter?

What are the key elements involved in working positively with parents?

The particular requirements of young babies in group and domestic care

THE EMOTIONAL AND SOCIAL NEEDS OF BABIES IN DAY CARE

The quality and character of children's early close relationships has for some time been recognised to be of central importance to their social and emotional development. This subject is covered in detail in Unit Four. The pioneering work of John Bowlby has continued to be influential. The theory of attachment and loss is that:

- babies and young children need to establish secure attachments with close carers
- the experience of such attachments is crucial to children's healthy social and emotional development
- separation from the person to whom they are attached can be distressing and damaging if the form of substitute care does not meet a baby's needs.

It follows that if babies and young children are to be separated during the day from the primary carers they have become attached to, they need to have a substitute carer to whom they can also become attached and from whom they can learn and therefore develop healthily.

THE EMOTIONAL AND SOCIAL NEEDS OF BABIES SEPARATED FROM THEIR PRIMARY CARERS

Research has shown that babies do not necessarily attach to those people who spend most *time* with them, but that attachments are more likely to be formed with those people who are most *sensitive* to the baby's needs. In order to develop an attachment, a baby needs:

- to experience a warm, continuous, loving relationship
- carers who will respond sensitively to them
- interaction to occur between the baby and carer(s)
- carers who will stay with the baby most of the time
- communication to develop between the infant and carers
- carers who give loving physical attention and affection.

It follows, therefore, that those who work with babies in day care must provide for babies in a way that meets these needs.

Attachment theory has had a great influence on both the provision and organisation of day care in the UK, and formed the basis of the guidance for the provision of day care in the Children Act 1989, with its emphasis on low ratios and rooms allocated specifically for babies.

In order to meet babies' needs when organising a baby room it is not however enough for a day nursery to provide a room with low staff ratios; the *quality* of the care given is of greatest significance to the babies' experience, development and happiness.

THE PROVISION OF DAY CARE FOR BABIES IN THE UK

Attachment theory was and still is widely influential. However, it was interpreted most strongly in the UK, partly because John Bowlby lived and worked here.

As a result of this theory, from the 1950s to the 1970s, mothers were strongly discouraged from working and it was regarded as bad practice to place young children in day care. For many years local authorities in the UK actively discouraged the placement of babies in any nursery, either in social services' nurseries or in the very few private nurseries that then existed. Full-time day care for older children was also strongly discouraged, although part-time nursery classes and playgroups were regarded as acceptable. If child care was required, childminders were used, in the hope that they would act as mother substitutes.

However, as equal opportunities attitudes and laws gained more ground, and as the economy experienced labour shortages that could be met by encouraging women back to work, it became more acceptable for mothers of young children to work and it was then that the private nursery market began to flourish.

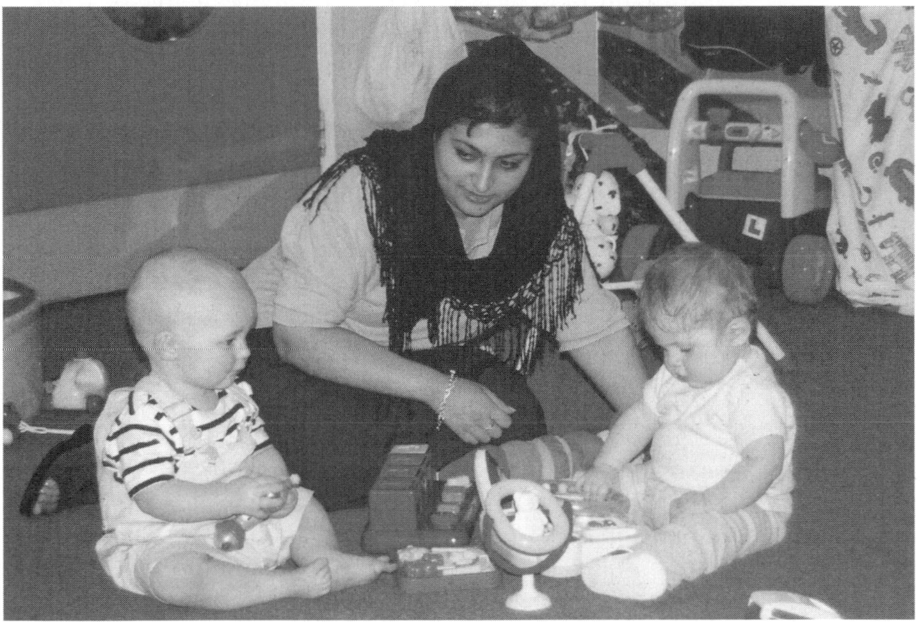

Babies in group care

Day nurseries

In 1989 the Children Act was passed; this acknowledged the need for child care, but, strongly influenced by attachment theory, insisted on guidelines concerning ratios of adults to babies of 1:3 for children aged 2 and under. The problem with this is that the level of staffing required to meet these ratios is very high and this has made day nursery provision in the UK very expensive, particularly when compared to some other countries. As a result costs in the private sector can only be met by paying low wages and/or charging high fees. The private nursery market has nevertheless expanded from its very low base to outstrip the public sector tenfold in the last 10 years and many babies are now cared for in these nurseries.

Childminders

Childminders have always been a popular child-care choice for parents of very young children. Since 1997, government policies have recognised the need for high quality and affordable child care as a factor in enabling parents to participate in the world of work and thus make their contribution to the economy. A number of initiatives have supported this. One of these has been to encourage, with a variety of incentives, the training and registration of many more childminders. This recognises that some parents will prefer to make a relationship with an individual childminder and will choose for their children to be cared for in a domestic, rather than a group care environment. Registration requirements that determine the number of children of particular ages that a childminder can care for, and usually limit the number of babies under a year to 1, mean that this experience will more closely resemble a family group, comprising children of various ages and one constant carer.

Nannies

Some parents will find that the demands of their employment and in particular the long hours and trips away from home that are expected of many managerial/professional workers mean that their child-care needs are difficult to meet. A nanny, who may be employed on a daily or live-in basis, can provide the flexible child care that is required here. The baby will benefit from the attention of one adult to whom they can make an attachment in the familiar environment of the home and parents will have regular, ongoing contact with their child's carer. Disadvantages of this option are, as with any option, that the nanny may decide to move on and the baby will be left to make another attachment to the replacement carer.

The key worker system

It is in the context and tradition of attachment theory and also within the tight regulatory framework of the Children Act 1989, that advice on day care for babies is usually given. One of the most comprehensive attempts to define good practice for young children is offered by Elinor Goldschmied and Sonia Jackson in their influential book *People Under Three: Young Children in Day Care* (Routledge: London, 1994). In their view, day care should try to be like a home environment, although they realise it is impractical to regard the nursery as a home. They recommended that children be age-grouped because it is then easier to meet their developmental needs. Within this age grouping, they recommend a '**key worker**' system, that is one person 'who holds responsibility for making relationships with a particular child, whenever possible greeting her on arrival, settling her in, subtly arranging, guiding and responding to her activities and attending to her physical needs'. If the key worker is not available substitute care should be arranged to minimise disruption. If this is provided, a baby should experience the conditions necessary to form an attachment.

> **key term**
>
> **Key worker**
> works with, and is concerned with the care and assessment of, particular children

THE ADVANTAGES OF THE KEY WORKER SYSTEM

In their literature Sure Start (an area-based government initiative – see Chapter 34 for more details) recommend having a key worker who is the main carer, especially for babies, because they need the security of a consistent carer.

The advantages of the key worker system are as follows:

- A baby cannot express his or her needs verbally, so a carer must tune into them by observing the baby's own rhythms of sleeping and feeding, and through exchanging information with the parents. This can be achieved if a close personal relationship is formed within the setting, which will help babies to separate from their home environment and enable them to cope better with the day care provision. For this reason children should belong to a key group and within that group they should be allocated a key worker. If two staff work together in a group, they can cover the key person role for each other and both will become familiar with all the children.

- Children will get to know their key worker and be able to use that relationship to develop a secure base within the setting to gain confidence and develop independence.
- The key worker will also take responsibility for ensuring that the child's documentation is up to date, including observations and assessments, and for developing a relationship with the family, which includes the regular exchange of information.

This arrangement does not mean that the key worker is the only adult who works with a child, but it is expected that they will spend some time of the day together, particularly around arrival, going home and mealtimes. For example, a baby should be greeted, fed, changed and settled into sleep by their key worker. This will enable the infant to develop and sustain the secure attachment necessary for their well-being.

Case study . . .

. . . the benefits of a key worker system

Pam had just been appointed senior nursery nurse in the baby room of a large day nursery. On most days, there were between seven and nine babies under one year, with three staff. Over the first week or so she observed the staff and babies during the daily routines and, in particular, the babies' responses. The babies were well cared for physically and staffing ratios met legal requirements. Babies were washed and nappies changed quickly, at set times during the day, by whoever was on bathroom duty. They were also fed at set times; sometimes a child-care worker would spoonfeed two weaned babies together, with two bowls and two spoons. Pam noticed, however, that the babies were sometimes fractious, noticeably during changing and feeding times.

Pam decided that she should make some changes and she called the staff together to discuss this. She explained that, in her opinion, the babies were having to relate to too many adults during the day and a result the staff did not have enough contact with individual babies during which they could really get to know each other.

They decided that they would introduce a key worker system so that each baby would be linked to a particular member of staff for most of their time in the nursery. Each worker would also pair with another worker so that they would cover shifts and staff holidays between them. The key worker would then be the main point of contact for parents and would be responsible for maintaining the baby's records.

When the system was in place the babies' key workers always spent some one-to-one time every day with their particular children and they got to know them really well. In addition, after discussing it with the staff, Pam reorganised some of the baby room routines and encouraged the staff to relax, not rush and make the most of the opportunities for close communication that feeding and changing routines particularly presented. Babies were now changed when necessary, rather than according to the clock and this was done, whenever possible, by their own key worker. They were also fed, as often as possible, by their own key worker when the babies were hungry and always one at a time.

After a few weeks, the staff met to discuss what they'd gained. They all agreed that the babies had benefited from the new system; they seemed happier and more relaxed. The staff felt that they had benefited too; they appreciated having time to get to know their 'own' babies and felt more able to anticipate their needs. They also felt that, because of their greater understanding of their individual babies, the contact they had with parents and the exchange of information with them each day had improved.

What do you think the problem was when Pam took up her post?

What did the introduction of a key worker system provide?

Why do babies need to have someone particular to relate to in a group care situation?

Why is it important to make the most of routines to interact with babies?

What do you think the benefits of these changes were to the baby room staff and to the parents of the babies?

THE DISADVANTAGES OF THE KEY WORKER SYSTEM

The disadvantages of the key worker system, making it difficult to operate in practice, stem from the organisation of day nurseries in the UK. This is for the following reasons:

- Fees are high, which results in many children attending nursery on a part-time basis. Nurseries, however, need to be full to be economically viable and accept as many children as possible, often on a part-time basis. This can make the allocation of workers difficult.
- Unlike in many European countries, nurseries usually remain open throughout the year to facilitate parental 'choice' and to accommodate the demands of the labour market, but this means that staff must take holidays throughout the year and may be away when their key children are present.
- The requirement of the 1:3 ratio for under 2s, together with varying numbers of children, means that staff will be frequently moved to cover in rooms if the ratios are short because of fluctuating numbers of children, staff holidays, absences, or any other contingency.
- The long nursery day and the consequent shift system of staff means that the child's key worker may not be there for the whole time. This may be an issue for parents who would like to speak to the same carer at the beginning and end of the day.
- Although there are regional variations, staff turnover is generally high in the private nursery sector. This means that the baby may have to make a number of new attachments.

In principle, the key worker system is in place in the UK but in practice, because of some of the factors outlined above, it can fail to operate as intended.

Progress check

How has the introduction of the key worker system been influenced by attachment theory?

What are some of the advantages of the key worker system?

Why is it helpful to the child and to the parents if there is more than one child-care worker in each key group?

List some of the disadvantages of the key worker system.

How babies learn through everyday interactions with their carers

Research has shown that the first year of life is a crucial time for the development of the infant brain and that the quality of the environment and, in particular, the interactions babies have with their carers are critical in ensuring babies' progress. Those who care for babies need to consider how they are meeting these needs in the routines and experiences they provide (Murray, L. and Andrews, L. *The Social Baby: Understanding Babies' Communications from Birth*, The Children's Project: London, 2000).

INTERACTIONS WITH BABIES

Babies are naturally social and seek out contact with those around them. They are likely to receive this contact from adults and older children, not from other babies. They need carers who recognise and are responsive to these early attempts at communication. If there is no response, babies will give up and the impetus to communicate and opportunities to learn that this provides will be lost.

The following points are suggestions for ways to support early learning and communication:

- Provide a calm atmosphere that allows the baby to pick out familiar sounds and voices. This does not mean silence but acknowledges that baby cannot make sense of a very noisy environment.
- A key worker system ensures that the babies are handled by those who are familiar. The key worker will know the individual baby's likes and dislikes and will be able to use this to build from.
- Use care routines as opportunities for communication with babies. Physical care may take up much of the baby's wakeful time. Changing and washing are good opportunities for close contact and chatting with a baby. Babies respond

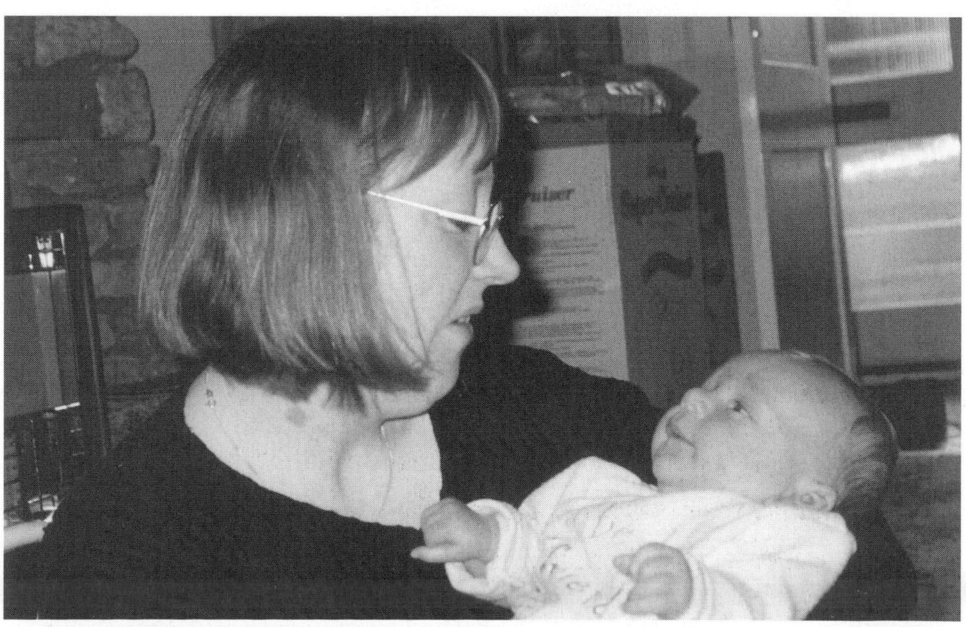

Communicating with baby

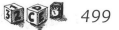

to the splash of the water and the feel of the cream on their skin. Time should be taken over these activities and a conveyor belt approach, where babies are whisked through the procedure as quickly as possible, should *never* be employed.

- Ensure that feeding is relaxed and pleasurable. Bottlefeeding should be a one-to-one experience and there should always be time for a cuddle. When babies are being weaned, the spoon should be offered at a pace that suits the baby, not the child-care worker. It will not be a pleasurable experience for anyone concerned if the child-care worker is spoonfeeding more than one baby at a time.
- Carers need to give babies their full attention. Babies thrive on this and will lose interest if the carer's attention is elsewhere.
- Take advantage of any opportunity to stimulate babies' curiosity about the world. Alert them to and talk to them about the birds perching on the fence, the rain gushing out of the drainpipe.
- When planning activities for babies, have realistic expectations about how they will respond and what they will get out of them. Handprinting on paper will be a meaningless task to an 8 month old. She will be far more interested in tasting the paint and smearing it all over her body.

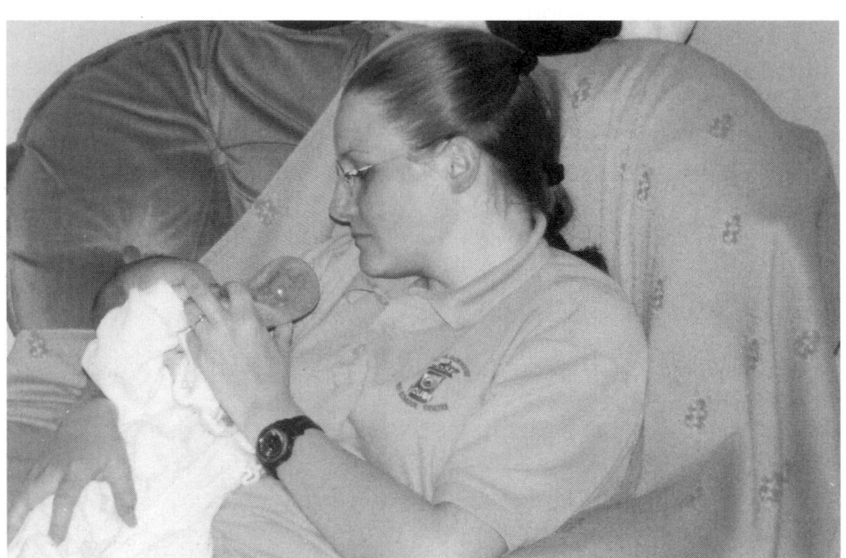

Feeding a baby should be a one-to-one experience

TIPS FOR TALKING WITH BABIES

> **key terms**
>
> **Motherease or parentease**
> term used by researchers to describe the enabling, focused language interaction, typically observed between mother and infant

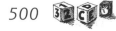

Babies love to communicate, but for those who have had no previous experience of working with babies, talking with babies can be daunting. Researchers use the term **motherease** (or **parentease**) to describe the close, enabling style of communication that encourages babies' early language development. But you don't have to be the parent to be 'tuned in' to the baby! Think about the following:

- Get close to the baby. Babies love faces and respond to smiles.
- Use short phrases and ordinary words, not baby talk.
- Consider the tone and modulation of your voice. Babies respond to a slightly higher pitch than usual and to expressive speech.

- Remember that you are talking *with*, not at the baby.
- Pause and listen so the baby can reply. This rhythm should reflect the pattern of normal conversation – babies don't appreciate monologues!
- Repetition of the same or similar phrases is helpful but don't overdo this.
- Follow the baby's lead and allow her to initiate the conversation. See what she's looking at or pointing to and respond.

Progress check

Why is it important to communicate with babies from the earliest stage?

How can care routines provide opportunities for worthwhile interaction between baby and carer?

What should child-care workers do to make mealtimes pleasurable for babies?

How can the child-care worker encourage curiosity in babies?

What are some of the features of motherease?

Now try these questions

What is the best way to establish positive relationships with parents?

How has attachment theory influenced the provision of day care in the UK?

What are the relative benefits of placing a baby in a day nursery, with a childminder or employing a nanny?

What are some of the key factors to remember when communicating with babies?

key terms

You need to know what the key terms and phrases in this chapter mean.
Go back through the chapter and find out.

Unit 8: Preparation for Employment

In this unit you will learn about the structure of a range of work settings and the role of the early years care and education worker within them. You will learn about how to prepare for employment in early years care and education and how to work as part of a team. This unit builds on Chapter 4 Professional Practice in the Support of a Positive Care and Education Environment.

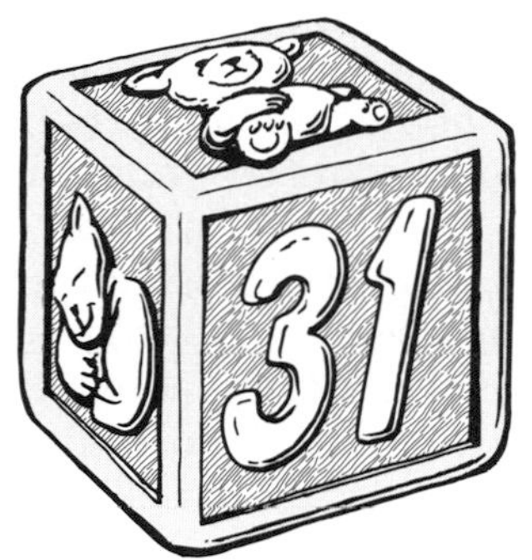

STRUCTURES OF ORGANISATION AND WORK SETTINGS AND THE JOB ROLE

This chapter will cover the following topics:

- *work settings and the job role*
- *structures of organisation and job role*
- *the responsibilities of a professional child-care worker*
- *how teams work*
- *preparing for employment.*

Work settings and the job role

key term

Statutory sector care establishments provided by the state

Patterns of employment change over time. Child-care workers now work in a wider range of settings than ever before. While some opportunities in the **statutory sector** remain static, or have declined, there are increasing opportunities within the private and **voluntary sectors**, both in establishments such as private day nurseries and in play facilities linked to leisure opportunities. Due to the expansion in tourism, many tour operators employ child-care workers abroad in holiday destinations.

key term

Voluntary sector
care establishments provided by voluntary organisations

key term

Inclusive
organised in a way that enables all to take a full and active part; meeting the needs of all children

key term

Multi-disciplinary
made up of different professionals

Disabled children are now more likely to be included in all settings. Consequently, there are more employment opportunities for child-care workers to support an **inclusive** approach to their care and education.

THE NATIONAL CHILD-CARE STRATEGY

The UK government is committed to enabling parents and carers to take up training and employment. The National Child-Care Strategy seeks to encourage the development of affordable, accessible child-care, including out-of-school care. This is likely to increase the opportunities for child-care workers. In addition the Early Years Development and Child-Care Partnerships and initiatives such as Sure Start provide opportunities for experienced child-care workers to be involved in developing a wide range of early years education and child-care services. These roles may involve working in innovative ways as part of a **multi-disciplinary** team.

NANNIES AND CHILDMINDERS

Opportunities for employment of nannies in private families continue to increase, both for residential and daily nannies. Many families choose childminders to care for their children but a decline in the number of registered childminders, particularly in some areas, limits this choice.

It is important that those working in isolation seek ways of accessing feedback on their practice, support and professional development. Discussion with others in a similar role can be supportive. There are a number of nannying networks and childminder networks developing in various parts of the UK. Opportunities for updating and further training should be considered.

Child protection

Working in isolation, just as in any child-care setting, you may become aware of possible child abuse. Without immediate recourse to colleagues it is vital to think out in advance how you would deal with any suspicion or disclosure, including how to refer to the appropriate agency, i.e. police, social services department or the NSPCC. You can contact the social services department for advice and guidance. Do not ignore or keep to yourself any disclosure or suspicion of possible child abuse.

Structures of organisation and job role

A work setting may be owned and managed by a statutory, voluntary or private organisation. This will influence its aims and objectives and the structure, including staff roles and line management.

AIMS AND OBJECTIVES

Each work setting is likely to have its own specified aims and objectives to influence and inform its practice. These, together with supporting policies and procedures, should be underpinned and influenced by the rights and needs of young children.

Policies, procedures, practices and guidelines

Within your workplace there are likely to be policies and procedures (codes of practice) concerning the following:

- equal opportunities – this means that no adult or child receives less favourable treatment on the grounds of their gender, race, colour, nationality,

ethnic or national origins, age, disability, religion, marital status or sexual orientation
- admissions
- financial arrangements
- premises and health and safety
- medical emergencies
- child protection
- health, nutrition and food service
- staff rights and responsibilities, qualifications, management, training and development
- ratio of staff to children
- record-keeping
- partnerships with parents
- liaison with other agencies
- emergency evacuation
- managing behaviour
- children with special educational needs
- off-site visits
- administration of legal drugs
- liaison with other professionals.

The responsibilities of a professional worker include familiarising yourself with the implications of these and understanding how they are influenced by statutory requirements.

Statutory requirements

Some policies and procedures result from statutory requirements (i.e. they are laid down in legislation). Aspects of the following legislation (laws) will have implications for policy and practice within all establishments:

- Children Act (1989)
- Education Act (1988)
- Education Reform Act (1993)
- Race Relations Act (1975)
- Sex Discrimination Acts (1975, 1986)
- Equal Pay Act (1970)
- Employment Protection Act (1978)
- Disabled Person's Act (1986)
- Offices, Shops and Railway Premises Act (1963)
- Health and Safety at Work Act (1974)
- Food Safety Act (1990)
- Food Hygiene Regulation (1970)
- Food Hygiene Amendment Regulation (1990).

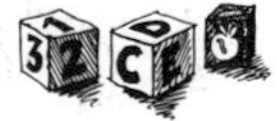

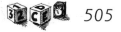

In addition, settings may have internal quality assurance systems to ensure policies and procedures are in place and adhered to, and to encourage continuous improvement in practice. These may be tied in to the external inspection of child-care settings put in place in September 2001 by the Office for Standards in Education (OFSTED).

Progress check

Why are there now increased employment opportunities for child-care workers?

What areas can policies and procedures cover?

What determines and governs statutory requirements?

The responsibilities of a professional child-care worker

Policies can increase awareness, but will not, in themselves, change attitudes or practice. Good practice will depend on staff commitment to the needs and rights of children, and to their ability and willingness to carry out their duties in a professional way. The responsibilities of a professional child-care worker include understanding and putting the following into practice:

- confidentiality
- responsibility
- reliability
- accountability
- planning and reviewing
- working in partnership with parents/carers
- commitment to equal opportunities and anti-discriminatory practice.

These aspects are all covered in detail throughout this book, particularly in Chapter 4.

PERSONAL DEVELOPMENT AND FURTHER TRAINING

As a professional child-care worker, you will want to receive further training, and be open to suggestions for changing your methods of working. You should find that your self-awareness increases through the supervision you receive from experienced workers. In-service staff development and further training will also help to keep you up-to-date with new developments and improve your working practice.

How teams work

WHAT MAKES A TEAM EFFECTIVE?

Effective teams will have the following:

- clearly defined aims and objectives (clarified and redefined regularly) that all members can put into words and agree to put into practice

key term

Prescribed roles duties laid down by others

- flexible roles that enable individuals to work to their strengths, rather than in **prescribed roles** where they must conform to pre-determined or stereotyped expectations (for example, the teacher always does story time, the child-care worker always clears up)
- effective team leaders who manage the work of the team, encourage and value individual contributions and deal with conflict
- members who are committed to:
  - developing self-awareness
  - building, maintaining and sustaining good working relationships
  - demonstrating effective communication skills, expressing their views assertively rather than aggressively
  - understanding and recognising their contribution to the way the group works
  - carrying out team decisions, irrespective of their personal feelings
  - accepting responsibility for the outcome of team decisions.

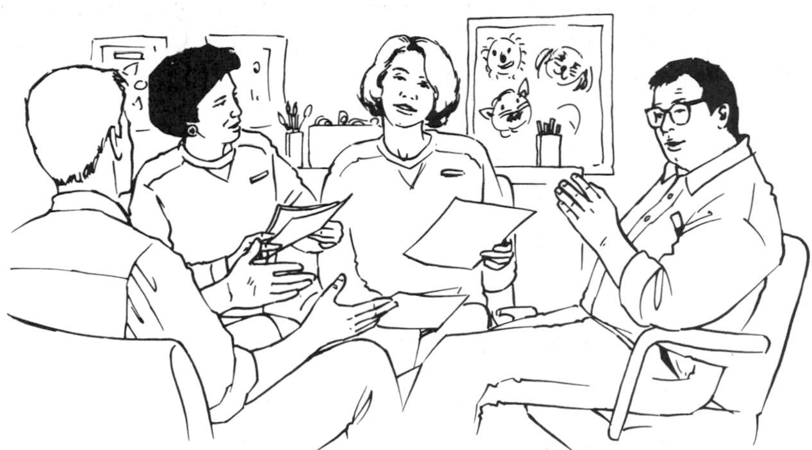

In the workplace, child-care workers usually work with colleagues as part of a team

STRESS AND CONFLICT WITHIN TEAMS

Within any team there is likely to be conflict. It is important to deal with this constructively rather than try to ignore it. The following guidelines for behaviour are likely to encourage the resolution of conflict:

- Join with the other person so that you can both 'win': people in a conflict often tend to be against rather than with each other. Keep a clear picture of the person and yourself, separate from the issue. The issue causing the conflict may be lost by the strength of bad feeling against the other person. You need to be committed to working towards an outcome that is acceptable to both parties.
- Make clear 'I' statements: take responsibility for yourself and avoid blaming the other person for how you feel and what you think.
- Be clear and specific about your view of the conflict and what you want, and listen to the other person's view.

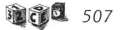

- Deal with one issue at a time: avoid confusing one issue with another and using examples from the past to illustrate your point. Using the past or only telling part of the story to make your own point can lead to a biased version of what happened. The other person is likely to have forgotten or may remember the incident very differently.
- Look at and listen to each other: deal directly with the difficulty.
- Ensure that you understand each other: if you are unclear about the issue, ask open questions and paraphrase back what you think you hear.
- Pool your ideas for creative ways of sorting out the conflict: make a list of all the possible solutions and go through them together.
- Choose a mutually convenient time and place: it is useful to agree on the amount of time you will spend.
- Acknowledge and appreciate one another: think of the other person's attributes separately from the conflict issue, and acknowledge and appreciate them.

PARTICIPATION IN TEAM MEETINGS AND GROUPS

Within the work setting there will be many groups meeting formally and informally: staff team meetings, groups of parents/carers, children and other professionals. Groups can be very effective at stimulating new ideas, managing projects, making decisions, monitoring and reviewing progress, and supporting group members. However, they can also be unproductive. It can help group members to consider their behaviour and the characteristics that may enhance or detract from the aims of the team.

Behaviour and characteristics of team members

Positive behaviour:

- *initiating* – getting and keeping things going
- *informing* – volunteering information, ideas, facts, feelings, views or opinions
- *clarifying, summarising or paraphrasing* – helping the group to sort things out, bring things together or round things off
- *confronting* – an important function if groups are to be effective, but requiring some skill and concern for the feelings of others
- *harmonising* – working to reconcile disagreements, to relieve tension, and helping to explore differences
- *encouraging*
- *compromising* – admitting an error or modifying a view or position
- *time-keeping* – ensuring the group keeps to time.

Negative behaviour:

- *aggressive* – attacking others, belittling their contribution or putting them down
- *blocking* – preventing the group from getting on with the task
- *dominating* – interrupting, asserting authority or interfering with the rights of others to participate
- *avoiding* – preventing the group from facing issues
- *withdrawing* – displaying a lack of involvement.

Progress check

What do the following need to do in order to facilitate effective teamwork:
(a) the team collectively? (b) members individually? (c) the leader?

What do team members need to be committed to in order to function effectively?

In dealing with conflict, what is the desirable outcome?

Preparing for employment

The same considerations apply to seeking and obtaining work with young children as for any other profession. Child-care workers need to avoid sentimentality and glamorising the role.

FIND OUT WHAT IS AVAILABLE

Employment opportunities may be advertised in magazines, journals, local newspapers or national newspapers, in the Job Centre or in some areas by the local authority in a job sheet. Alternatively, employment may be sought through an agency.

Remember to use all channels open to you to find out about possible employment opportunities. Your family and friends and the staff and students where you have undertaken training are all useful contacts.

CONDITIONS OF EMPLOYMENT

One of the most crucial aspects of obtaining and retaining employment is ensuring clarity of expectation on the part of the employer and the job seeker. Employment by a statutory, private or voluntary organisation is likely to be covered by a job description and conditions of service outlining the role and responsibilities of the child-care and education worker. A person specification may have been drawn up to indicate the requirements of the employer, the qualifications, experience, skills, knowledge and attitude required in any applicant. However, this is less likely to be the case when seeking employment as a nanny in a private family.

APPLYING FOR EMPLOYMENT

The information that follows is necessarily brief and in summary form. If possible, seek expert help with the process of applying for employment. At each stage in the process you will need to make the most of yourself, your qualifications, experience, skills and knowledge, if you are to move successfully to the next stage and ultimately obtain employment.

Preparing an accurate and representative curriculum vitae (CV)

The following guidance (from *A Practical Guide to Child-care Employment* by Christine Hobart and Jill Frankel, Stanley Thornes, 2000), outlines the main points:

- The CV should be typed (or word processed) tidily on white A4 paper.
- Some people think an imaginative and unusual presentation will have more impact. It may, but it could put as many people off as it interests. Ask friends, colleagues or tutors for their response.
- Spelling and grammar must be correct (have it checked).

- Keep it brief. It should be no more than two pages long.
- Avoid solid blocks of script.
- Use space to emphasise points and make sections stand out.
- Get a tutor or friend to check it for any ambiguity. It may be clear to you but muddled to an outsider.
- Update it regularly.

Your basic CV should include:

- personal details
- education and qualifications
- work experience and career history
- personal interests and hobbies
- other relevant details.

Completing an application form

You may be required to complete an application form instead of sending a CV. Read any information sent with it thoroughly. Ensure it is completed neatly and clearly. All questions should be answered honestly. Use your CV as a guide.

Covering letter

Use the information sent by the prospective employer to guide you. Again, ensure it is neat and legible, brief and to the point.

Statement of suitability for the post

This may be requested separately. Try to draw out points from your CV to match the job description.

INTERVIEW TECHNIQUES

Preparation and practice for interview are vital. Prepare by learning about the specific post and about interviews in general. This can be achieved through reading text, accessing Information and Learning Technologies, and through training programmes. Practise your communication skills in formal and informal settings. Undertake a mock interview with feedback from the interviewers. The following questions give a general idea of what might be asked at interview, but you will need to think through what an employer might want to know about you and why:

- Why do you want this job?
- What are you strengths and weaknesses?
- Describe how you have worked as part of a team.
- How would you encourage positive relationships with parents?
- What are the most important considerations in working with young children?
- How would you promote equality of opportunity and anti-discriminatory practice?
- If you were appointed, what would your training and development needs be?
- What questions would you like to ask us?

Finding out about the post

As well as a potential employer finding out about you, you will need to check out that you actually want the employment offered. You will obviously need to consider the terms and conditions, but you should also ensure that you are in agreement with the aims and objectives of the setting. You should also seek to find out the style of management that you would have to work with. Is the service run on democratic lines where decisions are made by the team? Are all the decisions made by managers without the team being consulted? Is there strong direction evident or does there appear to be a lack of leadership? If you do not know the setting, read any information sent to you and request a pre-visit.

Case study . . .

. . . Helen's first job

Helen was delighted to be the first student in her group to get a job. She had seen an advertisement in the local paper. It sounded great – own room with *en-suite* and use of a car. She had to share a room at home and couldn't wait to leave. The children's parents seemed really nice. They were too embarrassed to talk about money and hours, but she thought they would sort all that out when she started.

Helen came back to visit her tutor at college 6 months later. When her tutor asked how she was getting on, Helen said she had left. She explained that while the eldest child was at nursery, they had expected her to do more and more housework. They were so busy themselves that she couldn't say no. All that training to do the housework!

Then they expected her to babysit without any notice and told her to take time off in the day, when it suited them. She ended up doing split shifts and could never plan anything. The home was in the middle of nowhere and the last bus back was at 7p.m.!

The money was OK, but she never got chance to go out and spend any of it! She was really lonely. The parents did their best, but they were a lot older than her. She said she actually enjoyed sharing a room when she finally came home.

She got really attached to the children though and, when she said she wanted to leave, she felt really guilty for leaving them. The family offered her more money to stay, but it wasn't the money that was the problem. She wanted to make a clean break and finally just packed her bags and left without warning the parents. She felt she could never go back now even to visit and didn't think they would give her a reference.

How could this situation have been avoided?

What should Helen have clarified and asked for, before accepting the job?

What was wrong with the job as far as Helen was concerned?

How will the family feel now? What may the children have thought and felt?

Draw up a job description and a contract for this post.

CONDITIONS OF EMPLOYMENT

Contracts of employment

The Employment Protection Acts require that all employees who work for more than 16 hours a week have a contract of employment – a document stating their terms and conditions of employment.

Rights and responsibilities

Once employed, both you and your employer will have entitlements and responsibilities laid down in employment law. You will need to consider your responsibility for paying income tax and National Insurance contributions. You may also want to contribute towards a retirement pension.

THE ROLE OF TRADE UNIONS AND PROFESSIONAL ASSOCIATIONS

You may wish to consider joining a union and/or a professional association. You will need to research and be clear about the role of each and what membership entails.

Trade unions and professional associations may offer the following to their members:

- access to legal protection
- negotiation of pay and conditions
- inexpensive insurance cover
- collective efforts to improve working conditions
- protection of its members through health and safety practices, pension and entitlements issues.

Progress check

Where may employment opportunities be advertised?

What does a person specification indicate?

What should be included in a basic CV?

How can you prepare for an interview?

What will you need to know about the post you are applying for?

What should be included in a contract of employment?

What are the advantages of belonging to a trade union/professional association?

Now try these questions

In practice, how can child-care settings encourage partnership with parents?

Describe and explain six aspects of professional practice.

What are the needs and rights of young children?

Explain the advantages of working with colleagues in a team.

How can staff deal with conflict in the workplace?

Describe the behaviours and characteristics that make groups effective.

key terms

You need to know what the key terms and phrases in this chapter mean. Go back through the chapter and find out.

Unit 9: *The Provision of Services and the Protection of Children*

This unit is designed to give you an overview of the area of legal and social relationships as they affect the family. It will also give you an understanding of how to protect children from the possibility of abuse, and how to support children who have been abused.

The way that society works has an important effect on how child care and education workers do their jobs. They need to understand the structure of the family lives of the children they work with. They also need to understand the provision of services and the legal framework for England, Wales and Northern Ireland as they affect the lives of children and their families.

On successful completion of this unit you should understand the structure of family life; the sources of disadvantage in society; the policies and legislation that affects the provision of services for children and their families. You should be able to identify signs of abuse; understand the principles of protecting children from abuse; identify the procedures that follow suspicion or disclosure of abuse; identify ways of supporting children and families. You should be able to understand the role of the child care and education worker.

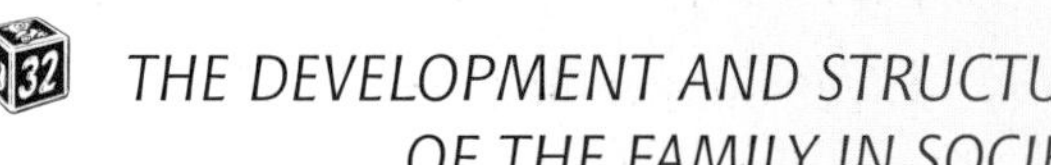
32 THE DEVELOPMENT AND STRUCTURE OF THE FAMILY IN SOCIETY

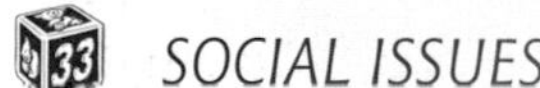
33 SOCIAL ISSUES

34 THE ROLE OF THE STATUTORY, VOLUNTARY AND INDEPENDENT SERVICES

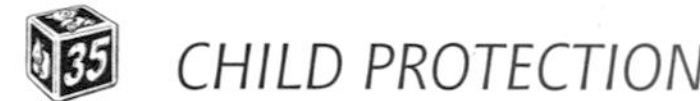
35 CHILD PROTECTION

36 FORMS OF ABUSE AND THE EFFECTS OF ABUSE

37 CHILD PROTECTION PROCEDURES

38 CHILD PROTECTION: RESPONDING TO CHILD ABUSE

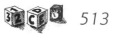

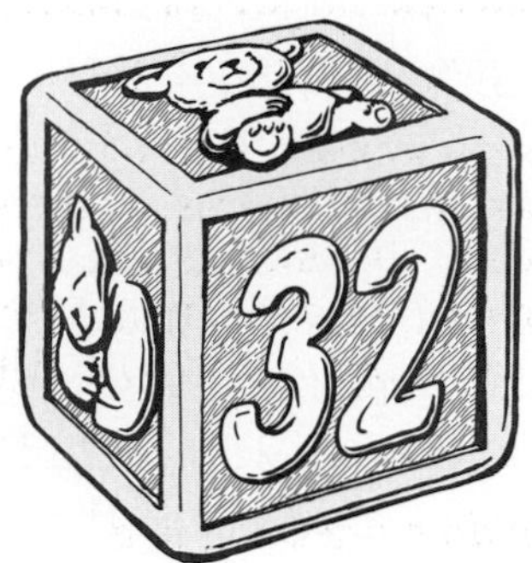

THE DEVELOPMENT AND STRUCTURE OF THE FAMILY IN SOCIETY

Children are totally dependent at birth. In order to survive and develop during this period of dependency they need care, security, protection, stimulation and social contact. In most societies and at most times during history children have been nurtured and cared for within their families. The family is therefore of the greatest significance to children's development. There are many different definitions of what constitutes a 'family'. Families of different types have many functions in common, but there are many differences in their structures and the way that they carry out their tasks.

This chapter will cover the following topics:

- *the diverse range of family structures*
- *the structure of the family*
- *family life, care and protection: the alternatives*
- *changing patterns of family life and roles*
- *legislation relating to children and their families*
- *legislation relating to child care in the UK*
- *working with children and their families.*

The diverse range of family structures

WHAT IS A FAMILY?

It is surprisingly difficult to define what a family is, but it can be said that:

- all families have things in common
- all families are different.

One all-purpose definition is: 'a group of related people who support each other in a variety of ways, emotionally, socially and/or economically'.

 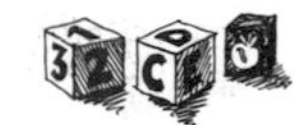

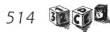

Case study . . .

. . . different families

In a busy nursery class the teacher is aware of the personal details of some the children who attend. Anna lives with her grandmother, her mother is dead and her father is unknown. Royston and his half-sister live with his mother, who is a lone primary carer. Jamil lives with his grandparents, parents, uncle, aunt and cousins. Jasmin lives with her mother and her mother's female partner. Tom lives with his father, his father's new partner and her older daughter.

1. *According to the definition above, which of these children are living in a 'family'?*
2. *Are there any reasons that some people might say that any of these children are not living in a family?*

WHY STUDY THE FAMILY?

Family life in some form is basic to the experience of most children. The family has a strong influence on every aspect of a child's life and development. For this reason, child-care workers need to:

- understand the importance of the family to children's development
- know the particular family background of the children in their care
- understand the possible influences and effects of different family circumstances on children.

> **key term**
>
> **Function of the family**
> the things the family does for its members

THE FUNCTIONS OF THE FAMILY AND THE SIMILARITIES BETWEEN FAMILIES

The **functions of the family** are the things the family does for its members. Families all perform similar functions to a lesser or greater extent. These functions are:

- socialisation
- practical care and protection
- emotional and social support
- economic support.

Families do however have different traditions, customs and ways of carrying out these functions.

> **key terms**
>
> **Culture**
> the way of life, the language and the behaviour that is acceptable and appropriate to the society in which a person lives
>
> **Values**
> beliefs that certain things are important and to be valued, for example a person's right to their own belongings
>
> **Norm**
> developmental skill achieved within an average time-scale

Socialisation

Families provide the basic and most important environment where children learn the **culture** of the society of which they are a part. The family consciously and unconsciously teaches children the main aspects of any culture. These are shared **values**, **norms** and a language.

The peer group, schools and the media have a strong influence as children grow older, but children learn the foundations of culture within the family.

Practical care and protection

The family is very effective in providing practical day-to-day care for its dependent members – children, those who are sick or have disabling conditions and those who are old. Caring for people outside the family is much more expensive, and often less effective.

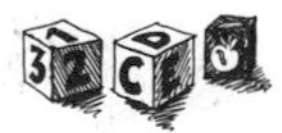

Emotional and social support

Families perform a very important role. They give a baby a name and initial position in society. (When we hear of an abandoned baby, we immediately wonder who the child is and where the child comes from.) The family gives a child an identity, a sense of belonging and a feeling of being valued.

A child's family is able to provide a positive feeling of worth that is fundamental (basic and very important) to healthy emotional development. It meets the basic need for love and affection, company and security. In a busy and crowded life, people are less likely to find this support outside their family where contacts are more impersonal. Foster care, or adoption (that is, a substitute family), is now the usual provision in the UK for children who lose their families. This is because the experience of family life is regarded as very important for emotional and social well-being.

Economic support

The extent of economic support that families provide varies between cultures. The family is still an economic unit in many ways. However, in the UK and other European countries, family members are no longer totally dependent on each other for survival. The state now provides an economic safety net, through for example social security benefits, which prevents the starvation and destitution that people experienced in the past when they were dependent on their families.

Progress check

What is a value and what is a norm?

What are the main functions of the family?

The structure of the family

Although there are many similarities between families, there are many variations in their structure and size. These differences can significantly affect the way families carry out their functions and, therefore, the lives of children.

key terms

Nuclear family
a family grouping where parents live with their children and form a small group with no other family members living near them

Family of origin
the family a child is born into

THE NUCLEAR FAMILY WITH TWO PARENTS

The **nuclear family** is a family grouping where parents live with their children and form a small group. They have no other relatives living with them or close by. This type of family has become increasingly common in modern societies like the UK, where many people move for work or education and leave their **family of origin** (that is, the one a person is born into).

In countries where there is an agricultural economy and people work on the land, they are much more likely to remain near their family of origin.

Social and cultural variations in nuclear families

Nuclear families are more common in higher **socio-economic groups**, that is, among those employed in managerial, administrative and professional jobs (such as business managers, teachers or lawyers). These families are more likely to move around geographically in order to obtain education and employment. The fact

key term

Socio-economic group
grouping of people according to their status in society, based on their occupation, which is closely related to their wealth/income; another way of referring to someone's social class

that they may then earn higher incomes make it both possible and worth doing. In some nuclear families, parents have developed a system of sharing family responsibilities. This is called a *democratic system*, because each partner shares earning money, child care and domestic jobs.

Life in a nuclear family

Children who grow up in a small nuclear family may:

- experience close relationships within the family
- receive a lot of individual attention
- have more space and privacy.

They may, however:

- feel a sense of isolation
- experience intensity of attention from parents
- have fewer people to turn to at times of stress
- suffer if their parents have no support system to care for them at times of illness or need.

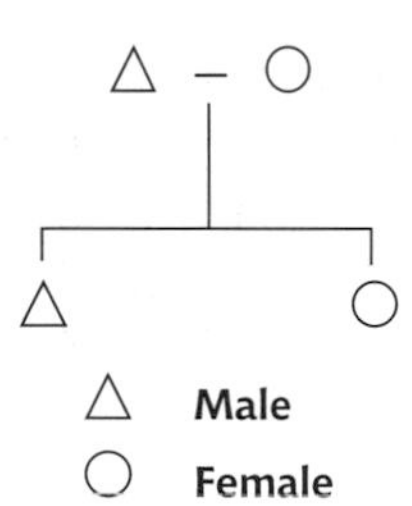

An example of a nuclear family

THE NUCLEAR FAMILY WITH A LONE PRIMARY CARER

The terms 'one-parent family' or 'lone-parent family' are also used to describe families with dependent children that are headed by a lone primary carer; of these, roughly 10 per cent are headed by men and 90 per cent by women. Of the women, about 60 per cent are divorced or separated, 23 per cent are single and 7 per cent widowed.

Social and cultural variations in one-parent families

An increasing number of children in the UK (one in every eight) are born to women who are not married. The incomes of most lone parents are lower than those of most two-parent families. Many receive state benefits and their lifestyle is affected, as there is little spare money for luxuries. Both lone parents and their children are also vulnerable at times of difficulty, such as illness, if they do not have an extended family (see below) nearby to support them. The publicity given to the Child Support Agency has focused attention on the government's attempts to make fathers more financially responsible for their families following separation.

Only a small minority of lone parents are well off economically and receive incomes that enable them to work and to afford day care for their younger children. Most lone mothers are less likely to work, than those who have partners. However, the government now has a clear policy to support them with their child-care costs, and to encourage them not to be dependent on welfare benefits. Most lone parents are divorced or separated; a smaller number are single parents. A high proportion is in the lower socio-economic groups.

key term

Matriarchal family
a family in which women are important and dominant

Although there are many married couples in the African-Caribbean community, there is also a tradition of single parenthood. This was one of the outcomes of slavery in the Caribbean, where the nurturing of children by their fathers was forbidden. Subsequent high unemployment rates, both in the West Indies and in the UK, have perpetuated this tradition of low involvement by some fathers. Many African-Caribbean families, therefore, tend to be **matriarchal**, where women are important and dominant.

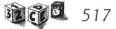

Life in a one-parent family

Children who grow up in a one-parent family:

- may establish a close, mutually supportive relationship with the parent they live with
- may maintain a close relationship with their other parent and his or her family.

However, they may:

- have experienced a period of grief and loss when their parents separated
- lose contact with their other parent
- experience lower material standards than children in a two-parent family
- have less adult attention at times when their parent is coping with practical and emotional difficulties.

> **key term**
> **Extended family** a family grouping that includes other family members who live either together or very close to each other and are in frequent contact with each other

THE EXTENDED FAMILY

An **extended family** extends beyond parent(s) and children to include other family members, for example grandparents, uncles and aunts. A family is usually referred to as extended when its members:

- live either together or very close to each other
- are in frequent contact with each other.

Many people who live at a distance from their relatives gain a great deal of emotional support from them, but distance makes the practical support offered by a close extended family difficult. When an extended family includes only two generations of relatives such as uncles, aunts and cousins, it is referred to as a *joint family*.

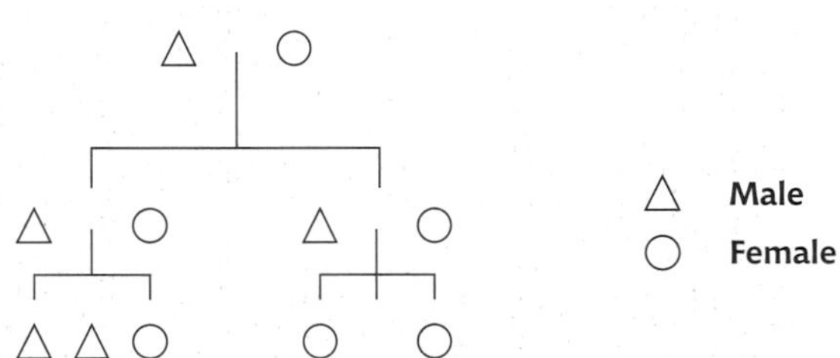

An example of an extended family

Social and cultural variations in extended families

People in lower socio-economic groups involved in semi-skilled or manual jobs are less likely to move from their locality for work or education. This means that they are more likely to be part of a long-established extended family system. This is evident in white, working-class families, where there is a tradition of women staying close to their mothers and a matriarchal system is common. Roles within the family are likely to be divided, with men traditionally the breadwinners and women in charge domestically, although they may also work part or full time outside the home.

Families who came originally from India, Pakistan and Bangladesh have maintained a tradition of living in close extended families. Many came from rural areas where this was traditional. Their cultural and religious background also

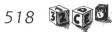

key term

Patriarchal family
a family in which men are dominant and make the important decisions

places a strong emphasis on the duty and responsibility to care for all generations of the family. These extended families are usually **patriarchal**, where men are dominant and make the important decisions. On marriage, a woman becomes a part of her husband's family and usually lives with or near them.

Families whose origins are in Mediterranean countries, such as Cyprus and Italy, also tend to have a strong extended family tradition. Family members frequently meet together for celebrations. Daughters tend to stay close to their mothers on marriage, but the man has considerable authority in the family.

Life in an extended family

Children who experience life within an extended family:

- have the opportunity to develop and experience a wide variety of caring relationships
- are surrounded by a network of practical and emotional support.

However, they may:

- have little personal space or privacy
- feel they are being observed by and have to please a large number of people
- have less opportunity to use individual initiative and action.

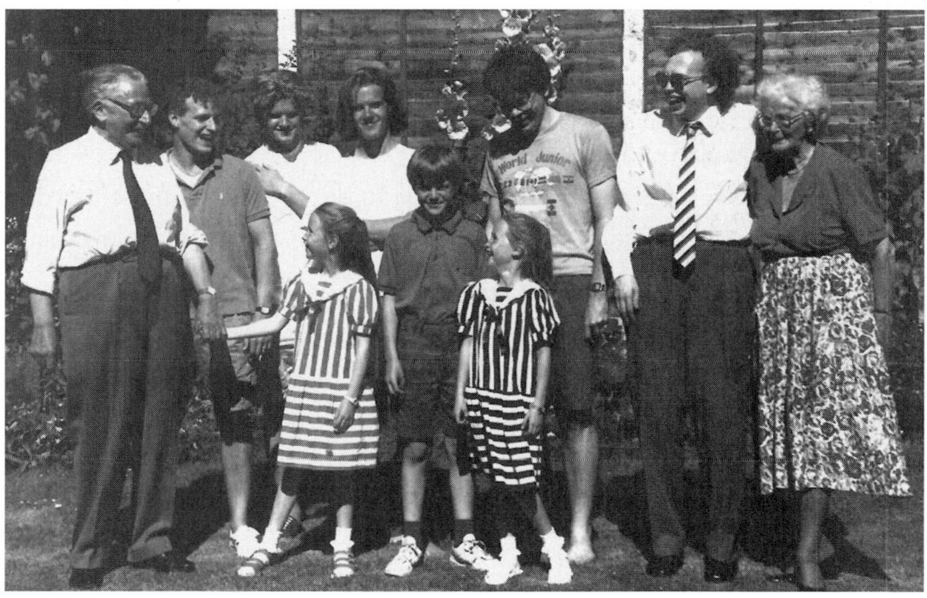

An extended family enables children to develop a variety of caring relationships

key term

Reconstructed family
a family containing adults and children who have previously been part of a different family

THE RECONSTRUCTED FAMILY

The **reconstructed family**, or reorganised family, is an increasingly common family system, since an increasing number of parents divorce and remarry. A reconstituted family contains adults and children who have previously been part of a different family. The children of the original partnership usually live with one parent and become the stepchildren of the new partner and stepsiblings of the new partner's children. Children born to the new partnership are half-siblings. Such families vary in their size and structure, and may be quite complicated!

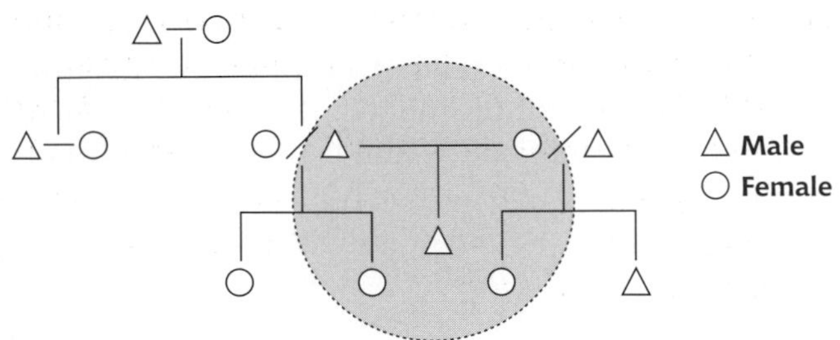

An example of a reconstructed family

Social and cultural variations in reconstructed families

Reconstructed families are more common among people who accept divorce. This could include people who have no religious beliefs, and Protestant Christians. Muslims do not forbid divorce, but are committed to family life and divorce is less common.

Reconstructed families are less common among people who have a strong belief in the family and who disapprove of divorce, usually because their religious doctrines are against it. These include Hindus, Sikhs and Roman Catholics to whom marriage is sacred and should not be dissolved.

Life in a reconstructed family

This can be a positive experience for a child because:

- their parent may be happier, more secure and have greater financial resources
- the child gains a parent and possibly an extended family.

However, they may:

- have difficulty relating to a step-parent and stepbrothers and sisters
- have to compete for attention with children of their own age
- feel a loss of attention because they have to share their parent
- have to accept the birth of children of their parent's new relationship.

Progress check

What is a nuclear family?

What is an extended family?

What is a reconstructed family?

Why are there an increasing number of reconstructed families?

PARTNERSHIP ARRANGEMENTS

Adults have a wide variety of arrangements for the way they form partnerships. These provide different care environments for children.

Partnership arrangements include the following:

- *Monogamy* – the marriage between heterosexual partners (one partner of each gender); this is still popular in the UK, although the rate of marriage has declined since the 1960s.

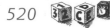

- *Polygamy* – the marriage of a person of one gender (usually a man) to a number of others (usually women) at the same time; it is illegal to enter into this arrangement in the UK, where it is called *bigamy*. It has been very common in other countries, especially those with Muslim cultures.
- *Serial monogamy* – a term used to describe one person of either gender having one partner followed by another over a period of time, each followed by separation or divorce.
- *Cohabitation* – partners live together without the legal tie of marriage; this is increasingly common in the UK, where about 30 per cent of partners cohabit.
- *Homosexual partnerships* – especially between women, are increasingly viewed as an acceptable base for the rearing of children. As recently as the early 1980s, women who left their husbands to live with a woman often lost the custody of their children; such an arrangement was thought unsuitable. In June 1994, two women from Manchester became the first lesbian couple to be made the joint legal parents of the child of one of them. This was made possible by the Children Act 1989 because it enables parental responsibility to be shared by a range of people. All the research carried out since the 1960s shows no differences in the social and emotional development of children of lesbian and heterosexual partnerships, or to their gender orientation.

Case study . . .

. . . family life

Mr and Mrs Jameson were married 26 years ago. They have three children, Sylvia, Roy and Belinda. Sylvia divorced her husband and now lives with her new partner in a house in the same road as her parents and sees them frequently. She has two daughters and he has a son, all of whom live with her. Sylvia's ex-husband has remarried and now has a baby son. Roy is also married, to a woman who has a child but was never married; they have one son, but live many miles away. Belinda lives locally with her female partner and their two daughters, each from previous relationships that have ended in divorce.

1. *Which family members are monogamously married?*
2. *How many of their original marriages ended in divorce?*
3. *Which people are living as part of an extended family?*
4. *Are any people in this case study not living in a family?*
5. *Draw a family tree and try to include all these people!*

Family life, care and protection: the alternatives

The family, both in the past and present, is by far the most common environment for bringing up children, both in the UK and in other countries. The family is probably the most common arrangement for child care because it the most practical way to meet both children's and parents' needs. However, there are circumstances and places where alternatives to family life have been either necessary or thought to be preferable.

THE MOST SIGNIFICANT ALTERNATIVES TO FAMILY LIFE

These are children's homes, communes and kibbutzim.

Children's homes

Large children's homes, sometimes called orphanages, existed in the past in the UK. Children whose parents were either dead or unable to care for them were cared for in large groups. This type of institutional children's home is no longer provided for this purpose in the UK. Where there is a need, children are mainly cared for in foster homes or small residential units. Some large children's homes have been redesigned to provide respite care (now known as 'short-term breaks') in small units for children with special needs. Large institutions do, however, still exist in some parts of Europe, especially in some former communist countries, where, as formerly happened in the UK, some children of very poor parents, children with disabilities and orphans are left in state care.

Communes

Occasionally people live together in communes. Adults share tasks and bring up their children collectively. This arrangement was popular among a small minority of people in the 1960s and 1970s in the US and the UK.

Kibbutzim

Some people in Israel live on kibbutzim. A kibbutz is a place where people live and work together for the economic benefit of the whole community. Children are cared for together, in units separate from their parents, leaving parents free to use their time and energy for work. This system still exists but the separation of children and parents is now often modified.

Progress check

Why is the family the most common environment for child care?

What are the main reasons that children have been and still are cared for in institutions?

Where do large institutions still exist?

What is a kibbutz?

Changing patterns of family life and roles

FAMILY SIZE AND FAMILY ROLES

The average number of dependent children per family in the UK is now a little less than two children This has gradually fallen since the middle of the 19th century when it was about six children. The most significant reasons for this change are:

- the increased availability of contraception and legal abortion
- a rise in the standard of living, together with the fact that children are costly to support and they start work later than in the past
- changes in women's roles, attitudes and expectations; many women regard child-rearing as only a *part* of their lives and want to do other things as well.

Although the average family has two children, there are of course larger families. Children from large families have some differences in their life experiences. Research shows that on average their life chances are not as good as children from small families.

Many children grow up in families where they are the only child. These children are more successful, but there are possible social disadvantages for them.

CHANGING GENDER ROLES WITHIN THE FAMILY

There is evidence that, in families across a range of social and cultural groups in the UK, the traditional role of male as 'provider and breadwinner', and female as 'carer and homemaker' have changed. Men are increasingly involved in the care of their young children, and women are more likely to work outside the home. Research shows, however, that women still have the major responsibility for either doing or organising domestic work, whatever their social or cultural background.

Women and employment

Nearly half the workforce in the UK is female. Although an increasing number of women with dependent children work outside the home, the younger their children are, the less likely they are to work either full-time or part-time. The growth of affordable child-care provision for young children is leading to an ever-increasing number of working mothers, and the government is encouraging this trend by supporting the expansion of child care. In some European countries, there is a much higher level of provision and a much higher proportion of mothers working outside the home.

Working parents

When both parents of young children work outside the home, they have to make arrangements for the care of their children. An increasing choice of day care alternatives is now available partly as a response to this demand and also in response to government initiatives. Research shows that children's needs can be met satisfactorily if they are provided with good day care.

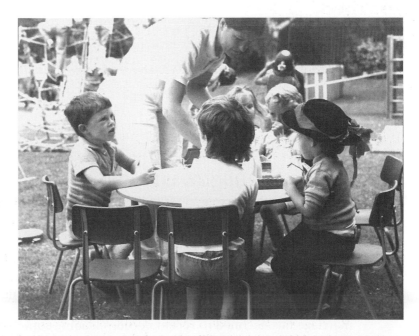

Children's needs can be met satisfactorily if they are provided with good day care

Case study . . .

. . . changing family roles

Wendy is married to John and they have a baby, Chloe, who is 9 months old. Chloe has attended a day nursery for five days a week since she was 6 months old, when her mother returned to work full-time as a pharmacist. Wendy and John share all household tasks, including looking after Chloe, shopping and cooking. John's mother, Mary, sometimes visits and helps them out, but she has worked full-time for the past 10 years so gets little spare time even for her own household tasks, though she does have a cleaner. She is a little concerned about her son and daughter-in-law's lifestyle, and often reminds them of how different things were when they were children. Wendy gets a bit annoyed when Mary reminds them of how she gave up work when her children were young and only returned part-time when they went to school. Wendy's grandfather, however, expresses very strong feelings about his granddaughter's lifestyle. He remembers the time when his wife gave up work and became a housewife as soon as they were married. When Wendy, in her annoyance, once said to him 'What for?', he replied 'To look after me, that's what for. I went out early and she needed to be there to cook my breakfast'. Wendy decided not to respond to this, as it was so different to her own experiences!

1. *What are the major changes in child-care practice that can be seen over these three generations?*
2. *How do these three generations reveal the changing role of women and paid work?*
3. *What changes can you see in men's and women's domestic roles?*
4. *Why do you think Wendy decided not to respond to her grandfather's statement?*

Progress check

What is the average number of dependent children per family in the UK?

What are the most significant reasons for the reduction in family size?

Why do an increasing number of mothers work?

Legislation relating to children and their families

MARRIAGE

Marriage is a legal contract between two people. It places on partners certain duties to behave reasonably and to support each other. It also gives certain rights to both partners, including the right to live in the marital home and to have equal parental responsibility for their children. The majority of people in the UK still marry but there are signs that marriage is gradually declining in popularity. The rate of marriage has declined in recent decades leading some people to predict that in the 21st century marriage could become a minority experience.

COHABITATION

Cohabitation (common law partnerships) is the arrangement between partners who live together without the legal tie of marriage; this is increasingly common in the UK, where about 30 per cent of partners cohabit; although many later marry their partner, especially after they have children. This arrangement is now acceptable among many social groups who would have previously seen it as a disgrace. Not all European countries have as high a cohabitation rate as the UK; those with a strong Roman Catholic religious tradition such as Ireland, Spain and Italy still have high marriage rates. Families of Asian origin also tend to have a high marriage rate and low cohabitation rate.

FAMILY BREAKDOWN: SEPARATION AND DIVORCE

The rate of divorce and separation has continued to rise in the UK since the dramatic increase began at the beginning of the 1970s following new divorce legislation. If current trends continue, around 40 per cent of marriages being presently formed will end in divorce. Britain and Denmark have the highest rates in Europe, but these are lower than the US.

It is not often appreciated that the law does not protect women who cohabit, or 'common law wives' as they can be referred to, in the same way as if they were married; on separation the courts do not have the power to redistribute the wealth of the man to her, however good a 'wife' she has been. A woman who has given up a career to have children and care for them, has no claim on the man for herself. The children will always have a claim for child support against their father and in certain circumstances can claim capital to provide for their housing while they are dependent. While this may help the mother provide a home for the children when they are young, it leaves her homeless when they become independent. A woman could be financially vulnerable in the event that the relationship breaks down, particularly so, if she has children and stops work to look after children.

Grounds for divorce

The sole grounds for divorce following the Divorce Reform Act 1969 is the 'irretrievable breakdown' of a marriage. The evidence that can be used to prove breakdown is:

- adultery
- unreasonable behaviour
- desertion for 2 years
- partners living separately for 2 years and each agreeing to a divorce
- partners living separately for 5 years.

In 2001, attempts to change the law and introduce 'no fault divorces' that could be settled in 3 months by agreement, were not successful.

Children usually experience the breakdown of the partnership between parents as stressful, whether their parents are legally married or not. Children can feel a deep sense of loss, and even blame themselves.

An unmarried father has no legal rights over his children following separation, unless he has acquired parental responsibility.

Children and divorce – the Children Act 1989

When a partnership breaks down there can be disagreements between parents about where a child should live and how often each parent should see the child. In such a dispute, parents can apply to the court for orders under the Children Act

key term

Section 8 Orders passed by a court when there is a dispute about who a child should live with, who they can have contact with, and some of the steps and decisions adults can take about them

1989. This Act replaced orders that previously concerned custody and access with four new orders known as **Section 8 Orders**, which together with a Family Assistance Order, determine with whom a child should live, whom they can have contact with, and some of the steps and decisions adults can take.

Section 8 Orders (Children Act 1989)

The four Orders are:

- *a Residence Order*, stating whom the child is to live with; it can be made in favour of more than one person and state how much time the child should spend with each person
- *a Contact Order*, requiring the person with whom the child lives to allow the child to have contact with the person named on the Order; parents, grandparents and other family members may apply for this if they are being denied contact with a child
- *a Prohibited Steps Order*, applied for if someone objects to something that a parent is doing concerning a child; the order aims to restrict the way that a person exercises their parental responsibility, for example, whether they can take a child abroad
- *a Specific Issues Order*, aiming to settle disputes about a child's care and upbringing; it can make a specific order, for example concerning education or medical treatment.

The *Family Assistance Order* aims to provide short-term help to a family who cannot overcome their disagreements concerning their children following separation.

Progress check

What are monogamy, polygamy and cohabitation?

What are the sole grounds for divorce?

What are the four main Section 8 Orders?

What does a Family Assistance Order aim to provide?

Legislation relating to child care in the UK

THE IMPORTANCE OF THE CHILDREN ACT 1989

The Children Act 1989 is a major piece of legislation. Previous laws affecting children, passed during the 19th and 20th centuries, overlapped and were sometimes inconsistent. This caused confusion and difficulty. The Children Act aims to provide a consistent approach to child protection both by bringing together and changing previous laws.

There was also a concern that recent law, passed before the Children Act, could be used too easily to take rights and responsibilities away from parents. This was thought to be neither in the interests of children nor parents. One of the main aims of the 1989 Act was therefore to balance the needs and rights of children, and the responsibilities and rights of parents.

THE RIGHTS AND RESPONSIBILITIES OF PARENTS

Parents' rights

In the past parents had the right of ownership of their children. This right, supported by the law, allowed parents to do more or less as they wished with their children. The law has gradually changed, and it now limits considerably parental rights and powers. It makes the rights of parents to bring up their children and make decisions on their behalf dependent on them carrying out their duties and responsibilities towards their children.

The law gives them the right to be involved throughout any child protection enquiry, as long as this is consistent with the welfare and protection of the child. They have the right, for example, to attend a case conference. Research shows that greater parental involvement leads to more purposeful and creative work with families, but that disagreement, real or perceived, between social workers and parents greatly hinders the achievement of positive outcomes for children following an enquiry.

Parents' responsibilities

The law includes the idea that parents have rights but that they also have certain duties and responsibilities towards their children.

The Children Act uses the phrase 'parental responsibility' to sum up the collection of duties, rights and authority that parents have concerning their children.

The idea of parental responsibility is a principle that is at the centre of the Children Act 1989. The law does not say precisely how adults should exercise their parental responsibility; it recognises that there is a great variety of ways that they can do this. It emphasises that parents have a duty to care for their children and raise them 'to moral, physical and emotional health'. In this way, the law imposes minimum standards for the care of children and protects their welfare.

The 1989 Act recognises that both parents have the responsibility towards their children for the following:

- caring for and maintaining them
- controlling them
- making sure that they receive proper education.

Parents also have the authority to:

- discipline them
- take them out of the country
- consent to medical examination and treatment.

The people who may have parental responsibility for a child

People have different rights over children at their birth – some people automatically have parental responsibility, others have none but they may acquire (or gain) parental responsibility during the child's life.

These people automatically have parental responsibility for a child at birth:

- a woman and man who were married at the time the mother gave birth to the child
- separated or divorced parents – parental responsibility is legally unaffected by the separation or divorce, but there may however be Section 8 Orders in force that say who a child should live with and who can have contact with the child (see above)
- an unmarried mother.

These people might acquire parental responsibility during a child's life:

- an unmarried father – he does not have it automatically; he must either make formal 'parental responsibility agreement' with the mother, or he may apply to court for an order that gives him parental responsibility
- a non-parent who applies for a Residence Order and can show that they have established a close relationship with the child and are in a position to undertake the role of parenthood, for example a stepfather
- people who are appointed as guardians if a child's parents die
- carers, following an Adoption Order or a Residence Order
- a local authority, when a court makes a Care Order or an Emergency Protection Order.

Parents do not now lose parental responsibility for their children (except when they are adopted, or if someone with parental responsibility applies to end the parental responsibility of an unmarried father). They continue to have responsibility even if a court order is made that removes a child from their care.

Case study . . .

. . . parental responsibility

James was born when his mother Emma was 17 and unmarried. After he was born, Emma made a formal parental responsibility agreement with his father Barry, who was 18, but she and James had no contact with Barry after he moved away when James was 1.

Emma and James continued to live with her parents for 4 years, after which she married her husband, Steven. James is now 8 and has been living with Emma and Steven since he was 4. Steven, with Emma's agreement, wishes to acquire parental responsibility for James, and intends to apply for a Residence Order to achieve this. At the same time, Emma intends to apply for Barry's parental responsibility to be brought to an end.

1. *Did Emma have parental responsibility for James when he was born, and why?*
2. *How did Barry acquire parental responsibility for James?*
3. *Why is it likely that Steven will acquire parental responsibility for James?*
4. *Why is it possible that Barry will lose parental responsibility for James?*

Progress check

In what fundamental way have parental rights changed significantly over the last 200 years?

What are some of the duties and responsibilities of parents?

What rights does the mother of a child automatically have in law?

Does an unmarried father have the same rights?

LOCAL AUTHORITY CARE

Under the Children Act 1989, local authorities have a responsibility to provide a range of services to safeguard and provide welfare for 'children in need' in their area. They can do this by providing advice, assistance and services to families, including day care. They may also 'look after' children by providing accommodation for them on a full-time basis, in foster homes or community homes.

Looked-after children – provision of accommodation

Sometimes the most appropriate help a local authority can give a family is to provide accommodation for a child under a voluntary arrangement with the child's parents. This might be offered:

- to give parents respite (a break) from looking after a child who is difficult to care for – this can be a particularly valuable service for families with a child who has disabilities
- when a family situation makes it very difficult for parents to meet the needs of a child, through illness or severe family problems.

Parents may take their children home at any time under this voluntary arrangement, and they are encouraged to have regular contact with them.

Looked-after children – Care Orders

Local authorities aim to keep children and parents together, and to promote the care of children within their own families. There are, however, situations when a child's welfare can only be protected by removing them from their family. To do this, the local authority must obtain a court order. These Orders are described in Chapter 37. The Orders include:

- an Emergency Protection Order
- a Child Assessment Order
- a Care Order.

Alternatively, the authority may be given the power to supervise a child compulsorily while they remain at home. To do this, the local authority needs:

- a Supervision Order; or
- an Education Supervision Order, which places a school-age child under the supervision of the local authority if the court decides that the child is not attending school properly.

TYPES OF SUBSTITUTE CARE

A local authority will provide the type of care for a child that is most appropriate to the child's needs. The type of care is not necessarily linked to whether the child is looked after by being provided with accommodation under a voluntary agreement, or is the subject of a court order. Children may be placed in a foster home, a residential children's home or, in some circumstances, with adopters.

Foster care

Foster parents are people from all backgrounds who are recruited by a local authority to take children into their homes for short or longer periods of time. They can be single or married couples. They are interviewed at length concerning their suitability to look after children; they need a range of qualities to meet the demands of looking after children whose behaviour may be disturbed by their life experiences. They may also have contact with the children's parents.

Once the foster parents are approved, they are paid a weekly allowance for children placed with them. Foster care is now considered the most appropriate form of substitute care for children who cannot be with their families. Local authority social services departments usually produce leaflets for the public to encourage them to apply to become foster parents or adopters.

Residential care

Residential care is the term used to describe children's homes, often referred to as *community homes*. They usually consist of small units, often houses within the community. They are staffed by residential social workers. They are generally considered to be unsuitable for the care of young children, except in special circumstances, such as emergencies, or if their behaviour is initially very difficult to manage. They are more likely to be used to accommodate older children, larger families, or to assess children's developmental needs.

Adoption

Adoption is a legal process whereby the parental rights and responsibilities for a child are given up by one set of parents and taken on by another. Adoption must be arranged through a recognised adoption agency and an order made in court. All local authorities must provide an adoption service. Adopters go through a similar interview and selection process as foster parents. In recent years, the number of babies placed for adoption has declined, from 2,649 in 1979 to 895 in 1991. Many adoptions now involve older children. Children have a right to make their wishes known at an adoption hearing. The current trend is towards open adoption, where some form of contact between a child and their birth parents or relatives is maintained. Attention is also given to the need to place children in families of the same ethnic origin.

Progress check

When might a child be 'looked after' by a local authority?

How can a child be removed from home compulsorily?

Why is foster care considered to be the most suitable form of substitute care for young children?

Who is residential accommodation most likely to be provided for?

What is adoption and in what circumstances may adoption be more suitable for a child than long-term foster care?

Working with children and their families

GOOD PRACTICE FOR CHILD-CARE WORKERS

There are some important points for anyone working with children and their families to remember:

- The family forms a central part of any child's life.
- Children come from a variety of family types and structures.
- Each child's family is important and meaningful to that individual child.

- Some children may be looked after in substitute families or establishments.
- We tend to be very self-centred in our view of families, seeing our own family as 'normal'.

IMPROVING WORKING PRACTICE

- Try to increase your awareness and understanding of different family patterns. You can do this by observing people around you, talking to them, reading books and articles, watching programmes on the television, films and videos. It is important to be open and willing to learn.
- Be aware of the alternative provisions for the care of children in the community.
- Inform yourself, when appropriate, of the family circumstances of each child in your care. Remember that confidentiality is essential, both in what you say to others and how you keep records.
- Assess the individual needs of each child. This is the only way that you can ensure equality of opportunity for each child. People who say that they 'treat all children the same' are denying children equality by not recognising and providing for their differences and particular needs.
- Plan the best way to meet children's individual needs and provide appropriate attention, care and stimulation.

Progress check

Why does our view of families tend to be self-centred?

How can a worker increase their understanding of different types of families?

What is the best way a worker can meet children's individual needs?

Now try these questions

What are the most significant differences between the experience of life for a child in a nuclear, extended or reconstituted family?

Why have changes in women's roles, attitudes and expectations been one of the reasons for a fall in the number of children in the average family?

What might be the particular needs of only children and children from large families when they start at nursery?

What are the differences between the tasks that men and women do now compared to those in the past?

What should good substitute day care provide in order to meet the all-round developmental needs of young children?

key terms

You need to know what the key terms and phrases in this chapter mean.
Go back through the chapter and find out.

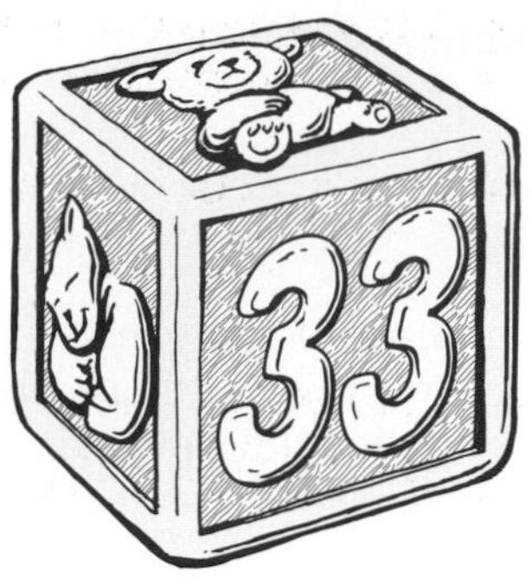

SOCIAL ISSUES

There are many things that affect the way that individuals and families live and experience life. Some of these are personal issues concerning their health, intelligence and personality, but others are social issues influenced by their education, wealth and position in society. Everyone experiences pressures in their life, but people have different practical, emotional and social resources to deal with these pressures. This can explain in part why people respond differently to problems and why some people are able to provide a good environment for their children despite considerable pressures, while others find it more difficult.

This chapter will cover the following topics:

- *what is society?*
- *economic and social policy – the legal framework*
- *the effects of social and economic deprivation.*

What is society?

One view is contained in the statement made in 1987 by Margaret Thatcher, then prime minister of the UK: 'There is no such thing as Society. There are individual men and women, and there are families.' Many people have since commented on this statement.

In contrast to this, many people believe that society *does* exist. They perceive that individuals and families do not live in isolation, but are part of society and are strongly affected by their social and legal environment.

Society can be described as people living together within a framework of shared laws and customs that have been created over a period of time. Society provides the social, cultural, economic and physical environment for people's lives.

key term

Multi-cultural society
a society whose members have a variety of cultural and ethnic backgrounds

A MULTI-CULTURAL SOCIETY

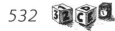

All societies include different social groups. Many societies, including the UK, also include different cultural groups. A **multi-cultural society** is one that includes a variety of cultural groups who may have some differing social customs and rules. This can provide a varied and positive social environment. Sometimes the customs of one group become known and adopted by another group. In this way, people's lives are enriched. A simple example of this in the UK is the enjoyment by many people of the traditional foods of different cultural groups, for example Asian, Chinese and Italian.

For a multi-cultural society to work positively and be of benefit to all its members, it is essential that:

- certain laws are shared and respected by all
- there is mutual acceptance and tolerance of differences in customs
- no group has, or is thought to have, more power, status and resources than another.

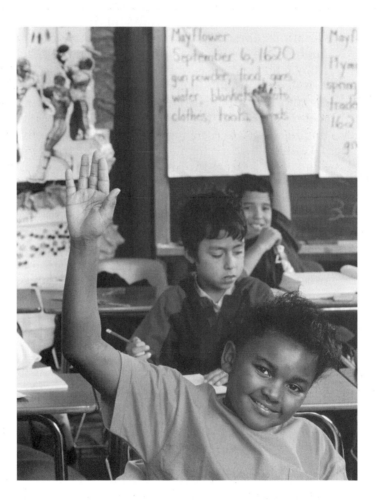

A multi-cultural society can provide a varied and positive social environment

Economic and social policy – the legal framework

The UK, like every democratic society, has a set of laws. These laws have been passed in parliament by elected representatives and apply to everyone. They form a framework of rules and laws that:

- cover the rights of citizens to be treated fairly and equally and to be protected from harm

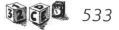

- include the approach by government to economic and social policy, and an outline of citizens' rights to certain services and welfare benefits, together with how these will be funded
- include the duty citizens have to behave in certain ways and the penalties and punishments an individual will incur if they break the law, including the illegal claiming of welfare benefits.

THE POSSIBLE EFFECTS ON FAMILIES OF SOCIAL AND ECONOMIC DEPRIVATION

The pressures caused by social and economic deprivation can have a powerful effect on families and their children. The strong influence of the social and economic background of a child's family becomes obvious when reading the published examination results of individual schools in the UK. With slight variations, the children from schools that are in areas where a large proportion of families are from lower socio-economic groups achieve lower results than children from schools in areas where most families are from higher socio-economic groups.

It would seem that, despite the introduction, in recent decades, of **equal opportunities policies** and comprehensive schools, the achievement of **social mobility** through the education system is still very limited for the children of families who are socially and economically disadvantaged.

Children inherit their social position from their family of birth. The day care and education system provides them with a real opportunity to broaden their experience and, if they wish, to change their social position as adults. The attitudes of their family of origin are very important in determining whether children make use of the opportunities provided for them through the care and education system. There is much evidence to show that only a minority of children at present overcome the effects of social and economic disadvantage. Current government policy, including the formation of the Social Exclusion Unit and the Sure Start programme, aims to counteract such disadvantage.

key terms

Equal opportunities policies
policies designed to provide opportunities for all people to achieve according to their efforts and abilities

Social mobility
the movement of a person from one social group (class) to another

Case study . . .

. . . social mobility

The grandparents of Leroy and Sam were born in Jamaica and were encouraged to come to the UK in the 1950s to work on public transport. Their mother and father were originally left in the Caribbean until their parents were established, and they joined them in their early teens.

Leroy and Sam's mother became a nurse and their father worked in service industries. They lived in a flat in an inner-city area. Both boys attended their local schools. Leroy and Sam were bright children and their parents were very keen for them to do well. They encouraged them to work hard, listened to them read, and made sure that they did their homework. Their teachers encouraged them, and Leroy and Sam passed their exams at school well. Leroy went to university and studied law. He now works as a solicitor. His brother, Sam, did teacher training and now teaches in a local primary school.

1. *Why have Leroy and Sam been successful within the education system?*
2. *What factors might have worked against this happening?*

THE SOCIAL PRESSURES AND DISADVANTAGES FACED BY SOME CHILDREN AND THEIR FAMILIES

Personal and social pressures and problems

All adults are likely to face some kind of difficulty, problem or pressure in their lifetime. If they are parents, their children will probably be affected in some way by their experiences.

Some problems can be referred to more accurately as 'personal', others as 'social'. The source of personal problems lies very close to the circumstances of an individual person's life. Examples of personal problems are difficulties with or loss of relationships, bereavement, mental and physical ill health. Other problems are usually referred to as 'social' when their source is mainly in the way the social and physical environment is organised. Examples of 'social problems' are urban decay or rural decline, racial and social discrimination, poverty, unemployment, bad housing and homelessness. Many families are multiply disadvantaged and the term 'social exclusion' is used to describe the effects of this disadvantage.

There are often close links between personal and social problems; the experience of social problems often causes personal problems. For example, the experience of long-term poverty can cause stress, worry and feelings of uselessness; social problems can then lead to anxiety, depression and ill health or domestic violence, drug and alcohol misuse.

Sources of social disadvantage and pressure

People can be described as disadvantaged if they do not have an equal opportunity to achieve what other people in society regard as normal. This may be because they are experiencing poverty, unemployment, inadequate housing, homelessness, racial discrimination, an impoverished environment, or are sick or disabled.

POVERTY

Lack of money and the long-term experience of poverty is often experienced as a major problem for families. A family is considered to be living in poverty if their income is less than half the national average weekly wage. This is called the *poverty line*. A Department of Social Security (DSS) report published by the government in 1994 revealed that 14 million people in the UK were living below the poverty line; 4 million of them were children. This is three times the number recorded in 1979.

Poverty is now usually described as being **relative**. This means that people are considered to be poor 'if their resources fall seriously short of the resources commanded by the average individual or family in the community' (Peter Townsend, *Poverty in the United Kingdom*, 1979). In past centuries in the UK there were many people living in **absolute poverty**, that is, they did not have 'enough provision to maintain their health and working efficiency' (Seebohm Rowntree, *Studies of Poverty in the City of York*, 1899).

> **key terms**
>
> **Relative poverty**
> occurs when people's resources fall seriously short of the resources commanded by the average individual or family in the community
>
> **Absolute poverty**
> not having enough provision to maintain health and working efficiency

Causes of poverty

The main causes of poverty are low wages or living on state social security benefits. The people who are most likely to be poor are those who are:

- unemployed
- members of one-parent families
- members of black and other minority groups
- sick or incapacitated
- elderly
- low paid.

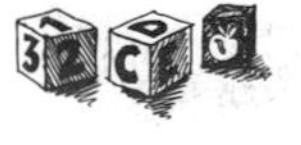

The effects of poverty on the family

Poverty can affect every area of a family's life. There may not be enough money for a nutritious varied diet, adequate housing, transport, household equipment, leisure activities or toys. It can cause stress, anxiety, unhappiness and lead to poor physical and mental health. People are limited in their ability to go out, to entertain others, and to have outings or holidays. Family relationships can become strained. People are aware, through the media, especially television, that others have a much higher standard of living. All this can result in a feeling of hopelessness and of being outside (excluded from) the mainstream of society.

Some sociologists refer to people living in extreme and continuous poverty as the 'underclass' – a group of people who feel they have no hope of improving their situation. The Social Exclusion Unit works at the centre of government to bring socially excluded people back into society.

> **key term**
>
> **Poverty trap**
> experienced by people if they are receiving state benefits and they find that by earning a small amount more they lose most of their benefits and become worse off

Many people experience the **poverty trap** if they are receiving state benefits – they find that, by earning a small additional amount, they lose most of their benefits and become worse off. They are trapped in their position. This is of great concern to the government, which now aims to get people out of this trap by welfare reforms that enable people to keep more of any increase in earnings they achieve.

UNEMPLOYMENT

Unemployment rates have always varied. It was high in the 1980s and since then it has both fallen, risen and fallen again. While full employment is unlikely to be achieved, if only half a million unemployed people are registered in Britain at any one time, this is considered very low unemployment. Unemployment has affected every section of the population, but some people are more vulnerable to it than others. These are:

- people without skills or qualifications
- manual workers
- young people and old people
- women
- people who generally suffer discrimination in society – these include people from ethnic minority groups and people who have disabilities, people who have suffered mental illness or have been in prison.

The effects of unemployment on the family

Unemployment can have profound effects on individuals and families. Those experiencing long-term unemployment are more likely to be living in poverty and suffering its effects. They may also have feelings of shame, uselessness, boredom and frustration that can affect their mental and physical health. Family relationships can become strained, and provide an unhappy or even violent environment for children. Whole communities can become demoralised and run down.

INADEQUATE HOUSING

Despite the fact that there has been a massive slum clearance and rebuilding programme since the 1950s, many people still live in accommodation that is damp, overcrowded and unsuitable for children. Some of the high-rise flats that were built to rehouse people in the 1950s and 1960s were very badly built. They contributed to a wide range of personal and social problems. Some of this accommodation has since been demolished or redesigned, although examples still remain in some urban areas.

There are obvious links between people being poor and living in poor housing conditions. Those who have money buy accommodation that suits their needs. Those who are poor usually have to take whatever is available to them.

The effects of inadequate housing on the family

Damp, inadequate and dangerous housing can lead to bad health, illness, accidents, the spread of infection and poor hygiene. It is difficult to improve broken-down houses or keep them clean. Adults may blame each other or feel depressed and worried. This, together with lack of play space, creates an unsuitable environment for children to grow up in.

HOMELESSNESS

There is a national shortage of accommodation at affordable prices. This was a result in part, in the 1980s, of the Conservative government's policy of giving council tenants the right to buy their houses, while not allowing councils to use the money from sales to build more houses. Private owners have been reluctant to let accommodation to families because legislation makes it difficult subsequently to evict them. There is a growing number of homeless people; they mainly become homeless when:

- their relatives are unwilling or unable to continue to provide them with accommodation
- they are evicted for mortgage or rent arrears
- their marriage or partnership breaks up.

The majority of homeless people are young, either single or with young families, on low incomes.

Accommodating homeless people

The local authority has a legal duty to accommodate homeless families. The shortage of accommodation means that an increasing number are placed in temporary bed and breakfast hotels. The conditions for families in bed and breakfast hotels are totally unsuitable. The accommodation can often be overcrowded, dangerous and unhygienic. There is usually a lack of cooking, washing and other basic amenities. There is little privacy or play space. People often suffer isolation from family and friends. In addition, their access to education, health and other services is disrupted. Families can spend several years in this type of accommodation.

The effects of homelessness on the family

Living for a long period in cramped and unsatisfactory conditions can have a very bad effect on family relationships between adults and children. Parents who experience this degree of stress in their everyday existence may have little energy to provide more than the basic necessities for children. It is often difficult for people to maintain good standards of hygiene and the provision of nutritious food can be a problem if there are little or no cooking facilities. The lack of play space can lead to children being under-stimulated and having little access to fresh air and exercise. Every aspect of their development can be affected. The provision of day care can be of great value for children living in bed and breakfast accommodation.

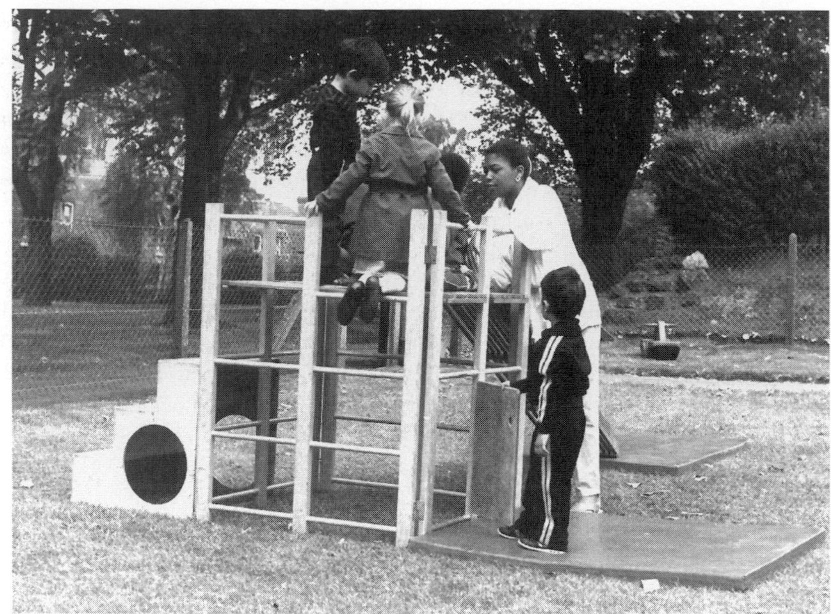

The provision of day care can be of great value for children living in bed and breakfast accommodation

RACIAL DISCRIMINATION

> **key terms**
>
> **Ethnic group**
> a group of people who share a common culture
>
> **Ethnic minority group**
> a group of people with a common culture, which is smaller than the majority group in their society

Race is difficult to define, but the term is used describe a group of people who share some common biological traits. **Ethnic groups** are people who share a common culture. **Ethnic minority groups** are groups of people whose number is smaller than the majority ethnic group in the society in which they live.

There are many ethnic groups in the UK. Some attract little attention, for example the many people of Italian, Polish and Irish origin who live in some parts of the country. The groups that receive the most attention are those who are noticeable because their culture, dress or skin colour makes them stand out, particularly those of African-Caribbean, Indian, Pakistani and Bangladeshi origin. They are commonly referred to as black and/or Asian.

The Race Relations Act (1965)

This Act made it illegal to discriminate against people, because of their race, in employment, housing and the provision of goods and services. Discrimination occurs when people are treated less favourably than others, either intentionally or unintentionally. In 1976 the Commission for Racial Equality (CRE) was given greater powers to take people to court for both direct discrimination (i.e. practised openly) and indirect discrimination (i.e. 'hidden', for example rules that exclude particular groups).

> **key term**
>
> **Migration**
> the movement either to or from a country

Patterns of migration

Historically the pattern of **migration** (the movement either to or from a country) in the UK has been that:

- there has been a steady flow of people emigrating (leaving)
- there have been noticeable waves of people immigrating (coming in).

Overall the numbers have more or less balanced each other, although some people express racist ideas about being 'overwhelmed' by numbers of immigrants that has no basis in fact.

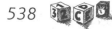

There is a growing issue concerning the treatment of asylum seekers in Britain. The attempt to disperse people to different parts of the country has not met with success overall, so the deployment of such families has more impact in some areas than others, particularly in the south of England and London.

The problems faced by families from ethnic minority groups

Ethnic minority families, particularly those that are very visible, may still experience discrimination, prejudice and intolerance, stereotyping and scapegoating as part of their everyday life. Black and Asian people experience discrimination particularly in:

- *employment* – they are more often found in low-status, low-paid jobs with less chance of promotion and more shift work than white people; black people are also more vulnerable to unemployment and poverty
- *housing* – differences between ethnic groups are very noticeable; Asian families have tended to buy their homes, but often the cheaper houses in inner-city areas; people of African-Caribbean origin have been more likely to live in poorer private or council accommodation
- *racial harassment and attacks* – there has been an alarming rise in racial attacks in the UK, some resulting in death; the experience of racial attack can be devastating for an individual and a family. The police are introducing programmes to counteract racism among police officers and to encourage a policy of quicker response to racist attacks.

THE URBAN ENVIRONMENT

Many inner-city areas in the UK are characterised by environmental pollution and decay, lack of play space and higher crime rates. They have attracted a lot of publicity in recent years. This has resulted in a number of government-funded and voluntary-funded schemes aimed at improving the environment and the quality of people's lives. The success of these initiatives is varied, partly because of the difficulty of knowing exactly what the problems are.

The UK's inner cities have suffered a loss of population in recent years. Many people have chosen to move from urban centres to the suburbs to have gardens and for cleaner air. This was made possible by the development of public and private transport. There has also been a loss of industry and employment opportunities in inner cities, and poor planning has contributed to impersonal environments and decay.

In most cases, therefore, with the exception of some 'sought-after' city centre areas, people who have material resources choose not to settle in the centre of towns, but to live on the outskirts. This leaves a concentration of people in inner cities who have fewer resources, including people experiencing:

- poverty, unemployment and housing stress
- physical and mental illness
- discrimination because of their ethnicity or disability
- social isolation, such as being members of one-parent families
- family problems, including violence and abuse.

There are also more people involved in crime, drug abuse and prostitution in inner-city areas.

In addition, demands on the health and social services tend to be higher, and because of this the quality of these services tends to be poorer.

key term

Multiple disadvantage the concentration of social problems in one area

One way of understanding inner-city problems, therefore, is through the idea of **multiple disadvantage**, which emphasises the fact that urban deprivation is not a single problem, but a number of problems concentrated in one area.

The effects on the family of living in a deprived urban environment

It is important to remember that an urban environment is *not necessarily* a negative experience for all residents. There are many people who live happy and fulfilled lives and who rear their children successfully in cities and towns. Disadvantage is, however, more common than in suburban areas. The lives of some children and their development may be adversely affected in a variety of ways by living in such an environment.

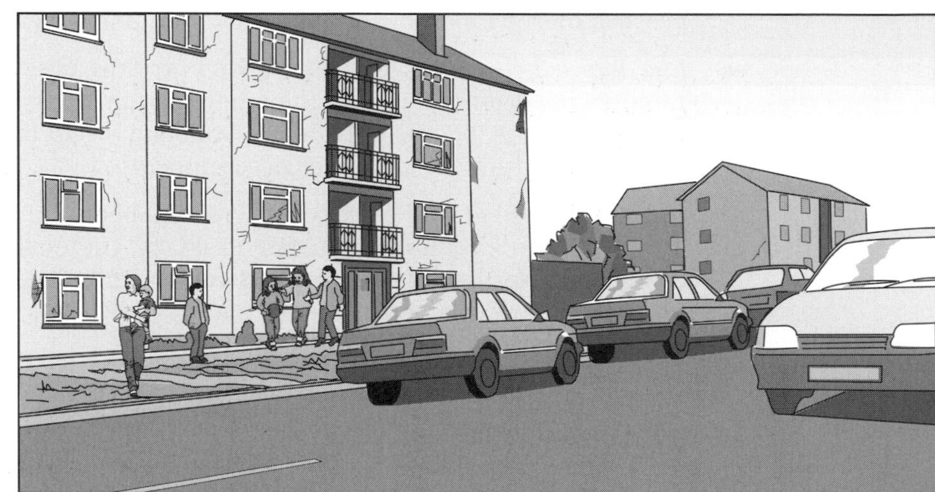

Many of the UK's inner cities are characterised by environmental pollution, decay and lack of play space

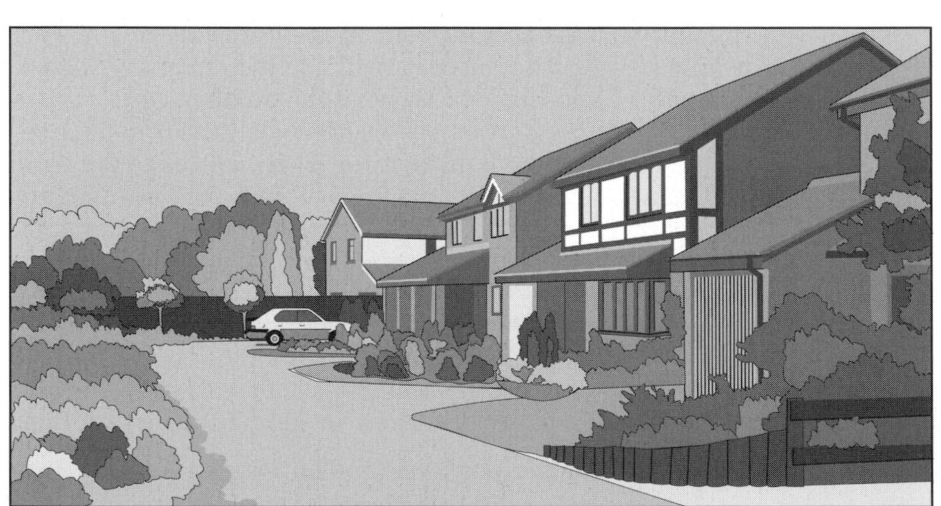

In most cases people who have material resources choose not to settle in the centre of towns, but live on the outskirts

THE RURAL ENVIRONMENT

Much less publicity is given to the problems faced by families in rural areas. The UK has a proportionately smaller rural population than many European countries. Some people who live in rural areas are supported by a high income and this buys them desirable housing, land and private transport. Others, for example farm workers, have incomes well below the national average. They may suffer from poverty and unemployment and all the effects that this can bring. They can find housing and transport very difficult to obtain. Their housing may be tied to their job so that they can lose both at the same time.

The effects of a rural environment on the family

Families living in a rural environment can be subject to similar pressures to those of an urban family if they have low incomes. The lack of public transport, and distance from support and advice centres can further exacerbate their experiences.

OTHER SOURCES OF PRESSURE FOR FAMILIES AND THEIR CHILDREN

Sources of pressure that can also have a negative effect on children's development and health include the misuse of drugs and alcohol by carers, domestic violence and mental illness.

Drugs and alcohol misuse

It is important not to generalise about this, but a parent's practical caring skills may be adversely affected by substance abuse, some of which can put children at risk of neglect, physical injury and emotional abuse. Misuse of alcohol by parents can result in physical abuse of children. Children can be particularly vulnerable if their parent is withdrawing from drugs, or if the misuse is chaotic or out of control. Parents may find it difficult to put the needs of their children first. The drain on a family's finances reduces the money available to meet basic needs, or may draw the parents into criminal activity. Children may suffer the risk of physical harm through their exposure to drugs and needles.

Domestic violence

This can affect children in many ways and prolonged exposure can affect a child's development in every area, but particularly emotionally and physically. They may become caught up in the violence directed at their parent and emotionally suffer great distress in witnessing this. Their parent's ability to care for them may be profoundly affected by their experiences, particularly when violence is combined with the misuse of drugs or alcohol. Prolonged exposure to parental conflict can have a serious effect on children's well-being, even when not combined with physical violence.

The mental illness of a carer

This does not necessarily have an adverse effect, especially if it is short term and mild and does not lead to parental conflict. It can, however, have an impact on a child's experiences. Mental and physical illness may restrict a child's activities and may put the child in a caring role at too young an age. In some cases a child's needs may be neglected or they may be vulnerable to physical assault.

Progress check

Which people are most likely to be poor in the UK today?

How can unemployment affect people?

Why is it very difficult for people to bring up children in bed and breakfast accommodation?

In what ways may people from ethnic minority groups experience disadvantage?

What multiple disadvantages can be experienced by people living in inner cities?

How can a family be disadvantaged by living in a rural location?

Name some other sources of stress for children within some families.

Case study . . .

. . . multiple disadvantage

Sharon is 7 years old and lives with her mother and father and two younger brothers in a fifth-floor flat of a six-storey block on an inner-city housing estate. The area around the flats is run down. Piles of rubbish accumulate regularly and graffiti covers many walls and doors. The lifts to the flats, even when working, are inhospitable. Sharon's mother, Sandra, works some shifts in a local factory, but as her father is unemployed, most of the money she earns is deducted from their income support. Sandra is often tired and depressed; her husband gets angry with her and sometimes hits her. Sharon's younger brothers are 3 and 4 years old, and regularly wet the bed at night. Washing and drying are difficult and, when their mother is at work, the boys sometimes remain unwashed and unfed. Sharon is mature for her age and helps her mother all she can, but she is often tired in the day and her concentration at school is poor.

List the problems that this family face.

Why is it difficult for the family to get out of the poverty trap?

What progress is Sharon likely to make at school, and why?

What sources of help might improve things for this family?

What are your thoughts about this situation?

The effects of social and economic deprivation

THE DIFFERING RESPONSES OF PEOPLE TO THE PRESSURES CAUSED BY DISADVANTAGE

One of the dangers of describing social problems and the way that people are affected by them is that not *all* people respond to them or are affected by them in the same way. It can be puzzling that some people cope with pressures and others are affected severely by them. We can only say that people *may* respond to pressures, or *might* be affected by them in certain ways. Differences in responses to the experience of disadvantage can be explained partly by:

- how severe, intense and long term the pressure is – many people cope reasonably well with *short-term* pressures in every day life, but are more tested by those which are long term and severe
- differences in the practical, social and emotional resources that people have to cope with life.

RESOURCES

Resources are the practical, social and emotional sources of help and strength that people have in varying degrees to help them to cope with life, and bring up their families. Some people have fewer resources to cope with everyday life than others.

This means that:

- at times of stress and difficulty they are very vulnerable and can be overwhelmed
- they are less able to protect their children from pressures and problems
- they may at times be unable to provide adequate care for their children. This does not mean, however, that they are irresponsible or lack affection for their children.

Lack of practical resources

Practical resources include reserves of money, material assets, managing skills and mobility. The stress caused by social conditions such as poverty, unemployment or poor housing may affect the capacity of a person to care for their children, either temporarily or permanently. People who have no savings, who worry constantly about money and who endure poor environmental conditions probably experience a higher level of stress in their everyday lives than those who have no such worries.

key term

Social isolation
people experience social isolation when they have no close family or friends to care about them.

Lack of social resources

Social resources include a supportive family, friends, a close social network and being a member of a group. People experience **social isolation** when they have no close family or friends to care about them. It means there is no one to share troubles and anxieties with. There is a saying 'A trouble shared is a trouble halved'. Parents who have warm and caring personal relationships, and have the support of others, may be better able to cope at times of stress and difficulty.

Lack of emotional resources

Emotional resources include having had the experience of stable and caring relationships, having high self-esteem, the ability to cope with stress and frustration, being able to recognise and deal with extreme feelings, and having a positive view of life and the ability to trust and give.

Many things may reduce a person's emotional resources. A range of personal issues such as low self-esteem, mental ill health, difficulties with relationships, bereavement, illness, incapacity or other previous life experiences. These issues can profoundly affect a person's view of life and make them vulnerable to stress. This may in turn affect parenting skills.

PROVISION FOR CHILDREN AND FAMILIES IN THE UK

There are many statutory, voluntary and private organisations that can help people at times of need. A nursery can help to meet the all-round needs of a child and help to compensate for any disadvantage the child may experience. Provision for children and families is detailed in Chapter 34.

Progress check

Why do people respond differently to pressures?

What varying resources do people use to cope with pressures?

How can day care help to compensate for the disadvantage a child may experience?

Now try these questions

What kinds of deviant behaviour might affect a family's ability to care for their children and what effect might this have?

With slight variations, the children from schools that are in areas where more families are from higher socio-economic groups achieve higher results than children from schools in areas where most families are from lower socio-economic groups. Why do you think this is?

How do people get caught in a poverty trap?

Describe how social pressures and a lack of resources can affect the healthy development of a child.

key terms

You need to know what the key terms and phrases in this chapter mean. Go back through the chapter and find out.

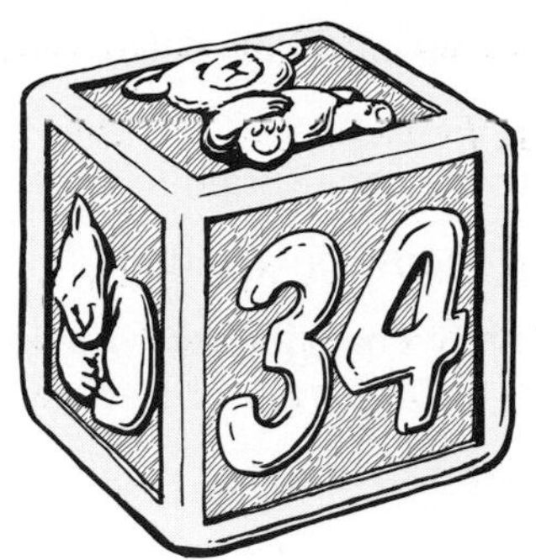

THE ROLE OF THE STATUTORY, VOLUNTARY AND INDEPENDENT SERVICES

The vast majority of children are brought up within their family. Child-care workers have differing contact with the parents of the children in their care, varying according to the setting in which they work. A thorough knowledge of both child-care legislation and the different types of child-care provision and support services available to children and families is essential to those who work with children and their families.

This chapter will cover the following topics:

- *main relevant legislation concerning the rights of children*
- *the role of statutory, voluntary and independent services in relation to children and families*
- *the range of services for children and families*
- *the political structure for service provision in the UK*
- *child-care and education services*
- *personal social services*
- *housing*
- *social security*
- *health.*

Main relevant legislation concerning the rights of children

THE CHILDREN ACT 1989

The Children Act 1989 came into force in October 1990. It aims to protect children in every situation, whether in their homes, in day care, or full-time care. It provides extensive guidance on the regulation of services for children and families. It is based on a number of important **principles** that are embodied in the Act. These principles include:

> **key term**
> **Principle**
> a basic truth, which underpins an activity

- Children are entitled to protection from neglect, abuse and exploitation.

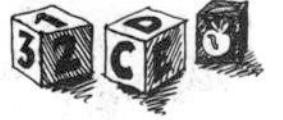

- The welfare of the child is the first consideration.
- Wherever possible, children should be brought up and cared for by their families.
- The child's wishes should be taken into account when making decisions.
- Unnecessary delay in procedures or court action should be avoided.
- A court order should only be made if it positively contributes to a child's welfare.
- Professionals should work in partnership with parents at every stage.
- Parents whose children are in need should be helped to bring up their children themselves.
- Although the basic needs of children are universal, there can be a variety of ways of meeting them. Patterns of family life differ according to culture, class and community. These differences should be respected and accepted.

THE UNITED NATIONS CONVENTION ON THE RIGHTS OF THE CHILD

Children's rights are most fully described in the United Nations Convention on the Rights of the Child. Created over a period of 10 years with the input of representatives from different societies, religions and cultures, the Convention was adopted as an international human rights treaty on 20 November 1989. It entered into force in record time on 2 September 1990. It contains a comprehensive array of rights, bringing civil and political, economic, social and cultural rights, as well as humanitarian rights, together for the first time in one international instrument. Overall, the Convention serves as a landmark in the promotion of the rights of the child, placing children alongside other population groups whose rights necessitate protection by way of an international treaty. It is based on the belief that all children are born with fundamental freedoms and the inherent rights of all human beings. This is the basic premise of the Convention on the Rights of the Child, an international human rights treaty that is transforming the lives of children and their families around the globe. People in every country and of every culture and every religion are working to ensure that each of the 2 billion children in the world enjoys the rights to survival, health and education, to a caring family environment, play and culture, to protection from exploitation and abuse of all kinds, and to have his or her voice heard and opinions taken into account on significant issues.

The role of statutory, voluntary and independent services in relation to children and families

There is a wide range of statutory, voluntary and private services that support children and their families in the UK today. The UK has a welfare state that provides statutory services both through the local authority and central government. The government introduced this during the 1940s. The aim of the welfare state is to ensure that all citizens have adequate standards of income, housing, education and health services. The welfare state and the services provided by it have changed a great deal since they were introduced. Recent governments have supported the growth of private and voluntary provision to supplement state services provided by local authorities and central government.

The range of services for children and families

Care and education services for children and their families are provided either by:

- the state, through either local authorities or central government departments organised in regions – these are referred to as **statutory services**
- volunteers or voluntary groups – referred to as **voluntary services**
- private individuals or companies – referred to as **independent or private services.**

key terms

Statutory service
a service provided by the government after a law (or statute) has been passed in Parliament

Voluntary services
services provided by voluntary organisations, which are founded by people who want to help certain groups of people they believe are in need of support

Private services
services provided by individuals, groups of people, or companies to meet a demand, provide a service, and make a financial profit

STATUTORY SERVICES PROVIDED BY EITHER LOCAL AUTHORITIES OR CENTRAL GOVERNMENT DEPARTMENTS

What is a statutory service?

A statutory service is one provided by the government after a law (or statute) has been passed in parliament. Such laws say that either:

- a service *must* be provided (i.e. there is a duty to provide it), for example education for 5 to 16 year olds; *or*
- a service *can* be provided (i.e. there is a power to provide it if an authority chooses), for example local authority day nurseries.

What do statutory services provide?

Statutory services provide for, among other things, education, health care, financial support, personal social services, housing, leisure services and public health. Government provision is sometimes referred to as 'the state sector'. Local authorities are mostly involved in the provision of education, social services, housing, public health and leisure services. Central government provides social security benefits and the National Health Service.

How are statutory services financed?

Statutory services are financed by the state, which collects money through local and national taxation and National Insurance. There may be some fund-raising activities and charging for services (for example, prescription charges and charges for outings in schools). There has been increasing pressure on state services to be more accountable financially and to be run more like private organisations and give 'value for money'. This philosophy has affected the way that both state hospitals and state schools are funded and organised.

How are statutory services staffed?

Most of the people who work in statutory organisations are trained and paid for their work, but volunteers may carry out some tasks (for example, parent-helpers in schools, WRVS workers in hospitals).

VOLUNTARY SERVICES

What are voluntary services?

Organisations are referred to as 'voluntary' when they are founded by people who want to help certain groups of people who they believe are in need of support (i.e. they are formed *voluntarily*, like Barnados and the NSPCC). The basic difference between voluntary and statutory organisations is that, unlike a statutory organisation, no legislation has to be passed in order for a voluntary organisation to be set up. The government is very positive about some services being provided by 'the voluntary sector', but it does pass laws to regulate them, requiring certain of them to register, so that the services they provide can be inspected by government officers in order to protect the people who use them (for example, playgroups and childminders, under the Children Act 1989).

What do voluntary services provide?

There is a long and varied tradition of voluntary work in the UK and as a result there is a wide variety of voluntary organisations. In some European countries the church has been the only source of voluntary activity. Voluntary organisations have a number of different functions. Some organisations combine more than one of these functions. They:

- act as information and campaigning bodies (for example, Shelter and the Pre-School Learning Alliance or PLA)
- provide money to help people in particular circumstances – these are sometimes called benevolent funds or charities (for example, the Family Welfare Association)
- help and support some people who have health conditions or impairments (for example, Scope, Royal National Institute for the Blind or RNIB)
- support and care for families and children, and other individuals (for example, Barnados and NCH day centres and family centres, Mencap, Relate).

How are voluntary services financed?

Money for voluntary organisations comes from a variety of sources that include donations, fund-raising, grants from central or local government, lottery grants and fees for the services they provide.

How are voluntary services staffed?

Some people do work without pay and have no qualifications (for example, in self-help groups), and this is the reason that most people think they are called 'voluntary'. However, many people who work for voluntary organisations are professionally trained and qualified and receive a salary (for example, inspectors in the NSPCC or workers in NCH family centres). Some voluntary organisations may pay one person who then organises many unpaid volunteers (for example, Homestart), or pay several people a small amount (for example, playgroup workers). They may be run by a voluntary management committee, as is the case for many playgroups and community groups.

INDEPENDENT OR PRIVATE SERVICES

What are independent services?

Independent services are usually private services provided by individuals, groups of people or companies to meet a demand, provide a service, and make a financial profit. As with voluntary organisations, the government is also positive about certain services being provided by 'the private or independent sector'.

What do independent services provide?

Independent services usually aim both to provide a service *and* to make a financial profit for their owners. They therefore need to be what is called 'financially viable', i.e. not run at a loss. They provide, among other things, nursery care, education, health care, counselling services, housing and leisure services. Nannies and childminders are part of the private sector.

How are independent services financed?

The financing of private services comes both from private investment by people wishing to make a return on their investment and from the fees that they charge for their use. In some cases the state may pay the fees for someone to use a private service. This happens when it has a duty to provide a service for a particular client but there is a lack of provision within the state sector in a particular area (for example, paying for day care with a childminder for a child who is considered to be 'in need' under the Children Act 1989).

How are independent services staffed?

Independent services are staffed according to the need of the organisation. In regulating some services the state may, for example, demand they employ a certain proportion of professionally qualified staff. Some users may also demand qualifications, for example, those using qualified nannies.

Progress check

Define 'statutory services' and give an example of one.

Define 'voluntary services' and give an example of one.

Define 'independent or private services' and give an example of one.

Which Act of Parliament covers the procedures for registering and inspecting the private and voluntary organisations that care for children?

The political structure for service provision in the UK

Statutory, voluntary and private services for children and their families are provided within the political structure of a country. Political structures vary between countries and there are therefore differences between the UK and other European countries in their provision. In the UK, although some service provision is administered centrally, other provision depends on the choices made by politicians in different local authorities. Services may therefore vary from one area to another. Political parties change and services may be modified as a result.

POLITICAL ATTITUDES AND THE LEVEL OF SERVICE PROVISION

Differences in levels of service provision, like that of state-run day nurseries, may reflect the political beliefs of the party in power in a local area or centrally in a country. A simple way of understanding why this is so is to look at the basic ideas behind opposing political beliefs. These basic ideas may be described as either 'right-wing' or 'left-wing'.

Right-wing beliefs

Right-wing beliefs include ideas such as the following:

- People should be responsible for themselves and their own families.
- The money the state collects in taxes should be kept to a minimum.
- Spending by the state on services should be kept to a minimum.

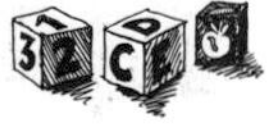

- People should pay little in tax and be free to keep and spend their money on which services they choose.
- It is better if certain services are provided by private or voluntary bodies, and that the people who want them should pay for them themselves.

Left-wing beliefs

Left-wing beliefs include ideas like the following:

- The state has responsibilities for the welfare of all its citizens.
- Sufficient money should be collected in taxes; more should be collected from those who have the highest incomes.
- The government should spend taxpayers' money to provide services.
- The state should provide services free for everyone who needs them, regardless of whether they have contributed towards them through taxes or insurance.

STATUTORY SERVICES: CENTRAL GOVERNMENT PROVISION

Some statutory services are provided by central government, through different departments. The *political process* that leads to this provision involves the following:

- In a general election, citizens elect politicians, called Members of Parliament (MPs). MPs make policy decisions about the services they want to provide, based on their political beliefs. They then pass laws (statutes) to say which services should be provided.
- MPs employ officers to put their policies into practice. These officers are called civil servants and are paid out of taxes. These officers work in central and regional offices throughout the country.
- The Department of Health, the Inland Revenue, and the Department of Social Security are all organised as central government departments with regional offices.

STATUTORY SERVICES: LOCAL GOVERNMENT PROVISION

Local government, through a local authority, also provides some statutory services. The organisation of local authorities in the UK is varied and complicated. The main differences are as follows:

- Some areas of the country have two tiers (or layers) of local government, both of which have elected councils, which are:
  - a district council, which may represent a borough, city or district
  - a county council, which will contain several districts.

In such areas the provision of services is divided between the two authorities.

- Others areas have just one tier (or layer) of local government and only one elected council. These are called *unitary authorities*, because *one* body provides all local services.

The *political process* that leads to the provision of services involves the following:

- Citizens vote for and elect councillors in district and county council elections. These councillors then form the local council. The party that has the greatest number of councillors takes charge (this is called the democratic process). The powers of local councils are given to them by Acts of Parliament and through passing local by-laws.

- Councillors appoint officers to put their policies into practice and to organise and provide services in that area. These are called local government officers and they are paid out of local and central taxation. These officers work in town halls, civic centres and other offices in the area. Some schools and other education services, social services, leisure services and housing are provided in this way by local government departments.

THE STATE IN RELATION TO INDEPENDENT AND VOLUNTARY SERVICES

The extent to which the state encourages independent or voluntary provision depends on its political outlook. Conservative governments have traditionally been associated with support for the independent, private sector. However, it is a fact that recent governments of both political persuasions have increasingly encouraged the provision of private and voluntary services. In order to protect the people who use them, the state passes laws requiring these services to reach certain standards, to register and to be inspected by government officials (for example, childminders and private day nurseries, under the Children Act 1989).

Apart from this, independent services can charge the amount that they believe people are prepared to pay for a service. They meet the demands of 'the market place'. Voluntary providers are usually controlled by some form of committee that decides who should be helped by their service. This may mean that services users may have to subscribe to a certain belief, or be 'deserving'. This is in contrast to state provision, which is available as a right to citizens if they are eligible.

Progress check

Why may levels of service provision differ depending on the political party that is or has been in power?

What is a right-wing political belief?

What is a left-wing political belief?

Who is selected in a general election?

Who appoints civil servants and what do civil servants do?

Who appoints local government officers and what do local government officers do?

What are unitary authorities?

Child-care and education services

STATUTORY PROVISION OF CHILD-CARE AND EDUCATION SERVICES

The state is required by law to ensure that all children, including those with disabilities, receive education if they are of **statutory school age**. This means from the beginning of the term after their 5th birthday, until the end of the school year in which they have their 16th birthday.

key term

Statutory school age

the ages at which a child legally has to receive education: from the beginning of the term after their 5th birthday, until the end of the school year in which they have their 16th birthday

Early Years Education

The structure of primary school provision varies between areas. Primary education may be provided for children in:

- *one* primary school until the age of 11
- an infant school until the age of 7, then a junior school until the age of 11
- a first school until the age of 8, followed by a middle school from 9 to 13 years.

Local management of schools

key term

Local management of schools (LMS)

enables a head teacher and the governors of a school to decide how to spend their money and staff a school

Local education authorities now give a large proportion of their education budget directly to schools. The head teacher and the governors of a school decide how to spend this money and how to staff the school. They are responsible for the financial and overall management of their school. This system is called the **local management of schools (LMS)**. Most people in education view this as a successful a policy that has given power and discretion to schools to manage their own budgets.

The National Curriculum and the Early Learning Goals

All state schools are now required by law to follow the National Curriculum. This is to ensure that all children follow a broad-based and balanced curriculum. The content of the National Curriculum and arrangements for testing it have been amended several times. Any setting in which children are funded by the state for the Foundation Stage, that is from 3 years old to the end of the reception year, is required to work towards the Early Learning Goals.

Nursery schools and classes

Local authorities have had the power to provide pre-school education for many years, but they have not used this power uniformly across the country or within their own area. As a result state provision of nursery schools and classes varies nationally. Some councils provide separate nursery schools, others provide nursery units attached to a primary school, while others provide very little. Education in these is usually part time. The government now funds pre-school education for all 4 year olds, but parents can choose whether this is in the state, voluntary or private sector. It has extended this funding to some 3 year olds and aims to fund all 3 year olds. To obtain funding, settings have to be inspected and judged to be offering provision that will satisfactorily promote the Early Learning Goals. There is still a strong emphasis on play and exploration in all nursery education. State nursery schools are more often found in areas of highest social need.

Most European countries provide more nursery education than the UK but their statutory school age is usually older. For example, in France and Germany there is a legal entitlement to a place in a kindergarten for every child from 3 to 6 years old. In Italy, 92 per cent of children attend pre-primary education as part of the state system from 3 to 6 years; this figure is 95 per cent in Belgium. In Sweden, all parents who work or study are entitled to a place for their children in a publicly funded centre from the age of 1 year.

key term

Children in need

a child is 'in need' if they are unlikely to achieve or maintain a reasonable standard of health or development without the provision of services, or if they are disabled

Day nurseries and family centres

The social services department (SSD) of a local authority has the power to provide day care for children in day nurseries and family centres, and a duty under the Children Act 1989 to provide for **children in need** in its area. Many of these powers in England have now been transferred to the Department for Education and Employment (DfEE), which has done much of the work in developing policies for Early Years Development and Childcare Plans and Partnerships and for setting up the first Early Years Excellence Centres.

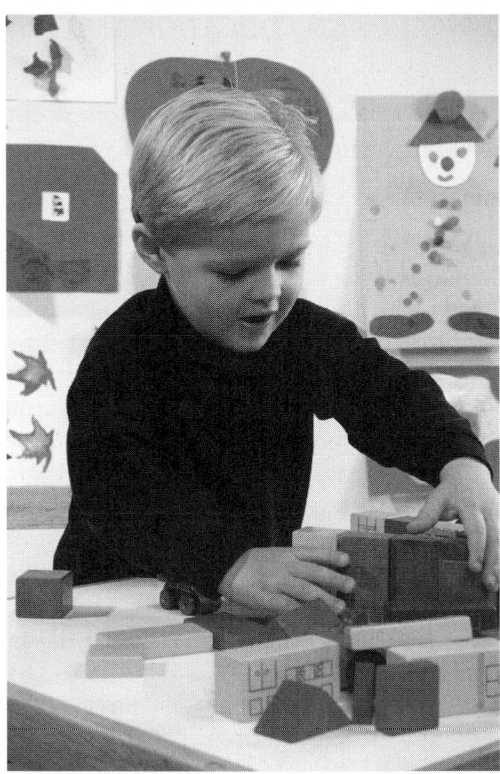

There is a strong emphasis on play and exploration in nursery education

GOVERNMENT INITIATIVES

Sure Start

Sure Start is an area-based government initiative. Launched in 1999 it aims to improve the health and well-being of families and children before and from birth, so children are ready to flourish when they get to school. Sure Start programmes are concentrated in neighbourhoods where a high proportion of the children are living in poverty and where it is hoped Sure Start can help them to succeed by pioneering new ways of working to improve all services for children and their families.

Sure Start is the responsibility of seven government departments working together. Programmes are run locally by partnerships, including voluntary and community organisations, health, local government, education and, most significantly, local parents.

Minimally, Sure Start programmes provide the following, but exactly how they do so depends on local circumstances and needs:

- outreach and home visiting
- support for families and parents
- support for good quality play, learning and child care
- primary and community health and social care
- support for children and parents with special needs.

Sure Start programmes work according to the following key principles:

- co-ordinate and add value to existing services
- involve parents, grandparents and other carers in ways that build on their existing strengths
- avoid stigma by ensuring all local families are able to use Sure Start services
- ensure lasting support by linking to services for older children
- be culturally appropriate and sensitive to particular needs
- promote the participation of all local families in the design and working of the programme.

key term

National Childcare Strategy
a strategy introduced by the UK government in May 1998 to ensure good quality, accessible, affordable child care for children aged up to 14

The National Childcare Strategy

The development by the Labour government of a **National Childcare Strategy** is also taking place in the DfEE. In May 1998 the government unveiled its plans to spend more than £300 million on funding child-care places over the following 5 years. Its aim is to ensure good quality, accessible and affordable child-care for children aged up to 14 years in every neighbourhood in England. Its strategy includes measures to make child care more affordable, by including tax credits for working families, and more accessible, by increasing the number of places and encouraging diversity in provision to satisfy the preferences of parents. A similar strategy is in place for Wales.

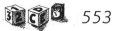

VOLUNTARY SECTOR PROVISION OF CHILD-CARE AND EDUCATION SERVICES

Pre-school playgroups

The playgroup movement in the UK began in the 1960s with the formation of one group by a parent. The movement spread rapidly through the country. Over the years it has filled a much needed gap in pre-school provision, but recent changes in funding and rise in provision by other sectors has led to a fall in the number of playgroups nationally.

To form a pre-school playgroup, local people usually group together, rent premises and form a committee that organises and appoints workers. Parents sometimes help on a rota at sessions. There are usually a number of part-time sessions available a week; a charge is made for each child, but 3 and 4 year olds may be funded. Pre-school playgroups have traditionally provided play facilities and social contact, but if they take funded 3-year-old or 4-year-old children they must demonstrate to OFSTED inspectors that their programme would enable children to achieve the Early Learning Goals by the end of the Foundation Stage. The OFSTED inspection process has been very demanding for some pre-school playgroups; staff are relatively low paid and may lack professional qualifications. Playgroups also had to register with and be inspected by the social services department. However, both arms of this inspection process were brought together under OFSTED in September 2001.

Parent and toddler groups sometimes use the same facilities as playgroups. Parents and carers bring children from babies upwards, but supervise them while they play.

The PLA

The Pre-school Learning Alliance (PLA) is a national educational charity with many years' experience in the field of pre-school education and care. It offers a national training programme for parents and pre-school staff, and publishes educational materials and advice for pre-school playgroups.

Nursery and family centres in the voluntary sector

Voluntary organisations that were once more traditionally involved in providing residential care now fund many nursery and family centres in areas of high social need. Organisations including Barnados and NCH Action for Children have diverted their resources into providing community day care and family support for those who are experiencing difficulties.

PRIVATE SECTOR PROVISION OF CHILD-CARE AND EDUCATION SERVICES

Childminders

Childminders are people who look after other people's children in their own homes. They have a legal duty to register, previously with the SSD, but now with the DfEE, and must conform to standards in the guidance to the Children Act 1989 and the new Care Standards. They must be of good health and character and have non-discriminatory attitudes. The Standards cover safety, floor space and for child-minder:child ratios according to the different ages. Childminders are free to fix their own charges. They are sometimes paid by a social service department to care for children in need.

The National Childminding Association (NCMA) is an influential body concerned with providing information and training, and acting as a pressure group for childminders.

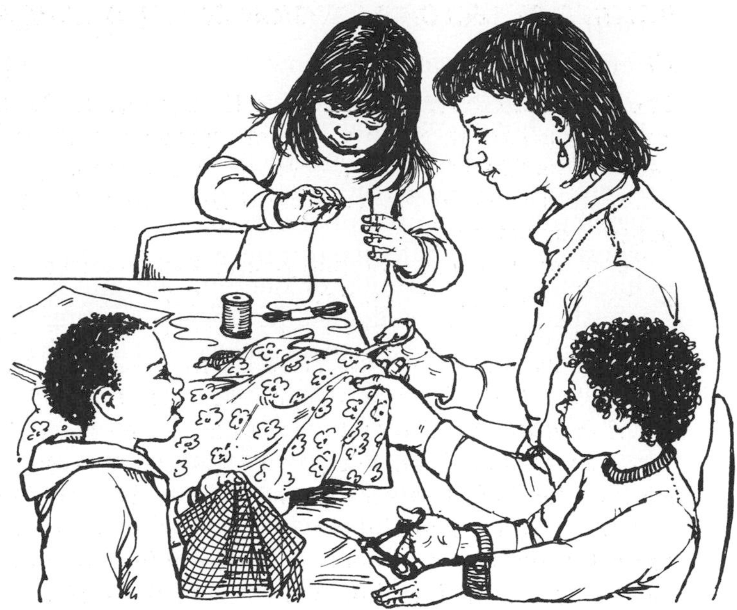

Childminders are people who look after other people's children in their own homes

Private day nurseries

Private day nursery provision more than trebled in the period from 1987 to 1997, when there were an estimated 6,100 day nurseries in England, providing 194,000 places. Private day nurseries occupy many types of premises including purpose-built nurseries and those in converted buildings; they vary in size. They all have to register with OFSTED for a specific number of children and conform to standards in the same way as childminders and to national regulations about qualified staffing levels. They provide full or part-time care and education for children under school age and many provide for babies. Some also provide before and after-school care and care during the school holidays. Charges vary and to some extent they reflect what people in an area can afford to pay. The National Day Nurseries Association (NDNA) aims to promote quality in the private sector.

Out-of-school clubs

Out-of-school clubs are provided in school, nursery or other premises and have had considerable financial backing from government in recent years. They provide invaluable support for the children of working parents in the periods between working hours and school hours. In 1997 the number of clubs was 2,600, providing places for 79,000 children from 5 to 7 years – a rise of 13 per cent over the previous year. These numbers are set to rise still further.

Private nursery schools

Private nursery schools exist to meet a demand from parents who want their children to be educated in the private sector. They are often part of a private school for children up to the age of 11 years. These schools provide full and part-time education for children from 3 years old during school hours; they may also provide before and after-school care. Their fees vary. Small class sizes are a key feature of this provision. Schools have to register with the DfEE and meet certain standards. If they are providing nursery education for funded children they have to register and be inspected by OFSTED.

Nannies

Nannies are privately employed by parents to look after children in the family home. Nannies may live in or out of the home. They negotiate their contract, which includes hours, pay and duties, with their employer. They do not have to be qualified; registration is only required if they are looking after the children of three or more families at the same time. There has been a call for nannies to be registered under a national system. This raises numerous problems, and some experts believe that registration would be unworkable and not serve to protect children. The Federation of Recruitment and Employment Services (FRES) has published a set of guidelines for anyone wanting to employ a nanny. It provides a ten-point list for prospective employers to help them to choose the right nanny.

Workplace nurseries

Provision of day care at places of work is fairly uncommon. In 1998 only 25 of 500 top companies provided a workplace nursery. Ten companies had reserved places at nurseries and 15 had after-school clubs. When asked, 88 per cent of the companies said they did not think that working mothers were less reliable staff members than employees in general and 65 per cent agreed they should do more to help working parents. Employers may increasingly recognise a strong business case for investing in child care, with more mothers with young children returning to work.

Case study . . .

. . . child care and education for children of working parents

Rose, Anne, Stephanie and Aisha are four friends who met at antenatal classes. They have remained in touch as their babies have grown older and sometimes discuss their concerns about making the right decisions about child care and education for their children. They all live with working partners but agree that, although they have made joint decisions, they are the ones who feel most responsible for arranging child care for their children. None of them has any close relatives living nearby. They all agree on the need for a flexible system that enables them to fulfil their work commitments, but gives their children good care in a suitably stimulating environment.

- Rose has a child of 18 months. She works from home and has some flexibility in her hours, but nevertheless most days she aims to complete 6 hours' work a day in her office.
- Anne has a baby of 6 months and one of 20 months. She has just returned to work part time for one whole day and three half-days a week in a departmental store.
- Stephanie has a 19 month old and a 3 year old, and works full-time as a nursery nurse in a primary school.
- Aisha has three children of 18 months, 4 and 7. She works as a clerk in a busy solicitors office.

1. *Outline what you think would be the most suitable, practical child-care arrangements for each of these families. Give reasons for your choices in each case.*
2. *Suggest an appropriate alternative for each family.*

Progress check

What child-care and education services are provided by the state sector?

What child-care and education services are provided in the voluntary sector?

What child-care and education services are provided by the private sector?

Personal social services

STATUTORY PROVISION OF SOCIAL SERVICES

Care for children in need

Local authorities provide personal social services through their social services department (SSD). The Children Act 1989 gave them a duty to provide services for 'children in need' in their area to help them to stay with their families and be brought up by them.

A child is defined as 'in need' if:

- the child is unlikely to achieve or maintain, or to have the opportunity of achieving or maintaining, a reasonable standard of health or development without the provision of services
- the child's health or development is likely to be significantly impaired, or further impaired, without the provision of such services
- the child is disabled.

The SSD tries to keep families together by offering them support in the community. It may provide social work support and counselling, practical support in the home, family centres, short periods of relief care, help with providing essential household needs and welfare rights advice. In certain cases it may look after children in need by providing them with foster care or residential accommodation and respite care (now known as a 'short-term break') for children who are disabled.

Children at risk

The SSD has a duty to investigate the circumstances of any child believed to be at risk of harm and take action on their behalf to protect them by using child protection procedures. It also provides care in residential or foster homes for children who are made the subject of care orders by a court.

Looked-after children

The SSD provides accommodation for children who, with the agreement of their parents, need a period of care away from their family. Foster carers, whom the department approves and pays, will often look after such children. It also provides community homes for some children. All SSDs provide an adoption service for children who need new, permanent parents.

Special needs

There is also a range of services that are provided for children with disabilities alongside those provided by the health and education authorities.

The National Health Service and Community Care Act 1990 placed on local authorities the responsibility for assessing the needs of individual clients who, for a variety of reasons, need help to enable them to continue to live in the community.

Case study . . .

. . . children 'in need'

Jeanette was 17 when her first child was born. The child's father was not named on the birth certificate. She subsequently had two more children by different fathers, the last of whom lived with her, but he was sometimes violent towards her and little involved with the children. Jeanette found it very difficult to manage. Her partner gave her little money and the children were sometimes unfed and poorly cared for. The health visitor called but never seemed to find them in. A neighbour referred them to the local social services office because she considered the children were being neglected.

After an enquiry and a case conference, the children's names were put on the child protection register because of the neglect and the presence of a potentially violent male in the household. The protection plan included recommending nursery centre places for her 2 and 3 year old. These were provided on a part-time basis, but this was on condition that Jeanette stayed with them for two mornings each week to learn about play and physical care. The 5 year old had a place in a local primary school. This school had a partnership with social services to provide before-school care, including breakfast, for some referred children. A social worker visited Jeanette and befriended her, helping her with advice and guidance. She also discussed her taking up a place with a local training agency to undertake some training for work.

A year later Jeanette had matured into a much more confident and mature young woman. She told her partner to leave, took control of her finances and embarked on a part-time course. Her children were thriving and noticeably more happy.

1. *Why was Jeanette referred to the local social services?*
2. *Why could her children be defined as being 'in need' in terms of the Children Act 1989?*
3. *What help did social services give after the children were placed on the child protection register?*
4. *Why do you think that, a year later, her children were thriving and noticeably more happy?*
5. *Why is this called preventive work?*

Finding information about services

Information about local social services departments can be obtained from their offices, which are listed in the telephone directory and at local libraries. The SSD will have leaflets to inform the public about their services.

VOLUNTARY PROVISION OF SOCIAL SERVICES

National voluntary organisations

There is a wide range of voluntary organisations that help to support families and children; some of these are shown in the following table. These organisations supplement the work of the social services department. Addresses and further information can be obtained from telephone books, from *The Charities Digest* published by The Family Welfare Association, available in public libraries, and at a volunteer bureau.

NATIONAL VOLUNTARY ORGANISATIONS

AFRICAN-CARIBBEAN, INDIAN, PAKISTANI COMMUNITY CENTRES

Exist in areas where there are numbers of people of Caribbean and Asian origin. They offer a range of advice and support services for local people. There is also a wide range of local organisations that aim to meet the needs of other minority communities. Some of these provide nurseries.

BARNADOS

Works with children and their families to help to relieve the effects of disadvantage and disability. It runs many community projects, including day centres where young children who are at risk can be cared for and their families supported. It also provides residential accommodation for children with special needs. It carries out research into areas of need and publishes the results of research.

CHILDLINE

Provides a national telephone counselling helpline for children in trouble or danger. It listens, comforts and protects. Its freephone number is 0800 1111.

THE CHILDREN'S SOCIETY

Offers child-care services to children and families in need. It aims to help children to grow up in their own families and communities.

NATIONAL ASSOCIATION OF CITIZENS' ADVICE BUREAUX

Provides free, impartial (not biased), confidential advice and help to anyone. It has over a thousand local offices that provide information, advice and legal guidance on many subjects. These include social security, housing, money, family and personal matters.

CONTACT-A-FAMILY

Promotes mutual support between families caring for disabled children. It has community-based projects that assist parents' self-help groups, and runs a national helpline.

FAMILY SERVICE UNITS

Provide a range of social and community work services and support to disadvantaged families and communities with the aim of preventing family breakdown.

FAMILY WELFARE ASSOCIATION

Offers services for families, children and people with disabilities. It provides financial help for families in exceptional need, social work support and drop-in centres.

GINGERBREAD

Provides emotional support, practical help and social activities for lone parents and their children.

JEWISH CARE

Provides help and support for people of the Jewish faith and their families. Among other facilities, it runs day centres and provides social work teams and domiciliary (home) assistance.

MENCAP

Aims to increase public awareness of the problems faced by people with mental disabilities and their families. It supports day centres and other facilities.

MIND

Is concerned with improving services for people with mental disorders and promoting mental health and better services.

NATIONAL VOLUNTARY ORGANISATIONS CONTINUED

THE NATIONAL CHILDREN'S HOMES (PREVIOUSLY NCH ACTION FOR CHILDREN)

Provides support for children who are disadvantaged and their families. It runs many schemes, including family centres, foster care and aid and support to families. It also carries out and publishes the results of research.

NATIONAL DEAF CHILDREN'S SOCIETY

A national charity working specially for deaf children and their families. It gives information, advice and support directly to families with deaf children. It helps them to identify local help and support.

NATIONAL SOCIETY FOR THE PREVENTION FOR CRUELTY TO CHILDREN (NSPCC)

Has a network of child protection teams throughout England and Wales. The RSSPCC works similarly in Scotland. Central to the NSPCC's services is the free 24-hour Child Protection Helpline – 0800 800500 – which provides counselling, information and advice to anyone concerned about a child at risk. It investigates referrals and also offers support in family care centres. It is very involved in research and publication, and provides information and training for other professionals. It also campaigns to change attitudes towards children and their care.

PARENTLINE

Offers a telephone support helpline for parents who are having any kind of problem with their children – 01702 559900.

PLAYMATTERS: THE NATIONAL TOY LIBRARIES ASSOCIATION

Exists to promote awareness of the importance of play for the developing child. Libraries are organised locally, loaning good quality toys to all families with young children.

RELATE (FORMERLY THE NATIONAL MARRIAGE GUIDANCE COUNCIL)

Trains and provides counsellors to work with people who are experiencing difficulty in their relationships. People usually make a contribution to this service according to their means.

THE SAMARITANS

Provides confidential and emotional support to people in crisis and at risk of suicide. The Samaritans is available 24 hours a day. Local branches can be found in the phone book under S, or phone 0345 909090.

In most areas there are local voluntary organisations that have grown up to meet the needs of the local population. They are often listed and co-ordinated by a local Council for Voluntary Service (CVS). They are also listed under 'Voluntary organisations' in *Yellow Pages* telephone directories. There is a wide range of these organisations. Some are self-help groups, others meet the needs of people from a variety of ethnic and national backgrounds. They may provide specific information services, advice and support.

INDEPENDENT PROVISION OF PERSONAL SUPPORT SERVICES

Some support services can be purchased privately, for example personal and family therapy, different forms of counselling, domestic and care assistance. These services tend to be expensive and financially impossible for many people, but they can provide a very useful service for many people in need of personal support with family matters.

Progress check

Which Act of Parliament gave the local authority a duty to provide services for children in need in their area?

Who is a 'child in need'? Try to put the definition in your own words.

Which Act gave local authorities the responsibility for assessing the individual needs of clients?

What do the NSPCC, NCH and Barnados provide?

Which voluntary societies provide telephone helplines for the public?

Which private support services can people purchase themselves?

Housing

STATE PROVISION OF HOUSING

Local authorities act as enablers in the provision of housing and are expected to take a strategic approach, encompassing all housing issues in their area. They encourage new house building by others in the private and voluntary sector, and have a duty to ensure that families in their area are not homeless. They first provided council housing at the beginning of the 20th century, but the demand for council housing has always been greater than the supply, and has always therefore been limited to certain categories of people. There was a massive slum clearance and rebuilding programme after the Second World War, and local authorities continue to have a duty to rehouse certain families displaced by slum clearance or redevelopment schemes.

Local authorities are expected to maintain the condition of their existing housing stock, but the amount of council housing is constantly declining, since the Conservative government introduced the 'right to buy' policy in the early 1980s. People have been encouraged to buy their council houses, but councils were not allowed by law to build new houses with the money gained from sales. As a result, there are fewer houses available for families. The sale of council houses has, in part, contributed to the rise in homelessness.

Homelessness

Local authorities have a duty to house homeless families but as they have insufficient accommodation they often have to place homeless families in hostels, of which there are few, or in bed and breakfast accommodation, which is very expensive and unsuitable, especially when there are young children.

Local councils pay Housing Benefit to people who need help to pay their rent.

key term

Housing associations non-profit-making organisations that exist to provide homes for people in need of housing from a variety of social and cultural backgrounds

VOLUNTARY PROVISION OF HOUSING

Housing associations

Large charitable trusts, such as the Guinness Trust and the Peabody Trust, have a long history of providing housing in some cities. More recently, other voluntary bodies have formed **housing associations**. The government has supported this movement, encouraging the growth of housing associations and providing money for them through the Housing Corporation, which is based in London.

Housing associations provide an alternative to council housing. They exist to provide homes for people in need of housing from a variety of social and cultural backgrounds; they are non-profit-making. They provide homes by building new units or by improving or converting older property.

Women's refuges

The local authorities help to finance refuges for women and their children, who are the victims of violent male partners. These refuges often act as half-way houses until they can reaccommodate the women. They are often staffed by a combination of volunteers and paid staff.

PRIVATE HOUSING PROVISION

Home ownership

About 65 per cent of housing in the UK is owner-occupied. There has been an enormous growth in owner-occupation during the 20th century. It is difficult for people on a low income to buy their own home, both because of the deposit required and the high cost of mortgage repayments.

Private renting

The number of properties available for private rental has declined enormously during the 20th century. This is especially so at the cheaper end of the market, where for a variety of reasons it is no longer very attractive to owners to let their properties to families. Nevertheless, nearly 10 per cent of all households live in privately rented accommodation. The law protects people with these tenancies from sudden eviction.

Progress check

Who does the state have a duty to provide accommodation for?

Why has there been a fall in the number of council houses available for renting?

Where might a homeless family be accommodated if there are no council houses available?

What is a housing association?

Where might a woman and her children go if they are the victims of violence?

In what way are private tenants protected?

Social security

STATUTORY SOCIAL SECURITY BENEFITS

The aim of statutory social security is to make sure that all adults have a basic income when they are unable to earn enough to keep themselves and their dependants. There is a range of financial benefits and allowances payable by the Department of Social Security (DSS) (central government) through its local Benefits Agency to people in a range of different circumstances. The Social Security Act 1986 set out the main changes, which were introduced in April 1988.

Logos of Social Security and the Benefits Agency

Changes to the system since 1998

In the spring of 1998 the Labour government announced major changes to the ways that state benefits are paid. This is part of its New Deal Welfare-to-Work programme. Its aim is to help and encourage people to work where they are capable of doing so, to support families and children, tackle child poverty, and to establish a flexible and efficient welfare system that is easier for people to use.

TYPES OF STATE BENEFITS

Contributory benefits

Contributory benefits include sickness, unemployment, disability and old age, maternity and widowhood benefits. These are paid to people in particular categories providing they have previously made a contribution (National Insurance contributions are deducted from a person's pay).

Non-contributory benefits

To receive non-contributory benefits a person has to be in a particular financial group or category, but does not have to have made a contribution beforehand. Non-contributory benefits fall into two groups:

- *Universal benefits* – given to all people in a certain category who claim them, whatever their income. These include Child Benefit, payable to all mothers, and Disability Living Allowance. Some politicians think that these benefits should be means-tested like those below.
- *Means-tested benefits* – only given to people in a certain category providing their income and savings are below a certain level. To claim, these people must fill in lengthy forms (tests) about their income (means), hence the phrase **means test**. This can discourage people from claiming them.

key term

Means test
an assessment of a person's income and savings, made by completing a form (test) about their income (means) to determine whether they are eligible to receive certain benefits

MAJOR BENEFITS FOR FAMILIES

Child Benefit

Child Benefit is seen as the cornerstone of the government's support for the family. It was formerly called Family Allowance. It is considered to be the fairest, most efficient and most cost-effective way of recognising the extra costs and responsibilities borne by all parents. Rises in the amount of benefits paid are often accompanied by the suggestion that the benefit paid to highly paid families should be taxed.

Income Support

Income Support is one of the main benefits in this group; it is payable to people who are not in paid employment, or who are employed part time, according to the DSS definition of 15 hours or below, and whose income falls below a certain level. Any income, whether from wages or from Child Benefit or Unemployment Benefit, is deducted from Income Support. The amount of money given in Income Support includes allowances for members of the family and for different needs. The level at which payments is set is a political decision. The government has for many years fixed this at the *poverty line*. This means that below this level of income people are accepted as living in relative poverty. This benefit is believed by some to be inadequate because those who live on Income Support for a long time are effectively living in poverty.

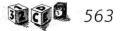

New initiatives to help unemployed claimants

key term

Job Seekers' Allowance benefits paid to people who are registered as unemployed

The Labour government is continuing the movement by the previous Conservative government to encourage people to work if they are able. It aims to rebuild the welfare state on the 'work ethic', and now calls benefits for those who are registered as unemployed the **Job Seekers' Allowance**. Its work-or-training scheme for 18 to 24 year olds, which became effective in April 1998, has been extended in many directions. In June 1998 the 225,000 people over 25 who had been receiving benefits for 2 years or more received a £75-a-week subsidy for employers to take them on; this was described by the government as a 'passport to work'. The New Deal also includes rights for up to 250,000 partners of unemployed claimants, 95 per cent of them women, who had previously been denied access to unemployment programmes. Lone parents looking for work have also been targeted for support.

WORKING FAMILY TAX CREDIT (WFTC)

Until October 1999 a previous benefit called 'Family Credit' was paid to families where a parent was in full-time work but their income was below a certain level. The government advertised this benefit, but many people who were eligible did not claim it. The claim form was long and completing it was difficult for some people. It also acted as a disincentive for people to earn more, because at a certain point they lost their Family Credit and were worse off. This prompted new initiatives with the aim of giving self-respect and dignity back to low-paid workers by allowing them to keep more of their earnings.

In the March 1998 Budget, effective from October 1999, hundreds of thousands of low-paid families were guaranteed a minimum income (£180 a week at that time) through the introduction of an American-style Working Family Tax Credit (WFTC), which replaced Family Credit. It is designed to lift the 'ceiling on the aspirations of men and women wanting to work their way up'. This reverses the situation where low-paid workers are sometimes forced to exist on state benefits because high rates of taxation make it uneconomic to work.

Under the WFTC, low-paid workers keep more of what they earn. Low-income families can also claim a tax credit, which provides a maximum of 70 per cent of their child-care costs up to a then ceiling of £150 a week; this, together with other initiatives, aims to ensure that 'all work pays'. Families are able to choose which partner receives the tax credit, which is either paid through the wage packet or directly to a non-working parent. Claimants must work a minimum of 16 hours a week, but those working more than 30 hours receive extra credit.

The government has also continued to reduce the amount of income tax paid by lower paid workers.

Social Fund

The Social Fund is a fund out of which payments are made to meet special needs not covered by Income Support. Most of this money is given in the form of loans to meet crisis and special household expenses. The criticisms of this benefit are that:

- it is discretionary (officers can chose whether to give it or not)
- it requires repayments by claimants who already have a low income
- there is a limited amount of money in the fund each year.

Finding out about benefits

There are many sources of information about the statutory benefits that are available to families and children, but people still remain unaware of some of the benefits to which they are entitled. It is for this reason that many people advocate the retention of non-means tested, non-contributory benefits such as Child Benefit, as the huge majority of people who are entitled to this receive it as they have to do very little to claim it.

Sources of information about benefits are available at all public libraries, health clinics, post offices and other public places. The benefits agency has help lines or people can call in person. Local authorities have welfare rights advisers whose phone numbers are available from the social services department. From time to time the benefits agency uses the media, including television, radio and newspapers to highlight a particular benefit, especially when it is newly introduced.

In the age of online services there is much information about benefits available on the internet (the author, using a major search engine, typed the words 'UK social security benefits' into it and obtained 115,000 hits in 1.54 seconds!) Access to the internet is a subject of political debate. Politicians are aware that groups of people in society may be disadvantaged by not having the means to access it. There is a commitment to providing access for all school children.

PROVISION OF FINANCIAL ASSISTANCE WITHIN THE VOLUNTARY SECTOR

Charities

There are many charities that give financial assistance to people in need in different situations. People need first to be aware of these and then to put in an application stating their case. Gaining awareness and making applications can both be difficult and people may need help with this. A further difficulty is that since the social security changes in 1988, the pressure on charities has been greatly increased and demand for their funds far exceeds money available. *The Charities Digest* gives the names of some charities with funds to help children and families.

THE INDEPENDENT PROVISION OF FINANCIAL SERVICES

Banks

People are at liberty to borrow money from private sources. Those who are already financially secure, with a job and a house, are more likely to be able to borrow from sources like banks and building societies, and to have credit cards.

Loan sharks

People who are less financially secure sometimes have to use less reputable sources if they need extra money; these include private companies and individuals (sometimes referred to as 'loan sharks'). People borrowing in this way may be charged higher interest rates and thus be put at a further disadvantage and slide deeper into debt. Some people believe that this form of lending should be subject to some form of legal control to protect people.

Progress check

What is a universal benefit?

What is a means test?

Who can claim Income Support?

What is the Job Seekers' Allowance?

What is Family Credit and what is the date of its abolition?

What is the Working Family Tax Credit?

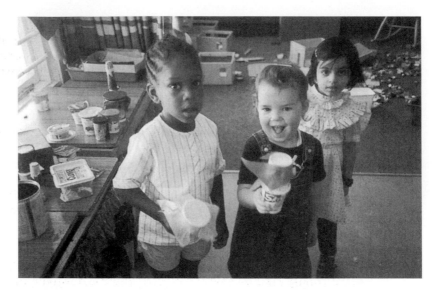

The National Childcare Strategy aims to ensure good quality, accessible, affordable child care for all children

Health

STATUTORY PROVISION – THE NATIONAL HEALTH SERVICE

The NHS was created in 1948 to give free health care to the entire population of the UK. Since it was founded:

- the general health of both children and adults has improved
- the demand for services has continued to increase, despite improvements in general health
- more expensive technology and treatments has meant that the cost of the service has increased enormously and is continuing to do so.

This increase in cost has resulted in a series of reforms over the years aimed at achieving greater efficiency, and contributing to what some regard as a decline in standards, for example the increase in hospital waiting lists, and the introduction and gradual increase in prescription charges.

Health Authorities

The Department of Health (central government) is in overall charge of policy and planning for the health service and social care. It gives powers and money to health authorities in Britain.

The role of each health authority is to:

- determine the full range of health needs of the local population, from vaccinations, to mending fractures, to treating cancer
- plan the shape of the services required, including the services of dentists, pharmacists and opticians
- purchase the services required to meet local health needs
- review their effectiveness and make any necessary changes.

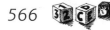

NHS trusts

More recently the concept of a 'market' for health care, introduced in 1990, has been modified, with health authorities co-ordinating groups of primary health care teams (GPs and community nurses) to commission the services that their patients need from NHS trusts. These are:

- primary care trusts (PCTs)
- community trusts, providing community services such as health visitors, midwives and clinics at health centres
- hospital trusts, providing a range of outpatient and inpatient services.

The work of the NHS trusts includes emergency and acute services, as well as meeting longer term needs in mental health and disability.

VOLUNTARY PROVISION OF HEALTH CARE

There is a long history of health care and provision through the voluntary sector in the UK. Many hospitals with voluntary status, however, including famous ones such as St Bartholomew's in London, became a part of the NHS when it was formed in 1948. Prior to this, people had to pay to see a GP, and if they could not afford this they sometimes went to a charitable hospital instead.

There are many voluntary organisations and self-help groups covering a very wide range of medical conditions and impairments that aim to help and support people, and to fund research.

The Sick Children's Trust is a national charity providing accommodation for the families of sick children at centres of specialist paediatric care. The trust owns houses in different cities in which it aims to provide homely accommodation to families at times of great stress.

PRIVATE PROVISION OF HEALTH CARE

There has been a large growth in private sector provision since 1979. Increasingly, people who are able to, and wish to, pay into private insurance schemes and then receive their treatment privately, or purchase care directly. This usually means that they do not have to wait for treatment, and the physical standards in private hospitals are usually better. However, not all services are provided in the private sector, including accident and emergency services. Some people believe that the presence of the private sector contributes to the growth of a two-tier health service, where those who can, pay for a good service, and those who cannot, make do with a poorer service by the NHS (similar to the effect of having private and state schools). It is possible that private health provision will begin to play a greater part within the NHS.

Progress check

When and why was the NHS created?

What do health authorities do?

What does the work of NHS trusts include?

What are self-help groups?

Why do some people choose to pay for private health care?

Now try these questions

What are the main differences between a statutory, a voluntary and an independent organisation?

How might differing political approaches affect the level of service provision in an area?

In what ways does the voluntary sector supplement the work of the state in providing services for children and their families?

What major new initiatives have there been in the area of social security provision for families?

key terms

You need to know what the key terms and phrases in this chapter mean. Go back through the chapter and find out.

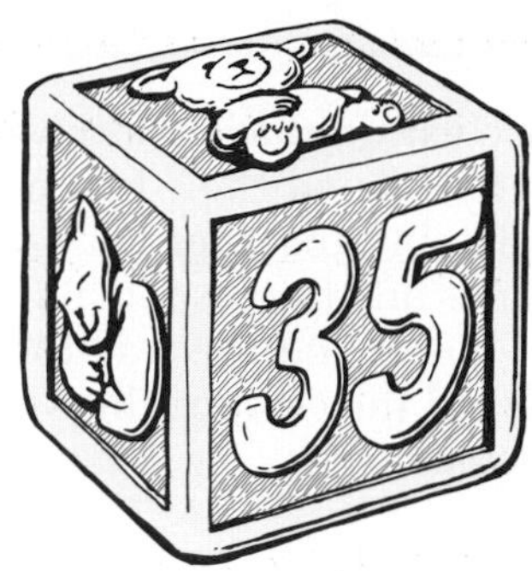

CHILD PROTECTION

Children of all ages, male and female, from all cultures and socio-economic groups are the victims of abuse. History reveals that it is not a new phenomenon. However, our awareness and understanding of child abuse and child protection within a society, such as the UK, that is legally and socially protective of children has only developed in recent decades.

One of the principles on which the Children Act 1989 is based is that the interest and welfare of the child must be of paramount (the most important) interest to all those who care for children.

This chapter will cover the following topics:

- *recognising abuse and working with young children*
- *the needs and rights of young children*
- *the assessment of abuse.*

Recognising abuse and working with young children

All those who work with young children have a unique opportunity and responsibility to:

- recognise the signs and symptoms of abuse
- know how to record and report their observations and follow the correct procedures if they suspect abuse
- listen to children, to deal with disclosure
- work to support abused children and their families. All workers have a responsibility to empower children, enabling them to develop the skills needed for self-protection
- be aware that abuse may be perpetrated within the institution in which they work and know the policies and procedures to follow to deal with this.

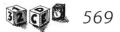

The needs and rights of young children

The view by any society of what constitutes child abuse within that society varies both between societies and within them at different stages in their history. In 19th- and 20th-century Britain that view evolved considerably, together with ideas about the needs and rights that children have as individuals and the responsibilities of parents towards them. In order to understand child abuse and the way to best protect children in the 21st century, we need to understand the current thresholds of what is considered to be abusive, and what leads to abuse.

THE RIGHTS OF CHILDREN – A HISTORICAL PERSPECTIVE

The unkind treatment by some adults of children has occurred throughout history. The novels of Charles Dickens paint a vivid picture of the lives of some children in 19th-century Britain. In *Oliver Twist*, for example, Dickens shows how cruelty and harsh punishment were both common and acceptable. Many children had to work long hours; they were often beaten and neglected.

key term

Rights of children the expectations that all children should have regarding how they are treated within their families and in society

The Earl of Shaftesbury was one of the people in the 19th century who initiated a series of social reforms that improved the lives of children. However, the amount of abuse that occurs in any society depends firstly on the view that that society has of what child maltreatment is, and this in turn determines the threshold at which society will take action against perpetrators. The 19th-century reformers would have had difficulty in recognising some 20th-century definitions of abuse, and when the state believes intervention to be appropriate. Laws passed since the 19th century have increasingly recognised the **rights of children** to be protected and to have their basic needs met, and the responsibilities of parents to protect children and meet those needs. The most recent major child protection law to be passed was the Children Act in 1989.

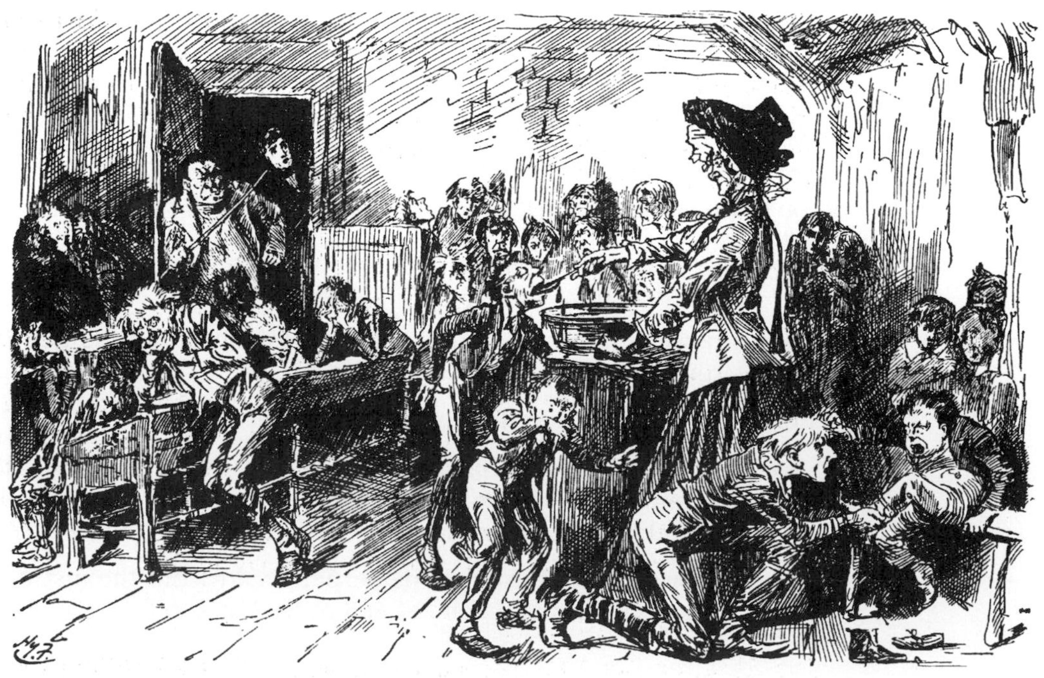

The novels of Dickens paint a vivid picture of the lives of some children in 19th-century Britain

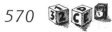

RECENT HISTORY

By the 1960s most people thought that the ill treatment of children was a thing of the past. Whenever cases came to light people thought that they were exceptional and explained them as **psychopathic events** carried out by people who lack the ability to put themselves in another person's place and empathise with how that person might be feeling. Such people also lack guilt about, and understanding of, the results of their sometimes violent behaviour.

There was an apparent lack of awareness of the widespread abuse taking place at a higher **threshold of acceptability**. The threshold of acceptability refers to the type of behaviour towards children that is believed to be acceptable by a society at a certain time. For example, at present in the UK parents giving their children a short, sharp smack is generally considered acceptable by the majority of people and it is not illegal, whereas the sustained beating of children that used to be acceptable is now both unacceptable and illegal. In other words, the threshold of acceptability has been lowered.

There remained also a commonly held belief that no one should interfere with the rights of parents over their children, especially the right to punish them. Consequently, the law still failed to protect children.

However, during the 1960s, some doctors and social workers began to develop a new awareness of abuse. They took a close interest both in the injuries that they observed in children and the explanations that carers gave for their children's injuries. They asked questions to try to find out whether some injuries were really accidental, and came to realise that certain kinds of abuse were more widespread and could not be explained as psychopathic. They began to develop an understanding of the social and environmental stresses that could prompt people to mistreat children. As a result, they discovered more and more cases of abuse.

In 1962, Dr C.H. Kempe wrote about 'the battered child syndrome'. This drew attention to the problem of 'non-accidental injury' of children by their carers both in the US and the UK, and the fact that some children were more vulnerable to abuse than others. During the 1970s and 1980s, awareness increased of a range of signs that might indicate deliberate injury to children, and also how certain social and psychological factors interact to predispose people to violent behaviour. Awareness of the occurrence and signs of sexual abuse also increased during the 1980s, followed by awareness of the activities of paedophiles and organised criminal abuse. Today, it is broadly accepted that a combination of social, psychological, economic and environmental factors play a part in the abuse or neglect of children.

key terms

Psychopathic events
actions by people who are unable to put themselves in another person's place and empathise with how that person might feel

Threshold of acceptability
the behaviour towards children that is believed to be acceptable by a society at a certain time

THE CHILDREN ACT 1989

The Children Act 1989 is a major piece of legislation. Previous laws, passed during the 19th and 20th centuries, overlapped and were sometimes inconsistent. This caused confusion and difficulty. The Children Act aims to provide a consistent approach to child protection both by bringing together and changing previous laws.

There was also a concern that recent law, passed before the Children Act, could be used too easily to take rights and responsibilities away from parents. This was thought to be neither in the interests of children nor parents. One of the main aims of the 1989 Act was therefore to balance the needs and rights of children and the responsibilities and rights of parents (see Chapter 34).

The needs of children

The Children Act 1989 recognises, however, that all children have certain needs that are universal. These basic developmental needs are the need for:

- physical care and protection

- intellectual stimulation and play
- emotional love and security
- positive social contact and relationships.

The rights of children

All children have certain rights. These include the right to:

- have their needs met and safeguarded
- be protected from neglect, abuse and exploitation
- be brought up in their family of birth wherever possible
- be considered as an individual, to be listened to and have their wishes and feelings taken into account when any decisions are made concerning their welfare.

Cultural differences in child-rearing patterns

The way that children are brought up varies a great deal between different social groups and different cultures. Families have different customs involving children. For example, some groups are traditionally more indulgent towards children, while others are stricter. Some use physical punishment more readily; others are more likely to use emotional forms of control. The Children Act 1989 acknowledges differences and values many of them. It recognises that a positive attitude to working in partnership with parents and understanding their perspective must underpin any action when working with families.

FURTHER PRINCIPLES INVOLVED IN THE PROTECTION OF CHILDREN

Adopting a professional approach

Despite the passing of legislation that makes children's rights and parents responsibilities clear, children are still neglected and abused in different ways. Child-care workers need to understand why this may happen in order to develop a

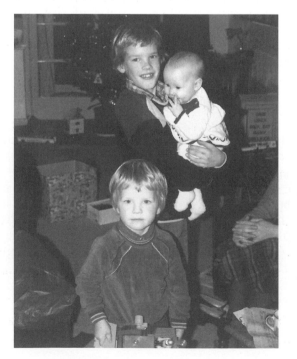

All children have the right to be brought up in their family of birth wherever possible

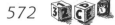

key term

Professional approach
how workers deal with and relate to people – they must not allow personal responses to affect their work

professional approach to parents and carers. Unless workers understand at least some of the factors that contribute to a case of child abuse, they may be in danger of behaving unprofessionally towards a carer and not treating them with consideration.

A professional approach includes:

- being considerate, caring and understanding
- having a non-judgemental attitude towards others
- not stereotyping individuals or groups of people
- respecting confidentiality appropriately.

key term

Partnership with parents
a way of working with parents that recognises their needs and their entitlement to be involved in decisions affecting their children

Working in partnership with parents

Child-care workers are increasingly involved in working with parents. **Partnership with parents** is one of the principles of the Children Act 1989. The Act recognises that parents are individuals with needs of their own, and are entitled to help and consideration. They are also entitled to be involved in decisions affecting their children.

key term

Predisposing factors
factors that make abuse or neglect more likely to occur – usually the result of a number of these factors occurring together

Avoiding judgemental attitudes in the assessment of abuse

An understanding of child abuse helps in planning for work with parents. There are many factors that contribute to parents being abusive to their children, these are sometimes referred to as '**predisposing factors**'. Understanding why abuse occurs increases a worker's ability to understand a carer's needs and to predict the prognosis (the most likely outcome) of working with a carer. The ability of the parent to respond to the support given may determine whether the parent is allowed to continue to care for their children.

Confidentiality

Personal information about children and families held by professionals is subject to the legal duty of confidence and should not be disclosed without the consent of the subject. Research and experience show, however, that keeping children safe from harm requires professionals and others to share information about children and their parents. The law therefore permits the disclosure of confidential information to safeguard a child in the public interest. Disclosure of information to other agencies and professionals should be justifiable in each particular case, and legal advice needs to be taken if there is any doubt. Social workers employed by a local authority or any other agency charged with protecting children, such as a day nursery, are not entitled to preserve confidentiality where this might risk the abuse of a child. Workers must guard against promising to keep confidences about disclosures of abuse.

Progress check

What has research shown about the occurrence of abuse?

Why do child-care workers need to know why abuse happens?

What does the Children Act 1989 recognise about parents?

What is a 'predisposing factor'?

What are the general principles regarding confidentiality in child protection?

The assessment of abuse

THEORIES OF ABUSE

There are various theories about why abuse happens and how it should be viewed. A combination of these perspectives is probably of the most use in understanding abuse:

- A medical model tends to look at the signs of abuse and concentrate on recognising these, and distinguishing them from accidental injuries or medical conditions. A concentration on this, rather than looking at the wider circumstances, occurred in the Anna Climbie case in 2000 and was one of the factors that contributed to her death.
- A psychological approach concentrates on the failure of attachments between carers and the children they injure. Many children who die are in fact killed by 'stepfathers', who have not been present to build up an early attachment to the child, but this does not give a complete explanation.
- A psychosocial approach emphasises the interaction between individuals and their social environments when looking for explanations of abuse.
- A social theory of child abuse emphases the role of social problems and social deprivation as a cause, but it is known that child abuse happens in all social classes and groups. However, stress caused by deprivation is a recognised factor in many cases.
- A feminist approach argues that abuse springs from the dominance of men in society and their need to assert their power over women and children.

PREDISPOSING FACTORS

Whatever the theory, research shows that abuse does not occur entirely at random, but is more likely to happen in some situations than others. There is a wide variety of predisposing factors that make abuse or neglect more likely to occur. Abuse is usually the result of a number of these factors occurring together. In each case, there will be a different combination of factors. The relative importance of each of them will also vary.

The danger in trying to understand abuse is that it might lead to a prediction that if certain characteristics are present abuse *will* happen, or that all people with those characteristics *will* become abusers. This is definitely not so. However, it is possible to look at certain factors, and find that a combination of them is usually present in many cases of abuse. These factors enable us to recognise, understand and work with families where there is a higher risk of abuse.

FACTORS THAT PREDISPOSE CHILDREN TO ABUSE

Researchers have identified five family types that illustrate the range of background characteristics to be borne in mind when abuse is suspected. They are multi-problem families, specific problem families, acutely distressed families, those with perpetrators from outside the family and those with perpetrators from inside the family.

Predisposing factors in many cases of abuse may include:

- factors in the adult's background and personality
- the presence of some kind of difficulty and stress in the adult's life or environment
- factors relating to the child.

Factors in an adult's personality and background

A combination of some of the following characteristics has been noticed in abusing parents (remember that non-abusing parents may also have some of these characteristics):

- *Immaturity* – some people have not developed a mature level of self-control in their reactions to life and its problems. Faced with stressful situations, an adult may lack self-control and react strongly just as a young child might, in a temper or with aggression.
- *Low self-esteem* – some people have a very poor self-image; they have not experienced being valued and loved for themselves. If they are struggling to care for a child, they may feel inadequate and blame the child for making them feel worse about themselves because they are finding it difficult.
- *An unhappy childhood where they never learnt to trust others* – parents who have experienced unhappiness in childhood may be less likely to appreciate the happiness that children can bring to their lives. They have not had a good role model to create a happy and caring environment for their children.
- *Difficulty in experiencing pleasure* – an inability to enjoy life and have fun may be a sign of stress and anxiety. This person may also have problems in coping with the stress of parenting and gain little pleasure from it.
- *Having unsatisfactory relationships* – when parents are experiencing difficulties in relationships, whether sexual or other difficulties, this can form an underlying base of stress and unhappiness in their lives. There may also be a general background of neglect or family violence within which there is little respect for any individual.
- *Being prone to violence when frustrated* – the damaging effects of long-term family violence on children has been recognised. Research shows that children who regularly see their mother beaten can suffer as much as if they had been frequently hit themselves.
- *Being socially isolated* – parents who have no friends or family nearby have little or no support at times of need; they have no one to share their anxieties with, or to call on for practical help.
- *Adults whose responses are low on warmth and high on criticism* – in such families, children can easily feel unloved and negative incidents can build up into violence.
- *Having a fear of spoiling the child and a belief in the value of punishment* – some people have little understanding of the value of rewards in dealing with children's behaviour; they think children should be punished to understand what is right; they think that responding to a child's needs will inevitably 'spoil' the child. They are more likely to leave a child to cry and not be warm and spontaneous in their reactions to them.
- *A belief in the value of strict discipline* – there are many variations in parenting styles, family structures and relationships; these are not necessarily better or worse than each other. They meet the needs of children in different ways. Some styles of discipline use punishment (both physical and emotional), rather than rewards. This is more likely, however, to lead to abuse when other stressful factors are present.
- *An inability to control children* – parents under pressure seldom have much time for their children and are more apt to lash out in a rage at the frustrations of everyday interactions.

- *Not seeing children realistically* – this involves having little or no understanding of child development and the normal behaviour of children at different stages; such adults are more likely to react negatively to behaviour that causes them difficulty, rather than accepting it as normal. They may punish a young child inappropriately for crying, wetting, having tantrums or making a mess.
- *Being unable to empathise with the needs of a child and to respond appropriately* – some people have difficulty in understanding the needs of children; they may react negatively when children make their needs known and demand attention.
- *Having been abused themselves as children* – these parents may have a number of unmet needs themselves and are therefore less likely to be able to meet the needs of a dependent child; they have also had a poor role model for parenting and family life.
- *Have experienced difficulties during pregnancy and/or birth, or separation from their child following birth* – research shows that difficulties during pregnancy and childbirth, or early separation of a mother from her child, can result in a parent being less positive towards a child. Faced with this child's demands, they may be less able to cope. They may lose their temper more quickly and resort to violence more easily.

DIFFICULTY AND STRESS IN THE ADULT'S LIFE AND ENVIRONMENT

Stress of some kind is found in many cases of abuse or neglect. Stress may be short or long term (sometimes referred to as acute or chronic). It may have many causes, some of which are set out below:

Causes of difficulty and stress in the adult's life and environment		
Social isolation – few friends/ no family	Chaotic lifestyles	Domestic violence – usually of a man towards a woman
The loss of relationships – especially through desertion	Mental illness or chronic unhappiness	Physical ill health
Misuse of alcohol and/or drugs	High levels of pressure in everyday life	Poor environmental conditions
Poverty/unemployment	Poor housing	Debt and money worries
Criminal behaviour within the family	The experience of discrimination	Bereavement

The experience of stress drains people's energy and leaves them with fewer resources available to cope with meeting the demands of children. The experience of multiple stresses can weaken a person's ability to cope, but it does not necessarily mean that they are irresponsible or lack affection for their children. It can, however, affect the capacity of a person to care for their children.

People who have constant worries and who have to endure long-term difficulties probably experience more stress than those without such worries. This can provide a background of unhappiness that may be significant if it is experienced in combination with other factors outlined in this section.

It does not necessarily follow that people who lack coping resources will abuse or neglect their children. In the majority of families they do not. The factors above can, however, help us to understand the different types of stress that may be present in any parent's life and may contribute to abusive situations.

FACTORS RELATING TO THE CHILD

In addition, some things about a child can make them less easy to love by some parents or carers. This does not mean that the child deserves ill treatment but, combined with other factors, it can be significant.

The significant factors about a particular child may include the following:

- *A crying child* – most people can sympathise with the stress created by a child who cries a lot; when a carer is tired, and other factors are present, the stress brought about by crying can make a child vulnerable to a violent response.
- *Interference in early bonding or attachment between carer and child* – there is a wealth of research from Bowlby onwards of the possible ill effects of early separation of parent and child. Early separation can result in a poor attachment of parent to child. There is evidence that a carer is more likely to abuse a child when the attachment to them is weak rather than strong; it is for this reason that modern antenatal and postnatal care aims to keep parents with their newborn babies and encourage the development of a strong bond between parent and child.
- *Children who are felt by their carers to be more difficult to care for at a specific stage of development* – some people find babies particularly demanding and difficult; others have more difficulty caring for toddlers or older children.
- *Children who 'invite' abuse* – these children have learned that the only attention they get is abusive; they learn to bring about certain negative reactions in their carers because this is preferable to having no attention at all.

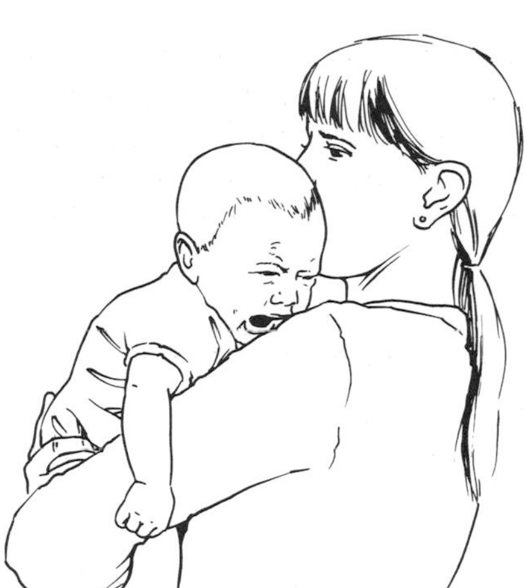

Most people can sympathise with the stress created by a child who cries a lot

Case study . . .

. . . vulnerable to abuse

Josey is the third daughter of Mr and Mrs Malik. Mrs Malik is 24 years old; Mr Malik is 10 years older than his wife. Mr Malik travels for his work and frequently spends several nights away from home at a time. This makes Mrs Malik anxious and unhappy. They live in an area where nobody has much to do with their neighbours, and she has no close friends. Mrs Malik sees very little of her family who live in the next town. She was unhappy at home as a child; her parents frequently argued and fought. She felt pleased to get away when she married. Although her husband's family lives nearby, she seldom sees them as they disapproved of their son's marriage to her as she is not from his community. Mrs Malik worries because she has never been very good at managing money or the house and her husband blames her for this. Before Josey was born they very much wanted a boy. Her two sisters are 2 and 4 years old. Mrs Malik had high blood pressure during her pregnancy; as a result of this Josey's birth was induced 4 weeks before term. During the birth she showed signs of foetal distress so a normal delivery was not possible and Josey was born by Caesarean section under general anaesthetic.

Mrs Malik was discharged from hospital 2 weeks before Josey. She found it very difficult to visit her during this time. When Josey came home, she was very unsettled and cried a lot. She took a long time to take her feed and the doctor diagnosed colic. In recent weeks Josey's mother has seen both her health visitor and doctor several times, and reported a series of minor ailments in the infant. Finally Mrs Malik called an ambulance following a long feeding session. They took the baby to the local casualty department: Josey's body was bruised and she was unconscious.

1. *What in Mr and Mrs Malik's lives and backgrounds may have contributed to the abuse that occurred?*
2. *What factors in the child may have contributed to the abuse?*
3. *What particular stresses may have contributed to the abuse?*
4. *When this case was discussed at a case conference, what plan of action do you think was agreed, bearing in mind the principles of the Children Act 1989?*

PREDISPOSING FACTORS IN CONCLUSION

There are many factors that can contribute to the abuse or neglect of children. An awareness of these can help professionals in their work with families and avoid judgemental attitudes. Such knowledge can also help workers' efforts to make the best possible decisions for a child in partnership with their parents.

Progress check

What are the needs and rights of children?

What is meant by the term 'predisposing factors'?

Name some significant stresses that can be experienced by parents of young children.

Now try these questions

Describe the development of society's awareness of child abuse.

What rights do children have and why?

What constitutes a professional approach when working with parents?

How is it possible to predict that some situations are more likely to result in a child being abused or neglected than others?

key terms

You need to know what the key terms and phrases in this chapter mean.
Go back through the chapter and find out.

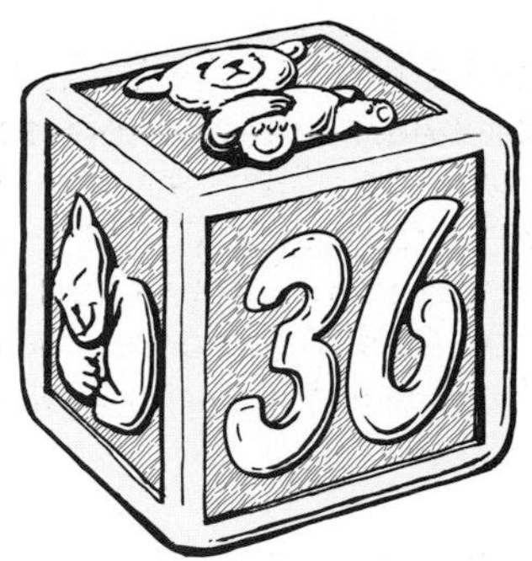

FORMS OF ABUSE AND THE EFFECTS OF ABUSE

A first step in protecting children from abuse involves workers facing up to the fact that it does happen, and then understanding the nature and types of abuse, and the signs and symptoms that may be present. A knowledge of the adverse effects of abuse on children serves to emphasise the duty of workers to make its prevention and diagnosis a key priority in their work.

This chapter will cover the following topics:

- *the effects of abuse*
- *types of abuse*
- *vulnerable children and abuse.*

The effects of abuse

The prolonged abuse or neglect of children can adversely affect all aspects of their development, their health and their feeling of well-being. It may be impossible for them to develop a positive self-image and healthy self-esteem, which can continue to affect their adult lives. Children may find it difficult to form and sustain relationships, to work or to be a good parent. The effects of abuse can be influenced for better or worse by the child's ability to cope and adapt, their previous experiences of family life, the support the child subsequently receives within the family and in the community, and the way that professionals respond.

THE IMPACT ON THE FAMILY AND COMMUNITY

The child's whole family may all be adversely affected by the abuse of a child in its midst; even if most of its members are innocent of abuse they may feel guilty for not having recognised the abuse and failing to protect the child. If a case is handled sensitively the outcome for the child and the possibility of remaining with their family is more likely to be positive.

There is recent evidence, highlighted in the media, that the presence of an abuser in a community can cause concern, particularly if the person has been convicted and imprisoned for sexual abuse. It can destabilise relationships in the community and lead to innocent people being mistakenly targeted for further punishment.

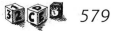

Types of abuse

Although the types of abuse are identified separately, children may be the victims of more than one type. The four types of abuse are:

- physical abuse and injury
- neglect
- emotional abuse
- sexual abuse.

PHYSICAL ABUSE AND INJURY

What is physical abuse and injury?

Physical abuse involves someone deliberately harming or hurting a child. It covers a range of unacceptable behaviour, including what some may describe as physical punishment. It can involve hitting, shaking, throwing, biting, squeezing, burning, scalding, attempted suffocation, drowning and giving poisonous substances, inappropriate drugs or alcohol. It includes the use of excessive force when carrying out tasks like feeding or nappy changing.

Physical abuse also includes Munchausen's Syndrome by Proxy. (Munchausen's Syndrome is a condition where a person presents themselves to medical staff for treatment of an illness that they do not have or have inflicted on themselves. They seek gratification from the subsequent medical attention, medical tests, care and treatment that they receive.) Munchausen's Syndrome *by Proxy* towards children occurs when a parent or carer receives gratification from the need for care or treatment by others after they have either feigned or deliberately caused illness or injury to a child.

key terms

Lacerations
tears in the skin

Weals
streak left on the flesh

Diffuse bruising
bruising that is spread out

Pinpoint haemorrhages
small areas of bleeding under the surface

Melanocytes
pigmented cells

Sacrum
base of the spine

Indicators of physical abuse

Early Years workers may be in a unique position to notice the signs and symptoms, also referred to as the indicators of child abuse. These include the following:

Bruises

Seventy per cent of abused children suffer soft tissue injury, such as bruises, **lacerations** or **weals**. The *position* of the bruising is important: bruises on cheeks, bruised eyes without other injuries, bruises on front and back shoulders are less likely to occur accidentally, as are **diffuse bruising**, **pinpoint haemorrhages** and fingertip bruises. Bruises occurring frequently or re-bruising in a similar position to old or faded bruising may also be indicators of abuse.

The *pattern* of bruises may also be an indicator: bruises reflecting the cause, for example fingertip, fist or hand-shaped bruising. Bruises incurred accidentally do not form a pattern.

It is very important that *mongolian spots* are not confused with bruises or arouse suspicion of abuse. Mongolian spots are smooth, bluish-grey to purple skin patches, often quite large, consisting of an excess of pigmented cells (**melanocytes**). They are sometimes seen across the base of the spine (**sacrum**) or buttocks of infants or young children of Asian, Southern European and African descent. They often disappear at school age. (See Chapter 5 for more on this.)

Diagnosis of child abuse is by professionals joining together to share information. It is rarely made on the basis of physical indicators alone.

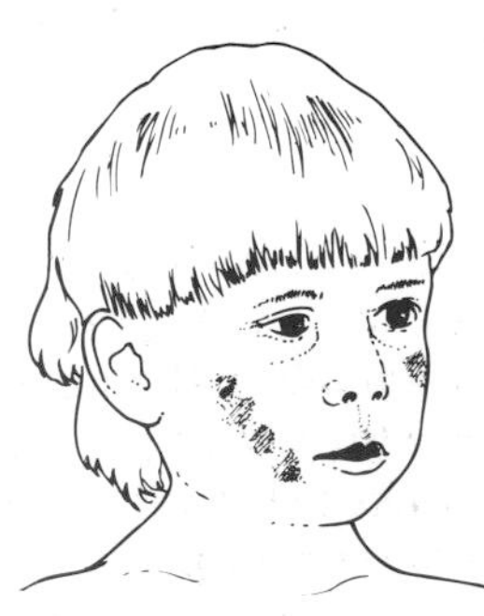

What might you suspect if you saw this pattern of bruising on a small child's face?

 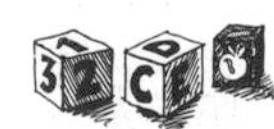

Burns and scalds

Around 10 per cent of abused children suffer burns. Examples are cigarette burns, especially when clear and round and more than one, and burns reflecting the instrument used, for example by placing a heated metal object such as an iron on the skin.

The pattern and position of scalds can be significant, showing whether hot water has been thrown deliberately or pulled down accidentally by the child. A child with scalds on the feet that are shaped like socks would imply that the child was placed in hot water and held there.

Fractures

In diagnosing non-accidental injury the following would be significant:

- the age of the child – immobile babies seldom sustain accidental fractures
- X-rays revealing previous healed fractures of differing ages
- the presence of other injuries
- the explanation given by child or carer (see Additional indicators of physical abuse, below).

Head, brain and eye injuries

Head, brain or eye injuries may indicate that a child has been swung, shaken, received a blow or been hit against a hard surface. A child's skull can be fractured and the brain damaged. Shaking a child or injuring the head can result in bleeding into the brain (a **subdural haematoma**). A child with even a small outward sign of head injury that is accompanied by irritability, drowsiness, headache, vomiting or head enlargement should receive medical attention urgently, as the outcomes can include brain damage, blindness, coma and death.

key term

Subdural haematoma bleeding into the brain

Internal damage

Internal damage, caused by blows, is a common cause of death in abused children.

Poisoning

Any occurrence of poisoning with drugs or liquids needs to be investigated.

Other marks

Other indicators of abuse may be bites, outlines of weapons, bizarre markings, nail marks, scratches and abrasions. A torn **frenulum** in a young child (the web of skin joining the gum and the lip) usually results from something being forcibly pushed into the mouth, such as a spoon, bottle or dummy. It hardly ever occurs in ordinary accidents.

key term

Frenulum the web of skin joining the gum and the lip

Behavioural indicators of physical abuse

As with any trauma, children's reactions to abuse vary. Being subjected to abuse can affect all aspects of children's development: physical, intellectual and linguistic and emotional and social. Perhaps the most significant effect of abuse is the long-term damage to a child's self-esteem, or self-respect, damage which may persist into adult life. To be abused is to be made to feel worthless, misused, guilty and betrayed. Children's feelings may be translated into observable behaviour patterns. This behaviour should be recorded in order to consider it alongside physical and additional indicators. It may help in diagnosis, but does not alone prove the existence of abuse:

- *fear and apprehension* – professionals working with abused children have described a particular attitude or facial expression adopted by abused children and labelled it **frozen awareness** or **frozen watchfulness**. This

key term

Frozen awareness/frozen watchfulness constantly looking around, alert and aware (vigilant), while remaining physically inactive (passive), demonstrating a lack of trust in adults describes a child whose eyes are constantly alert and aware (vigilant), while remaining physically inactive (passive), demonstrating a lack of trust in adults but a desire not to provoke attention

- inappropriately clinging to, or cowering from, the carer
- unusually withdrawn or aggressive behaviour (a sudden change in the way a child behaves may be particularly significant)
- the child's behaviour in role-play situations, including their explanation of how the injury occurred.

Martin and Beezley (1977) drew up a list of characteristic behaviour of abused children, based on a study of 50 abused children. The behaviour patterns may be regarded as indicators of abuse:

- *impaired capacity to enjoy life* – abused children often appear sad, pre-occupied and listless
- *stress symptoms*, for example, bed wetting, tantrums, bizarre behaviour, eating problems
- *low self-esteem* – children who have been abused often think they must be worthless to deserve such treatment
- *learning difficulties*, such as lack of concentration
- *withdrawal* – many abused children withdraw from relationships with other children and become isolated and depressed
- *opposition or defiance* – a generally negative, uncooperative attitude
- *hypervigilance*, or frozen awareness or watchful expression
- *compulsivity* – abused children sometimes feel or think they must carry out certain activities or rituals (sets of activities) repeatedly
- *pseudo-mature behaviour* – a false appearance of independence or being excessively 'good' all the time, or offering indiscriminate affection to any adult who takes an interest.

Children's reactions can be summarised as either 'fight or flight'. They may respond by becoming aggressive and anti-social (fight), or by becoming withdrawn and over-compliant (flight).

Additional indicators of physical abuse

Physical and behavioural indicators alone may be insufficient to diagnose child abuse. They should, therefore, always be considered alongside other factors. The presence of the following additional indicators increases the likelihood that injuries were sustained non-accidentally; they should be recorded alongside the physical indicators. Some of these additional indicators highlight the need to keep accurate, up-to-date records:

- an explanation by the parent or carer that is inadequate, unsatisfactory or vague, inconsistent with the nature of the injury, considering the age or stage of development of the child
- an unexplained delay in seeking medical attention, or seeking treatment only when prompted by others
- a series of minor injuries to a child, which may in themselves have satisfactory explanations
- a history of child abuse or neglect of this or other children in the family

- the existence of certain parental attitudes, such as a lack of concern, remorse or guilt over an accident, blaming others or the child for the injury, denying there is anything wrong or self-righteously justifying the infliction of injury during punishment. An example might be if a child aged 3 was found to have belt marks on their buttocks and lower back, and on being questioned the carer said, 'He deserved it. I warned him if he was cheeky once more I'd thrash him. Smacking does no good at all these days.'

Case study . . .

. . . dealing with possible physical abuse

A 2-year-old child often comes to the day nursery with fresh bruises on his arms and upper body. His mother explains these are the result of minor accidents while playing.

What might lead you to suspect that the child was being non-accidentally injured?

Explain how you would respond to the mother immediately.

Describe the procedure you would work through within the establishment, including how and what you would record.

The effects of physical abuse

Physical abuse can lead to physical injuries, neurological damage, disability and death. Children's development can be affected by the context of violence, aggression and conflict within which it takes place. It has been linked to aggressive behaviour, emotional and behavioural problems and educational difficulties.

Progress check

What is physical abuse? What does it include?

What is Munchausen's Syndrome by proxy?

What aspects of bruising are significant in cases of abuse?

What, together with a head injury, may drowsiness indicate?

Describe some possible effects of physical abuse.

key terms

Omission
not doing those things that should be done, such as protecting children from harm

Commission
doing those things that should not be done, for example beating children

NEGLECT

What is neglect?

Neglect involves persistently failing to meet the basic essential needs of a child, and/or failing to safeguard their health, safety and well-being.

Neglect involves acts of **omission,** that is not doing those things that should be done, such as not meeting a child's developmental needs or not protecting children from harm. This contrasts with other types of abuse that involve acts of **commission**, that is doing those things that should not be done, for example beating children.

Types of neglect (these areas will often overlap)

Physical neglect

Physical neglect involves not meeting children's need for adequate food, clothing, warmth, medical care, hygiene, sleep, rest, fresh air and exercise. It also includes failing to protect, for example leaving young children alone and unsupervised.

Emotional neglect

Emotional neglect includes refusing or failing to give children adequate love, affection, security, stability, praise, encouragement, recognition and reasonable guidelines for behaviour.

Intellectual neglect

Intellectual neglect includes refusing or failing to give children adequate stimulation, new experiences, appropriate responsibility, encouragement and opportunities for independence.

Indicators of neglect

The following signs and symptoms may be observed and should be recorded accurately and dated:

- constant hunger, voracious appetite, large abdomen, emaciation, stunted growth, obesity, failure to thrive (below)
- inadequate, inappropriate clothing for the weather, very dirty, seldom laundered clothing
- constant ill health, untreated medical conditions, for example extensive persistent nappy rash, repeated stomach upsets, chronic diarrhoea
- unkempt appearance, poor personal hygiene, dull matted hair, wrinkled skin, skin folds
- constant tiredness or lethargy
- repeated accidental injury
- frequent lateness or non-attendance at school
- low self-esteem
- compulsive stealing or scavenging
- learning difficulties
- aggression or withdrawal
- poor social relationships.

It is important to remember, however, that behavioural indicators may be due to causes other than neglect. Possible medical conditions that may account for the physical indicators observed will need to be ruled out. For this reason, workers need to be aware of the background of children in their care.

Case study . . .

. . . indicators of neglect

Rachel, aged 2, has just begun to attend an expensive private day nursery. Her parents, both solicitors, drop her off at 8a.m. Monday to Friday and are usually the last to pick her up when the nursery closes at 6p.m. On a number of occasions they have been as late as 7p.m. Rachel is underweight for her age, unable to manage solid food, preferring a bottle. She takes little interest in the activities of the nursery, preferring to sit alone sucking a toy and rocking rhythmically.

Her mother explains that Rachel was premature, and has never put on much weight, and that her husband's side of the family are all small anyway. Both parents resent being questioned about their child and offer extra payment, to cover the staff's inconvenience, when they are late to collect Rachel.

1. *Write a list of the indicators of neglect described in the case study.*
2. *Describe the kind of on-going records that should be available to confirm each indicator of neglect in this case.*
3. *Write a description of a child you have known to be physically neglected.*
4. *Why may the carers of the child you have described be neglecting their child's needs?*

Failure to thrive

The term 'failure to thrive' describes children who fail to grow normally. This can be for a variety of reasons. Some children are small because their parents are small. Others have a medical condition causing lack of growth. Children may be referred to paediatricians because of concern about growth. Growth charts (**percentile charts**) are used in the assessment of such children.

key term

Percentile charts/centile charts
specially prepared charts that are used to record measurements of a child's growth. There are centile charts for weight, height and head circumference

As a rough guide, any child falling below the bottom line on the graph (the third percentile) may be admitted to hospital for investigation. Most children admitted to hospital for medical reasons tend to continue to lose weight. If in hospital, with no specific treatment, the child gains weight at more than 50g a day, the failure to thrive is likely to be the result of neglect, particularly that the child has been given insufficient food.

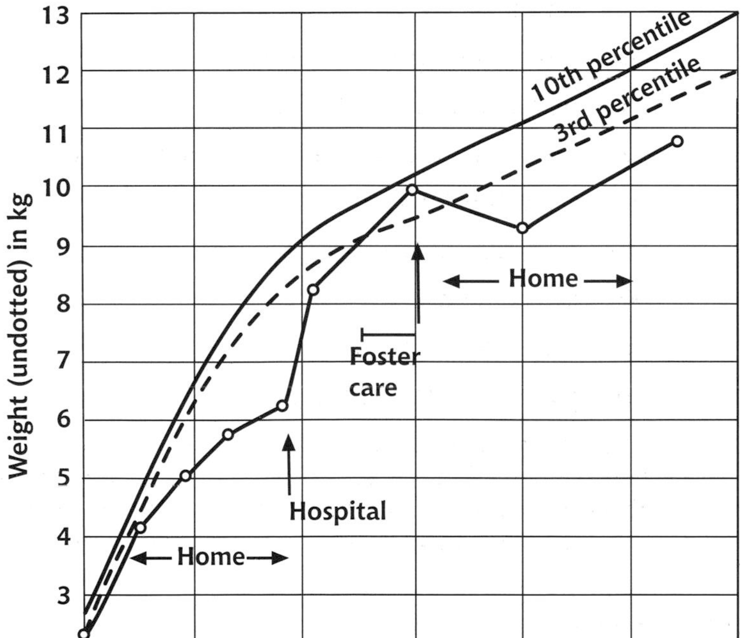

Chart showing a child's weight changes during stays in hospital, foster care and home

The effects of neglect

Severe neglect is linked to a major impairment of physical growth and intellectual development. If it persists it can lead to ill health and delayed development. Children may find social relationships difficult and their educational progress can be limited. In extremes it can result in death. Children who are neglected are more likely to be victims of other forms of abuse, such as emotional, sexual or physical abuse.

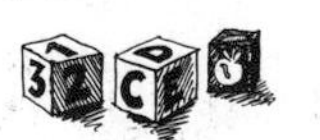

Progress check

What is neglect?

Describe three types of child neglect.

Describe the indicators of neglect.

What is failure to thrive?

Why is it important to know about the background of the children in your care?

EMOTIONAL ABUSE

What is emotional abuse?

Failing (omitting) to meet the needs of children emotionally will damage children's development. In addition, some adults commit acts of emotional abuse, such as harming children by using constant threats, verbal attacks, taunting or shouting. This category is usually used in diagnosis where it is the only or main form of abuse.

Emotional abuse includes the adverse effect on children's behaviour and emotional development as a result of a parent or carer's behaviour, including their neglect and/or rejection of the child. Domestic violence, adult mental health problems and parental substance misuse may be features in families where children are exposed to such abuse.

The effects of emotional abuse

There is increasing evidence of the adverse long-term consequences for children's development where they have been subject to sustained emotional abuse ('Working Together to Safeguard Children', Department of Health, 1999). Emotional abuse affects children's developing mental health, behaviour and self-esteem, and can be especially damaging to very young children. As an underlying factor its effects on a child may be as important as the other, more visible signs of abuse. Children may fail to thrive as a result of emotional neglect or abuse, as well as physical neglect.

Progress check

What does emotional abuse include?

What are some of the possible effects of emotional abuse?

Case study . . .

. . . indicators of emotional abuse and neglect

The Wilson family live in a well-maintained detached house in an expensive suburb. They have two children, James aged 6 and Sarah who is 4. Sarah is small for her age, with a thin, pale face. She looks sad and is wary of adults.

The nursery staff are concerned about Sarah, who seems to be failing to thrive and lacks confidence. Since starting nursery some 3 months earlier, she has been reluctant to join in structured activities and tells nursery staff that she is no good at anything.

When nursery staff invite the family in for an informal chat, Mrs Wilson constantly compares Sarah unfavourably with her brother, who looks on smugly and agrees with everything his mother says. Mr Wilson doesn't speak directly to Sarah at all, treating her as if she does not exist. In conversation with the staff he refers to her as 'just like her mother'.

The story unfolds that Sarah was premature, difficult to feed, did not put on weight, was slow to learn and was happy to be left alone to lie in her cot. Mrs Wilson often left her there as James was a rewarding child and demanded a lot of attention. Mr Wilson was away a great deal when Sarah was a baby.

Mrs Wilson made no effort to protect Sarah from the negative comments she was making, and said repeatedly to her that she was useless and hopeless, compared to her brother. James referred to Sarah as 'the dummy'. Mr Wilson said he couldn't understand what all the fuss was about, as she was only a girl.

1. *Write down the indicators of neglect in this case.*
2. *Describe how Sarah was being emotionally abused.*
3. *Describe the possible short-term and long-term effects on each aspect of Sarah's development.*
4. *How could staff in the nursery help to alleviate the effects of neglect or abuse?*
5. *How might the family be encouraged to adopt a different attitude towards Sarah?*
6. *Describe the roles of other professionals who may become involved with this family.*

SEXUAL ABUSE

What is sexual abuse?

Sexual abuse is 'the involvement of dependent, developmentally immature children and adolescents in sexual activities that they do not fully comprehend and are unable to give informed consent to, or that violate the social taboos of family roles' (Kempe, 1978). An example of a social taboo of family roles is incest.

Victims of sexual abuse include children who have been the subject of unlawful sexual activity or whose parents or carers have failed to protect them from unlawful sexual activity, and children abused by other children. Sexual abuse covers a range of abusive behaviour not necessarily involving direct physical contact. It often starts at the lower end of the spectrum, for example exposure and self-masturbation by the abuser, and continues through actual body contact such as fondling, to some form of penetration.

Who are the victims of sexual abuse?

Child sexual abuse is a universal phenomenon. It is found in all cultures and socio-economic groups. It happens to children in all kinds of families and communities. It is untrue that it is only found in isolated rural communities.

Both boys and girls experience sexual abuse. As far as we know, many more girls are abused than boys. There have been reported incidents of children as young as 4 months old being sexually abused.

Both men and women sexually abuse children. It is becoming clear that the majority of children who are sexually abused know the identity of the abuser, who is either a member of the child's family, a family friend or a person the child knows in a position of trust, for example a teacher or a carer.

How widespread is sexual abuse?

The prevalence of sexual abuse is largely unknown as it is under-reported and we are dependent on estimates. In a study of college students, 19 per cent of women and 9 per cent of men reported having been sexually abused as a child. Out of 3,000 respondents to a recent survey by a teenage magazine, 36 per cent said they had been subjected to a sexually abusive experience as a child.

Indicators of sexual abuse

Early recognition of the indicators of sexual abuse may prevent progression, by the abuser, from less to more abusive acts. If sexual abuse is not recognised in the early stages it may persist undiscovered for many years.

Physical indicators

> **key term**
> **Genital** sexual organs

The following are physical indicators of sexual abuse:

- bruises or scratches to the **genital** and anal areas, chest or abdomen
- bites
- blood stains on underwear
- sexually transmitted diseases
- semen on skin, clothes or in the vagina or anus
- internal small cuts (lesions) in the vagina or anus
- abnormal swelling out (dilation) of the vagina or anus
- itchiness or discomfort in the genital or anal areas.

In addition, there are signs that are specific to either boys or girls:

In boys:
* pain on urination
* penile swelling
* penile discharge

In girls:
* vaginal discharge
* urethral inflammation, urinary tract infections
* lymph gland inflammation
* pregnancy.

Behavioural indicators

> **key term**
> **Designated person** the person identified in an establishment to whom allegations or suspicions of child abuse should be reported

There may be no obvious physical indicators of sexual abuse, so particular attention should be paid to behavioural indicators. The following should be recorded accurately and discussed with the **designated person** in your establishment or a senior member of staff:

- what the child says or reveals through play with dolls with sexual characteristics, genitals, etc.
- over-sexualised behaviour that is inappropriate for the age of the child; being obsessed with sexual matters; playing out sexual acts in too knowledgeable a way, with dolls or other children; producing drawings of sex organs such as erect penises; excessive masturbation
- sudden inexplicable changes in behaviour, becoming aggressive or withdrawn
- showing behaviour appropriate to an earlier stage of development
- having eating or sleeping problems
- signs of social relationships being affected, for example becoming inappropriately clingy to carers; showing extreme fear of, or refusing to see, certain adults for no apparent reason; ceasing to enjoy activities with other children

 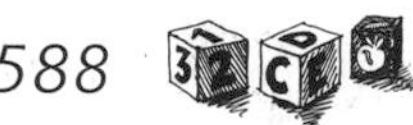

- saying repeatedly that they are bad, dirty or wicked (having a poor self-image)
- acting in a way that they think will please and prevent the adult from hurting them (placatory), or in an inappropriately adult way (pseudo-mature behaviour).

Progress check

According to Kempe's definition, what is sexual abuse?

What are the possible physical indicators and behavioural indicators of sexual abuse?

Who are the victims of sexual abuse?

Is the abuser likely to be known to the child?

Why is early recognition of the indicators of sexual abuse so important?

Case study . . .

. . . indicators of sexual abuse

Claire: During play in the nursery, Claire, aged 3 1/2, is observed to be pre-occupied with bedtimes and bathtimes. She places dolls, a teddy and herself into these situations again and again over a period of 2 weeks. She also acts out being smacked in the bath.

Rangit: When a group is asked to draw themselves for a display, Rangit draws himself with a huge penis and testicles, stating 'Boys have willies, girls have holes instead'.

Helen: Helen indicates that she is sore in the vaginal area. She has spent the previous weekend with her grandfather. Her grandfather was convicted of sexual abuse of the child's mother years ago.

Raymond: Raymond has been displaying over-sexualised play with other children. One 3-year-old boy states he is frightened of Raymond because he keeps asking him to hide and play 'sucking willies'.

Kearan and Liam: Kearan and Liam were playing together in water; both were lying naked on their stomachs. A staff member heard a lot of giggling and saw the boys doing press-ups in the water. When asked what they were doing, one boy said 'We're growing our tails'. Both boys had erections.

1. *For each of the cases above, decide whether the behaviour may be an indicator of sexual abuse or not.*
2. *Explain what influenced your decisions in each case.*

The effects of sexual abuse

Sexual abuse can lead to disturbed behaviour, inappropriate sexualised behaviour, sadness, depression and loss of self-esteem. The longer and more extensive the experience of abuse is, and the older the child, the more severe the impact is likely to be. Its effects can last into adult life. The child's ability to cope with the experience can be strengthened by the support of a non-abusive adult carer who believes the child, helps the child to understand, and offers help and protection. However, only a minority of children who are sexually abused go on to become abusers themselves.

Vulnerable children and abuse

All that has already been written about abuse applies also to disabled children and those with special needs and learning difficulties. These children are particularly vulnerable to all forms of abuse and have special need for protection.

WHY ARE DISABLED CHILDREN MORE VULNERABLE?

Some offenders abuse children because they are particularly attracted to their dependency. This, combined with society's negative attitude to disabled people, may increase the risk of disabled children, and those with learning difficulties, being abused. In addition disabled children:

- receive less information on abuse and may be less likely to understand the inappropriateness of it
- are often more dependent on physical care for longer and from different people – this increases their vulnerability
- may receive less affection from family and friends and so be more accepting of sexual attention
- may be less likely to tell what has happened (disclose) because of communication difficulties, fewer social contacts, isolation and the fact that they are generally less likely to be believed
- may have an increased desire to please because of negative responses generally, including rejection and isolation
- may lack assertiveness, vocabulary or skills to complain appropriately
- may find it difficult to distinguish between good and bad touches
- are likely to have low self-esteem and feel less in control
- are likely to have less choice generally, therefore less opportunity to learn whether to choose to accept or reject sexual advances.

Case study . . .

. . . a disabled child and abuse

Wayne Steadman, 7, has learning difficulties. He is looked after regularly by Philip, a long-standing friend of Mr and Mrs Steadman. They believe it is good for Wayne to meet older people and are glad of a break when Philip has Wayne to stay at his flat or minds him at home while the Steadmans go out.

Philip has been sexually abusing Wayne for a year. It started with Philip asking Wayne to show him his penis but has now progressed to mutual masturbation and oral sex. Philip gives Wayne sweets and tells him not to tell his parents or else he won't let Wayne stay up to watch TV with him.

Wayne tells a friend at school that he gets sweets from Philip and is allowed to stay up late watching TV if he lets Philip play with his 'willy'. Wayne's friend doesn't understand and asks Wayne to show him what Philip does. The boys are discovered in the library corner at school and asked to explain what they are doing. Wayne explains, but asks the staff not to tell his mother because she will be cross with him for staying up late.

1. *Describe how Wayne was being abused.*
2. *What indicators of sexual abuse may have been evident in this case?*
3. *Describe the possible short-term and long-term effects on Wayne of this abuse.*
4. *How could staff in school help to alleviate the effects of abuse?*
5. *Why was Wayne particularly vulnerable to abuse?*
6. *Suggest how Wayne could have been helped to protect himself and how the abuse could have been prevented.*

ABUSE BY A CHILD-CARE WORKER

Experience has shown that children can be abused in any and every setting by those who work with them. There should be clear written procedures in place in all settings to deal with such allegations, and these should be supported by the training and supervision of staff. All allegations of abuse should be taken seriously and the local child protection procedures should be used to investigate them. It is essential that all allegations are examined objectively by staff who are independent of the institution. ('Working Together to Safeguard Children', The Department of Health, 1999).

The Protection of Children Act 1999 requires child-care organisations proposing to employ someone in a child-care position to ensure that individuals are checked against a new 'Protection of Children Act List' and List 99 (DfEE) to ensure that they are not 'persons considered to be unsuitable to work with children'. It also enables the Criminal Records Bureau to disclose information about people who are included on the list along with their criminal records.

INSTITUTIONAL AND ORGANISED ABUSE

Institutional, organised or multiple abuse, including that which takes place across a family or community, involves one or more abusers and a number of related or non-related children or young people. The abusers may be acting together or in isolation, or may be using an institutional framework or position of authority to recruit children for abuse. There have been cases in recent years of this occurring in nurseries, residential homes and schools. It includes the growing use of the Internet by paedophile rings. Its investigation by police and social work staff is often very complex and difficult.

The effects of institutional abuse

This abuse is profoundly traumatic for children and its effects very disturbing. This is not least because when children are abused in institutional settings it is usually by the people they rightly expect to be there to care for and protect them. Children in foster homes and residential institutions may have been placed there to protect them from the abuse they have previously experienced at home. To be abused in these settings is a double trauma for them, leaving them with the belief that they can trust no one and think they have no one to turn to.

Progress check

Why are disabled children more likely to be abused?

What is institutional abuse?

Why is abuse in institutions potentially so damaging?

Now try these questions

Describe the main forms of child abuse.

Describe the indicators of physical abuse.

Describe the possible behavioural signs of sexual abuse.

Explain what failure to thrive means.

Explain the link between emotional abuse and all other forms of abuse.

key terms

You need to know what the key terms and phrases in this chapter mean. Go back through the chapter and find out.

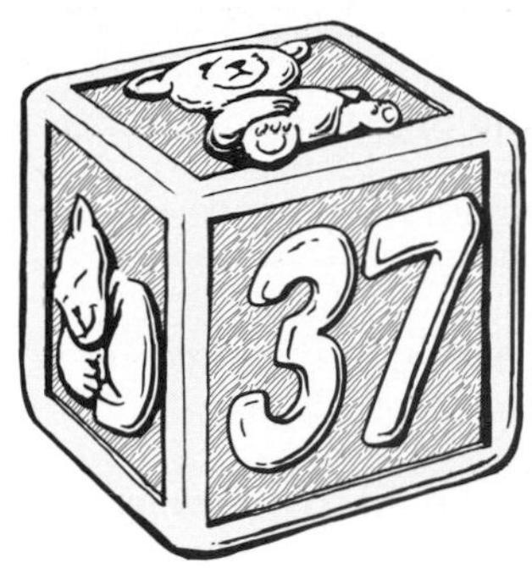

CHILD PROTECTION PROCEDURES

In the UK, as in many other countries, there are laws that aim to protect children from abuse and neglect. We have already seen that the Children Act 1989 is the most recent comprehensive piece of child protection legislation to be passed in the UK. It is based on a number of principles. One of the most important of these principles is that, when considering any action to protect a child, the welfare of the child is of the first, or paramount, importance. The Children Act 1989 also provides guidance to all local authority areas about the steps that should be taken if abuse or neglect is suspected. It requires them to agree and publish these steps, called procedures, and ensure that everyone who works with children in that local authority area is aware of them. Procedures are step-by-step instructions for action for the referral of abuse.

This chapter will cover the following topics:

- *the procedures for the protection of children*
- *referrals of suspected abuse*
- *the role of the child-care and education worker in recording the indicators of abuse*
- *dealing with disclosure*
- *procedures for the investigation of suspected abuse.*

The procedures for the protection of children

key term

Area Child Protection Committee writes, monitors and reviews the child protection procedures for its area, and promotes co-ordination and communication between all workers

Child abuse is a social and health problem that occurs among people of all social backgrounds, cultures and races. It affects both disabled and non-disabled children. It can take place in a variety of settings including the family, day care settings and residential homes. The Children Act 1989 recognises the need and right of children from every background and in every setting to be protected from abuse. The Act makes clear recommendations about how this should be done, and requires every local authority to form an **Area Child Protection Committee (ACPC)** to write the procedures for protection for that area.

The child protection procedures for any area include:

- a description of the signs and symptoms of abuse
- information needed by each agency about how to refer a concern
- details of the enquiries and protective measures that may follow a referral.

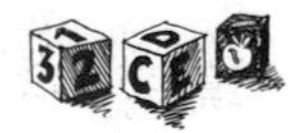

THE AIMS OF THE PROCEDURES

Child protection procedures aim to:

- protect all children from risk of abuse in any kind of setting
- give clear instructions for action to anyone involved in the care of children if they suspect that a child is at risk
- give details of how agencies, that is social services, the police or NSPCC, should deal with referrals
- promote co-ordination and communication between all workers by providing support and an understanding of their different roles.

The Area Child Protection Committee

The Area Child Protection Committee (ACPC) consists of representatives of all organisations that may be involved in protecting children. This includes the social services department, police, probation, education, the health service and representatives of voluntary organisations, including the NSPCC. The committee promotes a close working relationship between all professionals. The role of the ACPC is to write, monitor and review the child protection procedures for its area, and to promote co-ordination and communication between all workers. To do this, it uses the guidelines provided by the Children Act 1989 (see Chapter 34 for more on this).

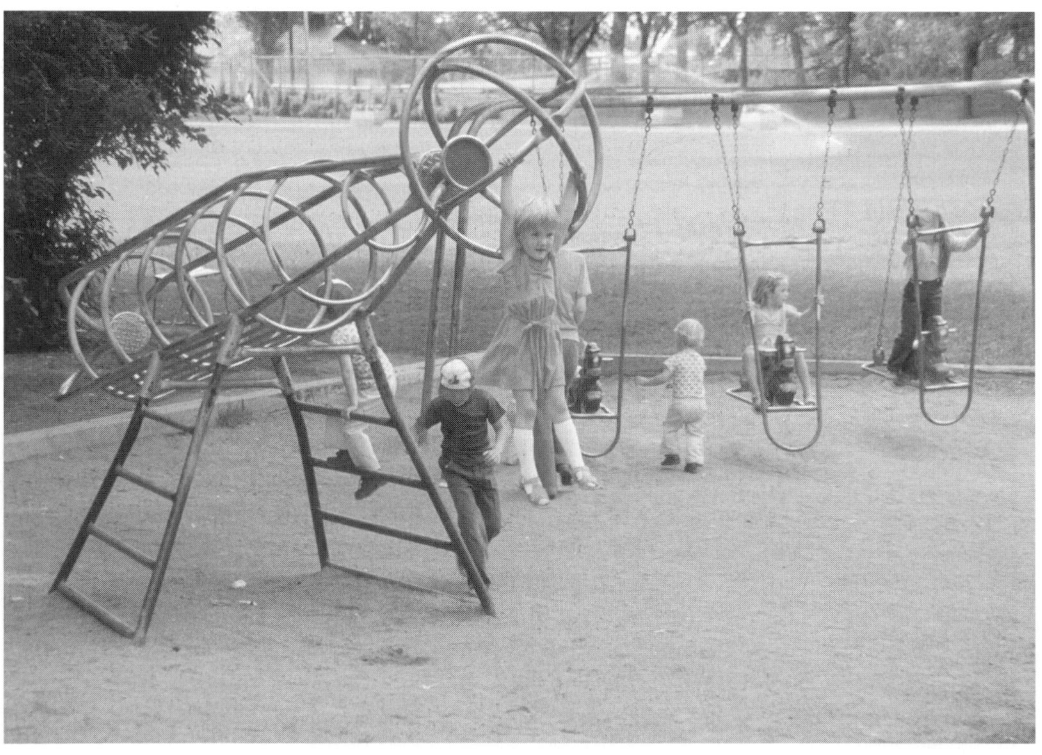

Child protection procedures aim to protect all children from all possible kinds of abuse in any setting

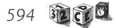

Progress check

In what settings can child abuse occur?

What are procedures?

What is the principle aim of child protection procedures?

What is the ACPC?

What is the role of the ACPC?

What is one of the most important principles underlying the Children Act 1989?

ORGANISATIONS AND PROFESSIONALS INVOLVED IN CHILD PROTECTION

All people who have contact with children have a duty to protect them. This includes people who work with children in schools, day care and health care. Certain agencies and professionals have a key role in child protection work.

THE RESPONSIBILITIES OF CHILD PROTECTION AGENCIES

Making enquiries

The only agencies with the legal (statutory) power to make enquiries and intervene if abuse is suspected are the social services department, the police, the National Society for the Prevention of Cruelty to Children (NSPCC) and the Royal Scottish Society for the Prevention of Cruelty to Children (RSSPCC). The basis for an effective child protection service must be that all professionals and agencies:

- work co-operatively on a multi-disciplinary basis
- understand and share aims and objectives, and agree about how individual cases should be handled
- are sensitive to issues associated with gender, race, culture and disability.

Promoting equality of opportunity

The Children Act 1989 makes it very clear that although discrimination of all kinds is a reality, every effort must be made to ensure that agencies do not use discriminatory practices or reinforce them. All people have a right to good, non-discriminatory services and equality of opportunity, and in some cases workers may need to take advice about how to achieve this. Child-care workers must take account of gender, race, culture, linguistic background and special needs throughout their working practices. In the opening stages especially, workers involved in child protection must keep an open mind about whether abuse has or has not taken place and avoid making any stereotypical assumptions about people. Here are some ways to increase equality of opportunity:

- Anyone who interviews a child or parent needs to use appropriate language and listening skills.
- It may help when black families are being investigated to involve a black worker, or at least someone with appropriate cultural knowledge and experience.
- It may be necessary to make arrangements for children and parents to be interviewed in their home language.

- If a parent or child has communication difficulties, for example a hearing impairment, assistance must be given during interviews.
- Remember that children and parents with disabilities have the same rights as any other person.
- The gender of those being interviewed needs be taken into account: it may be better to involve a worker of the same gender. This is especially true in cases where the victim of suspected sexual abuse is female and the alleged perpetrator is male.

THE SOCIAL SERVICES DEPARTMENT

Prevention

Social services departments have a wide range of statutory duties and responsibilities to provide services for individuals and families. The child protection work of social services departments is only a part of its child-care services. Social workers are also involved in prevention, by providing services such as referral for day care, and giving advice, guidance and support to families with children and other client groups. They have a broad awareness of the facilities that are available to help and support all families, and prevent neglect and abuse.

Making enquiries following a referral

Local authorities, through their social services departments, have a statutory duty under the Children Act 1989 to investigate any referral of a situation where there is reasonable cause to suspect that a child is suffering or is likely to suffer significant harm. They take the leading role both in enquiries, in child protection conferences, and keeping the child protection register (all described in more detail below). To fulfil this role, some social services departments have appointed social work specialists to advise and support other social workers in child protection work.

Social services departments also have a system for people to refer their concerns about individual children to them. They provide a telephone number for the public and children to contact them.

Working in partnership with parents

Local authorities must now involve parents throughout the child protection process, as long as this is consistent with the welfare and protection of the child. They must:

- give parents full information about what is happening
- enable parents to share concerns openly about their children's welfare
- show respect and consideration for parents' views
- involve parents in planning, decision-making and review.

THE NSPCC (RSSPCC IN SCOTLAND)

The National Society for the Prevention of Cruelty to Children is the only voluntary organisation that has statutory powers to investigate and to apply for court orders to protect children. To do this, it has teams of qualified social workers, called *child protection officers*. The society works in close liaison with the social services departments in the areas in which it is active.

The NSPCC is involved in the prevention of abuse, working with vulnerable children and their families, and in research and publication.

THE POLICE

Police officers have a duty to investigate cases of suspected child abuse that are referred to them. Their focus is to determine and decide whether:

- a criminal offence has taken place
- to follow criminal proceedings if there is sufficient evidence
- to prosecute if that is in the best interests of the child and the public
- to consider the best way to protect a child victim.

The police share their information with other agencies at child protection conferences. Co-operation and understanding at this level are essential.

The police also have a unique emergency power to enter and search premises and to detain a child in a place of protection for 72 hours, without application to a court.

THE ROLE OF OTHER WORKERS IN CHILD PROTECTION

Guardian ad litem

> **key term**
> **Guardian ad litem**
> person appointed by the courts to safeguard and promote the interests and welfare of children during court proceedings

The Children Act 1989 recognises that children can find it difficult both to speak for themselves in court and to understand the decision-making process. A **guardian ad litem** will help with both of these. They also provide a valuable second opinion in court about what outcome is likely to be in the best interests of a child.

Guardians are people appointed by the courts to safeguard and promote the interests and welfare of children during court proceedings. The guardian is an independent person, usually with training in social work. They have a number of powers, including being able to instruct a solicitor to legally represent a child in court if necessary.

The probation service

Probation officers have responsibility for the supervision of offenders. Through this, they may become involved in cases of child abuse, for example if an offender is released from prison. They will inform social services if they are concerned about the safety of a child who is in the same household as an offender.

The health service

Prevention

> **key term**
> **Referral**
> the process by which suspected abuse is reported by one person to someone who can take action if necessary

All health service workers are committed to the protection of children. They play an important role in supporting the social services department and provide ongoing support for children and their families. General practitioners and community health workers play an effective part in the protection of children. They identify stresses in a family and signs that a child is being harmed; they may make an initial **referral** and attend a child protection conference. Health visitors and school nurses record and monitor children's growth and development. They are in a good position to identify children who are being neglected and harmed or who may be at risk.

Treatment and examination

Where a child's health is the immediate issue, in an emergency the first duty of a doctor is to give treatment to the child as a patient. However, in situations where abuse is alleged or suspected, but there is no immediate medical emergency, a doctor's role is to examine a child who has been referred and record evidence that may be used in any legal proceedings. This is a skilled task and best undertaken by a designated doctor with a specialist knowledge of child abuse. Parents may try to prevent such an examination, but if they do, steps can be taken to protect the child, for example by calling on the police to use their powers.

The education service

Prevention

Schools may also be involved in prevention through a personal and social education programme. They can help children to increase their personal safety by developing assertiveness skills, raising their self-esteem and giving them an understanding of unacceptable adult behaviour.

Observation and referral

Teachers and other staff in schools have daily contact with children. They are therefore in a good position to observe both physical and behavioural signs of abuse. The education service is not an investigative agency; it must refer any suspicions to the social services department. All school staff need to know the referral procedures within their setting. Each school should have a trained senior member of staff who is given specific responsibility for referral and liaison with social services. This person is called the designated teacher.

Schools should be notified of any child whose name is on the **child protection register** (see below). This alerts them to observe the child's attendance, development and behaviour.

Educational welfare officers and educational psychologists also have important roles to play. They help and support the child in the school and home environment. They may contribute at child protection conferences.

> **key term**
>
> **Child protection register** lists all the children in an area who are considered to be at risk of abuse or neglect

Other voluntary organisations

There is a wide range of national and local voluntary organisations that provide services to support children and their families. National voluntary organisations, such as Barnados, the Children's Society and NCH Action for Children, all provide and run family support centres. Parentline and ChildLine provide telephone counselling and support services for parents and children.

There are many voluntary organisations that are locally based. Some of these specifically support families and children from ethnic minority groups.

Progress check

Which three agencies have the power to make child protection enquiries?

Name three things that a guardian ad litem may do.

Why may a doctor with specialist skills be needed in a child protection investigation?

What important role do child-care workers in schools have?

What is a designated teacher responsible for?

Referrals of suspected abuse

REFERRALS

Referral is the process by which suspected abuse is reported by one person to someone who can take action if necessary. Referrals of suspected abuse come from two main sources:

- *members of the public, including family members* – just over 51 per cent of all enquiries begin by someone, usually the child or member of the family, disclosing their concerns to a professional
- *the identification by professionals who work with children in a range of settings* – about 39 per cent of enquiries begin in this way.

The remaining 10 per cent of enquiries are suggested during unrelated events, such as home visits or arrests.

Referrals by members of the public

Members of the public are entitled to have their referrals investigated. If any person either knows or suspects that a child is being abused or is at risk of harm, that person should inform one of the agencies with a statutory duty to intervene (that is the police, social services department or the NSPCC/RSSPCC).

Referrals by professionals

Professionals including child-care and education workers have a duty to refer any case of suspected abuse. In order to be able to respond to signs of abuse and make referrals, professionals need:

- appropriate training to recognise the signs of abuse and neglect
- to know the procedures for the setting in which they work, including their own role, how to respond and their responsibility for referral, also whether it is appropriate either to report this to a designated person or to refer it themselves
- to be aware of the local procedures that will follow a referral of suspected abuse
- to be able to recognise and evaluate the difference between different sources of evidence, and the relative value of these including: directly observed evidence (i.e. evidence they see or hear themselves), evidence from reliable sources (i.e. the evidence of other professional colleagues), opinion (i.e. what people think, which must be used very cautiously), **hearsay** (i.e. evidence that is second-hand or more and may have been changed when passed between people).

> **key term**
> **Hearsay**
> what you are told by others

The role of the child-care and education worker in recording the indicators of abuse

> **key term**
> **Designated member of staff**
> the person identified in an establishment to whom allegations or suspicions of child abuse should be reported

If a child-care worker notices any indicators of abuse, their responsibility will include describing and recording them. They may be used for referral to, and liaison with, appropriate professionals. Records should be accurate and dated, and should clearly distinguish between direct observation and hearsay. The position of the injury, including any pattern, should be recorded as well as the nature of the injury. Physical indicators may be recorded on to a diagram of a child's body to make the position clear and accurate and to avoid misunderstanding.

All staff in an establishment need to use similar methods of recording and to share the responsibility of this task. Workers are in a good position to notice possible indicators of abuse, they must know who to report to in the establishment, i.e. **the designated member of staff.** They, or a senior colleague, should always be informed immediately in an appropriate way.

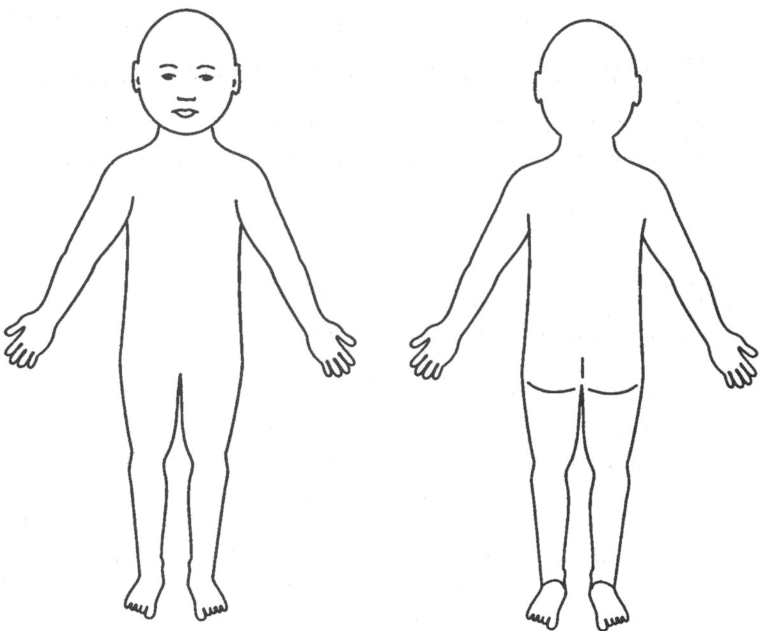

Physical indicators may be recorded on to a diagram of a child's body

Workers must be clear about the rules in their establishment concerning information sharing and confidentiality, and the circumstances under which these may be breached. If they are unsure about something they see or hear, they should discuss it with the designated person or a senior member of staff and not keep it to themselves.

Case study . . .

. . . working in a family and nursery centre

Jaswinder is a child-care worker in a busy family and nursery centre. Leanne, a 3-year-old child in her group, is giving cause for concern partly because of her irregular attendance.

Leanne's young mother, Carly, has been attending the centre and until recently staff had been pleased with the gradual maturing of her parenting skills. However, recently she started bringing Leanne late or not at all. She has also begun to make excuses about why she cannot stay on the mornings there are parenting classes. Jaswinder observes and records that Leanne now seems very hungry at mealtimes, she eats quickly and wants more, she falls asleep sometimes while playing, and is wearing small summer dresses into the late autumn. The manager of the centre has already contacted the child's health visitor who is concerned about Leanne's recent weight loss.

One morning her mother arrives late and obviously has a bruised eye herself. Leanne clings to her and cries, but Carly leaves her quickly saying she bumped into a cupboard. Another mother, Marie, is in the room at the time. She tells Jaswinder that Carly has a new boyfriend, and that the whole street knows about him because he plays loud music late into the night and is abusive to anyone who complains. She says that apparently he was in prison until earlier this year and neighbours say it was for assault. She says she thinks he is knocking Carly around and taking her money.

Jaswinder makes a full record of all she has seen and heard, and signs and dates it. She reports all her evidence and concerns to the manager.

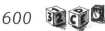

1. *What are the main causes for concern in this case?*
2. *Why is it important that the child-care worker signs and dates her report?*
3. *Give an illustrated example from this case study of observed evidence, evidence from a reliable source, opinion and hearsay evidence.*

Dealing with disclosure

WHAT IS DISCLOSURE?

key term

Disclosure (of abuse)
when a child tells someone they have been abused

In any day care setting, it is possible that children will tell a worker that they are being abused. In other words they will **disclose.** This could either happen in a full and open way, or through hinted words or behaviour. Disclosure may be partial, indirect or hidden. This may happen at inappropriate or pressured times and in awkward situations. Adults need to be prepared to respond sensitively and appropriately, both immediately, at initial disclosure, and later on. This section deals with the initial response.

THE ROLE OF THE CHILD-CARE WORKER IN RESPONDING TO DISCLOSURE

It is not possible to say exactly what a child-care worker should say when children tell them they have been, or are being, abused. Workers will need to draw on their communication skills and adapt their approach according to the age and stage of development of the child. The points below are only guidelines:

- Listen and be prepared to spend time and not hurry the child. Use active listening skills. Do not interrogate them and avoid using questions beginning Why? How? When? Where? or Who?
- Do not ask leading questions, putting words into children's mouths, for example, 'This person abused you, then?'.
- Reassure them truthfully. Tell them they are not odd or unique; you believe them; you are glad they told you; it is not their fault; they were brave to tell; you are sorry it happened.
- Find out what they are afraid of, so you know how best to help. They may have been threatened about telling.
- Be prepared to record what the child tells you, as soon as possible (within 24 hours), comprehensively, accurately and legibly, with the date of the disclosure.
- Let the child know why you are going to tell someone else.
- Consult your senior (designated person), your agency's guidelines or an appropriate professional you think will be able to help. If you are working in isolation, for example as a nanny, this may be a social worker, a health visitor, a police officer, or an NSPCC child protection officer. If you are a child-minder, you might first speak to an under 8's officer.
- Seek out support for your personal emotional reactions and needs from an appropriate colleague or professional.

Do not attempt to deal with the issue by yourself. Disclosure is a beginning, but by itself will not prevent further abuse.

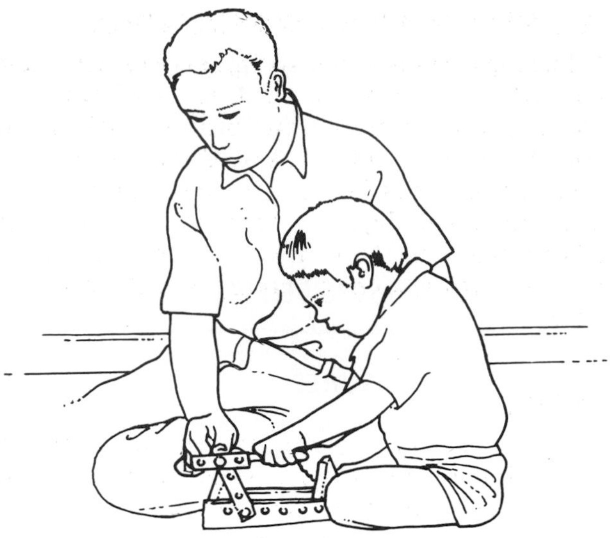

Listen and be prepared to spend time and not hurry the child

THE POSSIBLE PATH OF CHILD PROTECTION PROCEDURES

Medical emergencies

Any member of staff who discovers that a child has an injury, whatever its cause, should first decide whether the injury requires immediate medical treatment or not. If it does, the child must be taken to the accident and emergency department of the local hospital. It is better to have parental permission and involvement, although it may be appropriate in child protection cases to consult social services about gaining this.

Progress check

What do professionals have a duty to know and do in any case of suspected abuse?

Why are well-kept records essential?

What should a member of staff who discovers that a child has an injury first decide?

Why is it important to make records at least within 24 hours?

What does disclosure mean?

What does partial disclosure mean?

What are some of the important things to remember when communicating with children who tell you they have been abused?

Procedures for the investigation of suspected abuse

The procedures for the investigation of suspected abuse involve a series of steps, as outlined below.

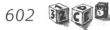

THE FIRST ENQUIRY – CONSULTATION

Following a referral, the social services department, the NSPCC and the police will consult one another, according to whom the referral was made. Records are checked, other agencies and professionals involved with the family are contacted, and the register will be checked. Those involved at this stage will decide whether there are grounds for further investigation and agree their respective roles in any subsequent **enquiry**. This first enquiry may be undertaken without the knowledge of the parents. Of the 160,000 referrals received in 1992, 40,000 resulted in no further investigation or enquiry (*Child Protection – Messages from Research*, HMSO, 1995).

> **key term**
>
> **Enquiry (into suspected abuse)**
> a local authority has a duty to carry out an enquiry if there are reasonable grounds to suspect that a child is suffering or is likely to suffer significant harm

ENQUIRY

Following a referral and consultation, if there are reasonable grounds to suspect that a child is suffering or is likely to suffer significant harm, a local authority has a duty to carry out an enquiry.

The aims of the enquiry are to:

- establish the facts
- decide if there are grounds for concern
- find out the source of the risk and assess how great it is
- decide what action, if any, to take to protect the child.

The enquiry must establish in particular whether there is an emergency and whether the police or the authority needs to exercise any of its powers under the Children Act to protect the child from any person or situation.

In order to establish the facts, social workers will make a home visit – approximately 120,000 home visits were made in 1992. They will interview the child, the parent(s), carers, anyone who has a personal interest in the child and any appropriate agencies and professionals. This may include a medical examination by a designated doctor. This is when the enquiry becomes public and the effect of this on a family can be devastating. Parents can be shocked, scared, and confused. Real care needs to be taken to work in partnership with them. Accurate recordings of any interviews are made. As with any records, the difference between fact, hearsay and opinion must be very clear. New provisions under the Criminal Justice Act 1991 allow a video recording of an interview with a child to be used as a child's main evidence in criminal proceedings.

If cause for concern is established during an enquiry, an initial child protection conference will be held. This should take place within 8 days of the initial referral, but in practice may not happen for a month.

Case study . . .

. . . the home visit

Aneka attends her local infants school. Her teacher is concerned about a recent decline in her general appearance. Her clothes and her body are frequently unwashed. At milk time she seems very hungry and asks for biscuits. Her mother's neighbour has recently been bringing her to school and implies that all is not well in the family.

The class teacher discusses Aneka with the designated teacher who decides to refer their concerns to social services. Social workers make an initial enquiry and establish that staff at the older children's school are also concerned. They decide to proceed with the enquiry and to visit the family. A social worker makes a home visit and tells Aneka's mother of the referral. She learns that Aneka is one of three young sisters who live with their mother. Her father has recently left the family home. Her mother is a shy woman, slow to tell anyone about her difficulties, but since the loss of her husband she has found it hard to cope, and this has led to some neglect of the children's physical needs. A decision is made not to refer the family to a case conference, but the social worker is able to suggest some services that will offer them help and support.

1. *Why were staff at the school concerned about Aneka?*
2. *What were the causes of the problems?*
3. *Why do you think that social services decided not to refer the case to a conference?*

POLICE PROTECTION

If it is considered that there is an emergency, the police can take a child into police protection. They can remove a child to suitable accommodation (for example, foster care or a community home), or ensure that the child remains in a safe place (for example, a hospital).

Police protection cannot last for longer than 72 hours. During this time, an officer who has special training (a designated officer) will enquire into the case. The officer must inform the child, those with parental responsibility, and the local authority of the steps taken. An appropriate court order (for example, an Emergency Protection Order, see below) must be obtained if the child continues to need protection.

Emergency Protection Order

> **key term**
> **Emergency Protection Order** a court order that enables a child to be removed to safe accommodation or kept in a safe place

If it is decided that a child needs further protection during an enquiry, the police or the local authority can apply for an **Emergency Protection Order**. To make this order, a court must be satisfied that:

- the order is in the child's best interests
- the child is likely to suffer significant harm if not removed from their present accommodation.

This order enables a child to be removed to safe accommodation or kept in a safe place. The court can also say who is allowed to have contact with the child while the order is in force.

An Emergency Protection Order lasts for a maximum of 8 days. An authority can ask a court to extend the order for a further 7 days if it needs more time to investigate. If the parents of a child were not in court when the order was made, they can, after 72 hours, put their own point of view to the court and apply for the Emergency Protection Order to be removed. The court may appoint a guardian ad litem to protect a child's interests during this period. In 1992, (the last year for which official figures are available) approximately 1,500 emergency separations were made.

Child Assessment Orders

If during the investigation a child is not considered to be in immediate danger, but the authority wish to make an assessment of the child's health, development, or the way the child has been treated, the authority can apply to the court for a Child Assessment Order, providing that:

- the parents or carers of a child are uncooperative during the investigation
- there is sufficient concern about the child

 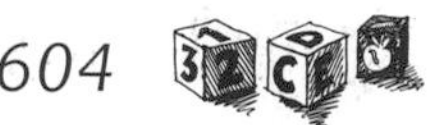

- the authority believes that the child may suffer significant harm if an assessment is not made.

The authority has to convince the court that they have made reasonable efforts to persuade parents or carers to co-operate with an assessment.

A Child Assessment Order has to say on which date the assessment will begin. It will then last for a maximum of 7 days. The court may appoint a guardian ad litem to protect the child's interests during the period of the order. Children can refuse to undergo any assessment or examination (providing they have sufficient understanding to make an informed decision about this).

key term

Initial child protection conference brings together the family, professionals concerned with the child and other specialists to exchange information and make decisions

THE INITIAL CHILD PROTECTION CONFERENCE

Following an enquiry, if there is enough cause for concern, an **initial child protection conference** is called. The Guidance to the Children Act 1989 says that this should be held within 8 working days, and *must* be held within 15 days. However, research shows that the average interval between referral and conference is 34 days.

The initial child protection conference brings together the family, professionals concerned with child protection (social services, health, the police, schools, probation), and other specialists who can give advice (psychiatrists, psychologists, lawyers). It enables them to:

- exchange information in a context within which sensitive information can be shared
- make decisions about the level of risk
- decide whether the child needs to be registered and how best to protect the child
- agree a child protection plan for the future and ensure that vulnerable children are subject to regular monitoring and review.

One of the ways that child-care workers may contribute to the protection of children is by providing information to other professionals at a child protection conference. This may take the form of a general report about a child's development, or a more specific report of something you have observed or witnessed.

WORKING WITH PARENTS

The principle of working in partnership with parents must form the basis of the child protection conference. Parents and carers will, as a matter of principle, be included in conferences. There may, however, be occasions when parental involvement may not promote the welfare of the child and they will be excluded from all or part of the proceedings. Research shows that in practice nearly a third of parents do not attend or are not invited to attend a conference. Children are encouraged to attend conferences if they have sufficient understanding. They can take a friend to support them.

The conference must assess risk and decide whether a child is suffering or likely to suffer significant harm. The conference may decide to register the child. It will appoint and name a key worker and also recommend a core group of professionals to be involved in a child protection plan. The key worker will be from the social services department or the NSPCC. However, it may agree that other workers from the core group will have more day-to-day contact with the child and family. Of the 40,000 cases that went to a conference in 1992, 25,000 were placed on the child protection register. In 96 out of 100 cases the children remained at home with relatives.

Case study . . .

. . . reporting to a case conference

Jackie is 3 years old and attends a local authority family and nursery centre. Her grandmother has made a referral to social services claiming that Jackie's mother's partner shouts at her a lot and that he makes her spend long periods locked in her room. An enquiry has resulted in a decision to call an initial child protection case conference. Marcia, her key worker at the centre, has been asked to present a written factual report about Jackie to the conference. The manager of the centre will be giving an overview report of the child, including facts about the family. Marcia is told that her factual report should be based primarily on her recorded observations of the child's development, and that it should also include:

- how long the child has been with her
- how often the child is with her during the week
- a description of the child when she arrives and leaves the nursery, including her physical and emotional state
- how the child responds when leaving and greeting her mother
- the stage of the child's physical, intellectual, language, emotional and social development
- the nature of her contact with the child's parents or carers
- whether she works alongside the parents in the nursery
- any special cultural, gender, physical or educational needs of the child.

1. *Why has Marcia been asked to write this report?*
2. *What will she base her report on the child's development on?*
3. *Why should she be able to describe accurately how the child responds to her mother, and what will she base this on?*
4. *What should she avoid including in her report?*

THE CHILD PROTECTION REGISTER

The child protection register lists all the children in an area who are considered to be at risk. A child's name is only registered following agreement at a child protection conference. The register must be kept in each social services area office. The four main categories of registration are:

- neglect
- physical injury
- sexual abuse
- emotional abuse.

But other labels are also used, including:

- failure to thrive
- a child living in the household of a previous abuser.

Following a decision to register, a child's name will be put on a central child protection register. Professionals see the register as an essential tool that gives a case conference a focus, and encourages co-operation between agencies. The registration of a child means:

- the protection plan for the child will be formally reviewed at least every 5 months
- that if a concerned professional believes a child is not being adequately protected, or that the plan needs to be changed, they can ask the social services department (or the NSPCC) to call a child protection review
- any professional who is worried about a child can quickly refer to the register to see if the child is registered and therefore considered to be at risk, and if there is a protection plan in force.

Case study . . .

. . . the child protection register

As a nursery officer in a day nursery, you have observed a child being reluctant to go home with her mother. She clings to you at home time, and you hear her mother speaking aggressively to her when leaving the nursery. A few weeks later you notice the child sitting astride a broom handle and rubbing herself and also touching herself inside her pants. You record these incidents and discuss them with colleagues. The next day you notice some fingertip bruising on the child's upper arms. You know that they were not there the day before. You report the matter to your officer-in-charge. She tells you that she will follow the child protection procedures and refer the matter to the social services department. She instructs you to write a factual report about everything you have heard and seen, and to draw on a diagram where the bruises are. Following an enquiry, the child is referred to a case conference. Investigations and discussions reveal that the mother has had a succession of male partners, and has poor parenting skills. The child is placed on the child protection register and an initial child protection plan is agreed.

1. *What were the signs that made the staff of the nursery concerned?*
2. *Why do you think the officer-in-charge decided to refer the matter to the social services department?*
3. *Why was the child placed on the child protection register?*

INITIAL CHILD PROTECTION PLAN

The initial child protection plan that is made by the core group of professionals after the conference will:

- include a comprehensive assessment of the child and the family situation
- form the basis for future plans of work with the child and family.

A CARE ORDER

If a conference concludes that a child is at risk, the social services department may apply to a court for a Care Order. If made, this places the child in the care of the local authority. It also gives the authority parental responsibility, in addition to the parents. A Care Order gives the local authority the power both to care for the child and to determine the extent that parents can be involved with their child. A child may either be placed in the care of foster parents or in a children's home.

AN INTERIM CARE ORDER

If assessments are not complete enough to decide on making a full Care Order, the court may make an Interim Care Order. This cannot last initially for more than 8 weeks; a subsequent order can only last for 4 weeks to avoid extending the decision-making process.

A SUPERVISION ORDER

If it is considered that a Care Order is not necessary, the court may make a Supervision Order. This gives the local authority the right to supervise, advise, befriend and direct the care of a child who remains at home. It is effective for a year.

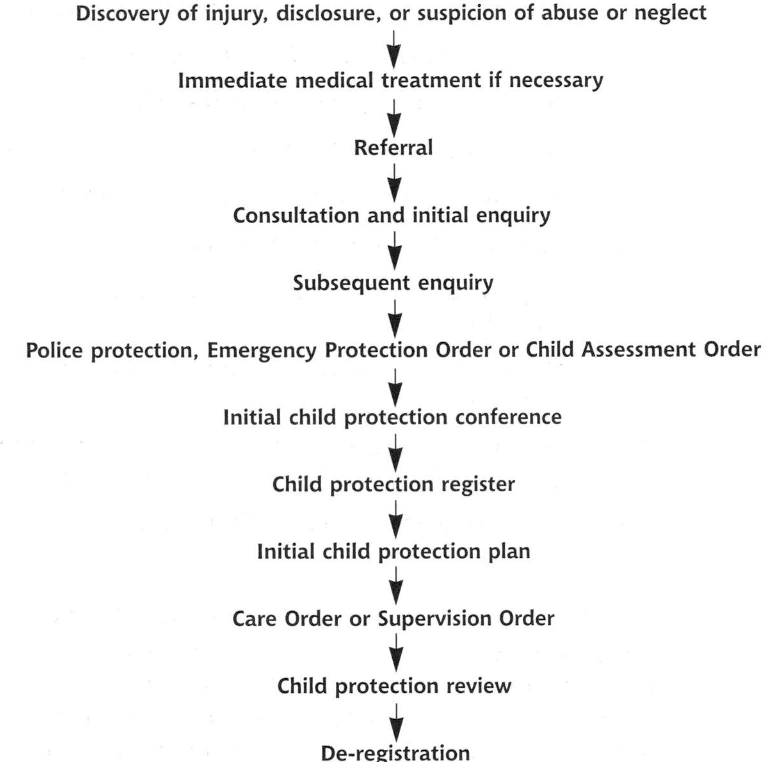

The possible path of child protection procedures

A CHILD PROTECTION REVIEW

To ensure that registered children continue to be protected from abuse, and that their needs are met, a review of the child protection plan by those involved must be held regularly, at least every 6 months.

De-registration

De-registration (the removal of a child's name from the child protection register) should be considered at every child protection review. Alternatively, a conference can be called by any agency to consider de-registration. The grounds for de-registration are:

- the original factors that led to registration no longer apply, the home situation may have improved or the abuser has no further contact with the child

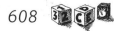

- the child and family have moved to another area (when this happens the other area will have to accept the responsibility for the case)
- the child is no longer a child in the eyes of the law: this follows an 18th birthday or marriage before this age
- the child dies.

THE PROCEDURES FOR REPORTING AND INVESTIGATING INSTITUTIONAL ABUSE

Where allegations of abuse are made against a staff member or volunteer, the procedures listed below should be followed.

1. The matter should be referred to the social services department. Social services should always discuss the case with the police at the first possible opportunity if a criminal offence may have been committed against a child.

   Any investigation may have three strands:

   - child protection enquiries related to the safety and welfare of the child
   - a police investigation into a possible offence
   - disciplinary procedures in the setting.
2. The risk of harm to children should be evaluated and managed.
3. The person involved should be supported and treated fairly and honestly and kept informed.
4. Affected parents should be given information about the concerns and of the outcomes.
5. The investigation must be open to looking at patterns that suggest it might be more widespread than at first reported.
6. If an allegation is substantiated, the lessons learned should be used to guide future practice.

Investigations of organised, institutional or multiple abuse

Each investigation of institutional abuse will be different, but all will require good planning, inter-agency working and attention to the welfare and needs of the child. In addition to the guidance above it is important that local procedures reflect the need to bring together a trusted and vetted team of police and social workers to conduct major investigations, and that any investigation involves senior mangers using appropriate resources. As with all cases, records must be safely and securely stored. Workers and the investigating team may need support and counselling.

Confidentiality

The subject of confidentiality is covered in Chapter 35, on page 573.

WAYS THAT CHILD-CARE WORKERS CAN PROTECT THEMSELVES FROM ALLEGATIONS OF ABUSE

There may be times when child-care workers are themselves accused of abuse. Sadly, although rare, there are occasions when these allegations are founded. All those who work directly with children need to consider how to avoid unfounded allegations. There may already be guidelines in the establishment in which you work. If so you should ensure that you know what they are and follow them. If not, the following common-sense ideas, from *The Kidscape Training Guide* may be used to help you to draw up guidelines for your own workplace:

- In the event of any injury to a child, accidental or otherwise, ensure that it is recorded and witnessed by another adult.
- Keep records of any false allegations a child makes against you. Record dates and times.
- Get another adult to witness the allegation, if possible.
- If a child touches you in an inappropriate place, record what happened and ensure that another adult knows (do not make the child feel like a criminal).
- On school trips, always have at least two members of staff.
- Do not place yourself in a position where you are spending excessive amounts of time alone with one child, away from other people.
- In residential settings, never take a child into your bedroom.
- Do not take children in your car by yourself.
- If you are involved in a care situation, try to have someone with you when changing nappies, clothing or bathing a child.
- Never do something of a personal nature for children that they can do for themselves, for example wiping bottoms.
- Avoid going on your own to the toilet with children.
- Be mindful of how and where you touch a child. Consider using a lap cushion with young children or disabled children who may need to sit on your knee.
- Be careful of extended hugs and kisses on the mouth from children. This may be particularly relevant to those working with children with learning difficulties.
- Always tell someone if you suspect a colleague of abuse.

Progress check

What takes place at the initial enquiry stage?

What is a case conference?

What is the child protection register?

What is institutional abuse?

What are some of the main ways that workers can protect themselves from allegations of child abuse?

Now try these questions

Describe the particular powers of the social services department, the NSPCC and the police in protecting children that are not shared by other organisations.

Describe the role of designated person for child protection in a work setting.

What are the differences between observed evidence, evidence from reliable sources, opinion and hearsay evidence?

Describe a situation that might lead to a child being referred to a case conference.

What are the possible outcomes of referrals of suspected abuse or neglect to social services departments?

key terms

You need to know what the key terms and phrases in this chapter mean.
Go back through the chapter and find out.

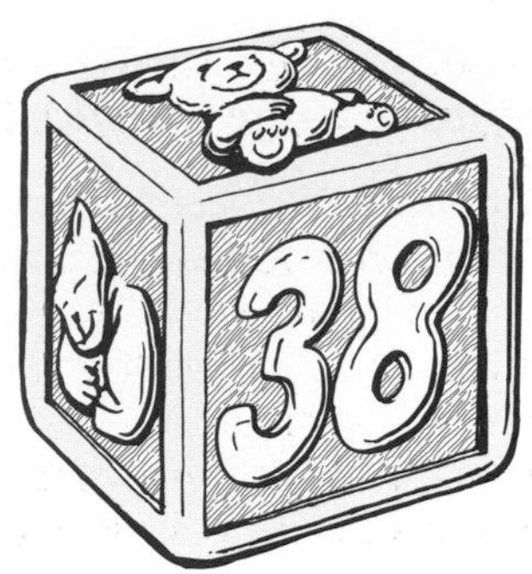

CHILD PROTECTION: RESPONDING TO CHILD ABUSE

Parents, professionals and even politicians share responsibility for the protection of children and the prevention of child abuse. Part of this responsibility involves teaching children to protect themselves. This alone will not prevent all abuse, just as teaching children about safety will not prevent all accidents. Nevertheless, it would be negligent for those concerned to fail in this responsibility. Many adults are reluctant to tackle the subject of protection from abuse because they:

- *are reluctant to recognise there is a danger*
- *feel embarrassed or ashamed*
- *want to maintain the innocence of childhood*
- *do not want to introduce the subject of sex in a negative way or frighten children*
- *are unsure how to tackle the subject.*

This chapter will cover the following topics:

- *self-protection*
- *supporting children who have been abused.*

Self-protection

PRINCIPLES OF HELPING CHILDREN TO PROTECT THEMSELVES

Much insight into the area of self-protection for children in the UK has come from the work of the Kidscape Campaign for Children's Safety and subsequently as part of the NSPCC's 'Full Stop' campaign.

Basic concepts involved in helping children to protect themselves are as follows:

- Children should understand that they have a right to be safe and how they can enhance their personal safety.
- Children should develop awareness of their bodies and an understanding that their bodies are their own and that no one should touch them inappropriately.
- Children should learn to recognise, trust and accept their own feelings.

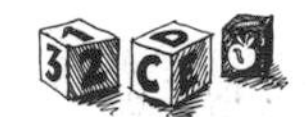

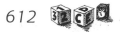

- Children's self-confidence and assertive skills should be promoted.
- It should be recognised that children need to be able to talk, to share their worries, to be listened to and believed. They need to learn that kisses, hugs and touches should never be kept secret, even if they feel good.

These concepts, together with the skills that children need to put them into practice, can be taught through the existing curriculum in schools. They can also be incorporated into themes and topics in pre-school settings. If taught well, they will promote children's confidence, assertiveness and communication skills, as well as contributing to their protection. They are relevant to all children, including disabled children and children with learning difficulties, who may be especially vulnerable.

The right to be safe

Children need to understand that they have a basic human right to be safe and to be protected from danger. They can learn that adults have a responsibility to protect them and keep them safe. The NSPCC suggests various activities to emphasise this idea, including some that increase children's understanding of who keeps them safe, how to play safely and what to do if something worrying happens. Kidscape has compiled an advice list for children's personal safety that includes not answering the door if at home alone, nor telling anyone they are alone if they ring, always telling carers where they are going, going to a safe place like a shop if lost or frightened, running away if attacked, knowing their phone number, and never going anywhere with a stranger, even if they tell a believable story.

An awareness of their bodies and their rights over them

Children can develop an awareness of their own body through curriculum activities. They need to be able to name their body parts and understand their functions at a level that is appropriate to their development. Topics such as 'All about me' will

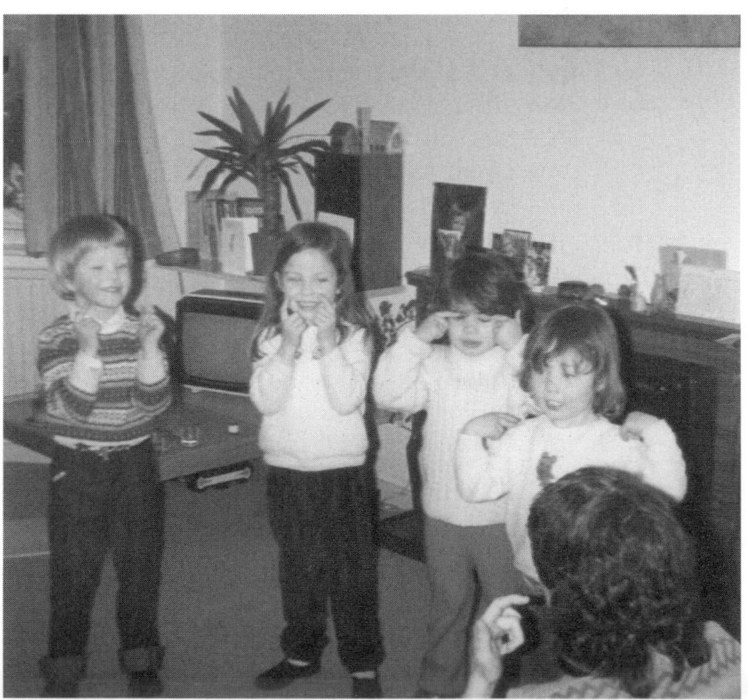

Children need to be able to name their body parts and understand their functions at a level that is appropriate to their development

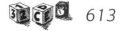

help them to understand growth and development, and activities about 'Me', for example, can help explore ideas about different rates of development and the relationship between people's size and their power. An activity about 'Me and my body' can be used to develop their understanding that their bodies are their own, that they have the right to say what touches are acceptable or unacceptable, that no one should touch them inappropriately or against their wishes. Children can think and talk about touches that feel good, safe and comfortable, and touches that feel bad, unsafe or are secretive.

Learning to recognise, trust and accept their own feelings

Children can explore their feelings and thoughts about a variety of experiences; this may include feelings about anything, but include things they don't like. They can learn to talk about 'yes' and 'no' feelings. This will help them to recognise and learn to trust and accept their own feelings.

Promoting children's self-confidence, assertive skills and body awareness

key term

Self-esteem
liking and valuing oneself; also referred to as self-respect

In order to promote children's assertive skills it is important to enhance their feelings of **self-esteem** and self-worth. Adults working with children also need to:

- contradict the usual messages they give children about always listening to adults and behaving in the ways that adults request, learning that there are times when the rules of being polite do not apply
- help children to learn how to say 'no', practising doing this in an assertive way through role play and simulations
- teach children that in some circumstances they may even need to say no to someone they love, but that if it is not possible to say no, because of fear or the threat of violence, other caring adults will understand and support them
- ensure they know the difference between safe secrets and unsafe secrets, and understand the difference between presents and bribes
- show them how to get help and adult assistance when someone tries to take away their rights, for example through abuse or bullying, and differentiate between telling tales to get someone into trouble and getting help when someone is threatening their safety.

Recognising that children need to be able to talk, be listened to and believed

Children can be encouraged to talk through devising a list of 'What if . . . ?' questions for the children in their care to encourage discussion of potentially dangerous or abusive situations. Some examples of such questions are, 'What if you were being bullied by someone who made you promise not to tell?' or 'What if a grown up told you to run across the road and there was a car coming?'.

Adults must provide situations and the time for children to talk to them. It is vital to listen to children and believe what they say.

Resources for developing awareness and protection skills

There are a large number of books and resource materials concerning protection (for example, children's books and videos) that are available to use with children. In general, they will need to be used in an interactive way with adult support if they are to be truly effective. They need to be part of a programme offering children the opportunity to discuss the issues raised. Child-care workers must be prepared for handling children's fears and worries or any disclosure of abuse.

 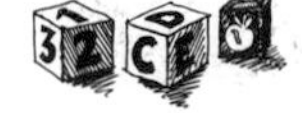

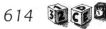

Progress check

Who is responsible for child protection?

Why are many adults reluctant to tackle the subject of protection with children?

What are the principles of child protection?

Supporting children who have been abused

DAY CARE PROVISION FOR CHILDREN IN NEED

The Children Act 1989 identifies the duty of local authorities to provide a range of services that are appropriate to the needs of children in their area who are 'in need'. These are children who are 'unlikely to achieve or maintain a reasonable standard of health or development without the provision of services'. Children who have been abused are considered to be children 'in need'.

For children who live with their families the local authority should provide family centres to work both with children and their parents and carers. They may also consider providing day care for under-5s and out-of-school provision for school-age children. A local authority may also provide particular care for young children with registered childminders. Child-care workers may work in any of these settings with young children, some of whom may have been abused.

THE ROLE OF THE CHILD-CARE WORKER

Child-care workers need to develop particular skills to help support children who have been neglected and abused. Children may tell workers or show them how they were abused.

Child-care workers may have to *observe* and *monitor* abused children, help to alleviate the effects of abuse and manage difficult behaviour. They may have regular contact with families, including those members who commit abuse.

They will probably have to record their observations for *referral* to other agencies and professionals, and *liaison* with staff, parents and carers.

To practise in a professional way it is essential to:

- recognise your own reaction to child abuse issues
- put the needs of children and their families before your own needs
- acknowledge the physical and emotional stress of working in these situations
- make provision to receive support
- form good working relationships with staff team members
- talk about and share your feelings with appropriate people.

Many of the skills required in these situations can be learned and developed during practice, supervised by experienced professionals.

ALLEVIATING THE EFFECTS OF ABUSE

The effects of abuse do not generally make children appealing. Abused children may be very difficult to like. Often they do not attract the love and affection they so desperately need. Alleviating the effects of abuse requires a professional response

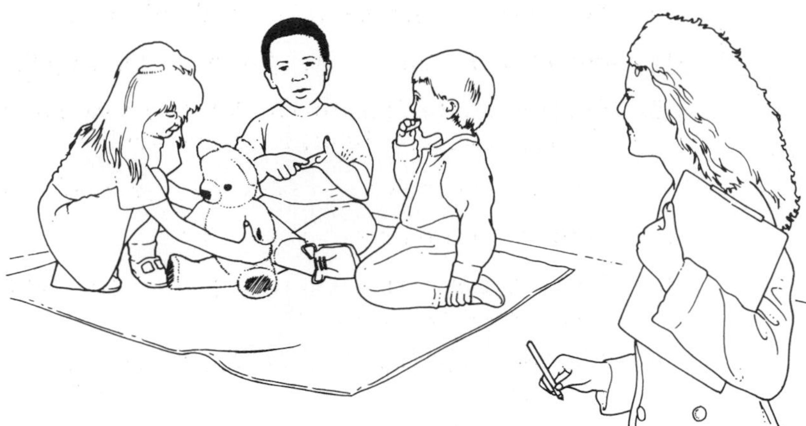

Observation skills are invaluable

that puts the needs of children before your own. Caring for abused children may provide you with a deep sense of satisfaction, but abused children are not there to provide this for you. Love and affection should be offered to even the most unattractive, unresponsive personalities. Abused children need consistent, caring adults they can rely on, who will provide unconditional love and affection.

Perhaps the most significant effect of abuse is the long-term damage to a child's self-esteem, or self-respect, damage that may persist into adult life. To be abused is to be made to feel worthless, misused, guilty, betrayed. Children's feelings may be translated into observable behaviour patterns (outlined in 'Signs of abuse' in Chapter 36).

Improving children's self-image

In order to help abused children, you need to have a good understanding of the development of self-image or self-concept. You will need to contribute to the development of a positive self-image, and enhance children's self-esteem. How you do this in practice will vary according to their age or stage of development.

Twenty golden rules for enhancing children's self-esteem:

1. From the earliest age, demonstrate love and give children affection, as well as meeting their all-round developmental needs.
2. Provide babies with opportunities to explore using their five senses.
3. Encourage children to be self-dependent and responsible.
4. Explain why rules exist and why children should do what you are asking. Use 'do' rather than 'don't' and emphasise what you want the child to do, rather than what is not acceptable. When children misbehave, explain to them why it is wrong.
5. Encourage children to value their own cultural background.
6. Encourage children to do as much for themselves as they can, to be responsible and to follow through activities to completion.
7. Do not use put-downs or sarcasm.
8. Give children activities that are a manageable challenge. If a child is doing nothing, ask questions to find out why. Remember that they may need time alone to work things out.
9. Give appropriate praise for effort, more than achievement.

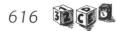

10. Demonstrate that you value children's work.
11. Provide opportunities for children to develop their memory skills.
12. Encourage children to use language to express their own feelings and thoughts and how they think others feel.
13. Provide children with their own things, labelled with their name.
14. Provide opportunities for role play.
15. Give children the opportunity to experiment with different roles, for example 'leader, follower'.
16. Provide good flexible role models with regard to gender, ethnicity and disability.
17. Stay on the child's side! Assume they mean to do right rather than wrong. Do not presume on your authority with instructions such as 'You must do this because I'm the teacher and I tell you to', unless the child is in danger.
18. Be interested in what children say; be an active listener. Give complete attention when you can and do not laugh at a child's response, unless it is really funny.
19. Avoid having favourites and victims.
20. Stimulate children with interesting questions that make them think.

Encouraging expression of feeling

Abused children benefit from involvement in activities that enable and encourage them to express their feelings in an appropriate, acceptable way. There are many activities that child-care workers can plan to help children to understand feelings and express them in positive and safe ways. Those who work with abused children need to understand the link between feelings and behaviour. They need to be able to see beyond presenting behaviour to children's underlying feelings, and to respond to these rather than to the unacceptable behaviour they may demonstrate.

Observation skills are invaluable in this respect. Information from observations should be carefully recorded and available to all those involved with the care of an abused child. It is not always possible to be certain about children's feelings. The behaviour observed should always be recorded as well as what you think the child was feeling (the evaluation or interpretation).

Managing anger and difficult behaviour

Emotional damage may well show itself in anti-social behaviour. Even if you understand the reason for abused children's feelings, it may not be easy to cope with their behaviour. The way you respond to difficult behaviour will affect children's self-image and self-esteem. Appropriate responses can help to alleviate the effects of abuse.

It is impossible to give detailed advice about how to respond to all the situations that you may encounter. The table below summarises the underlying principles for managing difficult behaviour. They may be difficult to live up to in practice, but it is important to set high standards. Abused children may already have suffered considerable emotional damage at the hands of an adult in a position of trust.

We all respond more to praise and encouragement than punishment. If punishment cannot be avoided, keep it as low-key as possible. Seek to make punishment a removal of attention from the child, rather than a drama that they will want to repeat because it brings them attention.

PRACTICAL POINTS FOR MANAGING ANGER AND DIFFICULT BEHAVIOUR

DO	DON'T
• Reward positive or acceptable behaviour • Routinely give praise, time and attention • Remain calm and in control of your feelings • Respect the child • Reassure the child that you will go on loving them • Recognise how the child's behaviour makes you feel • Restrain the child gently if necessary • Reason with the child • Respond consistently to similar events	• Punish aggressive behaviour with violence • Presume that a child's behaviour is aimed at you personally • Pretend that everything is all right if it is not • Presume that you are always right • Promise what you cannot do

It is important to remember that a child's feelings of anger, frustration or distress can lead to aggressive behaviour. It is not helpful for children to bottle up their feelings, or be told they are naughty and be punished for them. Children need to learn to direct their aggression in a way that gives them some relief without harming themselves or others. Play with malleable and natural materials such as dough, clay, sand and paint can help a child to do this and to talk about how they feel.

Play therapy and the use of anatomically correct dolls

Some abused children will need expert professional counselling or play therapy in order to alleviate the effects of abuse. This may be with a child psychologist, a psychiatrist, a counsellor or a play therapist. You may be involved in liaising with these professionals. Under their direction you may be involved in the use of **anatomically correct dolls** with children who have suffered sexual abuse.

> **key term**
> **Anatomically correct dolls** dolls with accurately reproduced body parts including sexual organs

Use of the dolls can be helpful because they:

- ease the anxiety involved in discussing sexual matters for the adults as well as the children
- act as an ice-breaker to get discussion going, possibly by establishing names for describing the sexual organs and their characteristics
- appeal to a wide age range of children
- maintain a child-oriented atmosphere
- give the child permission to discuss sexual matters and understand what is natural.

The dolls can be used to:

- give children an opportunity to act out, through the dolls, their feelings about what has happened to them
- educate children about sexual matters generally
- describe and demonstrate the events involved in the abuse

- facilitate group or individual play therapy sessions, involving other family members.

They may also be used to encourage and enable disclosure in the investigation of suspected abuse and to obtain evidence of actual abuse. In these contexts their use may be videoed.

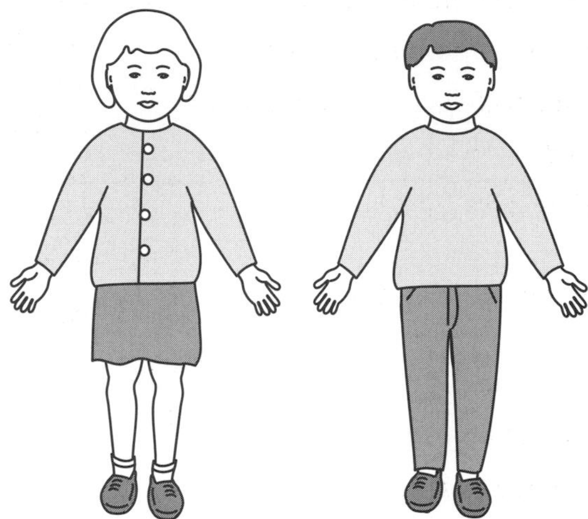

The use of anatomically correct dolls may ease the anxiety involved in discussing sexual matters

Partnership with parents and carers

Part of your responsibility may include working with parents. Your aim will be to enhance, not undermine, the relationship between abused children and their parents or carers. Support and encouragement should be given to parents or carers to motivate them to emulate good methods and practices in relation to their child, rather than to judge and alienate them.

It may be necessary to help particular children to develop positive relationships with their parents or carers. This role will require sensitivity and a real understanding of the importance of the relationship between parent or carer and child. It will require a genuine commitment to partnership with parents.

Progress check

Why may abused children be difficult to like?

Why do abused children desperately need unconditional love and affection?

Take each of the 20 golden rules listed on pages 616–17 and explain why they are likely to enhance children's self-esteem and contribute to the development of a positive self-image or self-concept.

How does the way you respond to difficult behaviour affect children's self-image or self-esteem?

How can appropriate responses help to alleviate the effects of abuse?

Why is praise and encouragement more effective than punishment?

How can dolls be used to help abused children?

What activities help children to express strong feelings safely?

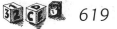

Now try these questions

Describe the ways that the effects of abuse can be alleviated.

How can the difficult behaviour demonstrated by abused children be managed?

key terms

You need to know what the key terms and phrases in this chapter mean.
Go back through the chapter and find out.

Unit 10: Anti-discriminatory/Anti-bias Practice

In this unit you will learn about the rights of children and their families and the causes and effects of discrimination. You will learn about legislation, charters and policies designed to promote equal opportunities and the role of the child-care and education worker in promoting anti-discriminatory and anti-bias practice.

Throughout this book the balance of rights and responsibilities of individuals and families is explored, e.g. in the context of child protection. In this Unit they are explored in the context of ensuring equality of opportunity.

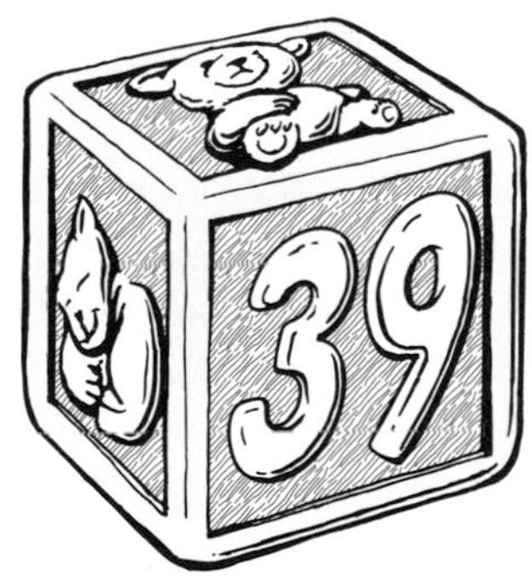

THE RIGHTS OF CHILDREN AND THEIR FAMILIES

Although the principles of rights, equality of opportunity, anti-discriminatory and anti-bias practice are dealt with separately in the following chapters, they should be seen as integral to all the work you do in child care and education. As well as understanding the issues, you will need to develop self-awareness and a positive attitude that values diversity in order to work this understanding out in practice.

This chapter will cover the following topics:

- *the rights and needs of children*
- *the causes and effects of discrimination*
- *how society promotes equal opportunities.*

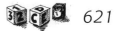

The rights and needs of children

The following statements, taken from *Young Children in Group Day Care: Guidelines for Good Practice* by the Early Childhood Unit of the National Children's Bureau, outline a challenging set of beliefs about the needs and rights of young children. They apply equally well to any care or educational setting:

- Children's well-being is paramount.
- Children are individuals in their own right, and they have differing needs, abilities and potential. Thus any day care facility should be flexible and sensitive in responding to these needs.
- Since discrimination of all kinds is an everyday reality in the lives of many children, every effort must be made to ensure that services and practices do not reflect or reinforce it, but actively combat it. Therefore equality of opportunity for children, parents and staff should be explicit in the policies and practice of a day care facility.
- Working in partnership with parents is recognised as being of major value and importance.
- Good practice in day care for children can enhance their full social, intellectual, emotional, physical and creative development.
- Young children learn and develop best through their own exploration and experience. Such opportunities for learning and development are based on stable, caring relationships, regular observation and ongoing assessment. This will result in reflective practitioners who use their observations to inform the learning experiences they offer.
- Regular and thorough evaluation of policies, procedures and practices facilitates the provision of high quality day care.

THE HUMAN RIGHTS ACT 1998

The European Convention on Human Rights was a treaty ratified by the UK in 1951 guaranteeing the various rights and freedoms in the United Nations Declaration on Human Rights, adopted in 1948. The Human Rights Act 1998, which came fully into force on 2 October 2000, gives people in the UK opportunities to enforce these rights directly in the British courts, rather than having to incur the cost and delay of taking a case to the European Court in Strasburg.

The causes and effects of discrimination

THE ROLE OF ATTITUDES, VALUES AND STEREOTYPED VIEWS IN INFLUENCING BEHAVIOUR

Attitudes and discrimination

It is important that child-care workers demonstrate positive attitudes towards the children and families that they work with. Children and their families need to feel that they are valued for themselves, for who they are. Negative attitudes on the part of child-care workers can lead to discriminatory practices, which affect feelings of self-worth. This may result in children failing to achieve their potential in later life and in families becoming disaffected with the child-care centre and its workers.

Positive and negative attitudes

Attitudes reflect our opinions. These can be both positive and negative. Our attitude to people affects the way we act and behave towards them. If we demonstrate a positive attitude towards someone, it enables that person to feel good, valued and have high **self-esteem**. A negative attitude towards a person is likely to lower their self-esteem and to make them feel worthless and rejected.

> **key term**
> **Self-esteem** liking and valuing oneself

Labelling and stereotyping

Stereotyping contributes to the development of negative attitudes. It involves making assumptions about people, without any evidence or proof, because, for example, they are of a particular race, gender or social origin. Stereotypes are harmful because they perpetuate negative, unthinking attitudes: they are limiting because they influence expectations.

> **key term**
> **Stereotyping** when people think that all the individual members of a group have the same characteristics as each other; often applied on the basis of race, gender or disability

We give specific names to some negative attitudes:

- Racism describes when people of one race or culture believe that they are superior to another.
- Sexism is the term used when people of one gender believe that they are superior to the other.
- Stereotypical assumptions are often made about people with disabilities, those in the lower **socio-economic groups**, gay men and lesbian women, and other minority groups.
- Where one group in society is powerful and holds stereotypical views about other groups, **discrimination** and **oppression** are likely to occur. This can reduce the choices, chances and, ultimately, the achievements of that group.

> **key terms**
> **Socio-economic group** grouping of people according to their status in society, based on their occupation, which is closely related to their wealth/income
> **Discrimination** behaviour based on prejudice, which results in someone being treated unfairly
> **Oppression** using power to dominate and restrict other people

INSTITUTIONAL DISCRIMINATION

Discrimination can occur even when individual workers have positive attitudes. If the institution does not consider and meet the needs of everyone involved in it and makes assumptions based on one set of values/stereotyped views, **institutional discrimination** can occur. This can happen when, for example:

- children with disabilities are not given access to the full curriculum
- the meals service does not meet the dietary requirements of certain religious groups
- a uniform code does not consider the cultural traditions of certain groups concerning dress.

Child-care workers are often not aware of how powerful the culture and institutionalised practices of their organisation are in discriminating against certain groups of children and their families. Institutional discrimination is not necessarily a conscious policy on the part of the organisation; more often it occurs because of a failure to consider the diversity of the community. Whether conscious or unconscious, institutional discrimination is a powerful and damaging force.

> **key term**
> **Institutional discrimination** unfavourable treatment occurring as a consequence of the procedures and systems of an organisation

THE EFFECTS OF DISCRIMINATION AND DISCRIMINATORY PRACTICES ON CHILDREN'S DEVELOPMENT

Children may suffer the effects of stereotyping and discrimination in a number of ways:

- Research by Milner (1983) shows that children as young as 3 attach value to skin colour, with both black and white children perceiving white skin as 'better' than black. This indicates that children absorb messages about racial stereotyping from a very early age. These messages are very damaging to the self-esteem of black children and may result in a failure to achieve their potential. Harm is done to white children too, and to society in general, unless this perception of racial superiority is confronted and challenged effectively. These findings underline the need for all settings, including those in all-white areas, to provide a positive approach that challenges stereotyping.

- Even very young children can hold fixed ideas about what boys can do and what girls can do. Observation of children's play shows that some activities are avoided because of perceptions of what is appropriate for girls or for boys. This can result in boys and girls having a very limited view of the choices available to males and females in our society. This is particularly significant when, despite advances in recent years, many women still under-achieve.
- Children with disabilities and their families are subject to many forms of discrimination. Even a caring environment may neglect the ordinary needs of the disabled child out of a concern to meet their special needs. This may mean that the disability is seen first, rather than the child, and that the child's development is affected because of limited opportunities and low expectations.
- Statistically, children from lower socio-economic groups under-achieve academically. As there is a strong connection between educational success and subsequent economic well-being, this is a worrying link which government policy is keen to address.

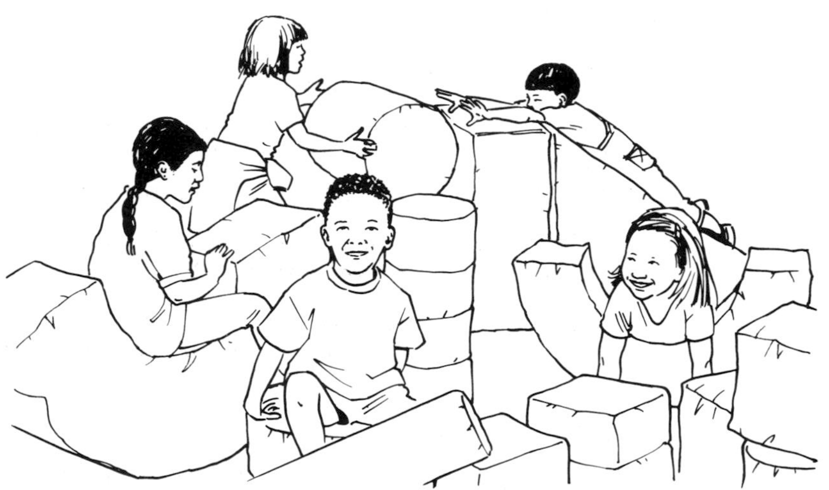

Child-care practice must meet the needs of a culturally diverse community

Progress check

Why is it important that child-care workers demonstrate positive attitudes towards the children and families that they work with?

What are the effects of stereotyping and discrimination?

What is institutionalised discrimination?

Which are the main groups that are likely to be affected by discrimination?

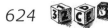

How society promotes equal opportunities

key term

Equal opportunities all people participating in society to the best of their abilities, regardless of race, religion, disability, gender or social background

Promoting **equal opportunities** means giving everyone an equal chance to participate in life to the best of their abilities, regardless of race, religion, disability, gender or social background. This will not be achieved by treating everyone the same, but by recognising and responding to the fact that people are different, and that different people will have different needs and requirements. If these needs and differences are not recognised, then people will not receive equality of opportunity.

Equality of opportunity is promoted in a number of ways:

- At government level, laws exist that are aimed at combatting oppression and discrimination.
- At institutional level, many organisations have policies and codes of conduct that promote equality.
- On a personal level, equal opportunities are addressed as the awareness of individuals is raised, and they examine their own attitudes and values.

GOVERNMENTAL LEVEL

The role of legislation

Laws in themselves do not stop discrimination, just as speed limits do not stop people speeding. However, the existence of a law does send out a very clear message that discrimination is not acceptable and that penalties exist for those who flout the laws.

Legislation to combat racism

- The Race Relations Act 1965 outlawed discrimination on the basis of race in the provision of goods and services, in employment and in housing. Incitement to racial hatred also became an offence under this Act.
- In 1976 the Commission for Racial Equality was given power to start court proceedings in instances of racial discrimination.
- The Children Act 1989 required that needs arising from children's race, culture, religion and language be considered by those caring for them.

Legislation to combat sexism

- The Equal Pay Act 1970 gave women the right to equal pay with men for work of the same value.
- The Employment Protection Act 1975 gave women the right to paid maternity leave.
- The Sex Discrimination Act 1975 outlawed discrimination on the grounds of sex in employment, education, provision of goods and services and housing.
- The Equal Opportunities Commission was set up in 1975 to enforce the laws relating to discrimination on the grounds of sex.

Disability legislation

- The Education Act 1944 placed a duty on local education authorities (LEAs) to provide education for all children, including those with special needs.

- The Disabled Persons (Employment) Act 1944 required larger employers to recruit a certain proportion of registered disabled people into their workforce.
- The Education Act 1981 laid down specific procedures for the assessment and statementing of children with special educational needs. This was superseded by the Code of Practice for Special Educational Needs, which was introduced as part of the Education Act 1993.
- The Chronically Sick and Disabled Persons Act 1970 and the Disabled Persons Act 1986 imposed various duties on local authorities towards disabled people.
- The Children Act 1989 defined the services that should be provided by the local authority for 'children in need'. Children who are disabled are included in this category.
- The Disability Discrimination Act 1995 was passed to ensure that any services offered to the public in general must be offered, on the same basis, to people with disabilities.

Although there appears to be a substantial amount of legislation here, it should be remembered that it is up to the person who feels that they have been discriminated against to make a case and start proceedings. Successful prosecutions are comparatively rare.

INSTITUTIONAL LEVEL

Policies and procedures

Many organisations have developed and adopted their own equal opportunities policies, which they apply to matters involving both staff and clients. Operating against the policy will often have serious disciplinary implications for staff involved. As with all policies, equal opportunities policies are only effective in promoting their aims if staff are committed to implementing them, if they are properly resourced and if they are regularly evaluated, reviewed and updated.

> **key term**
>
> **Anti-discriminatory practice**
> practice that encourages a positive view of difference, and opposes negative attitudes and practices that lead to unfavourable treatment of people

HOW INDIVIDUALS CAN PROMOTE EFFECTIVE EQUAL OPPORTUNITIES, ANTI-DISCRIMINATORY AND ANTI-BIAS PRACTICE

As individuals, people contribute to promoting effective equal opportunities, **anti-discriminatory** and anti-bias practice by:

- examining their own attitudes and values – this can sometimes be a difficult and disturbing experience
- challenging behaviour and language that is abusive or offensive
- increasing their knowledge and understanding of people who are different from themselves
- undertaking training to increase their ability to provide for the needs of all.

Progress check

What do you understand by the term 'equality of opportunity'?

Why is treating everyone the same unlikely to provide equality of opportunity?

Why is it important to have laws that deal with discrimination?

How can equal opportunities policies promote equality?

What can an individual child-care worker do to promote equality?

VALUING DIVERSITY

The first step in implementing anti-discriminatory and anti-bias practice is to recognise the diversity of our society and to value this diversity as a positive rather than a negative factor.

Valuing a variety of child-rearing practices

key term

Non-judgemental
not taking a fixed position on an issue

In order to be able to do this, child-care workers will need to adopt an approach that is **non-judgemental** when working with families. This means that differences in family style, beliefs, traditions and, in particular, ways of caring for children should not be judged as being better or worse but should be respected. Different families will provide for their children in a number of different ways and child-care practice that is **anti-discriminatory** will seek to meet the needs of all families within a framework that respects their individuality.

Case study . . .

. . . responding to difference

Dinh started at playgroup when he was 3. His family had recently moved to the small town where the playgroup was located. His mother and father spoke some English, but Dinh understood and spoke only Vietnamese. The playgroup staff had little experience of working with non-English-speaking children, but they contacted the local education authority who were able to provide them with some support from a peripatetic English as a Second Language teacher and access to some specialised resources. Together with the teacher, the staff were able to support Dinh who gradually gained competence and confidence in English, and was soon able to join in and enjoy all the playgroup activities.

1. *What were Dinh's needs?*
2. *What would have happened to Dinh if the playgroup staff had not responded to him in this way?*
3. *Think of some other situations where failing to respond to difference would result in needs not being met?*

THE WORKER'S ROLE IN RECOGNISING DISCRIMINATION AND DISCRIMINATORY PRACTICES

The clearest indication that child-care workers value diversity will be in a positive environment provided for the care and education of children. In this context, the environment comprises the attitudes and behaviour of everyone associated with the centre, as well as the physical environment of buildings, displays and equipment, and the day-to-day implementation of care and the curriculum. An approach that values diversity enriches the experience of all children and prepares them for adult life in today's society. The following should be considered:

key term

Positive image
an image that challenges stereotypes and that extends and increases expectations

- demonstrating, through a positive approach, that you value families and children for themselves
- providing resources, including books and displays, that present **positive images**, particularly of under-represented groups

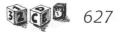

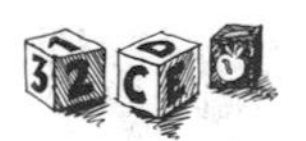

- ensuring that the environment and activities presented are accessible to all children in the group, including those with disabilities
- giving consideration to the wishes and customs of parents concerning the care of their children. This may include preferences concerning diet or dress or any other matter
- having an equal opportunities perspective as an integral element of curriculum planning
- encouraging all children to participate in a full range of activities that avoid gender and cultural bias
- taking **positive action** when one child or group of children seems to be at a disadvantage. Intervention and another approach will often solve the problem
- encouraging staff to question their own attitudes and values. Is rough play more readily accepted from boys than from girls? Do staff have lower expectations of children from some socio-economic groups, of children from ethnic minority groups or of children with disabilities?
- showing a commitment to monitoring and evaluating provision to ensure that it meets the needs of all groups.

key term

Positive action
taking steps to ensure that a particular individual or group has an equal chance to succeed

THE WORKER'S ROLE IN CONFRONTING AND COMBATING DISCRIMINATION AND DISCRIMINATORY PRACTICES

There are occasions when, despite taking the positive steps outlined above, childcare workers will have to deal with instances of discrimination. This is likely to be a difficult and challenging experience. It may be helpful to consider some strategies in advance:

- Challenge abusive behaviour or language. This could be the sexist joke you overhear in the lift or the racist remark someone makes in the staff room. If you allow the incident to go unchallenged, you will appear to be condoning it. If this occurs at work, you may need to discuss the incident with your manager.
- Take seriously any incidence of name calling or bullying. It is not enough to comfort the victim; the behaviour must be challenged and be seen to be unacceptable.
- Remember that language has a powerful influence in shaping children's self-esteem and identity. Be aware of the terms that you use. Sexist comments about 'strong boys' and 'pretty girls' reinforce stereotypes. Avoid terms that associate black with negative connotations, such as 'black mood', 'black magic', 'accident black spot', rather than in a descriptive way, such as 'black paint', 'black trousers', 'black coffee'. Challenge abusive words such as 'nigger', 'spastic' and 'cripple' when you hear them used by children and by adults.

Everyone who works with children is very influential in the formation of their attitudes and values. Children will take their cue from adult responses and reactions, and it is therefore important that staff do not skate over issues of equality.

Case study . . .

. . . responding to discriminatory behaviour

Luke and Callum both attended a busy inner-city nursery. They lived on the same street and were often dropped off at nursery together. The nursery staff were puzzled when they stopped playing together and, in fact, began to avoid one another. One afternoon it became clear what had happened. At home time, their mothers started arguing outside the nursery entrance. They had fallen out about one of them playing loud music late at night and disturbing the neighbours. The argument became very heated, culminating in Callum's mother shouting abuse and calling Luke and his mother a pair of 'black bastards'. The nursery staff heard what was going on and tried to calm things down by separating them and taking them into other rooms, away from the children. The teacher asked them both to come and see her the next day. When she spoke with Callum's mother, she made it clear to her why her remarks were unacceptable and asked for an assurance that it would not happen again or she would not be welcome on nursery premises in future.

1. *Why was this a difficult situation for the nursery staff to deal with?*
2. *How did they manage to defuse the situation?*
3. *What would the needs of the children be in this situation?*

Progress check

Why is it important to value diversity?

How can child-care workers show their commitment to promoting diversity?

What can child-care workers do to oppose discrimination?

Why is language an important aspect of anti-discriminatory practice?

Why should you always take a stand when you witness abusive or discriminatory behaviour?

Now try these questions

Why is a consideration of equal opportunities an important issue for child-care workers?

What laws exist to counter discrimination? Why are successful prosecutions rare?

As officer-in-charge, you are responsible for ensuring that the nursery reflects the cultural diversity of the community. How would you do this?

Within your day-to-day work as a child-care worker, how can you oppose discrimination?

What kinds of training activities do you think would be helpful for child-care workers who are committed to implementing anti-discriminatory practice?

key terms

You need to know what the key terms and phrases in this chapter mean. Go back through the chapter and find out.

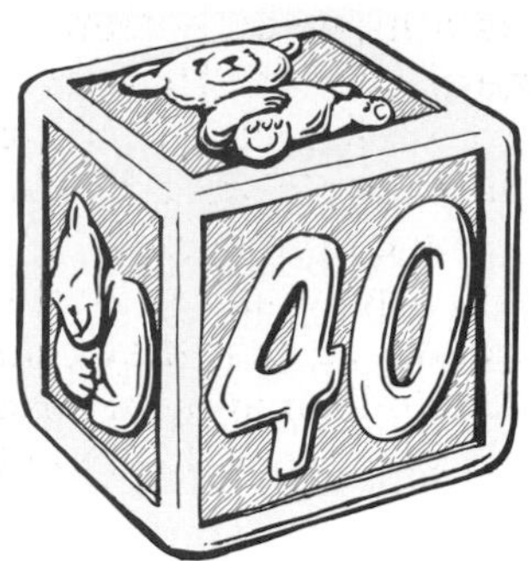

THE IDENTIFICATION OF DISABLED CHILDREN (CHILDREN WITH SPECIAL EDUCATIONAL NEEDS)

Understanding the needs of disabled children requires a thorough knowledge of child development. Unit Four provides detailed information on each aspect of children's development: physical development, language and cognitive development, and social and emotional development. All of this is relevant to the development of disabled children and their needs should be considered alongside those of all children.

The information given here cannot cover every aspect of disability. There are many condition- or impairment-specific organisations working with particular groups of disabled people that produce useful information and offer disability-awareness training. To be authentic, such information and training should include those most closely involved: disabled people themselves.

It is now more likely that disabled children will be included in all settings, such as nursery classes, schools, day nurseries, family centres or residential establishments. For child-care practice to be truly inclusive, the needs of disabled children and their families must be recognised and met.

This chapter will cover the following topics:

- *the causes and effects of discrimination*
- *how society promotes equal opportunities for disabled children*
- *the identification of children with special educational needs*
- *the special educational needs Code of Practice.*

The causes and effects of discrimination

key term

Disability
the disadvantage or restriction of activity caused by society that takes little or no account of people who have physical or mental impairments and thus excludes them from the mainstream of

THE ROLE OF ATTITUDES, VALUES AND STEREOTYPED VIEWS IN INFLUENCING BEHAVIOUR

Disability is generally seen as an undesirable condition experienced by other people that individuals hope will never happen to them. Disability in children is often regarded as a tragedy, eliciting pity for the 'victims' and their families. These and other attitudes, together with the environment, for example physical access to buildings, often cause unnecessary disability. Ignorance and fear can lead to separation, exclusion, prejudice and discrimination against disabled people.

This chapter aims to affect readers' attitudes as much as to increase their knowledge. Working with young children provides an ideal opportunity to influence attitudes. Children do not exclude or devalue each other until they are taught to do so by the unconscious or uninformed behaviour of adults.

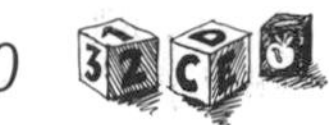

social activities. According to the social model, disability is defined as 'socially imposed restriction' (Oliver, 1981)

The implications of history

During the Industrial Revolution in Britain there was a move away from small, family-based cottage industry to employment in large factories. This served to discriminate against disabled people because they were no longer able to control their own surroundings nor their pace of work. Disabled people were forced into dependency and poverty, losing the status that comes from employment.

At about the same time, the influence of the medical profession was increasing. Doctors sought to treat people and cure their **impairments** so that they could fit into society. If this was not possible, disabled people were hidden away in hospitals and long-stay institutions out of sight; there was little contact with the outside world.

Progress check

How is disability often seen by society?

What causes unnecessary disability?

During the Industrial Revolution, what served to discriminate against disabled people?

What happened to disabled people at that time, if their impairments could not be cured?

key terms

Impairment
lacking all or part of a limb, or having altered or reduced function in a limb, organism or mechanism of the body. According to the social model, impairment is defined as 'individual limitation' (Oliver, 1981)

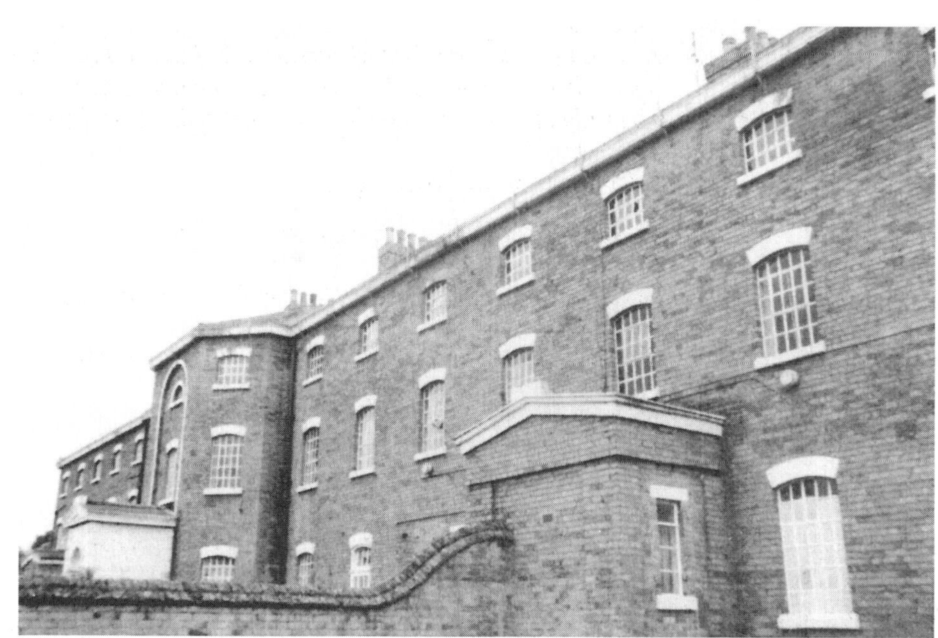

Children with disabilities used to be hidden away in long-stay institutions

MODELS OF DISABILITY

key term

Medical model
a view of disability as requiring medical intervention

The medical model

The result of the past is that society has become conditioned to treat disabled people according to a **medical model** (also known as the personal tragedy model). Society separates and excludes incurably disabled people as if they are somehow not quite human. Disability is viewed predominantly as a personal tragedy needing medical intervention. This encourages a negative view, focusing on what a person cannot do, rather than what they can. Disability is seen as a problem to be solved or cured, rather than as a difference to be accepted. It is all too easy, within this medical model, to see disabled people themselves as problem individuals who should adapt themselves to fit into society.

key terms

Social model a view of disability as a problem within society

Condition medically defined illness

The social model

Disabled people, however, are no longer prepared to accept the medical model of disability. Through organisations such as the Disability Movement, they are campaigning for acceptance of a **social model** of disability. They want people to see impairment (the medically defined **condition**) as a challenge, and to change society to include disabled people whether or not they are cured. This will involve responding to their true needs.

The social model views disability as a problem within society rather than within disabled people. It maintains that many of the difficulties disabled people face could be eliminated by changes in people's attitudes and in the environment. According to the social model, a mobility problem, for example, is seen to be caused by the presence of steps rather than by an individual's inability to walk; a deaf person's difficulty with accessing information is seen to be caused by other people's lack of skill in British Sign Language rather than by an individual's hearing loss.

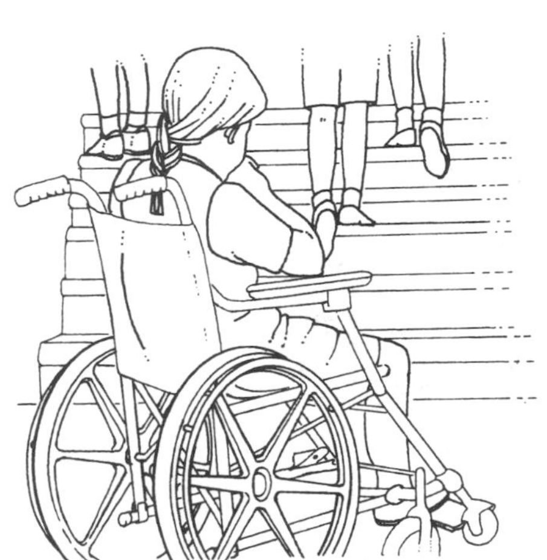

A mobility problem is seen to be caused by the presence of steps, rather than by an individual's inability to walk

Disabled people have taken the social model a stage further and defined disability as a **social creation**, a problem created by the institutions, organisations and processes that make up society. This model of disability has led to disabled people coming together to campaign for their rights, for social change and to fight against **institutional oppression**.

One example of this was the Campaign for Accessible Transport: mass attempts were organised for wheelchair users to get on buses and tube trains in London. This direct action was intended to draw attention to public transport systems that serve only non-disabled people and discriminate against disabled people.

Progress check

Define the medical and social models of disability.

key terms

Social creation brought about by society

Institutional oppression the power of organisations brought to bear on an individual to keep them in their place

THE IMPORTANCE OF TERMINOLOGY

Why is terminology important?

Terminology reflects and influences the way disability is viewed by society, including disabled people themselves. It also influences people's perceptions and attitudes, which subsequently affect the provision of resources and services.

Over the years, disabled people have been referred to and labelled using many different terms, usually conferred on them by non-disabled professionals. These have included general classifications that dehumanise, like 'the infirm' and 'the handicapped', or even 'the disabled'.

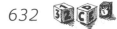

In addition, people have been referred to in such a way that they become their impairment: 'Jane is a spastic', 'John is an epileptic', 'Our Down syndrome child', 'Paul is a wheelchair case'. Many of these terms are patronising and contemptuous

of disabled people. Some terms are used as a form of abuse amongst non-disabled people, for example 'cripples', 'dummies', 'spazzies', 'idiots', 'mongols', 'invalids', and worse.

There are many different conditions or impairments that disabled people have; when the condition or impairment is known, the correct name should be used for it. This is particularly true for disabled children, who are often denied accurate information about themselves.

Explaining terminology to young children, both non-disabled and disabled, provides an opportunity to teach basic information about such topics as bodies, health or illness. This is not a taboo topic to young children who need, and like, to know the truth. It provides an opportunity to dispel some of the myths and fears surrounding disability, and to influence attitudes at a formative stage.

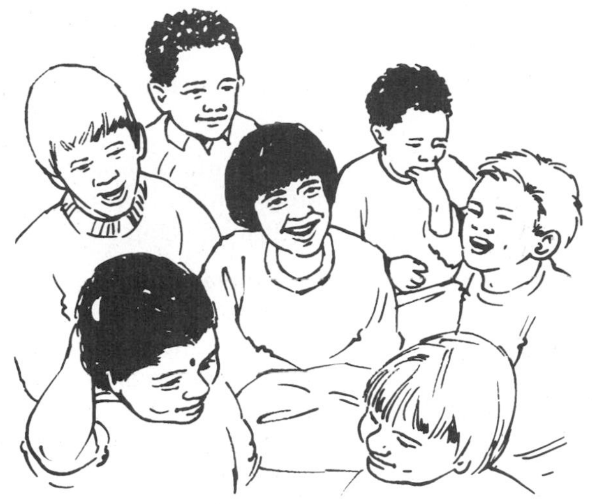

Children do not exclude or devalue each other until they are taught to do so by the unconscious or uninformed behaviour of adults

Definitions of disability

The definitions used in this book seek to respect the views of disabled people and promote good practice in the use of terminology. They were devised by the Union of the Physically Impaired Against Segregation in 1976. They are widely accepted by the Disability Movement and those working on disability equality issues.

Impairment may be described as lacking part or all of a limb, or having altered or reduced function in a limb, organ or mechanism of the body. Oliver (1981) defines impairment as 'individual limitation'.

Disability may be described as the disadvantage or restriction of activity caused by contemporary social organisation (society), which takes little or no account of people who have physical or mental impairments and thus excludes them from the mainstream of social activities. Oliver defines disability as 'socially imposed restriction'.

It is important to remember that disabled people are individuals with names. However, using the above definitions, it is appropriate to refer to disabled people or disabled children. These terms enable individual disabled people to identify themselves as a group with a common struggle, to end oppression by a disabling society. The adjective 'disabled' is similar to the term 'black' in that it was a negative term, but now represents the pride people feel in their identity.

It follows from the above definitions that people may have physical impairments, sensory impairments, and/or learning impairments. There may, however, be preference for other terms within these groups of disabled people. For example, some adults who have lost their hearing in later life may refer to themselves as 'hard of hearing'. People born with a hearing loss may refer to themselves as 'deaf', 'partially hearing' or 'partially deaf'. Some people with learning impairments prefer to be referred to as 'having learning difficulties'.

Children with special needs

key term

Special educational needs
learning difficulties requiring special educational provision to be made

The term special needs (in full, **special educational needs**) is now in common usage, especially in educational settings, in relation to children. The 1981 Education Act introduced the concept of special educational needs. Children with special needs include those whose learning difficulties call for special educational provision to be made. The Act states that children have learning difficulties if they have:

- significantly greater difficulty in learning than the majority of children their age, or
- a disability that prevents or hinders them from making use of educational facilities of a kind generally provided in school, for children of their age, within the local authority concerned.

In the past children with special needs may have been categorised as 'handicapped' or 'subnormal'. Individual children may have been labelled as 'physically handicapped', 'visually handicapped' or 'mentally subnormal'.

Those who advocate use of the term special needs suggest that these other labels are unsatisfactory because they:

- focus on weaknesses, not strengths
- do not indicate the practical effects of the difficulty and so the measures that may support the child
- suggest that all 'handicapped' or 'subnormal' children are the same and need the same kind of support
- encourage people to focus on the condition and view children with particular difficulties in stereotypical ways; for example, children with Down syndrome are seen as sweet, innocent and lovable; deaf children are assumed to be slow on the uptake
- imply a clear-cut division between 'handicapped' and 'subnormal' children and other children.

Supporters of the term special needs seek to emphasise the similarities between children with special needs and children who are developing according to the norm. They hope that the change in terminology from 'handicap' to 'needs' will encourage the treatment of each child as a unique individual with their own personality, ideas, sense of humour and level of ability. However, the term 'special needs' still conforms to the medical model of disability.

The range of special educational needs

Within the term 'special educational needs', children can be considered to have:

- moderate to severe learning difficulties
- sensory impairment, that is hearing and/or visual impairment
- physical or neurological (linked to the function of the brain) impairment

- speech and language difficulties
- emotional or behavioural difficulties
- **specific learning difficulties** – this term is used to describe children's difficulties learning to read, write, spell or in doing mathematics. Such children do not have difficulty learning other skills.

Progress check

Define the terms impairment and disability.

Where is the term special educational needs in common usage?

How society promotes equal opportunities for disabled children

key term

Specific learning difficulties
difficulties in learning to read, write or spell or in doing mathematics, not related to generalised learning difficulties

key term

Legislation
laws that have been made

Legislation concerning the care and education of disabled children is regularly changed and updated. This section aims to explain the underlying principles contained in current legislation. You will need, however, to refer to the legislation itself for more detail, and to update yourself regularly on any changes.

THE EDUCATION ACT 1944

This was the first piece of legislation to describe and define special educational needs and provision. Doctors were central to the process, and children were assessed as having one of eleven 'disorders' before being placed in a specialist school.

At this time children with severe learning difficulties were not thought to be able to benefit from education, and were looked after in junior training centres run by health authorities.

THE WARNOCK REPORT 1978

This report reviewed the provision that was available to all children with special needs. The Warnock Report was very important because it informed the 1981 Education Act.

THE EDUCATION ACT 1981

The Education Act stated that local education authorities (LEAs) have a statutory duty to ensure that special educational provision is made for pupils who have special educational needs.

The Act aimed to shift the focus to individual children rather than on to their impairments. The term 'children with special needs' included those whose learning difficulties called for special educational provision to be made. The Act stated that children had learning difficulties if:

- they had significantly greater difficulty in learning than the majority of children of their age
- they had a disability that prevented or hindered them from making use of educational facilities of a kind generally provided in school, for children of their age, within the local authority concerned.

The identification of children with special educational needs

key term

Statutory duty duty required by law

STATUTORY ASSESSMENT PROCEDURES

The 1981 Education Act also stated that LEAs have a **statutory duty** to identify and assess children with special educational needs in order to determine the educational provision that will meet their needs. A multi-professional assessment procedure was to be set up.

LEAs are required to:

- respond to parents' requests for their child's assessment, as long as the request is reasonable (parents have the right of appeal to the Secretary of State for Education)
- involve parents in the assessment process.

A subsequent circular, 1/83, Assessments and Statements of Special Educational Needs, advised that assessments should follow the five stages laid down in the Warnock Report. The assessments should not be an end in themselves, but part of a continuous process involving regular reviews, to reflect the changing needs of the children as they get older. The assessments should include:

- direct representations from parents (verbal or written)
- evidence submitted either by the parent or at the request of the parent
- written educational, medical and **psychological** advice
- information relating to the health and welfare of the child from the district health or social services authorities.

key term

Psychological from the study of the mind

key term

Statement of Special Educational Needs a written report, setting out a disabled child's needs and the resources required to meet these needs

STATEMENTS OF SPECIAL EDUCATIONAL NEEDS

As a result of the statutory assessment procedures, a **Statement of Special Educational Needs** would be drawn up, which would describe in detail a child's needs and the resources that should be made available to meet these needs.

It was noted that, where possible, provision should be made within a child's local school.

Every statement should be in five parts:

- Part 1, introductory page, including factual information such as name, address, age, etc.
- Part 2, the child's special educational needs as identified by the professionals involved in the assessment.
- Part 3, the educational provision considered necessary to meet the child's special educational needs, specifying any facilities, teaching arrangements, curriculum and equipment needed for the pupil.
- Part 4, the type of school or establishment (for example, hospital) thought appropriate for the child.
- Part 5, any additional non-educational provision considered necessary to enable the child to benefit from the proposed educational provision, for example hearing aids from the health authority.

Note: An additional part now describes how a child will get the help described in Part 5.

Initially, the statement should be in draft form. It should be sent to the parents, with an explanation of their right to appeal. If the parent disagrees with any of the content, they have 15 days in which to put their views to the local education authority. Ultimately, the parents have right of appeal to the Secretary of State for Education, whose decision is binding on the parents and the local authority.

The confidentiality of the statements is crucial. In most circumstances, no disclosure from the statement can be made without the parents' consent. The statement is usually kept in the administrative offices of the local authority.

The progress of children who are the subject of a statement of special educational needs must be reviewed at least once every 12 months. This is called the Annual Review. Children, parents, professionals and all other interested parties are given the opportunity to contribute to these reviews. The review should consider any progress made and set new aims and targets for the coming year.

Progress check

In the 1981 Education Act, who was given responsibility for identifying and meeting the needs of children with special educational needs?

How does the 1981 Education Act define children with special educational needs?

What should be included in a statement of special educational needs?

What is the purpose of the Annual Review?

key term

National Curriculum
a course of study, laid down by government, which all children in state schools in the UK must follow

THE EDUCATION REFORM ACT 1988

The 1988 Act requires all maintained schools, including special schools, to provide the **National Curriculum**. For a child with a statement, it is not necessary to modify or exempt the child from the requirements of the National Curriculum, but it is possible if modification is in the child's best interests. The 1988 Act encourages inclusion rather than exclusion of children with special needs in the National Curriculum. Most importantly, it states that all children with special educational needs have a right to a broad and well-balanced education. This includes as much access as possible to the National Curriculum.

Progress check

According to the 1988 Education Reform Act, who must provide the National Curriculum?

What do children with special educational needs have a right to according to the 1988 Education Reform Act?

THE CHILDREN ACT 1989

The Children Act 1989 brings together most public and private laws relating to children. It includes the functions of social services departments in relation to disabled children. Disabled children are treated in the Act in the same way as all other children.

The Act defines a category of 'children in need' for whom the social services department should provide services. Disabled children are included in this category. The Children Act defines disability as follows: 'A child is disabled if he is

key term

Congenital deformity
a term used in the Children Act 1989; a disability evident at the time of birth

blind, deaf or dumb or suffers from mental disorder of any kind or is substantially and permanently handicapped by illness, injury or **congenital deformity** or such other disability as may be prescribed.'

Duties of local authorities

The Act places a general duty on the local authority to provide an appropriate range and level of services to safeguard and promote the welfare of 'children in need'. This is to be done in a way that promotes the upbringing of such children within their own families.

Underlying principles

The Children Act outlines the following principles for work with disabled children:

- the welfare of the child should be safeguarded and promoted by those providing services
- a primary aim should be to promote access for all children to the same range of services
- the need to remember that disabled children are children first, not disabled people
- the importance in children's lives of parents and families
- partnership between parents and local authorities and other agencies
- the views of children and parents should be sought and taken into account.

key terms

Domiciliary services
services provided in the home

Portage home teaching scheme
a scheme to help parents/carers to teach their children with learning difficulties in their own homes, by setting short-term, achievable goals

Services

In order to encourage families to care for disabled children at home, local authorities are encouraged to provide the following services, either directly or through voluntary organisations:

- **domiciliary services**, for example the **Portage home teaching scheme** (see Chapter 42 for more on this) and befriending schemes
- guidance and counselling or social work
- respite care – this would be provided in co-operation with district health care trusts, and may be in health service settings, or in settings run by voluntary organisations
- day care services, including family centres and childminding services – wherever possible these would be in day care settings available to all children rather than in separate or segregated settings
- services from occupational therapists, rehabilitation workers, technical officers, specialist social workers and provision of **environmental aids and adaptations**
- information on a range of services provided by other agencies
- **advocacy** and representation for children and parents
- help with transport costs to visit children living away from home
- holiday play schemes
- toy libraries
- support groups
- loans of equipment or play materials.

key terms

Environmental aids and adaptation
for example, a flashing light doorbell for deaf people, modified utensils and eating tools, bathing aids etc.

Advocacy
speaking on behalf of, or in favour of, disabled people

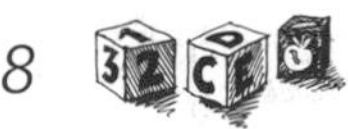

Other services for the disabled child and their family may include:

- identifying needs in their area and publicising services available
- working together with local education authorities and district health authorities
- compiling a register of children with disabilities in their area
- assessing, reassessing and reviewing children in need and planning for their long-term future
- planning services in partnership with parents and disabled children themselves.

key term

Accommodation away from home
a placement with a foster carer or in a residential setting arranged by the local authority social services department

Accommodation away from home

Disabled children may be **accommodated away from home** in foster care or residential settings. The Act provides new safeguards for them:

- their cases must be reviewed
- consideration must be given to their welfare
- they and their parents must be consulted before decisions are taken.

The Act requires local authorities to ensure that the accommodation they provide or that provided by education or health authorities for disabled children is suitable to the child's needs.

This means, in practice, that disabled children should have access to all the accommodation and the same rights to privacy as their non-disabled counterparts. Homes that accommodate disabled children must provide the necessary equipment, facilities and adaptations. The aim should be to integrate children into every aspect of life in the home. Health and safety aspects concerning disabled children must be considered.

Progress check

What laws does the Children Act 1989 bring together in one Act?

What is the LEA's responsibility towards 'children in need' according to the Children Act?

What services are local authorities encouraged to provide for disabled children and their families?

THE 1993 EDUCATION ACT

The 1993 Education Act builds upon and largely replaces the 1981 Education Act. It includes a Code of Practice giving practical guidance on how to identify and assess special educational needs.

The special educational needs Code of Practice

The 1993 Code of Practice for children with special educational needs revised the 1981 Education Act. Some terms from the old legislation, such as Statements of Special Educational Need, were retained.

The Code of Practice is a guide for schools and LEAs about the practical help they can give to children with special educational needs. Since 1 September 1994, all state schools should identify children's needs and take action to meet those needs as early as possible, working with parents.

Most importantly, under the Code of Practice, schools are given clearer guidance on how to identify and manage the needs of all children. Assessment of all children is now seen as a staged process and, within this, only some will reach a level where the local education authority will assess and issue a statement.

A staged approach

A staged approach to special educational needs might be as follows:

- *Stage 1* – the child's teacher identifies and records their concerns. Discussions take place with parents and action is taken in class.
- *Stage 2* – the Special Educational Needs Co-ordinator (SENCO) becomes involved, and an **Individual Education Plan (IEP)** is drawn up after consultation with the child's parents.
- *Stage 3* – specialist advice may be sought at this stage, and new individual education plans may be produced. Review meetings will be held. A decision will be made about whether to ask the LEA to make a statutory assessment
- *Stage 4* – the LEA is consulted, and a **multi-professional assessment** may be carried out.
- *Stage 5* – the LEA considers the information gathered from the assessment, and draws up a Statement of Special Educational Needs on the basis of the information.

> **key term**
> **Individual Education Plan (IEP)**
> an outline of short-term and long-term aims and objectives with targets for achievement of goals by children with special educational needs

> **key term**
> **Multi-professional assessment**
> a measurement of the child's performance by professionals from different backgrounds, e.g. health care, social work, psychology etc.

These stages are not seen as a one-way-street. Most children's needs will be fully met at Stages 1, 2 or 3, without the need for a Statement.

Once their problems have been identified and overcome, children are expected to drop back down the ladder. Only a small proportion will progress to Stages 4 and 5.

School policies and procedures

Schools must consider what the Code of Practice says when drawing up their policies for children with special educational needs. The school's policy will outline:

- the name of the teacher who is responsible for children with special educational needs (often called the Special Educational Needs Co-ordinator)
- the school's arrangements for deciding which children need special help, stage by stage
- how the school plans to work closely with parents.

Progress check

Describe the staged process laid down by the Code of Practice for identifying and managing the needs of all children.

What should be drawn up at Stage 2?

At what stage would outside specialist professionals be involved?

How can parents appeal against the assessment process or the provision made by the LEA?

The Code of Practice and parents

The Code of Practice gives new rights to parents, whose role is now seen as being much more central than it was before. Schools and other agencies must work in partnership with parents, and parents have the right of access to a new, independent tribunal if they feel the assessment or the provision made available by the LEA is flawed.

Now try these questions

Explain the implications of history for disabled people.

Describe a medical and a social model of disability.

Why is it important to use appropriate terminology to describe disabled people?

What are the advantages and disadvantages of the term special needs?

Outline the main requirements regarding children with special educational needs in the Education Act 1988.

Describe, in your own words, the underlying principles of the Children Act concerning disabled children.

What services may be required by families with a disabled child?

Describe the procedure in a school if a member of staff thinks a child in their class has special educational needs.

How has recent legislation safeguarded the welfare of disabled children?

How has recent legislation promoted partnership with parents of disabled children?

key terms

You need to know what the key terms and phrases in this chapter mean. Go back through the chapter and find out.

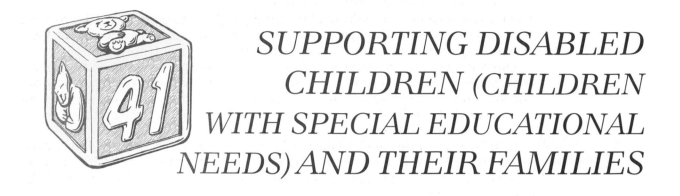

SUPPORTING DISABLED CHILDREN (CHILDREN WITH SPECIAL EDUCATIONAL NEEDS) AND THEIR FAMILIES

Understanding the needs of disabled children requires a thorough knowledge of child development. Working in partnership with parents extends to the parents of disabled children, and this chapter will help the child-care worker to empathise with their needs.

This chapter will cover the following topics:

- *disabled children's needs*
- *practical ways of working with disabled children (children with special educational needs).*

Disabled children's needs

UNDERSTANDING THE NEEDS OF DISABLED CHILDREN

Throughout this book it has been emphasised that development does not correlate with age. Children may reach stages, or milestones, of development at different ages. Individual children also proceed at different rates through the different stages of the developmental areas.

Disabled children are often made to feel that they are younger than they are because they have not reached so-called 'normal' milestones in all aspects of their development. If, for example, a disabled child needs to wear nappies at 5 years or ride a three-wheeler at 10 years, they may well be treated as younger than they are.

SPECIAL NEEDS OF DISABLED CHILDREN

key term

Specific therapeutic goal identifies objectives to counteract the effects of the condition or impairment

Another danger for disabled children is that their special needs override their ordinary needs. Following the medical model of disability, the implication is that there is something wrong, and that the child's efforts should be directed to **specific therapeutic goals**. This attitude may be encouraged through special programmes such as conductive education.

Disabled children may need physiotherapy, speech therapy or special learning programmes, but these should not always override their ordinary needs. All children need periods of self-directed play. Disabled children need adults who will facilitate, rather than always direct, play activities.

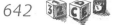

MEETING DISABLED CHILDREN'S NEEDS

Each disabled child is an individual with unique gifts and needs. In order to meet their needs, some knowledge of the causes and medical implications of their specific impairment or condition may be helpful.

This knowledge will be most helpful when combined with a positive attitude and a willingness to learn how to maximise individual children's potential. You can support your knowledge by further reading or talking to professionals, but remember that the full-time carer of each child may often be the best source of information and guidance.

In order to meet the needs of disabled children, attitudes and assumptions about disability need to be examined. Disability equality training (DET), led by an experienced DET trainer, and involving disabled people themselves, is one of the best ways of doing this.

> **key term**
> **Empower children** to enable children to take part in the world

Empowerment

Like all children, disabled children need to be enabled (**empowered**) to take part in the world effectively, but this needs to be on their own terms, rather than having to conform to the expectations of non-disabled people. This may be encouraged by doing the following:

- Responding to disabled children's expressed needs and initiatives. Disabled children may not find self-expression or communication easy. They need adults who will listen, wait and recognise the smallest indications that a choice has been made, or a need expressed. Adults may need to make guesses, try many alternatives and keep looking to see if they have judged correctly.
- Praising and rewarding effort rather than achievement. Children, especially disabled children, should not be compared to one another. It is better to compare their success and achievement to their own previous attempts.
- Responding positively to the things over which children have control, rather than to **innate ability** or attributes. Adults often praise young children for achievements over which the child has little control, for example their size, speed, or their cleverness and physical skill: 'Oh, she smiled at 3 days'; 'He's eating solids already!'; 'She never cries'; 'He started reading before he went to school'. This serves to devalue children who are small, slow, inept, and so on. Comments like 'Oh, that was a kind thing to do!' and 'You have worked really hard today' help to give value to the things over which children do have control.

> **key term**
> **Innate ability** natural ability

Progress check

Why are disabled children often treated as younger than they are?

Name two special educational programmes for disabled children.

How can disabled children be empowered?

Who is usually the best source of information and guidance about individual disabled children?

What is one of the best ways of examining attitudes and assumptions about disability?

DIAGNOSIS

When a child is born with a specific condition or impairment, or one is later diagnosed, parents or carers will react in their own individual way. Society predominantly views disability as a tragedy, and it is possible to recognise in many parents or carers a pattern of response similar to that experienced following other 'tragedies', such as bereavement.

This pattern of response is divided into four stages. Individuals may progress through these stages at different rates:

- *shock and disbelief* – 'This can't be happening to us'
- *a period of mourning and isolation* – 'We were grief stricken. We felt we were being punished. We didn't want to be with anyone who did not know about our child'
- *a period of adaptation* – 'We felt it was a challenge. We wanted information, help and understanding, and not to feel alone'
- *adjustment* – 'We are learning to cope, and enjoy our child. When we could face up to telling friends and relatives things became easier'.

As with bereavement and loss in other circumstances, some people do not move through the stages of 'grief' but may remain stuck at one particular stage.

THE NEEDS OF PARENTS AND CARERS

In common with all parents or carers, those of disabled children need to find pleasure in their child, and to feel confident and pleased with themselves as parents. In order to accomplish this they are likely to need:

- information about their child's condition or impairment, the social model of disability, the services available, new ideas, etc.
- emotional support, and help in finding pleasure in their child
- practical help, for example child-sitting, respite care, environmental aids and adaptations, domestic help, financial support
- contact with other parents or carers of disabled children, and opportunities to work together to obtain the services they need
- reassurance by service providers (of education and care), that their child is wanted and can be coped with
- contact with disabled adults for advice, support, information, etc.
- training in **self-advocacy** and getting what they need for themselves and their family
- time to be themselves and meet their own needs and the needs of other family members
- recognition that usually they are the ones who know their child best.

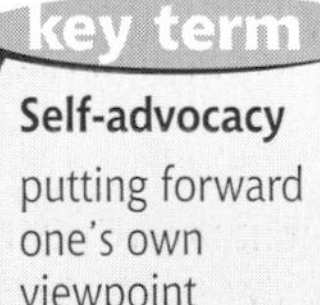

Self-advocacy
putting forward one's own viewpoint

The needs of siblings

It is impossible to generalise about the effects on siblings of having a disabled child in the family. Much will depend on factors such as the nature of the condition or impairment, the number of children in the family, their birth order and so on.

The need of brothers and sisters may be similar to the overriding need of parents or carers, that is to find pleasure in having a disabled sibling. In addition they may have the following needs:

key terms

Identification
making oneself the same as those who are significant to us

Inclusive
organised in a way that enables all to take a full and active part; meeting the needs of all children

- encouragement to express their feelings openly and honestly
- information with meaningful terms at a level they can understand
- preparation for the possible negative attitudes and behaviour of other people
- reassurance of their own and their disabled sibling's value and worth
- individual attention
- involvement in the care of the disabled child, without overwhelming responsibility.

While it is relatively easy to outline potential disadvantages, it is possible for siblings to benefit from growing up alongside a disabled child.

DISABLED PARENTS AND CARERS

Many disabled people are themselves parents or carers. Often they are not recognised by society as capable of being responsible, caring adults, with much to give. Their own understanding and experience of the possible effects of specific conditions or impairments may not be used by those around them.

In professional and non-professional roles, disabled adults may be willing to support the carers of disabled children. They may also be willing to act as role models for disabled children.

It is possible for young disabled children to grow up with little or no contact with disabled adults. This has implications for the process of **identification** and the development of self-image.

Disabled parents and carers are sometimes thought to disadvantage their own children. This has, on occasions, led to their children being accommodated away from home by a local authority. Often alternative measures such as help with domestic chores, environmental aids and adaptations or financial support could be used to overcome the difficulties.

Disabled adults sometimes find themselves excluded from the services provided for their children. **Inclusive** care and education will consider their needs alongside other service users. The emphasis on parents and carers as partners with professionals should include disabled carers as well.

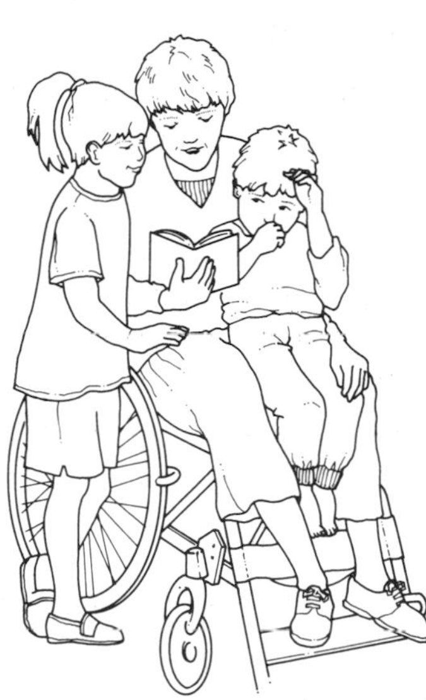

Many disabled people are themselves parents or carers

Case study . . .

. . . a baby just like me

My hearing friends were surprised when they asked me, 'Claire, do you want a boy or a girl?' and I said 'I don't mind, so long as the baby is deaf'. You see I'm profoundly deaf and the imminent prospect of becoming a parent myself has made me think about my own childhood again.

There was no getting away from the fact that I was a disappointment to my parents. A tragedy really. How could this have happened to them? What had they done wrong? Now, I can understand their reaction; then, I could only experience it.

Their determination that I would be just like any other child was well meaning, but impossible for me to achieve. My earliest memories are of seemingly endless waits in various clinics. The look of disappointment on my parents' faces. The speech training that seemed to go on for hours and hours, and when I produced my best efforts the look of total incomprehension on hearing people's faces!

Eventually they gave up the fight and sent me to the Deaf School. What joy! Other children just like me and adults who communicated at a remarkable speed using their whole bodies.

In the end, my parents started to learn British Sign Language and even came to the Deaf Club occasionally. My sister is training to be a sign language interpreter. I guess she's got me to thank for being bilingual.

If my baby is hearing, we'll cope, but naturally we all want a baby just like us!

1. *What do these thoughts tell us about Claire's childhood?*
2. *Why does she want a deaf baby?*
3. *Why did Claire's parents see sending her to a Deaf School as giving up?*
4. *How was Claire's sister affected by her deafness?*

Progress check

Describe the pattern or response that may be demonstrated by parents or carers when their child's disability is diagnosed.

What are the needs of parents or carers of disabled children following diagnosis?

What are the needs of the siblings of disabled children following diagnosis?

What can disabled parents or carers offer to disabled children?

PROVISION OF ALTERNATIVE CARE

Residential care

Recent legislation confirms that the best place for a disabled child to be brought up is within their own family. For many reasons, however, this may not be possible. Some disabled children need medical care and for this reason are accommodated in health service establishments. Some attend residential special schools where they may be weekly or termly boarders.

Disabled children in residential care are particularly vulnerable. There have been many incidents, some recorded in the biographies of disabled people, of long-term mistreatment in residential institutions. The Children Act 1989 aims to provide safeguards concerning the welfare of disabled children accommodated away from home.

Generally speaking, children should not be accommodated long term in National Health Service hospital settings. The intention of the Children Act is that disabled children in residential care, including independent schools, should not be forgotten and that social services departments should assess the quality of child care offered.

Accommodation away from home

If a child has to be accommodated away from home, their residential homes must be registered and regulated. Social services departments are empowered to enter a care home in order to find out if children's welfare is being satisfactorily safeguarded and promoted.

Foster placements

There has been an increase in the number of successful foster placements for disabled children over the last 10 years. Some national voluntary organisations provide specialist fostering programmes for disabled children.

Foster carers have to be willing to be involved in their disabled child's educational learning programmes, where appropriate, in assessments and reviews, and be willing to encourage the disabled child to make friends in the community.

Respite care

Caring for a disabled child, though often rewarding, can be exhausting. If the best place for a disabled child to be brought up is within their own family, the family is likely to need support and encouragement to enable them to go on caring. Respite care (now often referred to as a 'short-term break') provides one way of offering such support and encouragement.

There are four main types of respite care:

- residential care
- family-based care
- care in the child's own home
- holiday schemes.

These services are offered by different agencies, both statutory and voluntary, and groups of parents who have banded together for the purpose. The service may be provided by a voluntary organisation, while the cost is met by social services. Each service offers parents or carers time off, and has advantages and disadvantages. Rarely are all available to the parents or carers of disabled children; occasionally none is available.

Residential respite care

The disabled child goes to stay in approved accommodation for an agreed period of time. This accommodation is usually provided by an institution such as a hospital ward, a children's home or a boarding school.

The disadvantage is that it is usually institutionalised care, a complete contrast to family life at home. The advantages include the possibility of it becoming familiar to the child and that it does not depend on any one person offering the service.

Family-based respite care

The family of a disabled child is linked to another family (or single person), who is willing to take the disabled child into their home for periods of time. Such schemes are usually managed by social services or a voluntary organisation.

Respite care in a child's own home

This type of care is a specialised child-sitting service. It may be an extension of a home-help service, except that the 'family aid' cares for the child rather than the home.

Respite holiday schemes

There are holiday schemes for disabled children. Some provide for children only, others for the whole family. They are organised by a number of voluntary organisations and take a number of different forms, for example adventure holidays, foreign trips. Often parents or carers have to pay for this service.

Progress check

Where is usually the best place for a disabled child to be brought up?

Which Act aims to safeguard the welfare of disabled children accommodated away from home?

What must foster carers of disabled children be willing to do?

Identify four types of respite care.

Practical ways of working with disabled children (children with special educational needs)

Recent legislation encourages the involvement of disabled children in mainstream settings, both in education and care. It is therefore now more likely that disabled children will be in nursery classes, schools, day nurseries, family centres or residential establishments. Consideration of the needs of all children will be necessary if these settings are to be truly inclusive.

If settings adopt the social model of disability, they will want to review their provision to ensure that the environment, attitudes and practices do not disable children with identified conditions or impairments.

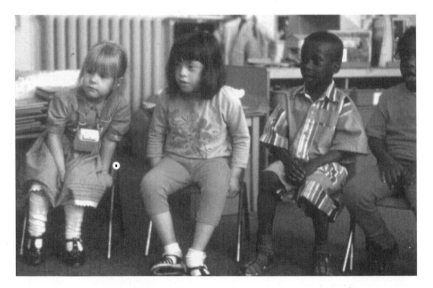

Recent legislation encourages the involvement of disabled children in mainstream settings

PROMOTING EFFECTIVE EQUAL OPPORTUNITIES, ANTI-DISCRIMINATORY AND ANTI-BIAS PRACTICE

Language

As with issues of race and gender, the setting should have a clear policy about the use of language to describe disabled children. This policy should be clearly explained to all users of the setting.

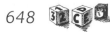

Images

Everything learned about images of other marginalised or minority groups applies to disabled children. In the past, nearly all images of disabled people were produced by non-disabled people, often on behalf of charities. Their aim was to evoke sympathy, pity, fear and guilt. This was justified as necessary to raise money for disabled people.

It is very difficult to find positive images of disabled children. Children's books have few disabled characters. The books available often focus entirely on the impairment, with titles such as *Mary Has a Hearing Loss* or *I Have Cerebral Palsy*. Rarely are disabled people portrayed as ordinary people. However, Letterbox Library now market some texts portraying positive images of disabled children and including disabled characters alongside their non-disabled peers.

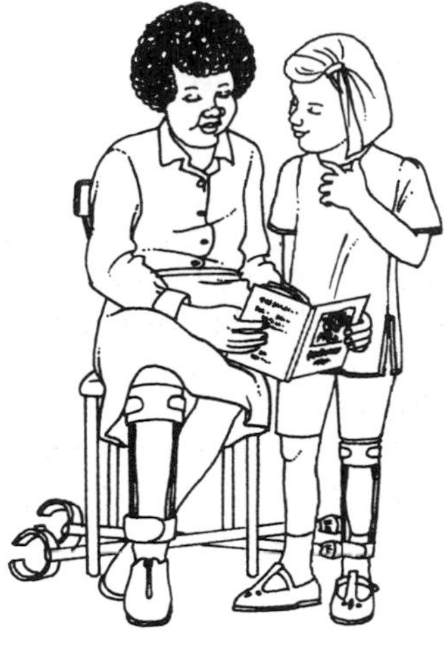

The involvement of disabled adults can provide positive role models for disabled children

Activities

Organised, directed activities should always seek to be inclusive. The needs of disabled children in the group should be considered at the planning stage. If a child cannot do something in the same way as most children, they may be consulted about what they could do instead.

In educational settings, teachers will aim to use differentiation in the tasks set. This means that individual or groups of children are given different tasks related to the aim of the lesson, at a level that provides a manageable challenge to them. This involves careful planning if disabled children are not to be segregated from the class. Special needs support assistants may be involved in this process at the planning and implementation stage (see Chapter 42).

Role models

The involvement of disabled adults, of all ages and at all levels, in care and education settings can provide positive role models for disabled children. Disabled adults can also help to raise the level of disability awareness in the setting.

Progress check

Where have most images of disabled people come from in the past? What were they produced for?

What play equipment should be available in an inclusive setting?

What is differentiation?

How can the involvement of disabled adults benefit any educational setting?

ACCESS

For an establishment to include disabled children, certain aspects need to be considered. Detailed information and training on inclusion of disabled children is available from condition- or impairment-specific voluntary organisations and self-help groups, but outlines of general principles for good practice are listed above. Establishments including disabled children need to provide:

- equipment that all children can use; much equipment produced for disabled people is inclusive: ramps, lifts, adjustable tables, automatic doors, long-handled taps, touch-sensitive controls, large print and grab rails can be used by all children

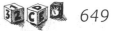

- a range of options such as tapes, Braille and print versions of documents
- a range of seat and table sizes and shapes
- empty floor space that is kept uncluttered
- flexible, adjustable equipment, for example a sand tray that comes off the stand, high- chairs with removable trays
- sturdy versions of 'ordinary' toys and furniture
- a range of scissors, knives and other implements
- soft play areas for activities such as crawling, jumping, climbing
- extra adult supervision to facilitate integration
- some equipment for individual children to facilitate integration; there should be discussions with the child and full-time carers about what to buy before expensive purchases are made
- spacious toilet facilities designed for wheelchair users that can then be used by all children
- private age-appropriate toilet or changing area
- disability awareness and equality training for all staff.

Access for children with sensory impairments

The following aspects need to be considered in order to include blind and partially sighted children. Establishments will need to provide:

- opportunities to explore the environment and people using touch, smell, hearing and any residual sight
- the opportunity for children to orientate themselves physically (this may involve visiting the setting when few people are present)
- stability and order, a place for everything and everything in its place; the child will need to be informed and shown any changes
- plenty of light
- a hazard-free environment, or an indication of hazardous things such as steps or sharp corners
- information about other children's needs, for example a child with a hearing loss who may not respond to them
- some specific items such as books in Braille, toys or board games, which are especially designed to be inclusive.

The following points need to be considered by an establishment including deaf and hearing-impaired children:

- hearing impairment is largely invisible; even a mild hearing loss is significant in a noisy crowded room
- a child with impaired hearing cannot tell you what they missed!
- hearing aids are not a replacement for hearing and may be of little use to some children
- deaf children's greatest special need is access to language and communication; complete access can only come about through universal use of language

and communication accessible to deaf children. This will often mean British Sign Language, which will need to be used by everyone in the setting

- deaf children need to communicate with other children as well as adults
- deaf children have a range of intellectual ability as all children do; if we deny them access to language we create a learning difficulty for them.

Case study . . .

. . . inclusive education

Lake View Primary School's brochure states that they provide education for all children in the locality aged 3 to 7 years. I don't think they realised what a challenge it would be, when they offered my daughter, Emily, a place in the nursery.

Before Emily started, we went to visit for a session. The other children were curious and asked me why Emily had a funny face and couldn't talk properly. After our visit, the staff decided to prepare the children before Emily started properly. They had to search hard for suitable books to read to the children, but finally found Letterbox Library. The staff were willing to learn; they asked me questions about Emily and had a couple of sessions with a disability equality trainer.

Emily was very clingy and demanding at first. Staff couldn't manage her with 35 other children, so the school employed a special needs support assistant for part of the time, to help Emily integrate with the other children. They approached the local college and a student with learning difficulties came to the school on work placement. Emily latched on to him and it seemed to increase his self-confidence, as well as Emily's.

Whenever the children ask what is wrong with Emily, staff explain that she has Down syndrome. They always answer the children's questions honestly, even when they are funny, like 'Is it catching?'.

The nursery staff say they have learned so much from having Emily and now do some things differently for all the children.

Why did Emily's parent want her to go to the local school?

How did the nursery staff prepare for Emily's admission?

Why did staff explain Emily's condition using the proper name?

Why did staff seek out a student with learning difficulties to help in the nursery?

Progress check

In what formats should written documents/information be produced to ensure their accessibility to parents/carers who may themselves be disabled?

What will be needed to facilitate children's integration in the setting?

How should a setting decide what to purchase to support a disabled child?

What should be provided for all staff?

What creates a learning difficulty for deaf children?

Now try these questions

How does the Children Act seek to safeguard the welfare of disabled children and encourage support for parent/carers to care for their disabled child in their own home?

How can disabled children and their families benefit from respite care?

Why is it important to have a thorough knowledge of child development in order to understand the needs of disabled children?

Explain why it is important to ensure that the special needs of disabled children don't overide their ordinary needs.

Describe the possible reactions of parents after their child is diagnosed with a particular condition or impairment.

What are the needs of disabled children's families?

Why is it important for child-care workers to have contact with disabled adults?

How does the Children Act seek to safeguard the welfare of disabled children and encourage support for parents/carers to care for their disabled child in their own home?

key terms

You need to know what the key terms and phrases in this chapter mean. Go back through the chapter and find out.

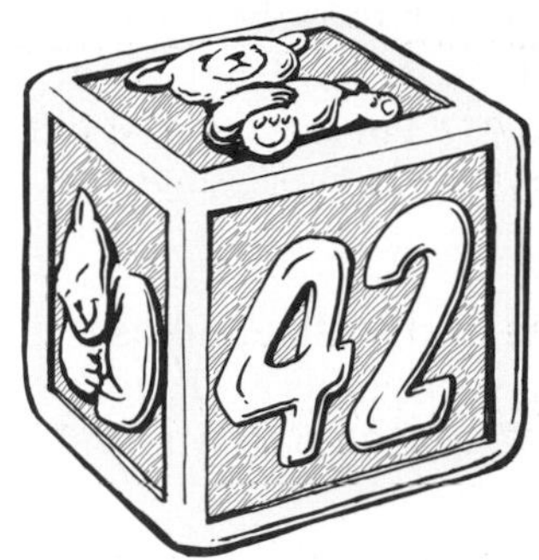

PROFESSIONALS WORKING WITH DISABLED CHILDREN (CHILDREN WITH SPECIAL EDUCATIONAL NEEDS)

There seem to be a baffling array of professionals involved with disabled children and their families. Their titles change from time to time. It is important that child-care workers can find their way around the statutory, voluntary and private sectors, and act as a signpost to disabled children and their families. They will need to have a basic knowledge and understanding of the roles of significant professionals.

For simplicity, the professionals described in this chapter have been identified as working within either health, education, social services or voluntary organisations. Of course, some may work for more than one. In some areas, a service that is provided by, for example, social services will, in another area, be provided by a voluntary organisation, on behalf of social services.

The information in this chapter should be used to support information you are able to find locally.

This chapter will cover the following topics:

- *health service professionals*
- *education service professionals*
- *social service professionals*
- *Social Security Benefits Agency*
- *voluntary organisations.*

Health service professionals

PAEDIATRICIANS

Paediatricians are doctors specialising in the diagnosis of conditions and impairments in children, and the medical care of children with these conditions and impairments. They may be the first health service professional to become involved with a disabled child in the maternity unit, the children's ward or outpatient department.

HEALTH VISITORS

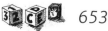

Every child under the age of 5 has a health visitor. Health visitors are qualified nurses with additional training. They work in the community attached to a clinic or general practice and usually undertake the routine developmental checks. The health visitor is often the health-care professional most closely involved with the family at home. They are able to provide a link with, and between, other professionals and services.

PHYSIOTHERAPISTS

Physiotherapists assess children's motor development and skills, and assess how well they can move and balance. They may work in schools as well as hospital clinics. They may demonstrate exercises and activities that parents and other carers will carry out themselves with their children.

key term

Independent life skills
skills needed to live and care for oneself

OCCUPATIONAL THERAPISTS

Occupational therapists seek to encourage **independent life skills**, such as dressing, eating and moving around independently. For this reason they may assess a child's fine motor skills. They can advise about any special equipment that may be helpful and arrange for it to be supplied. This may be done out in the community as well as in hospital clinics.

SPEECH AND LANGUAGE THERAPISTS

Speech and language therapists seek to develop all aspects of children's expressive and receptive communication skills and language development. As well as assessing speech, they also assess tongue and mouth movements, and their effects on eating and swallowing. Speech therapists will work out programmes of activities and exercises to help children to acquire language, understand concepts and use speech. Parents or carers may be involved in carrying these programmes out. Speech therapists may be based in schools, hospital clinics or in the community.

CLINICAL PSYCHOLOGISTS

Clinical psychologists are mainly concerned with children's emotional, social and intellectual development. Their assessment of children covers all aspects of their circumstances. They will have discussions with their families and other carers, as well as making direct observations of children's behaviour.

SCHOOL NURSES

School nurses often check children's weight, height, eyesight and hearing in school. They may pick up difficulties in any of these areas. They may be based full time in special schools where they supervise the routine medical care of disabled children.

PLAY THERAPISTS

Play therapists use play to help children handle particular feelings or experiences that may be hindering their development. The therapists need to have been trained for and supported in this task, as they are likely to be dealing with powerful emotions.

PLAY WORKERS

Play workers are usually trained nursery nurses, employed in some hospitals to play with children, both those visiting clinics and those admitted to the wards. They represent a non-threatening adult in a setting that may provoke anxiety for children. They may be involved in raising awareness and preparing children for a possible stay in hospital.

Progress check

Why may an occupational therapist assess children's fine motor skills?

Which professional may explain a disabled child's condition or impairment to parents following diagnosis?

What do speech therapists do to encourage children's language development?

What is the difference between a play therapist and a play worker?

Education service professionals

EDUCATIONAL PSYCHOLOGISTS

Educational psychologists advise the local education authority about the education of individual children. They will be involved in the educational assessment of disabled children, including the assessment that may lead to a statement of special educational needs. They may advise the professionals who are working directly with a disabled child about learning and behaviour modification programmes.

SPECIAL NEEDS SUPPORT TEACHERS

key term

Peripatetic travelling to see those they work with

Special needs support teachers, sometimes called specialist teachers or support teachers, are teachers who often have additional training and experience; they are often **peripatetic** and visit disabled children in different schools. They may specialise in one particular impairment, for example hearing loss or visual impairment. They are involved in the direct teaching of individual children, as well as in advising staff and parents of ways to maximise children's learning potential.

PRE-SCHOOL SUPPORT TEACHERS

These are special needs support teachers who work with disabled children and families before a child starts school. They visit children in their own home and devise small steps teaching programmes for parents/carers to follow with their child.

SPECIAL NEEDS SUPPORT ASSISTANTS

Special needs support assistants have many different labels, for example special assistants, education care officers, classroom assistants or special needs nursery nurses. They may be qualified nursery nurses or child-care workers, or they may have no formal child-care training.

They adopt a variety of different roles, depending on the school or nursery and the children they are employed to support. Some work with individual children who have a Statement of Special Educational Needs, others with groups of children with a variety of additional needs. The main focus of their work may be to provide medical or learning support. They may be involved in observing and monitoring children, liaising with other professionals and working under their direction. They may have regular contact with parents and carers.

SPECIAL NEEDS ADVISERS

Special needs advisers focus on the curriculum, teaching methods, materials, schemes and equipment used in schools. They have a role as inspectors to ensure provision of the National Curriculum.

EDUCATION WELFARE OFFICERS

Education welfare officers undertake welfare duties on behalf of children and their parents or carers. They will be involved with children whose attendance is irregular. They may arrange transport for disabled children to school.

Progress check

Who will be involved in the statutory assessment procedure for children with special educational needs?

What does it mean to be peripatetic?

Describe the role of a special needs support assistant.

How may an education welfare officer be involved with disabled children and their families?

Social service professionals

SOCIAL WORKERS

key term

Statutory child protection those aspects of protecting children that are covered by legislation

Social workers may be based in hospitals or in local area offices. Their work with disabled children includes **statutory child protection** duties. They may advise on the availability of all services in the area, such as health, education, welfare benefits or care, or they may put families in touch with appropriate agencies.

They may advocate on behalf of disabled children, for example enabling them to obtain the services to which they are entitled. Social workers may be involved in assessment for referral to day care, respite care, home helps and other domiciliary care, under the heading of family aids.

SPECIALIST SOCIAL WORKERS AND TECHNICAL OFFICERS

Specialist social workers and technical officers may have additional training and experience to work with children with particular conditions or impairments, for example deaf or blind children.

NURSERY OFFICERS

Nursery officers work in day nurseries and family centres. They may also visit family homes to liaise between home and nursery.

FAMILY AIDS/VISITORS

Family aids/visitors provide practical support for families in the families' own homes. The helpers may be involved in domestic duties, child care and other family needs.

RESIDENTIAL CHILD-CARE WORKERS

Residential child-care workers may work in long-stay or short-stay residential accommodation for disabled children. The worker may be a key worker for a disabled child accommodated away from home by the local authority.

Progress check

What statutory duties do social workers carry out?

In what capacity do nursery nurses work for social services?

Social Security Benefits Agency

The main role of the Social Security Benefits Agency is the provision of welfare benefits. There is a range of benefits available to disabled children and their families. These are frequently subject to change. The Citizens' Advice Bureau provides up-to-date advice and information about welfare benefits.

Progress check

What is the function of the Social Security Benefits Agency?

Which voluntary organisation can give advice about social security benefits?

Voluntary organisations

Collectively, voluntary organisations provide every conceivable type of support for disabled children and their families. Some are national organisations and others local. It is beyond the scope of this book to provide information about the services they offer, but information is available from local libraries.

In recent years, there has been an increase in the role and extent of involvement by voluntary organisations in the lives of disabled children. Many of these organisations work in a highly professional and pioneering way. Much of the innovative work with and on behalf of disabled people is done through voluntary organisations and self-help groups.

Progress check

What are the roles and functions of voluntary organisations who are concerned with disabled children and their families?

LEARNING AND THERAPY PROGRAMMES

Portage home teaching scheme

The Portage Guide to Early Education was originally developed in a rural area centred on the town of Portage in Wisconsin in the US. The schemes devised are used with children with moderate and severe learning difficulties, behaviour problems and developmental delay. Weekly home visits of 1 to 2 hours are made by a Portage home visitor. Home visitors come from a range of professions.

Most approaches have found that a short training programme is all that is initially required. The purpose of each visit is to help the parent or carer to select and set short-term goals for the child, expected to be achieved in 1 or 2 weeks, and to devise an appropriate way for the carer to teach these.

As well as short-term goals, each Portage home visitor sets, with the parent or carer, long-term goals for the child to work towards, so that the weekly visits and short-term goals can be seen as steps in a general progression towards the desired objective.

Workers are trained to use a developmental checklist, which covers development from birth to 6 years, in the areas of socialisation and language, cognitive, self-help and motor skills.

One of the aims of Portage is that parents and carers will become sufficiently skilled to enable the role of the Portage home visitor to change to consultant and supporter. The Portage method aims to enable parents and carers to become independent of the home visitor eventually, and to become the main worker with the child. Unfortunately, because of limited financial resources, some local authorities may see Portage as a relatively cheap solution to the needs of disabled children and their families, rather than as a service to offer alongside other services.

Bobath technique

The Bobath technique is a form of physiotherapy developed by Professor Bobath and his wife, aimed at enabling the best possible posture and mobility for children with cerebral palsy. It is important that skills are transferred from the therapist to the parents or carers and from them to anyone caring for the child. Treatment begins with an initial assessment at the Bobath Centre in London.

Doman-Delacato therapy (patterning)

Doman-Delacato therapy claims that it is possible to treat the brain itself. The theory is that undamaged portions of the brain are taught to take over the function of the damaged part. The basic assumption behind the therapy is that mobility can be achieved through movement. This movement cannot occur spontaneously and must be initiated from the outside by other people. Movement must be frequent, intense and repetitive. Teams of volunteers put the child through a set of movements for between 3 and 8 hours a day. Not surprisingly the child often protests at this and Doman-Delacato is consequently a controversial therapy.

Conductive education

According to Dr Mari Hari, a leading supporter of conductive education, it is 'a method of enabling "the **motor impaired**" to function in society without requiring special apparatus such as wheelchairs, ramps or other artificial aids'. It is based on the theory that, under the right conditions, the central nervous system will restructure itself.

Conductors (therapists) use **orthofunction**, a teaching method that involves the whole person physically and mentally and 'instils in children the ability to function as members of society, and to participate in normal social settings appropriate to their age'.

key terms

Motor impaired
an impairment of a function of movement

Orthofunction
a teaching method that involves the whole person physically and mentally, and 'instils in children the ability to function as members of society, and to participate in normal social settings appropriate to their age'

Conductive education offers a positive approach to a clear set of goals. It has produced results beyond the expectations of professionals and parents of children with cerebral palsy and spina bifida. It should be remembered, however, that the treatment places emphasis on adapting individuals rather than environments. It follows a medical, not a social, model of disability.

Progress check

Give brief explanations of the following learning and therapy programmes:

(a) Portage

(b) Bobath technique

(c) Doman-Delacato therapy

(d) conductive education.

Now try these questions

Choose either health, education or social services. Outline the roles and responsibilities of three professionals in that service.

What are the advantages and disadvantages of learning and therapy programmes?

key terms

You need to know what the key terms and phrases in this chapter mean. Go back through the chapter and find out.

In this unit you will learn how to recognise, value and respect parents as the primary carers and educators of their children. You will consider your role and responsibilities in relation to the parents of the children you care for, and you will analyse the factors that contribute to good communication with parents and ways of achieving this. You will also identify the variety of ways in which you can involve parents in the care and education you provide for their children.

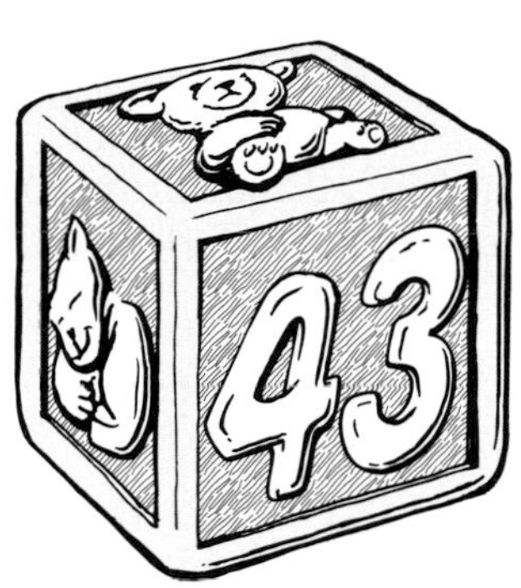

WORKING WITH PARENTS

All those who work with young children will recognise that the relationship between the child-care establishment and the parents (or primary carers) of the child is very important. A good relationship will benefit the child, the parent and those who work with the child. This chapter will look at issues surrounding working with parents, and will examine ways of establishing and maintaining an effective partnership between the child-care centre and parents.

It is recognised that not all children are cared for by their parents. This term has been used for ease of reading and includes others who take on the parenting role.

This chapter will cover the following topics:

- *why work with parents?*
- *good communication with parents*
- *parents and record keeping*
- *difficult situations*
- *getting parents involved.*

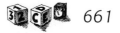

Why work with parents?

Until quite recently the practice of actively involving parents in the child-care setting was relatively uncommon. You may remember seeing notices that positively discouraged parents from crossing over the threshold into school or nursery. A notice that proclaims 'No parents beyond this point' is hardly likely to foster good relationships between parents and those who care for their children, and should be harder to find these days. There are a number of reasons why working with parents is considered to be important and necessary:

- Parents have the most knowledge and understanding of their children. If they are encouraged to share this with staff, the children will benefit.
- Children need consistent handling to feel secure. This is most likely to occur if there are good channels of communication between parents and staff.
- Recent legislation contained within the Education Reform Act 1988, the Children Act 1989, and the Special Educational Needs Code of Practice 1993, places a legal responsibility on professionals to work in partnership with parents. Services provided for children in the public, private and voluntary sector must take this into account.
- It is a condition of receiving public funding for educational provision for 3 and/or 4 year olds (known as nursery grant) that settings work in partnership with parents.
- Initiatives such as the Parents' Charter emphasise parents' rights to make choices and be consulted in decisions concerning their children's education.
- Research has demonstrated conclusively the positive effect that parental involvement in the education process has on the progress of children. If parents become involved early on in the child's education, they are likely to maintain this involvement throughout the the child's educational career.
- Children's learning is not confined to the child-care setting. An exchange of information from centre to home and from home to centre will consolidate learning, wherever it takes place.
- Parents have a wealth of skills and experiences that they can contribute to the child-care centre. Participation in this way will broaden and enrich the programme offered to all the children. Many groups rely on a parents' rota to complement their staffing.
- An extra person to work at an activity, to help out on a trip or to prepare materials can make a valuable contribution to a busy setting. Parents who are involved in this way will gain first-hand experience of the way that the centre operates and an understanding of the approach.
- Some centres may operate with regulations that require a parent representative on the management committee or governing body. The responsibilities here can be quite significant and will include financial management and accountability, selection and recruitment of staff, as well as day-to-day running of the centre.
- Parents who are experiencing difficulties with their children may be able to share these problems and work towards resolving them alongside sympathetic and supportive professionals.
- Child protection procedures may require that professionals in the child-care centre observe and supervise parents with children as part of access or

rehabilitation programmes. (Such situations need workers with experience and sensitivity.)

- Parents may experience a loss of role when their child starts nursery or school. Being involved and feeling valued may help them to adjust to this change.
- Provision for young children is often under-funded. Many centres have parent groups that organise social activities and raise funds. This enables parents who are not available during working hours to become involved.
- New initiatives such as Sure Start, which are targetted at improving opportunities and facilities for young children and their families, require communities to take an active part in deciding what is needed and how it should be provided. Parents of young children will play a key role in these developments.

All centres develop ways of working with parents, but naturally there are differences, depending on the emphasis of each particular establishment. For example, a family centre where many of the children are referred by social services, perhaps as a result of some crisis, will work with parents in ways that are quite different to those used in, say, a workplace day nursery that cares for children during parents' long shifts, or a playgroup where parents operate a daily rota. Nevertheless, there are general principles that will always apply:

- Be friendly and approachable. Remember that parents might feel uneasy in an unfamiliar setting and it is up to staff to make the right kind of approach.
- Be courteous and maintain a professional relationship.
- Encourage a meaningful exchange of information between the home and centre.

Progress check

Why is it important for child-care professionals to work with parents?

What legislation requires that professionals work in partnership with parents?

How does partnership benefit:

(a) children?

(b) parents?

(c) child-care workers?

Why do centres need to develop their own particular ways of involving the families that they work with?

Good communication with parents

It is the responsibility of those who work with children to do everything that they can to make parents feel welcome and valued. The needs and feelings of all parents should be considered. This may include some who have less than positive memories of their own childhood experiences and who need particular encouragement to feel comfortable. Parents who are unfamiliar with the methods and approaches used may require extra explanation and reassurance. Parents from some minority ethnic groups may be concerned that their child's cultural and religious background is understood. Provision should be made to ensure that parents who do not use the language of the setting are provided with the full range of opportunities to be involved in their children's care and education.

FIRST IMPRESSIONS

First impressions count for a great deal and can make the difference between a parent choosing a particular centre for the child or going elsewhere. Most establishments will recognise this and take particular care to make the way into the building clear, with signs directing visitors to an appropriate person. Noticeboards and displays in entrance halls and foyers give an immediate impression of the philosophy of the centre. Carefully mounted and imaginatively displayed children's work demonstrates professional standards and shows what the children do and that you value their work. Named photographs of staff and their roles give parents an indication of how the centre operates. A well-maintained noticeboard giving information about current activities and topics may attract a parent's attention and encourage them to become involved. The physical condition and upkeep of the building also creates an impression; no parent would choose a gloomy, unsafe or unhygienic environment for their child.

Perhaps even more important than the welcome communicated by the physical environment is the response of the staff. In most establishments there will be a particular person with responsibility for dealing with enquiries and settling in new children and families, but this does not mean that other members of staff should not be involved. Everyone should have time for a greeting and a smile while the required person is found. Remember that parents may feel ill at ease in an unfamiliar setting. Leaving a child for the first time is almost certainly going to be stressful and they will need your support. Remembering the following may help you to put parents at their ease:

- Smile or nod when you see a parent, even if they are making their way to another member of staff.

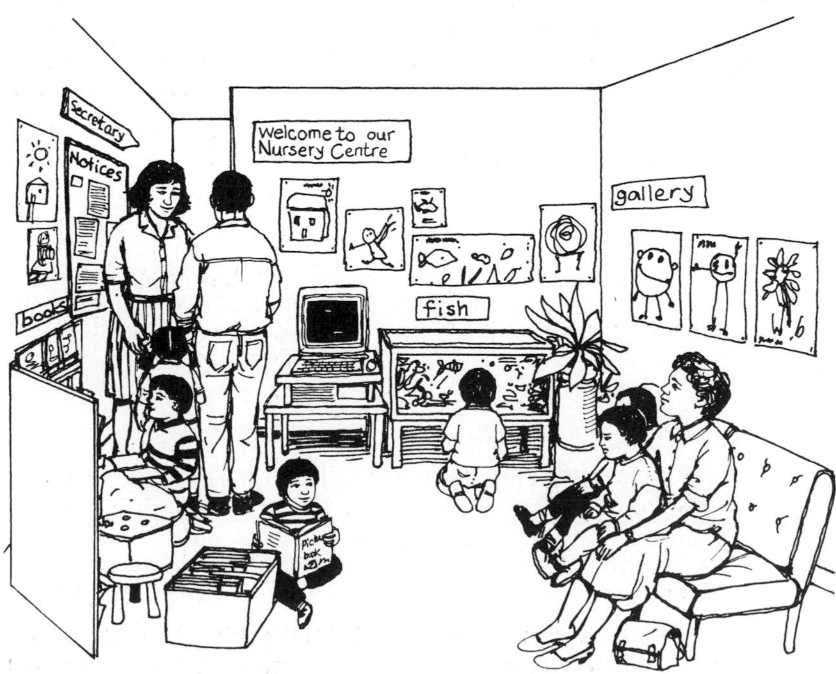

A welcoming entrance creates a positive impression

- Make time to talk with parents. If they have a concern that requires time and privacy, try to arrange a mutually convenient appointment.
- Try to call people by name. 'Ellie's mum' may do in an emergency but might not be the most appropriate way to address someone.
- Remember that there are many different types of families and that it is not at all unusual for parents to have a different surname from that of their child or of their partner. In our culturally diverse society, be aware that communities have their own naming customs and may not follow the Western naming custom of personal names followed by family names. Ask colleagues or consult records to find out parents' preferred forms of address. If you are unsure of the correct pronunciation, ask the parent.

Case study . . .

. . . a good impression

Marcia took a career break from her job when her daughter, Imogen, was born. When the time came for her to return to work, she visited a number of day nurseries that were conveniently situated between her home and workplace. Many of her friends had children at local nurseries, so she listened to what they had to say and chose some to visit. When Marcia telephoned the nursery that she eventually chose, she arranged a visit for a time when the senior nursery nurse would be free to show her around. She was encouraged to bring Imogen.

Marcia had no difficulty in finding the nursery. A sign directed her to the main door which opened into a bright entrance hall. It was clear that the nursery were expecting them as the member of staff who opened the door greeted her and Imogen by name. She was asked to sit down and wait in the hall while the senior nursery nurse was found. She had time to look at the displays of children's work and the prominent parents' noticeboard which was full of information about what was going on at nursery, alongside reminders for parents. Marcia and Imogen were taken on a tour of the nursery. The organisation of the rooms and the routine were explained and they were introduced to the staff. Imogen was shown the room that she would be based in and she met the staff who worked with that age group.

Marcia was offered a cup of tea in the nursery office and given an opportunity to ask about anything that she had seen and to raise any other points. She was given plenty of time and all of her questions were answered fully. As she left, she was given a copy of the nursery brochure and encouraged to get in touch if she had any questions or concerns.

What do you think made Marcia choose this nursery?

Why do you think the nursery encouraged Imogen to visit with her mother?

What might a parent want to find out on a first visit to a nursery?

SKILLS FOR TALKING AND LISTENING

Thinking about your own communication skills and how these might have an effect on your relationships with parents can be helpful. When talking with or listening to parents, consider the following points:

- Make eye contact but be careful – a fixed stare can be very off-putting.
- Don't interrupt and make comparisons from your own experiences. Encourage further conversation with phrases such as 'I see . . .', 'Tell me . . .'.

- Make sure that you are at the same level. Do not sit down if the parent is standing, or vice versa. This will make communication less equal.
- If the parent seems upset or wants to discuss something in private, find somewhere suitable to talk.
- Make the limits of confidentiality clear. Assure the parent that you will deal with any information shared professionally, but that you may have to pass some things on.
- Summarise the points that have been made during and at the end of a discussion. This recap will be particularly helpful if the parent has come to discuss ways of dealing with a problem.
- Keep your distance. Everyone needs a space around them. If you get too close, the person you are speaking to may feel uncomfortable. (On the other hand, people from some countries might have a different view of personal space and could interpret your distance as hostile.)
- You may feel that a parent is worrying over something quite unimportant. Do not dismiss these concerns as insignificant as the parent may be reluctant to confide in you in future. Try to be reassuring.

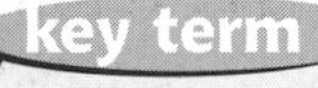

Jargon
terminology that is specific to a particular professional background

- Avoid using **jargon** (terms that only someone with your professional background would understand). This is off-putting and limits the effectiveness of your communication.
- If you have parents at your centre who do not speak English, try to organise someone to interpret for them. Some local authorities will provide this service or you might find someone locally. All parents, not just those who speak English, will want to share information and be consulted about their children's progress.
- Remember (particularly if you are a student) that you will usually need to discuss with colleagues and your line manager any requests that a parent might make. Don't make agreements that you might not be able to keep!

WRITTEN COMMUNICATIONS

All centres will have a brochure that they provide for parents that will give them initial information about the service offered. Of course, these will vary, though there will be common factors. These will probably include:

- location, including address, telephone number, person to contact
- the times that the centre is open and the length of sessions
- the age range of children catered for
- criteria for admission (for example, a workplace nursery may require the parent to work in the establishment; many social services establishments require children to be referred through a social worker or health visitor)
- information about meals and snacks provided
- information about the facilities and accommodation available
- schedule of fees (if any) to be charged
- reference to any policies, especially those relating to special educational needs and equal opportunities
- the qualifications of the staff and staff roles and responsibilities

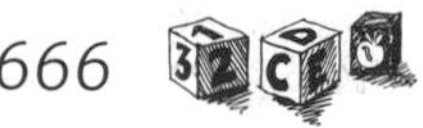

- an indication of the daily or sessional programme for the children
- what parents are expected to provide, for example nappies, spare clothing, sun cream
- details of any commitments the parent must make, for example rota days, notice of leaving, regular attendance
- details of any approach to learning followed such as learning through play, Highscope, Montessori and the curriculum followed
- information about the complaints procedure.

A brochure can provide the parent with a great deal of information that will also be useful for reference.

Parents can expect to receive a whole range of written communications once their child has started at a centre. Some centres produce their own booklets, for example, about their approach to reading or other areas of the curriculum, indicating to parents the part they can play in their children's learning. Parents might also receive regular newsletters, invitations to concerts, parents' meetings, requests for assistance and support, information about the activities provided for children, advance notice of holidays and centre closures, and so on. These will often be reinforced with notices and verbal reminders. It is important that these notices and letters communicate the information in a clear and friendly manner.

Sometimes there will be a need for a more individual exchange of information, for example if a child has an accident during the session. This might be written in a note to the parent or it might be explained at pick-up time. Parents need to know what has happened and someone needs to have responsibility for passing on this information.

Progress check

Why is it important that the entrance to a centre is welcoming and inviting to parents?

What should child-care staff do to ensure that their conversations with parents are positive and rewarding?

How can you ensure effective communication with parents who do not use English as their first language? Give examples.

What information should be included in the centre brochure?

What other kinds of written information might parents expect to receive?

What should you have in mind when preparing written information to circulate to parents?

Parents and record keeping

All establishments are required to keep records of the children and families that they work with. The content of these records will vary depending on the type of care that is being provided. They will always include personal data about the child supplied by parents. There will also be records that document the child's progress and achievements during their time at the centre and parents will be asked to contribute to these too.

INITIAL INFORMATION

Usually parents are asked to complete a form that includes the following:

- personal details about the child: full name, date of birth, etc.
- names, addresses and phone numbers of parents and other emergency contacts
- medical details that will include the address and telephone number of the child's doctor and any information about allergies and regular medications
- details about any particular dietary needs
- details about religion which might have a bearing on the care provided for the child.

Additionally, there may be sensitive information that is necessary for the centre to have; for example, are there any restrictions on who may collect the child from the centre? Are social services involved with the family?

Parents will need to be assured that such information will be confidential and stored securely. Centres need to make sure that this essential information is correct and up to date.

Other types of information will also be very helpful to staff. These might include the following:

- any comfort object the child might have
- food likes and dislikes
- any particular fears
- special words the child might use, for example for the lavatory.

It is particularly important that parents have confidence in staff and feel that they are able to pass on information about events at home that might affect the child. Illness in the family, a new baby or a parent leaving home will all have an effect on the child. The more that the exchange of this type of information is encouraged, the smoother the process of sharing care is likely to be. Some centres use a **key worker** system where one member of staff has responsibility for a particular group of children. This can be helpful to parents as they can build a relationship with their child's key worker.

Remember that some parents may have difficulty with filling in forms and with written information. They may not be literate, or they may be literate in another language and might need oral support or access to translated information.

key term

Key worker
works with, and is concerned with, the care and assessment of particular children

Case study . . .

. . . expressing concerns

Shamila had been coming to nursery for over a year. She was a bright and outgoing child who had plenty of friends and joined in with all the activities. One morning she came in looking very pale and tired. She spent the whole of the session curled up in the book corner, often with a rug over her, pretending to be asleep. At home time, the nursery nurse made a point of having a word with Shamila's mother and described her behaviour. Her mother seemed very upset. She explained that Shamila's grandmother, who lived with them, was seriously ill and had been admitted to hospital the previous day and the whole of the family had been affected.

What do you think was wrong with Shamila?

Why is it helpful for the staff to know what's upsetting her?

What opportunities do parents in your setting have to share this kind of individual information?

PROGRESS AND ACHIEVEMENTS

A great deal is to be gained from sharing record keeping with parents. This does not mean merely making children's records available to parents, but encouraging parents to contribute by offering their own observations of their children, thus putting the child into the wider context of home and community. Parents can be involved in the process of recording their children's progress and achievements in a number of ways:

- Parents will often help staff to compile a profile of their child at admission. This is usually organised around areas of development and shows what the child can do. It may also include space to refer to the child's preferences, for example 'likes painting', and any other related information, including concerns. These initial profiles serve as a starting point and will be added to as the child progresses and achieves new skills.
- An exchange of information about a child's achievements or concerns will usually take place on an informal basis at the beginning and end of sessions and can be very useful.
- Most settings and parents would agree that there is a place for a regular, more structured exchange of information where records can be updated by parents and by staff and progress discussed. This will give parents the opportunity to add to the records compiled by staff and supplement these with additional information from their own observations. Plans for continuing progress should also be discussed with parents, emphasising the partnership between parents and staff, and recognising the parents' key role in promoting their children's development.
- Checklists that detail skills and achievements in pictorial form, as shown below, are quick and easy to fill in. Children and parents will enjoy filling these in and recording progress together
- Diary-type booklets that are regularly written up and sent home with children for parents to read and comment on provide another useful channel for exchanging information, particularly for those parents who are unable to get to the centre on a regular basis.

Progress check

What kind of information will centres keep on the children they care for?

Why is it important that this information is stored securely and kept up to date?

How can child-care workers ensure that parents have an opportunity to share individual or sensitive information that concerns their children?

How can parents contribute to records of their children's progress and achievements?

Why is this beneficial to parents and to the staff?

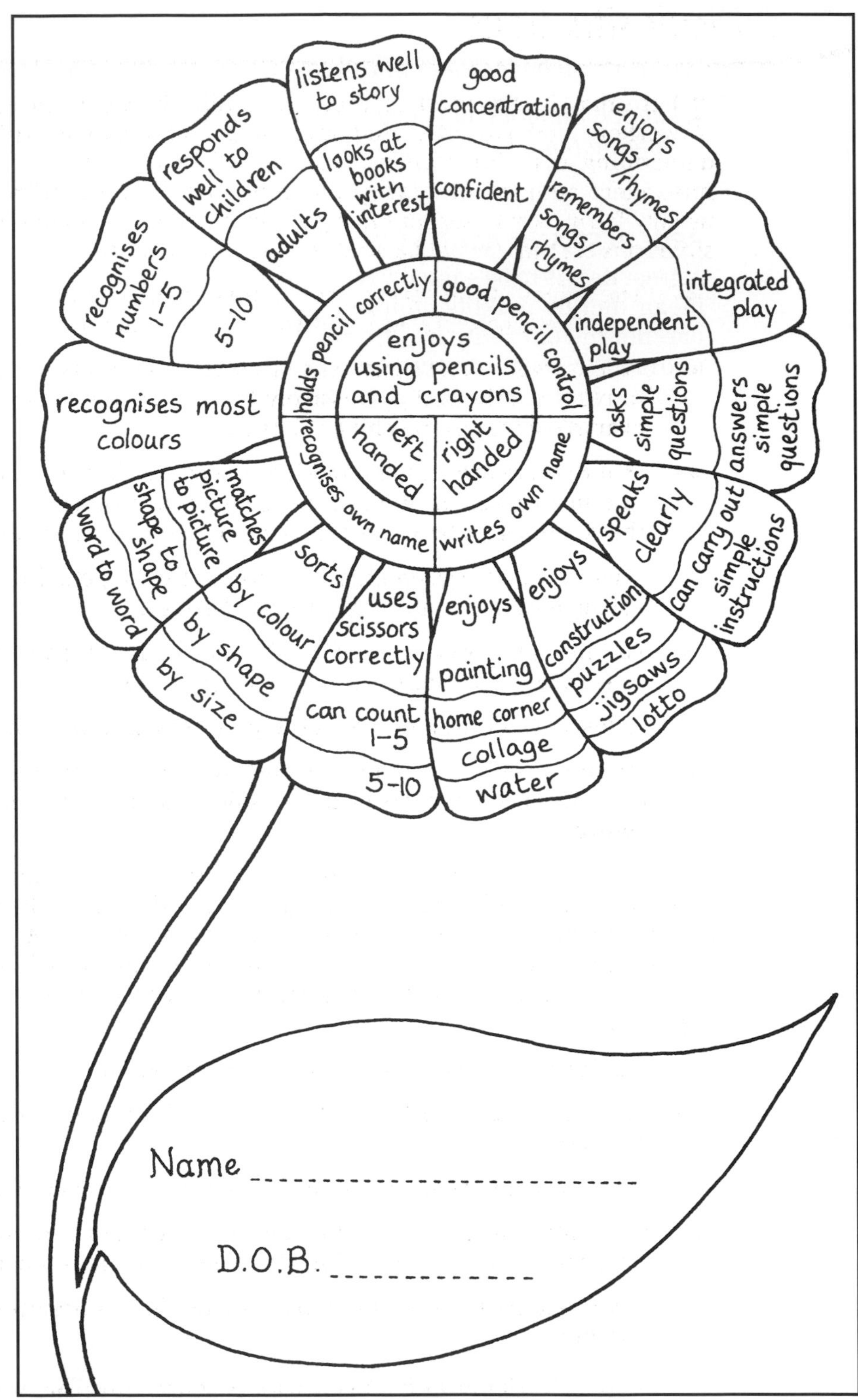

Parents and children will enjoy recording progress together

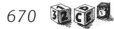

Difficult situations

There may be times when there is conflict between the child-care centre and workers and parents. Understanding and resolving this conflict can be a demanding task for staff to manage. Difficulties that arise out of a simple misunderstanding, for example a child coming home with the wrong coat, are usually fairly easy to sort out in a good-humoured way. Below are some examples of situations that might not be quite so straightforward:

- The values of the centre, for example methods of disciplining children, may sometimes be quite different from those at home.
- Parents who are experiencing stresses and strains in their lives may appear to react angrily and aggressively to what seems to be a minor incident, for example a tear in the child's clothes.
- Where there are child protection procedures in operation, and a centre has a role in monitoring and reporting on contact between parents and children, the relationship between child-care workers and parents may be strained.
- There may be agreements over, say, collecting children at the agreed time, paying fees in advance, that are not kept to.
- Parents may disagree with the methods of the centre, for example challenging a learning through play approach.
- Rules such as no smoking on the premises may be broken and challenged.
- Parents may have complaints and concerns directed at particular members of staff. This could result in an official complaint being lodged against the centre.

There is no magic formula for resolving difficulties of any type and there is a clear need for regular training to equip staff with the skills that enable them to cope with challenging and difficult situations. A centre that values its partnership with parents will work hard to maintain the confidence of parents by attempting to resolve difficulties to the satisfaction of all concerned. This is most likely to happen if:

- staff deal seriously and courteously with parents' concerns
- anger and aggression are dealt with calmly and not in a confrontational manner
- parents' skills, feelings and opinions are acknowledged and valued
- the centre has a consistent and well thought-out approach to the way that it works with parents, and all staff are aware of and supportive of it
- any concerns the staff have are communicated promptly and honestly with parents.

To sum up, to work most effectively with parents, child-care workers need to take a non-judgemental approach, that is one that recognises that parents have a great deal to contribute in the shared care of their children, and where professionals value and act on these contributions.

Case study . . .

. . . a difficult situation

Helen had been having a difficult time with her partner. Staff at the family centre who cared for her son, Liam, were aware that there were problems at home and had noticed how worn and tired Helen looked recently. One afternoon Helen stormed into the centre shouting abuse at Julie, Liam's key worker. When Julie asked her what was wrong, she grabbed Liam and then tried to leave the centre. Julie stood by the door and asked Helen to come and have a word with her in the office. Helen was reluctant but Julie remained calm and firm and eventually she agreed. Julie asked Helen what was wrong and Helen explained that she had arrived home to find that her partner had left her. She said that she'd been worried that he might try to take Liam away with him. Julie suggested what she might do and whom she should contact if she felt that there was a risk that Liam would be snatched. After she had calmed down, Helen apologised and said that she would stay with Liam for the rest of the session to put her mind at rest.

1. *Why did Julie feel that she needed to talk with Helen, rather than let her storm off?*
2. *What did Julie do to minimise confrontation?*
3. *Why was it helpful to go into the office?*

Progress check

What kinds of issues might give rise to conflict between the child-care centre and parents? Give some examples.

Why is it important that staff try to resolve these difficulties?

How can staff help to minimise the effects of this conflict?

Why is a non-judgemental approach important?

Getting parents involved

All parents will have some involvement with the centre that their child attends. Just what form this involvement takes depends on the type of centre, on the way that the staff interpret their brief to work with parents and on the parents themselves. The following are some examples of ways in which child-care centres can work together with parents to the benefit of their children.

SETTLING IN

Everyone recognises the importance of the settling-in period for both the child and the parent, and will encourage parents to play a full part. Centres will use some or all of the following to make this transition a positive experience.

- Parents will often stay with their child until, with the encouragement of staff, they feel comfortable about leaving. At this stage the exchange of information is vital: staff will want to know all about the child and parents will want to know all about how their child is doing during these early days. Parents who have full-time jobs may find it difficult to stay during these sessions but will be just as concerned; giving them plenty of notice of arrangements for starting may mean that they can organise other commitments and be there.

- Day nurseries who cater primarily for working parents will often have a programme for introducing parents and children to the setting, providing evening sessions where children and parents can meet staff and visit the building. When the child starts, there is usually someone at the end of a telephone to report back and reassure parents.
- Some centres will have their own pre-school (or pre-nursery) club where children come with their parents for a number of sessions before they start officially.
- Some centres will make home visits to families prior to their children starting nursery or school. Parents often feel more comfortable in their own homes rather than in a strange, perhaps intimidating environment.

It is important to remember that the settling-in period can sometimes be more stressful for the parents than for the child. Parents may take some time to adjust to a new role.

After the settling-in period, parents may be involved in a variety of ways.

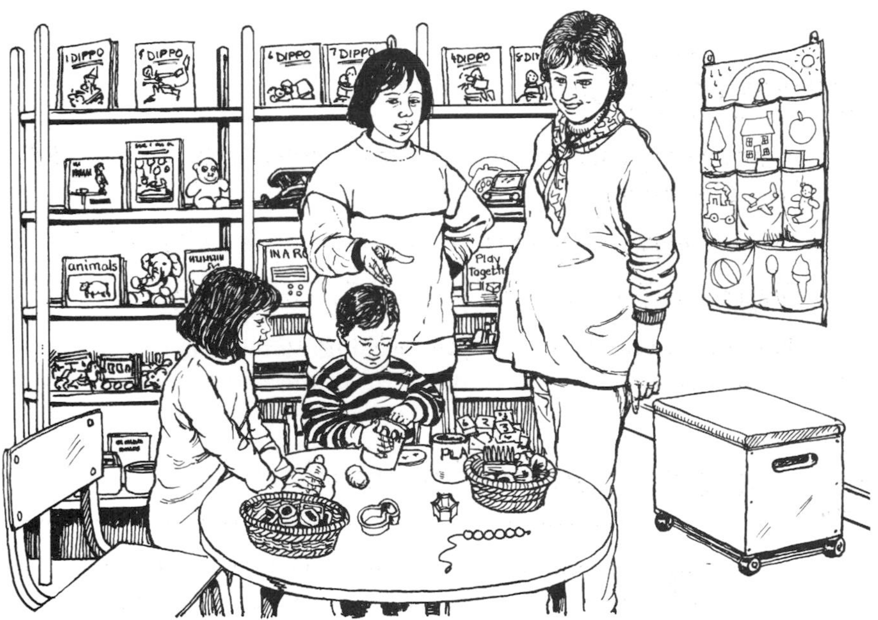

Stay and play sessions can be very popular

WORKING WITH THE CHILDREN

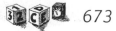

Here parents are encouraged to stay and become involved in activities with the children, sometimes committing themselves to a regular session – as with a playgroup rota – but more often on an occasional basis. The children benefit from the presence of another adult, parents have a chance to see the setting at work and the child is aware of the link between home and the centre. Cooking, craft and swimming sessions are often provided in this way and many schools rely on parent help for reading activities. Outings with groups of children would neither be possible nor safe without parent volunteers to accompany them. Parents might also be able to contribute in a more specific way, for example by talking about their job, telling a story in another language or playing an instrument.

Case study . . .

. . . giving a talk

The reception class had been working on a topic about 'Ourselves'. The children had examined their own features and compared them with those of their friends and taken part in many other linked activities. The school had a good relationship with its parents and they were often involved in classroom activities. At the beginning of every topic, class teachers displayed their plans on the parents' noticeboard and asked parents for contributions, either of materials or ideas. One parent noticed that some work was planned on joints and the skeleton. As a radiographer, she had access to X-rays that she thought might be useful for the project. After a chat with the class teacher, she was persuaded not only to donate the X-rays but also to come and give a talk to the class. Although she had some misgivings, she came along in her hospital uniform and talked to the children about her job. There were lots of questions after she'd finished, with many from children who'd had their own experiences of X-rays after accidents. When she came in next to pick up her children, she saw the follow-up work that the children had done after her visit was displayed on the classroom noticeboard.

1. *What do you think the children gained from this experience?*
2. *What do you think the parent gained from participating in this way?*
3. *Do you think all parents would be happy taking on this role? What would it depend on?*

WORKING BEHIND THE SCENES

Not everyone feels comfortable or is able to work alongside the children. Making, mending and maintaining equipment is a task that can involve parents. Also in this category of involvement will be the fund-raising and organisation of social events that many parent groups take responsibility for. These social events that bring together staff and parents are usually very successful in promoting good relationships and often raise funds too. Parents who are not available during the day may be able to become involved in these ways.

SPECIAL OCCASIONS

Most centres have occasions when parents are invited along to parties, concerts, sports, open days or stay and play sessions. Such events are usually very popular indeed. More parents will be able to take advantage of the invitation if other commitments are taken into account, for example if babies and toddlers are welcome at an afternoon concert, or if there are occasional evening events so that those who are out at work during the day can attend.

SUPPORT FOR PARENTS

In some centres the staff have a special brief to work with parents. This is probably because there is some difficulty in the family that affects the child and the parent needs some support. Staff work alongside parents and children in individual programmes. For this kind of work to be successful, it is crucial that the member of staff has the trust and confidence of the parent. Some centres might also offer 'drop-in' facilities and parents' groups as part of their programme.

TAKING THE CURRICULUM HOME

Most parents will expect to play a part in helping their children to read. Home–school reading diaries, in which parents and staff exchange comments on books and reading, provide a link and show children that everyone is involved in supporting their progress. Sometimes settings provide children and parents with activity packs or sheets suggesting ways to continue or consolidate what they have been working on during the session. This approach recognises and emphasises the important role that the home and parents have in children's learning.

OFFICIAL ROLES

Some parents will be involved with the child-care centre in an official capacity. All state schools will have parents, elected by other parents, on their governing bodies and they have an important role defined in law. Playgroups are usually run by a committee of parents for the benefit of the local community. Other types of settings may have parent representatives on their management committees. Sometimes parents may be reluctant to become involved in this way and need to be assured that they have a necessary and valuable contribution to make.

Progress check

Why is settling in a key time for involving parents?

Why is it important to be flexible when making arrangements for children to settle in?

Does being involved mean that the parent has to help out in the classroom? Explain your answer.

How can parents participate in the curriculum?

List ways in which parents can work 'behind the scenes'.

Now try these questions

Why is it important that child-care staff should work in partnership with parents?

How can you make it clear to parents that you welcome them and that you value their participation?

How might you meet the needs of:

(a) parents who are not fluent in English?

(b) parents who feel uneasy or intimidated in the setting?

Why is it helpful to children's progress if record keeping is shared with parents?

key terms

You need to know what the key terms and phrases in this chapter mean.
Go back through the chapter and find out.

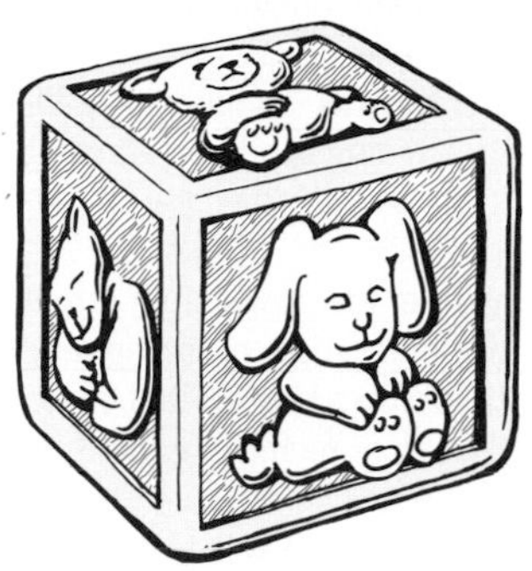

GLOSSARY

ABC of behaviour the pattern of all behaviour: Antecedent – what happens before the behaviour occurs; Behaviour – the resulting behaviour, acceptable or unacceptable; Consequence – the result of the behaviour, positive or negative

Absolute poverty not having enough provision to maintain health and working efficiency

Accessible easy to reach or approach

Accident book legal documentation of all accidents and injuries occurring in any establishment

Accommodation away from home a placement with a foster carer or in a residential setting arranged by the local authority social services department

Achievement the emotional need for the satisfaction gained from success

Active immunity the body's ability to resist a disease that has been acquired by having the disease or by having a specific immunisation

Advocacy speaking on behalf of, or in favour of, disabled people

Affection the emotional need to feel loved by parents, carers, family, friends and the wider social community

Almar grasp whole-hand grasp

Amino acid part of a protein

Amniocentesis a sample of amniotic fluid is taken via a needle inserted into the uterus through the abdominal wall; used to detect chromosomal abnormalities

Amnion the membranes that make up the sac containing the developing baby

Anaemia a condition in which the blood lacks adequate amounts of haemoglobin

Anatomically correct dolls dolls with accurately reproduced body parts including sexual organs

Animism the belief that everything that exists has a consciousness

Anterior fontanelle a diamond-shaped area of membrane at the front of the baby's head. It closes between 12 and 18 months of age

Anti-convulsant a drug that is given to prevent fits

Anti-discriminatory practice practice that encourages a positive view of difference, and opposes negative attitudes and practices that lead to unfavourable treatment of people

Antibody a substance made by white cells to attack pathogens

Apgar score a method of assessing the newborn baby's condition by observing the vital signs

Area Child Protection Committee writes, monitors and reviews the child protection procedures for its area, and promotes co-ordination and communication between all workers

Artificial ventilation mouth-to-mouth breathing to get oxygen into the lungs of the casualty

Assessment matching a child's reponses or performance against a standardised scale, measuring achievements (e.g. SATs) or norms of development

Associative play play begins with other children; children make intermittent interactions and/or are involved in the same activity although their play remains personal

Asthma difficulty in breathing, when the airways in the lungs become narrowed; triggered by allergies, infections, exercise and emotional upset

Attachment an affectionate two-way relationship that develops between an infant and an adult

Attainment targets the different elements of a curriculum area; for example, the attainment targets for English are speaking, reading and writing

Autism difficulty in relating to other people and making sense of the social world

Average a medium, a standard or a 'norm'

Baseline assessment required assessment of children's skills currently (January 2001) undertaken on entry to school. In future, likely to be applied at the beginning of Year 1

Bedtime routine a consistent approach to putting children to bed, which encourages sleep by increasing security

Behaviour acting or reacting in a specific way, both unacceptably and acceptably

Behaviour modification techniques used to bring about changes in unacceptable behaviour so that it becomes acceptable

Belonging the emotional need to feel wanted by a group

Bilingual speaking two languages

Biological theories our temperament, sociability, emotional responses and intelligence are determined by what we inherit genetically from our biological parents

Birth asphyxia failure of the baby to establish spontaneous respiration at birth

Booster an additional dose of a vaccine, given after the initial dose

British Sign Language (BSL) the visual, gestural language of the British deaf community

Bronchitis a chest infection caused by infection of the main airways

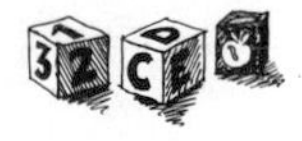

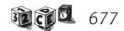

Bronchodilator (reliever) a drug that helps the airways to expand, used to treat asthma

Caesarean delivery of the fetus via an abdominal incision
Calorie a unit of energy
Capillaries very small blood vessels
Cardiopulmonary resuscitation (CPR) chest compressions and artificial ventilation to get oxygen circulating around the body
Central nervous system the brain, spinal cord and nerves
Cerebral palsy a disorder of movement and posture; part of the brain that controls movement and posture is damaged or fails to develop
Cerebro-spinal fluid the fluid surrounding the brain and spinal cord
Child protection register lists all the children in an area who are considered to be at risk of abuse or neglect
Child-centred with the child at the centre, taking into account the perspective of the child
Children in need a child is 'in need' if they are unlikely to achieve or maintain a reasonable standard of health or development without the provision of services, or if they are disabled
Chorionic villus sampling (CVS) A small sample of placental tissue is removed via the vagina; used to detect chromosomal and other abnormalities
Chronological age the age of a child in years and months
Cleft lip or palate a structural impairment of the top lip, palate or both
Co-operative play children are able to play together co-operatively; they are able to adopt a role within the group and to take account of others' needs and actions
Coeliac condition a metabolic disorder involving sensitivity to gluten; there is difficulty in digesting food
Cognitive development the development of thinking and understanding, which includes problem solving, reasoning, concentration, memory, imagination and creativity; also called intellectual development
Colostrum the first breast milk containing a high proportion of protein and antibodies
Compensatory education a programme or initiative that is offered to those who might be likely to experience disadvantage in the education system
Complementary feeds additional feeds as well as breast feeds
Complete protein a protein containing all the essential amino acids; also called first-class proteins
Concentration the skill of focusing all your attention on one task
Conception occurs when sperm fertilises a ripe ovum
Condition medically defined illness
Conductive deafness deafness caused by an interruption to the process of sounds passing through the eardrum and the middle ear
Conductive education a teaching method aimed at enabling motor-impaired children to function in society
Congenital a disease or disorder that occurs during pregnancy and is present at birth
Congenital deformity a term used in the Children Act 1989; a disability evident at the time of birth
Congenital disorders of the hip the hip joint is unstable or dislocated because it fails to develop properly before birth
Conscience the faculty by which we know right from wrong
Conservation an understanding that the quantity of a substance remains the same if nothing is added or taken away, even though it may appear different
Consistency provision and quality of interaction that is constant (remains the same) regardless of which adults the child is in contact with
Consistency the emotional need to feel that things are predictable
Continuity provision of activities and experiences in a logical sequence
Contract an agreement between an adult and child – the child agrees to behave in a particular way and the adult agrees to reward that behaviour when it occurs
Contraction involuntary, intermittent muscular tightenings of the uterus
Creativity the expression of ideas in a personal and unique way, using the imagination
Cultural background the way of life of the family in which a person is brought up
Culture the way of life, the language and the behaviour that is acceptable and appropriate to the society in which a person lives
Curiosity an inquisitive interest
Curriculum the content and methods that comprise a course of study
Customs special guidelines for behaviour, which are followed by particular groups of people
Cystic fibrosis an hereditary, life-threatening condition affecting the lungs and digestive tract

Day care the provision of care during the day in a variety of settings outside a child's own home with people other than close relatives, either full-time or part-time
Decentre being able to see things from another's point of view
Deep relaxing sleep (DRS) periods of unconsciousness during the sleep cycle
Demand feeding feeding babies when they are hungry in preference to feeding by the clock
Designated member of staff the person identified in an establishment to whom allegations or suspicions of child abuse should be reported
Developmental level the stage of development that a child has reached. This may or may not be consistent with the child's chronological age (age in years)
Diabetes a condition in which the body cannot metabolise carbohydrates, resulting in high levels of sugar in the blood and urine
Differentiate to distinguish and classify as different
Diffuse bruising bruising that is spread out
Digestion the process of breaking down food so that it can be absorbed and used by the body
Disability the disadvantage or restriction of activity caused by society that takes little or no account of people who have physical or mental impairments and thus excludes them from the mainstream of social activities. According to the social model, disability is defined as 'socially imposed restriction' (Oliver, 1981)
Disclosure (of abuse) when a child tells someone they have been abused
Discrimination behaviour based on prejudice, which results in someone being treated unfairly
Distraction test a hearing test carried out at about 7 months
Distress syndrome the pattern of behaviour shown by the children who experience loss of a familiar carer with no one to take their place

 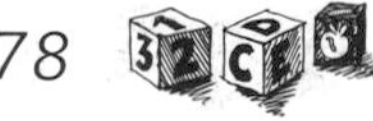

Domiciliary services services provided in the home
Dose the prescribed amount of medicine to be taken
Down syndrome a condition caused by an abnormal chromosome, which affects a person's appearance and development
Duchenne muscular dystrophy a condition involving progressive destruction of muscle tissue, only affecting boys

E number a number given to an additive approved by the EU
Early Learning Goals what most children will achieve in the six areas of learning, by the beginning of Key Stage One
Egocentric self-centred, from the words ego, meaning 'self' and centric, meaning centred on; seeing things only from one's own viewpoint
Embryo term used to describe the developing baby from conception until 8 weeks after conception
Emergency Protection Order a court order that enables a child to be removed to safe accommodation or kept in a safe place
Emergent writing an approach to writing that encourages children to write independently; also known as developmental writing
Emotional development the growth of the ability to feel and express an increasing range of emotions appropriately, including those about oneself
Empathy an understanding of how other people feel
Empower children to enable children to take part in the world
Encopresis deliberate soiling into the pants, on to the floor or other area after bowel control has been established
Endometrium the lining of the uterus
Enquiry (into suspected abuse) a local authority has a duty to carry out an enquiry if there are reasonable grounds to suspect that a child is suffering or is likely to suffer significant harm
Enuresis involuntary bed wetting during sleep
Environmental aids and adaptation for example, a flashing light doorbell for deaf people, modified utensils and eating tools, bathing aids etc.
Enzyme a substance that helps to digest food
Epidural anaesthetic injected into the epidural space in the spine to numb the area from the waist down
Epilepsy recurrent attacks of temporary disturbance of the brain function
Episiotomy a cut to the perineum to assist the delivery of the fetus
Equal opportunities all people participating in society to the best of their abilities, regardless of race, religion, disability, gender or social background
Equal opportunities policies policies designed to provide opportunities for all people to achieve according to their efforts and abilities
Ethnic group a group of people who share a common culture
Ethnic minority group a group of people with a common culture, which is smaller than the majority group in their society
Experiential achieving through experience
Extended family a family grouping that includes other family members who live either together or very close to each other and are in frequent contact with each other

Failure to thrive failing to grow normally for no organic reason
Family of origin the family a child is born into
Fat-soluble vitamin a vitamin that can be stored by the body, so it need not be included in the diet every day
Febrile convulsions a fit or seizure that occurs as a result of a raised body temperature
Femur the long bone in the thigh
Fetus the term used to describe the baby from the eighth week after conception until birth
Fine motor skills small finger movements and manipulative skills, hand–eye co-ordination
Flammable material that burns easily
Fluoride a mineral that helps to prevent dental decay
Food allergies reactions to certain foods in the diet
Forceps spoon-shaped implements to protect the baby's head and assist in the delivery of the fetus
Foundation Stage the introductory stage of the National Curriculum, for children from 3 until year 1 of Key Stage One
Frenulum the web of skin joining the gum and the lip
Frozen awareness/frozen watchfulness constantly looking around, alert and aware (vigilant), while remaining physically inactive (passive), demonstrating a lack of trust in adults
Function of the family the things the family does for its members

Gender being either male or female
Genital sexual organs
Glue ear where infected material builds up in the middle ear, following repeated ear infections
Gluten a protein found in wheat, rye, barley and oats
Grief feelings of deep sorrow at the loss, through death, of a loved person
Gross motor skills whole body and limb movements, co-ordination and balance
Guardian ad litem person appointed by the courts to safeguard and promote the interests and welfare of children during court proceedings
Guthrie test on the 6th day after birth, a sample of the baby's blood is taken, usually by pricking the heel, to test for phenylketonuria, cystic fibrosis and cretinism

Haemoglobin a red oxygen-carrying protein containing iron, present in the red blood cells
Haemophilia an inherited blood disorder, where there is a defect in one of the clotting factors
Head lag The baby's head falls back when pulled to sit
Health visitor a trained nurse who specialises in child health promotion
Hearing impairment either conductive deafness or nerve deafness; ranges from slight hearing difficulty to profound deafness
Hearsay what you are told by others
Hidden curriculum messages, often unintended, that are communicated to children as a consequence of the attitudes and values of the adults who deliver the curriculum
Housing associations non-profit-making organisations that exist to provide homes for people in need of housing from a variety of social and cultural backgrounds
Human chorionic gonadotrophin (HCG) a hormone produced by the implanted embryo, which is excreted in the mother's urine; its presence confirms pregnancy

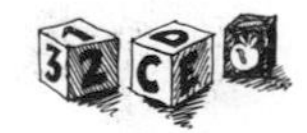

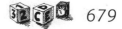

Hydrocephalus a condition involving an increase in the fluid surrounding the brain, often associated with spina bifida
Hygiene the study of the principles of health
Hypoglycaemia low levels of glucose in the blood
Hypothesis the provisional explanation or solution to a problem reached by assessment of the observed facts

Identification making oneself the same as those who are significant to us
Imagination the ability to form mental images, or concepts of objects not present, or that do not exist
Imitate to copy closely, take as a model
Immunity the presence of antibodies that protect the body against infectious disease
Impairment lacking all or part of a limb, or having altered or reduced function in a limb, organism or mechanism of the body. According to the social model, impairment is defined as 'individual limitation' (Oliver, 1981)
Implantation occurs when the fertilised ovum settles into the lining of the uterus
Inclusive organised in a way that enables all to take a full and active part; meeting the needs of all children
Incomplete protein a protein containing some essential amino acids; also called second-class proteins
Incubation period The time from when pathogens enter the body until the first signs of infection appear
Incubator an enclosed cot that regulates temperature and humidity
Independence the emotional need to feel you are managing and directing your own life
Independent life skills skills needed to live and care for oneself
Individual Education Plan (IEP) an outline of short-term and long-term aims and objectives with targets for achievement of goals by children with special educational needs
Induction starting labour by artificial means, for example by breaking the waters or giving hormones to stimulate contractions
Initial child protection conference brings together the family, professionals concerned with the child and other specialists to exchange information and make decisions
Innate ability natural ability
Instincts patterns of behaviour that are not learned
Institutional discrimination unfavourable treatment occurring as a consequence of the procedures and systems of an organisation
Institutional oppression the power of organisations brought to bear on an individual to keep them in their place
Insulin a hormone produced in the pancreas to metabolise carbohydrate in the bloodstream and regulate glucose
Internalise to understand the things that adults think are important and begin to believe and behave similarly

Jargon terminology that is specific to a particular professional background
Jaundice yellowing of the skin and whites of the eyes as a result of too much bilirubin in the blood
Job Seekers' Allowance benefits paid to people who are registered as unemployed

Key worker works with, and is concerned with the care and assessment of, particular children
Labelling giving a reputation (or label) to someone based upon a small part of their behaviour. For example, a child who is very noisy may be labelled as disruptive. This creates a prejudiced view of the child
Labour the process by which the fetus, placenta and membranes are expelled from the birth canal
Lacerations tears in the skin
Language Acquisition Device (LAD) the name Chomsky gives to our innate physical and intellectual abilities that enable us to acquire and use language
Language development the development of communication skills, which includes non-verbal communication, reading and writing, as well as spoken language; also called linguistic development
Lanugo the fine hair found on the body of the fetus before birth and on the newborn infant; mainly associated with pre-term babies
Layette first clothes for a baby
Learning outcome a statement of what the children/child will learn from the activity or experience
Learning theories children develop as they do because they have contact with other people and learn from them
Legislation laws that have been made
Lethargy lacking energy, tired and unresponsive
Light-for-dates a baby who is smaller than expected for the length of pregnancy (gestation)
Literacy the aspects of language concerned with reading and writing
Local management of schools (LMS) enables a head teacher and the governors of a school to decide how to spend their money and staff a school
Localising searching for and locating the source of a sound
Locomotion the developing ability to move from one place to another, usually by crawling, walking or running
Look and say an approach to reading that relies on recognition of the shape or pattern of a word
Low birthweight babies born prematurely (pre-term) or below the 10th centile for their gestation, usually weighing less than 2.5kg at birth

Makaton a system of simple signs used with people who have limited language skills
Maternal deprivation 'the prolonged deprivation of young children of maternal care' (Bowlby)
Matriarchal family a family in which women are important and dominant
Maturity being fully developed and capable of self-control
Independence the development of skills that lead to less reliance on other people for help or support
Means test an assessment of a person's income and savings, made by completing a form (test) about their income (means) to determine whether they are eligible to receive certain benefits
Meconium the first stool passed by the newborn – a soft, black/green motion present in the fetal bowel from about the 16th week of pregnancy
Medical model a view of disability as requiring medical intervention
Melanocytes pigmented cells
Menstrual cycle the process of ovulation and menstruation in sexually mature, non-pregnant women
Metabolic related to the process of digesting, absorbing and using food
Migration the movement either to or from a country

 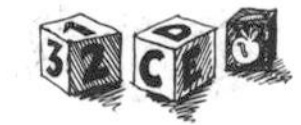

Milia 'milk spots' – small white spots on the noses of newborn babies caused by blocked sebaceous glands
Milk teeth the first 20 (deciduous) teeth
Mongolian blue spots smooth, bluish-grey to purple skin patches consisting of an excess of pigmented skin cells
Motherease or parentease term used by researchers to describe the enabling, focused language interaction, typically observed between mother and infant
Motor development the process of muscular movements becoming more complex
Motor impaired an impairment of a function of movement
Multi-ability society a society where people have a variety of differing abilities and disabilities
Multi-cultural society a society whose members have a variety of cultural and ethnic background
Multi-disciplinary made up of different professionals
Multilingual speaking many languages
Multiple disadvantage the concentration of social problems in one area
Multi-professional assessment a measurement of the child's performance by professionals from different backgrounds, e.g. health care, social work, psychology etc.

National Childcare Strategy a strategy introduced by the UK government in May 1998 to ensure good quality, accessible, affordable child care for children aged up to 14
National Curriculum a course of study, laid down by government, that all children between 5 and 16 in state schools in the UK must follow
National Literacy Strategy government guidance (1998) for the structure and content of a daily hour-long literacy lesson for children from Reception to Key Stage Two
National Numeracy Strategy government guidance (1999) for the structure and content of a daily 45-minute numeracy lesson for children from Reception to Key Stage Two
Nature–nurture debate discussion as to whether genetic factors (nature) or environmental factors (nurture) are more important in influencing behaviour and achievement
Negative self-image the child feels they are not worth while or valuable
Neonate a newborn baby
Nerve deafness deafness caused by damage to the inner ear, or to the nerves, or hearing centres in the brain
Neural tube cells in the embryo that will develop into the baby's spinal cord
Non-judgemental not taking a fixed position on an issue
Non-verbal communication non-spoken communication, for example, bodily movements, eye contact, gestures and facial expression; sometimes used to enhance or replace speech
Norm developmental skill achieved within an average time-scale
Normative measurements an average or norm against which any individual child's development can be measured
Norms the rules and guidelines that turn values into actions
Nuclear family a family grouping where parents live with their children and form a small group with no other family members living near them
Nursery grant public funds paid to settings in the private and voluntary sector for the education of 3 and 4 year olds
Nutrient a substance that provides essential nourishment

Object permanence an understanding that objects continue to exist when not in view
Objective free of personal feelings or thoughts
Observation a record of a child's response to an activity or situation, used by professionals to determine progress and needs
Oedema swelling of the tissues with fluid
Oesophagus the top of the digestive tract, leading from the mouth to the stomach
Oestrogen a hormone produced by the ovaries
Omission not doing those things that should be done, such as protecting children from harm
Oppression using power to dominate and restrict other people
Orientate to determine the position of things
Orthofunction a teaching method that involves the whole person physically and mentally, and 'instils in children the ability to function as members of society, and to participate in normal social settings appropriate to their age'
Otitis media an infection of the middle ear
Ovum egg produced by the ovary

Pancreas a gland that secretes insulin and enzymes that aid digestion
Parallel play a child plays side-by-side with another child but without interacting; their play activities remain personal
Paramount of first importance
Parasite lives on and obtains its food from humans
Partnership with parents a way of working with parents that recognises their needs and their entitlement to be involved in decisions affecting their children
Passive immunity the body's ability to resist a disease, acquired from antibodies given directly into the body, for example the antibodies passed on in breast milk
Pathogens germs such as bacteria and viruses
Patriarchal family a family in which men are dominant and make the important decisions
Pelvis the bones that make up the hip girdle
Percentile chart Specially prepared charts that are used to record measurements of a child's progress in growth or development. There are percentile charts to measure weight, height, head circumference and development
Peripatetic travelling to see those they work with
Personal identity one's own individuality, the characteristics that make us different and separate from others, our personality
Phagocytosis the process by which white cells absorb pathogens and destroy them
Phenylketonuria (PKU) a metabolic impairment that prevents the normal digestion of protein; recessively inherited
Phonics an approach to reading that is based on recognition of sounds
Physical development the development of bodily movement and control
Pincer grasp thumb and first finger grasp
Pinpoint haemorrhages small areas of bleeding under the surface
Placenta structure that supports the baby as it develops in the uterus

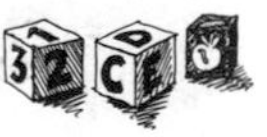

Portage home teaching scheme a scheme to help parents/carers to teach their children with learning difficulties in their own homes, by setting short-term, achievable goals
Positive action taking action to ensure that a particular individual or group has an equal chance to succeed
Positive images the representation of a cross-section of a whole variety of roles and everyday situations, to challenge stereotypes and to extend and increase expectations
Positive self-image a view of oneself as worth while and valuable
Posture position of parts of the body
Poverty trap experienced by people if they are receiving state benefits and they find that by earning a small amount more they lose most of their benefits and become worse off
Pre-term a baby born before 36 completed weeks of pregnancy; also referred to as premature
Preconception the time between a couple deciding they want a baby and when the baby is conceived
Predisposing factors factors that make abuse or neglect more likely to occur – usually the result of a number of these factors occurring together
Prejudice an opinion, usually unfavourable, about someone or something, based on incomplete facts
Prescribed roles duties laid down by others
Preventer drug given on a regular basis to prevent asthma attacks, often given by inhaler
Primary health care first-line health care and health promotion
Primary health-care team a group of professionals who are concerned with the delivery of first-line health care and health promotion
Primitive reflex an automatic response to a particular stimulus in a neonate
Primitive tripod grasp thumb and two finger grasp
Principle a basic truth, which underpins an activity
Private services services provided by individuals, groups of people, or companies to meet a demand, provide a service, and make a financial profit
Problem-solving the ability to draw together and assess information about a situation in order to find a solution
Procedure a pre-set agreed way of doing something
Process a continuous series of events, leading to an outcome
Professional approach how workers deal with and relate to people – they must not allow personal responses to affect their work
Progesterone a hormone produced by the ovaries
Prone lying face down
Psychoanalytical theory a mixture of biological and learning theories, involving the idea that a child's development can be badly affected if at any stage their needs are not met appropriately
Psychological from the study of the mind
Psychopathic events actions by people who are unable to put themselves in another person's place and empathise with how that person might feel
Pyloric stenosis a thickening of the muscle at the outlet of the stomach to the small intestine – milk cannot pass through the narrow outlet into the small intestine

Rapid eye movement (REM) periods of dream sleep
Ratio the numerical relationship or proportion of one quantity to another
Rationale the reason for providing an activity or experience
Reconstructed family a family containing adults and children who have previously been part of a different family
Recovery position safe position in which to place an unconscious casualty if they are breathing and have a pulse
Referral the process by which suspected abuse is reported by one person to someone who can take action if necessary
Reflective practitioners workers who think about what they have done/said, with a view to improving practice
Reflex an involuntary response to a stimulus
Regression responding in a way that is appropriate to an earlier stage of development
Regulations formal rules that must be followed
Reinforcement responding to an action or behaviour so that a particular consequence – a reward or punishment – is associated with the action and it is repeated (positive reinforcement) or not (negative reinforcement)
Relative poverty occurs when people's resources fall seriously short of the resources commanded by the average individual or family in the community
Residential care the provision of care both during the day and the night outside a child's home with people other than close relatives
Respite care short-term care for a child to receive training and assessment and/or to allow their family to have a break
Rights of children the expectations that all children should have regarding how they are treated within their families and in society
Role model a person whose behaviour is used as an example by someone else as the right way to behave
Role play acting out a role as someone else

Sacrum base of the spine
Safety legislation laws that are created to prevent accidents and promote safety
Sanction a negative outcome attached to a specific behaviour
Saturated fats solid at room temperature and come mainly from animal fats
Schema Piaget's term for all the ideas, memories and information that a child might have about a concept or experience
Screening checking the whole population of children at specific ages for particular abnormalities
Sebum an oily substance that lubricates the skin, it is produced by the sebaceous glands and secreted through the hair shaft
Section 8 Orders passed by a court when there is a dispute about who a child should live with, who they can have contact with, and some of the steps and decisions adults can take about them
Self-acceptance approving of oneself, not constantly striving to change oneself
Self-advocacy putting forward one's own viewpoint
Self-approval being pleased with oneself
Self-awareness a knowledge and understanding of oneself
Self-concept (or self-image) the image that we have of ourselves and the way we think that other people see us

 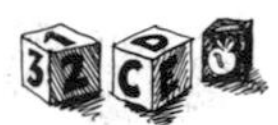

Self-esteem liking and valuing oneself; also referred to as self-respect
Self-reliance the ability to depend on oneself to manage
Self-worth thinking of oneself as having value and worth
Sensitive (or critical) period a period of time vital for the achievement of a particular skill
Sensory impairment hearing or sight loss
Separation distress infants becoming upset when separated from the person to whom they are attached
Serum alpha-fetoprotein (SAFP) a protein found in the maternal blood during pregnancy; a high level requires further investigation
Sickle cell anaemia an inherited condition of haemoglobin formation
Skill an ability that has been practised
Social approval when a person's conduct and efforts are approved of by others
Social creation brought about by society
Social development the growth of the ability to relate to others appropriately and become independent, within a social framework
Social emotions empathy with the feelings of others; the ability to understand how others feel
Social isolation people experience social isolation when they have no close family or friends to care about them
Social mobility the movement of a person from one social group (class) to another
Social model a view of disability as a problem within society
Social role a position in society that is associated with a particular group of expected behaviours
Social status the value that a society puts on people in particular roles
Socialisation the process by which children learn the culture (or way of life) of the society into which they are born
Socio-economic group grouping of people according to their status in society, based on their occupation, which is closely related to their wealth/income
Solitary play a child plays alone
Spatial awareness a developing knowledge of how things move and the effects of movement
Special educational needs learning difficulties requiring special educational provision to be made
Specific learning difficulties difficulties in learning to read, write or spell or in doing mathematics, not related to generalised learning difficulties
Specific therapeutic goal identifies objectives to counteract the effects of the condition or impairment
Sperm the mature male sex cell
Spina bifida a condition in which the spine fails to develop properly before birth
Spina bifida a condition in which the spine fails to develop properly before birth
Spiritual beliefs what a person believes about the non-material world
Statement of Special Educational Needs a written report, setting out a disabled child's needs and the resources required to meet these needs
Statutory child protection those aspects of protecting children that are covered by legislation
Statutory duty duty required by law
Statutory school age the ages at which a child legally has to receive education: from the beginning of the term after their 5th birthday, until the end of the school year in which they have their 16th birthday
Statutory service a service provided by the government after a law (or statute) has been passed in Parliament
'Stepping stones' indication of the steps children need to take from 3 years towards the early learning goals at 5+
Stereotyped roles pre-determined, fixed ideas to which individuals are expected to conform
Stereotyping when people think that all the individual members of a group have the same characteristics as each other; often applied on the basis of race, gender or disability
Sticky eyes a discharge from the eyes in the first 3 weeks of life
Stimulus something that arouses a reaction
Stools faeces, the product of digested food
Story sack an aid to story telling that contains puppets, games or other activities linked to the story
Stranger anxiety fear of strangers
Subconscious thoughts and feelings that a person is not fully aware of
Subdural haematoma bleeding into the brain
Substitute care the care given to children during periods of separation from their main carers
Sudden infant death syndrome (SIDS) the unexpected and usually unexplained death of a young baby
Suffocation stopping respiration
Supine lying on the back
Sweat liquid produced in the sweat glands and secreted through the pores on to the surface of the skin

Talipes an abnormal position of the foot, caused by the contraction of certain muscles or tendons
Term between the 38th and 42nd week of pregnancy
Theories of development ideas about how and why development occurs
Threshold of acceptability the behaviour towards children that is believed to be acceptable by a society at a certain time
Thrush a fungal infection of the mouth and/or nappy area
Toilet training teaching young children the socially acceptable means of emptying the bladder and bowels into a potty and/or toilet
Tokenistic a superficial representation of minority or disadvantaged groups, for example including a single black child in a school brochure, a single woman on the board of directors
Toxin a poisonous substance produced by pathogens
Transcutaneous nerve stimulation (TENS) an electronic device to help control pain in labour
Transition the movement of a child from one care situation to another
Trial-and-error learning the earliest stage in problem-solving. Young children randomly try out solutions to a problem, often making errors, until finding a solution or giving up
Triple test an antenatal blood test to measure levels of serum alpha-fetoprotein (SAFP), human chorionic gonadotrophin (HCG) and oestriol
Umbilical cord contains the blood vessels that connect the developing baby to the placenta
Unconscious showing no response to external stimulation
Undescended testicles when the testes remain located in the body, instead of coming down into the scrotum
Unsaturated fats liquid at room temperature and come mainly from vegetable and fish oils

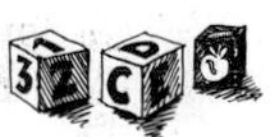

Uterus part of the female reproductive tract; the womb

Vaccine a preparation used to stimulate the production of antibodies and provide immunity against one or several diseases
Values beliefs that certain things are important and to be valued, for example a person's right to their own belongings
Vascular well supplied with blood vessels
Ventouse a suction cup applied to the fetal head to assist delivery
Ventral suspension when the baby is held in the air, face down
Vernix white creamy substance found on the skin of the fetus, in the skin creases of mature babies and on the trunk of pre-term infants
Viable capable of surviving outside the uterus
Visual impairment impairment of sight, ranging from blindness to partial sight
Voluntary action an intentional act that a child chooses to do
Voluntary sector care establishments provided by voluntary organisations
Voluntary services services provided by voluntary organisations, which are founded by people who want to help certain groups of people they believe are in need of support

Weals streak left on the flesh
Weaning the transition from milk feeds to solid foods

Zone of proximal development Vygotsky's term for the range of learning that the child is incapable of achieving alone but that is possible with assistance

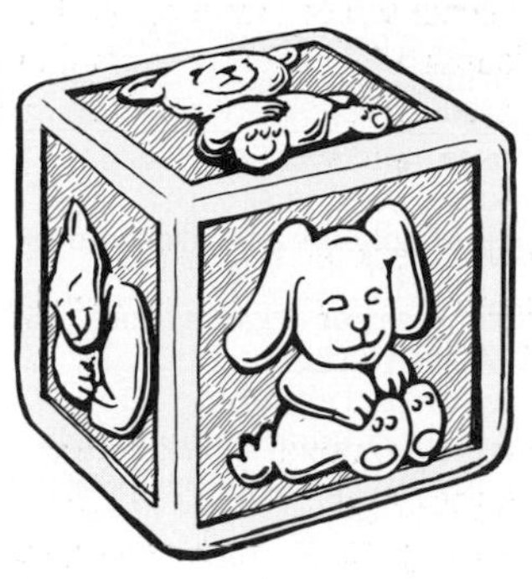

INDEX

Page references in *italics* indicate figures, tables or illustrations.

 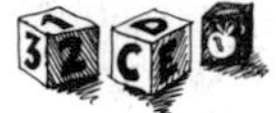

 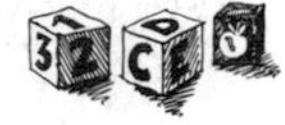

 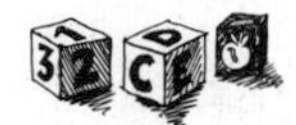

 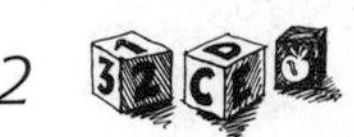